Rome II

The Functional
Gastrointestinal
Disorders

Senior Editor
Douglas A. Drossman, M.D.

Editors
Enrico Corazziari, M.D.
Nicholas J. Talley, M.D., Ph.D.
W. Grant Thompson, M.D.
William E. Whitehead, Ph.D.

Forewords by
Donald O. Castell, M.D.
Aldo Torsoli, M.D., F.R.C.P. (Edin.)

Degnon Associates
McLean, VA, USA

Rome II

The Functional Gastrointestinal Disorders

Diagnosis,
Pathophysiology
and Treatment:
A Multinational
Consensus

Second Edition

Second Edition

This book is the basis for a series of articles based on Working Team Reports, which was published in abridged form by BMJ Publishing Group in *GUT*.

Edited by Lou Ann Brower
Design and composition by B. Williams & Associates, Durham, NC
Printed by Allen Press, Inc., Lawrence, KS

Library of Congress Cataloging-in-Publication Data
Rome II : the functional gastrointestinal disorders : diagnosis, pathophysiology, and treatment : a multinational consensus / senior editor, Douglas A. Drossman ; editors, Enrico Corazziari . . . [et al.] ; forewords by Don Castell, Aldo Torsoli. — 2nd ed.
   p. cm.
Includes bibliographical references and index.
ISBN 0-9656837-1-0 (cloth : alk. paper). — ISBN 0-9656837-2-9 (pbk. : alk. paper)
1. Gastrointestinal system—Diseases. 2. Gastrointestinal system—Diseases—Psychosomatic aspects. 3. Irritable colon.
4. Gastrointestinal system—Diseases—Classification.
I. Drossman, Douglas A. II. Functional gastrointestinal disorders.
III. Title: Functional gastrointestinal disorders. IV. Title: Rome 2.
V. Title: Rome two.
   [DNLM: 1. Gastrointestinal Diseases. WI 150 R763 2000]
RC802R65 2000
616.3'3—dc21
DNLM/DLC
for Library of Congress   99-40667
                        CIP

Printed in the United States of America

First Printing

This book is dedicated
with love to our wives
and children for their
support, encouragement
and patience and to all
our friends and supporters
who have kept us going.

Contents

Members of Working Teams

Coordinating Committee for Functional Gastrointestinal Disorders

Douglas A. Drossman, M.D., Chair
Professor of Medicine and Psychiatry
Co-Director, UNC Center for Functional
    GI and Motility Disorders
The University of North Carolina at
    Chapel Hill
Chapel Hill, North Carolina, USA

Enrico Corazziari, M.D.
Cattedra di Gastroenterologia I
Clinica Medica II
Università "La Sapienza"
Roma, Italy

Nicholas J. Talley, M.D., Ph.D.
Professor of Medicine
University of Sydney, Nepean Hospital
Penrith, NSW, Australia

W. Grant Thompson, M.D.
Emeritus Professor of Medicine
University of Ottawa
Ottawa, Ontario, Canada

William E. Whitehead, Ph.D.
Professor of Medicine and Psychology
Co-Director, UNC Center for Functional
    GI and Motility Disorders
The University of North Carolina at
    Chapel Hill
Chapel Hill, North Carolina, USA

Functional Gastrointestinal Disorders Committees

Basic Science

Jackie D. Wood, Ph.D., Co-Chair
Professor of Physiology and Internal
    Medicine
Chairman Emeritus, Department of
    Physiology
The Ohio State University College of
    Medicine and Public Health
Columbus, Ohio, USA

David H. Alpers, M.D., Co-Chair
William B. Kountz Professor of Medicine
Washington University School of Medicine
St. Louis, Missouri, USA

Paul L. R. Andrews, Ph.D.
Professor of Physiology
St. Georges Hospital Medical School
London, UK

Physiology: Motility/Sensation

John E. Kellow, M.D., Chair
Associate Professor of Medicine
University of Sydney
St. Leonards, New South Wales, Australia

Michel M. Delvaux, M.D., Ph.D., Co-Chair
Gastroenterology Unit
University Hospital Rangueil
Toulouse, France

Physiology: Motility/Sensation (cont'd)

Fernando Azpiroz, M.D., Ph.D.
Associate Professor of Surgery
Chief, Digestive Systems Research Unit
Hospital General Vall d'Hebron
Barcelona, Spain

Michael Camilleri, M.D.
Professor of Medicine and Physiology
Mayo Clinic
Rochester, Minnesota, USA

Eamonn M. M. Quigley, M.D.
Professor of Medicine
Cork University Hospital
National University of Ireland
Cork, Ireland, UK

David G. Thompson, M.D.
Professor of Gastroenterology
Department of Medicine
Hope Hospital
University of Manchester
Manchester, England, UK

Psychosocial Aspects of Functional
Gastrointestinal Disorders

Douglas A. Drossman, M.D., Chair
Professor of Medicine and Psychiatry
Co-Director, UNC Center for Functional
  GI and Motility Disorders
The University of North Carolina at
  Chapel Hill
Chapel Hill, North Carolina, USA

Francis H. Creed, M.D., Co-Chair
Professor of Psychological Medicine
University of Manchester
Manchester, England, UK

Kevin W. Olden, M.D.
Senior Associate Consultant in Medicine
  and Psychiatry
Mayo Clinic-Scottsdale
Scottsdale, Arizona, USA

Jan Svedlund, M.D.
Head, Department of Psychiatry
Sahlgrenska University Hospital
Associate Professor of Psychiatry
Institute of Clinical Neuroscience, Section
  of Psychiatry
Göteborg University
Göteborg, Sweden

Brenda B. Toner, Ph.D.
Head, Women's Mental Health Research
  Program
Centre for Addiction and Mental Health
Associate Professor
Department of Psychiatry
University of Toronto
Toronto, Ontario, Canada

William E. Whitehead, Ph.D.
Professor of Medicine and Psychology
Co-Director, UNC Center for Functional
  GI and Motility Disorders
The University of North Carolina at
  Chapel Hill
Chapel Hill, North Carolina, USA

Functional Esophageal Disorders

Ray E. Clouse, M.D., Chair
Professor of Medicine and Psychiatry
Washington University School of Medicine
St. Louis, Missouri, USA

Joel E. Richter, M.D., Co-Chair
Chairman and Professor
Department of Gastroenterology
The Cleveland Clinic Foundation
Cleveland, Ohio, USA

Functional Esophageal Disorders (cont'd)

Robert C. Heading, M.D.
Department of Medicine
The University of Edinburgh
Edinburgh, Scotland, UK

Jozef Janssens, M.D.
Department of Gastroenterology
University of Leuven
Leuven, Belgium

Janet A. Wilson, M.D.
Professor of Otolaryngology, Head and
    Neck Surgery
Department of Surgery
University of Newcastle-upon-Tyne
Newcastle-upon-Tyne, England, UK

Functional Gastroduodenal Disorders

Nicholas J. Talley, M.D., Ph.D., Chair
Professor of Medicine
University of Sydney, Nepean Hospital
Penrith, NSW, Australia

Vincenzo Stanghellini, M.D., Co-Chair
Associate Professor of Internal Medicine
Department of Internal Medicine and
    Gastroenterology
University of Bologna
Bologna, Italy

Robert C. Heading, M.D.
Department of Medicine
Royal Infirmary
Edinburgh, Scotland, UK

Kenneth L. Koch, M.D.
Professor of Medicine
Gastrointestinal Division
Milton S. Hershey Medical Center
Hershey, Pennsylvania, USA

Juan-R. Malagelada, M.D.
Digestive System Research Unit
Hospital General Vall D'hebron
Barcelona, Spain

Guido N. J. Tytgat, M.D.
Professor of Gastroenterology
Chief, Department of Gastroenterology
    and Hepatology
Academic Medical Center
Amsterdam, The Netherlands

Functional Bowel Disorders and
Functional Abdominal Pain

W. Grant Thompson, M.D., Chair
Emeritus Professor of Medicine
University of Ottawa
Ottawa, Ontario, Canada

George F. Longstreth, M.D., Co-Chair
Chief of Gastroenterology
Department of Internal Medicine
Kaiser Permanente
Clinical Professor of Medicine
University of California San Diego
San Diego, California, USA

Douglas A. Drossman, M.D.
Professor of Medicine and Psychiatry
Co-Director, UNC Center for Functional
    GI and Motility Disorders
The University of North Carolina at
    Chapel Hill
Chapel Hill, North Carolina, USA

Kenneth W. Heaton, M.D.
Senior Research Fellow
University of Bristol
Bristol, England, UK

Functional Bowel Disorders and
Functional Abdominal Pain (cont'd)

E. Jan Irvine, M.D.
Professor of Medicine
McMaster University
Hamilton, Ontario, Canada

Stefan Muller-Lissner, M.D.
Professor of Medicine
Park-Klinik
Weissensee, Berlin, Germany

Functional Disorders of the Biliary
Tract and Pancreas

Enrico Corazziari, M.D., Chair
Cattedra di Gastroenterologia I
Clinica Medica II
Università "La Sapienza"
Roma, Italy

Eldon A. Shaffer, M.D., Co-Chair
Head, Department of Medicine
University of Calgary
Calgary, Alberta, Canada

Walter J. Hogan, M.D.
Professor of Medicine and Radiology
Division of Gastroenterology and
   Hepatology
Medical College of Wisconsin
Milwaukee, Wisconsin, USA

Stuart Sherman, M.D.
Associate Professor of Medicine and
   Radiology
Division of Gastroenterology and
   Hepatology
Indiana University School of Medicine
Indianapolis, Indiana, USA

James Toouli, M.D.
Gastrointestinal Surgical Unit
Flinders Medical Centre
Adelaide, Australia

Functional Disorders of the Anus
and Rectum

William E. Whitehead, Ph.D., Chair
Professor of Medicine and Psychology
Co-Director, UNC Center for Functional
   GI and Motility Disorders
The University of North Carolina at
   Chapel Hill
Chapel Hill, North Carolina, USA

Arnold Wald, M.D., Co-Chair
Professor of Medicine
University of Pittsburgh Medical Center
Pittsburgh, Pennsylvania, USA

Nicholas E. Diamant, M.D.
Professor of Medicine and Physiology
University of Toronto
Toronto, Ontario, Canada

Paul Enck, Ph.D.
University of Tübingen
Tübingen, Germany

John H. Pemberton, M.D.
Professor of Surgery
Mayo Clinic
Rochester, Minnesota, USA

Satish S.C. Rao, M.D., Ph.D.
Department of Internal Medicine
University of Iowa Hospitals and Clinics
Iowa City, Iowa, USA

Childhood Functional Gastrointestinal Disorders

Paul E. Hyman, M.D., Chair
Associate Clinical Professor of Pediatrics
University of California at Los Angeles
Director, Pediatric Gastrointestinal
    Motility Center
Children's Hospital of Orange County
Orange, California, USA

Andree Rasquin-Weber, M.D., Co-Chair
Professor of Pediatrics
University of Montreal
Montreal, Quebec, Canada

Salvatore Cucchiara, M.D.
Associate Professor Child Health
University Federico II School of Medicine
Naples, Italy

David R. Fleisher, M.D.
Associate Professor of Child Health
University of Missouri
Columbia, Missouri, USA

Jeffrey S. Hyams, M.D.
Professor and Vice Chair
Department of Pediatrics
Head, Division of Digestive Diseases and
    Nutrition
University of Connecticut School of
    Medicine
Hartford, Connecticut, USA

Peter J. Milla, M.D.
Professor of Paediatric Gastroenterology
    and Nutrition
Institute of Child Health
University of London
London, England, UK

Annamaria Staiano, M.D.
Associate Professor of Pediatrics
University Federico II School of Medicine
Naples, Italy

Design of Treatment Trials for Functional Gastrointestinal Disorders

Sander J. O. Veldhuyzen van Zanten, M.D.
    Ph.D.,Chair
Associate Professor
Queen Elizabeth II Health Sciences Center
Dalhousie University
Halifax, Nova Scotia, Canada

Nicholas J. Talley, M.D., Ph.D., Co-Chair
Professor of Medicine
University of Sydney, Nepean Hospital
Penrith, NSW, Australia

Peter Bytzer, M.D.
Consultant in Gastroenterology and
    Internal Medicine
Department of Medical Gastroenterology
Glostrup University Hospital
Glostrup, Denmark

Kenneth B. Klein, M.D.
President, International Drug
    Development Consulting
Bainbridge Island, Washington, USA

Peter J. Whorwell, M.D.
Consultant Gastroenterologist
Senior Lecturer in Medicine
Department of Medicine
University Hospital of South Manchester
Manchester, England, UK

Alan R. Zinsmeister
Consultant Statistician
Section of Biostatistics
Mayo Clinic
Rochester, Minnesota, USA

I. Foreword

In Delphi, in an olive-tree valley dominated by the remains of ancient temples, a tiny museum provides evidence of how the oracle's messages were released to travelers who had faced a long and perilous journey to obtain them. The message, often obscure or ambiguous, was not released as such, but only after the priests had meditated on it, discussed it together and finally made it clearer or univocal.

This is the first historical trace of a procedure, the so-called Delphic approach, which has been recently used in medicine in different ways—from the consensus conferences to our Working Team Reports (WTRs)—in the attempt to clarify topics either controversial or not easily settled by the usual scientific inquiry or literature review. The Working Teams, first organized in Rome in 1987 within the purview of an international congress of gastroenterology (ROMA88), were committees of experts from different countries, invited to an in-depth study of given topics on the basis of their own experience and of the pertinent literature. Approximately one year later, the experts submitted a preliminary individual report to the chairman who, after a two-day interactive meeting, amended the various reports and merged them in a final document to be published. The whole process required usually two years time [1]. It soon appeared that such study groups were suitable for analyzing topics such as the GI functional disturbances where a high prevalence is associated with the lack of those detectable anatomical or biochemical abnormalities which are traditionally seen by doctors as the necessary background of a real disease entity. Until 1994, in fact, when we were responsible for the Working Team organization, the number of reports dealing with functional GI troubles exceeded that of any other topic. Now that such organizational duty has passed into the hands of an International Committee, the same format continues to appear useful, as the present book shows.

The work of the Rome Coordinating Committee, chaired by Dr. Drossman, has had prestigious antecedents. S. Freud was probably the first to maintain that morbid manifestations may be independent of anatomical changes, and it is thanks to G. von Bergmann that, in the thirties, the concept of *funktionnelle Pathologie* was introduced in medicine, particularly in gastroenterology [2]. The Committee's work was inspired by the principle that both interpretation and treatment of GI functional disturbances might be facilitated by a preliminary symptom-based categorization of patient subgroups [3]; this conceptualization also testified to a significant change in the medical way of thinking. Symptoms are signals that bring patients to ask doctors for help, however they are not simply a subjective trigger leading doctors to search for what is believed to be really important, i.e., signs. Originating from physiological derangements, variations of individual sensitivity and/or particular psychological and relational situations, symptoms reveal to physicians an essential dimension of illness. Not appreciating this value means to tarry in a sort of neo-Hippocratic position, one that modern medical education tries to contrast when providing students with a biopsychosocial rather than a purely biomedical profile.

The conceptual view brought about by the Rome II project under the facilitation of Doug Drossman of a multinational collaborative effort has been very productive. We have only proposed an instrument which in his hands—we are sure—will continue to be a winning one.

Aldo Torsoli, M.D., F.R.C.P. (Edin)
Università "La Sapienza," Roma

1. Torsoli A et al. Working Team Reports. Gastroenterol Internat 1991;4:189–190.
2. Bergmann von G. Funktionnelle Pathologie. Berlin:Springer,1931.
3. Drossman DA, Richter JE, Talley NJ, Thompson WG, Corazziari E, Whitehead WE. The Functional Gastrointestinal Disorders: Diagnosis, Pathophysiology and Treatment: A Multinational Consensus. McLean,VA: Degnon Associates, 1994.

II. Foreword

The Maturation of the Rome Criteria

Since the seminal meeting of those investigators who assembled in Rome in 1988 to initiate a consensus process to develop criteria to define functional gastrointestinal disorders, the resulting "Rome Criteria" have evolved into a well-respected position in the field of gastroenterology. The initial Multinational Working Team Committees divided their deliberations into five major anatomical regions: esophagus, gastroduodenum, biliary, intestines, and anorectum. One of the major accomplishments of these working groups was to focus attention on the symptomatic presentation of this complex group of patients having functional GI symptoms in order to establish a working paradigm to better categorize these patients. These groupings have worked to simplify diagnosis and treatment and to help in selecting appropriate patients for research endeavors by avoiding the previous morass of lumping patients with varying symptom presentations (e.g., combining those with predominant diarrhea with those having predominant constipation) under the rubric of the irritable bowel syndrome. It would appear that the arduous efforts of the "Rome Group" have helped provide important clarity to this field and to clinical diagnosis, treatment algorithms, and outcomes research. The initial working team has had the foresight to expand their membership to include clinicians and clinical investigators from the international GI community having an interest in functional GI disorders.

Perhaps the most definitive indication that the "Rome Criteria" for functional GI disorders has succeeded is the publication of this second edition: *Rome II: The Functional Gastrointestinal Disorders: Diagnosis, Pathophysiology, and Treatment: A Multinational Consensus.* I am truly honored to have been asked to provide a foreword to this very worthwhile text, particularly considering the high quality of the international authorities who have contributed the information contained within its pages. Great credit must go to Professor Aldo Torsoli, who played a major role in initiating the first multinational working team committees to begin the consensus process. Douglas Drossman, as Senior Editor, and the other Editors, Enrico Corazziari, Nick Talley, Grant Thompson, and Bill Whitehead, however, deserve particular recognition for their willingness to "step up to the plate" and be the driving force to continue to breathe life into this project. The chapters contained within this second edition are excellent in their content and focus and provide outstanding clinically useful material relating to the approach to patients with functional GI disorders. This is balanced by exceptional discussions of basic mechanisms as in the chapter on "Fundamentals of Neurogastroenterology: Basic Science" and that on "Principles of Applied Neurogastroenterology: Physiology/Motility-Sensation." The additions of a chapter on these disorders in childhood and the excellent summary on Clinical Outcomes Conferences have brought this second edition to an exceptional level of value to both the investigator and the clinician interested in functional GI disorders. I applaud the authors for their excellent text material, and I hope that all those who take the time to read the material contained within this text will enjoy it as much as I have.

Donald O. Castell, M.D.
Past President, American Gastroenterological
    Association
Kimbel Professor and Chairman
Department of Medicine
The University of Pennsylvania
Graduate Hospital
Philadelphia, Pennsylvania

Preface to the
First Edition

Man should strive to have his intestines relaxed all the days of his life.
——Moses Maimonides, 1135–1204 A.D.

A good set of bowels is worth more to a man than any quantity of brains.
——Josh Billings (Henry Wheeler Shaw), 1818–1885 A.D.

For centuries, physicians and historians have recognized that it is common for maladies to afflict the intestinal tract, producing symptoms of pain, nausea, vomiting, diarrhea, constipation, difficult passage of food or feces, or any combination. When persons experience these symptoms as severe enough, or that they impact on daily life, they define the symptoms as an illness and may seek medical care. In modern times, the physician caring for these patients seeks to identify metabolic, infectious, neoplastic, and other structural abnormalities. If they are not found, the patient is (often by exclusion) considered to have a functional gastrointestinal (GI) disorder. This book is dedicated to helping the clinician and investigator to: (1) make a positive diagnosis of these disorders, (2) understand their pathophysiology and (3) make effective treatment decisions.

It is with great pleasure that we introduce the first edition of *The Functional Gastrointestinal Disorders*. This book, the culmination of over 7 year's effort by 30 internationally recognized investigators in the field, provides the first categorization of the 25 functional GI disorders from esophagus to anorectum. Also included is the most comprehensive discussion available of the epidemiology, physiology, psychosocial features, clinical evaluation and treatment recommendations for these disorders.

Perhaps the most unique component of this book is the inclusion of the symptom-based ("Rome") diagnostic criteria for the functional GI disorders. The efforts of seven multinational Working Team Committees have, through careful review of the literature and consensus, developed a standard for diagnosis that can be used in research and clinical care. In effect, the methods leading to these criteria (see Chapter 1) duplicate the processes that eventuated in the successful development of diagnostic classifications in psychiatry (DSM-III) and rheumatology (ARA Criteria). For easy retrieval of information, these criteria are listed not only in the chapters for each organ system, but are also compiled into a single section (Appendix A). We are hopeful that their inclusion in this book will encourage the use of standardized diagnostic methods for epidemiological surveys and clinical trials. We also expect that their use by physicians in practice will reduce the need for costly and unnecessary diagnostic studies occasionally done to "rule out organic disease."

Some additional features of this book are worth noting. First, it is well recognized that most studies in this field are methodologically flawed because of difficulties relating to patient selection, efficacy and outcome assessment, and statistical analysis. So, for investigators interested in clinical trials, we include a chapter that not only reviews the limitations of previous studies, but also makes recommendations for the optimal design of future protocols (Chapter 7). Second, we recognize the need for epidemiologists, health policy planners and clinicians to refer to population-based frequency data for these disorders. In Chapter 8, we include tabular data and summary information from a recently published U.S. national study using our recommended "Rome" criteria. This chapter includes information on the prevalences of all these disorders with breakdown by gender, age and other sociodemographic factors, as well as health care use and disability statistics. Finally, since these criteria were originally developed for physician assessment, they are not easily adapted to surveys or self-report questionnaires. Therefore, the authors have produced a matched set of question items (Appendix B) as used in the national survey for clinical investigators to use in their research.

We expect that as new scientific data about these disorders accumulate, there will be a need to revise the diagnostic criteria as well as information on pathophysiology and treatment. Therefore, we have set up a process for future committee meetings that will permit ongoing review and modification of our current recommendations. These changes and enhancements will be included in future editions of this book.

The editors would like to thank Professor Aldo Torsoli for his foresight and support of the Working Team process, the many committee members and reviewers who helped in the creation of these documents, Ms. Sandy Hall for her assistance in the preparation of the manuscript, and Ms. Lynne Herndon whose professional commitment and tireless efforts made the publication of this book a reality.

Douglas A. Drossman, M.D. and
The Working Team Committees
1994

Preface to the
Second Edition

It is with great enjoyment and anticipation that we offer this second edition of *Rome II: The Functional Gastrointestinal Disorders.* This book is the culmination, and most visible product of the ROME II project, a 4-year effort organized by a dedicated Coordinating Committee, and implemented with the assistance of over 50 international investigators and an equal number of reviewers, a tireless administrative staff, and the support and interest of many pharmaceutical sponsors and regulatory agencies.

This edition improves upon the first edition, published in 1994, in several ways: (1) All previous chapters (esophageal, gastroduodenal, bowel, biliary and anorectal disorders, design of treatment trials) have been completely updated and expanded to accommodate the rapid growth in the field of functional GI disorders; (2) Several new committees have been formed to contribute chapters on the physiological (motility/sensation), basic science (brain-gut), and psychosocial aspects of these disorders, as well as on a new classification system for the pediatric functional GI disorders; (3) We have added a historical piece ("The Road to Rome") that catalogues the evolution in thinking and process of the ROME I and II projects; (4) We include a summary and recommendations from the recent Clinical Outcomes Conference, held at the World Congress of Gastroenterology (Vienna) in 1998. This conference began the process of collaboration, among the ROME committee members, pharmaceutical companies, international expert advisors, and regulatory agencies; and (5) Finally, we provide new questionnaires and coding schemes for the ROME II criteria that can be used in clinical research or practice. The Modular Questionnaire (with investigator and respondent forms) was designed for clinical investigation and surveys. It allows the investigator to select out parts of the instrument as needed to key in specific diagnoses. The Integrative Questionnaire is designed primarily for epidemiological surveys, but can also be used for clinical investigation. The pediatric form can function as a diagnostic "checklist" for the clinician or investigator.

Possibly the most important component of the book is the inclusion of symptom-based diagnostic criteria for clinical investigation and practice. Since publication of the original criteria over five years ago, there has been enthusiastic support, and also well-founded criticism. The criticism relates to concerns that the criteria are not physiologically based; that they were determined by consensus ("Delphi" approach) rather than through validation studies; and that they are likely to change over time. With regard to the first concern, to date, no physiologic criteria have emerged to diagnose these disorders. In addition, these symptom-based criteria have stood the test of time. They have proved their value in clinical trials and, it is hoped, have reduced patient care costs by curtailing the tendency to order unneeded diagnostic studies to "rule out organic disease." Second, we recognize and accept the need for validation studies, and over the last few years several studies using factor analysis or clinical validation by experts have supported these criteria (primarily for IBS). In addition, we have set up a research fund and have awarded several grants to encourage clinical investigators to test the validity of these new criteria. Whatever the results, the information obtained will be used either to support or lead to modification of the criteria. Finally, we have also set up a rigorous, yet conservative, process for changes to the previous criteria (see Chapter 1). All prior criticisms against the inclusion of specific items, and recommendations for new items were collected and communicated to the committees so they could be addressed and commented upon. In some cases, this led to changes in the criteria. In addition, the peer review process for the criteria and the chapters was expanded to include external and internal academic reviewers, and had to be evidence-based, and/or acceptable to all parties. The changes made in the criteria in most cases do not eliminate the use of the previous criteria, but enhance them, and they are more consistent with the new knowledge in our pathophysiological understanding of these disorders.

This book is part of a larger effort by the ROME II Committees to help advance the field of functional GI disorders, and to legitimize these conditions for our patients. I would like to outline some of the projects underway:

Publication of GUT supplement. The September 1999 publication of the Rome II criteria and an abridged version of the these chapters in a supplemental issue of GUT is a way to communicate our findings and recommendations to a much larger audience. This book provides a more in-depth treatment of the topic.

Formation of an International Resource Committee. We have formed a committee of pharmaceutical sponsors and regulatory agencies, and have met biennially to address the shared interests and concerns relating to the design of treatment trials. One outcome of this group has been the Clinical Outcomes Conference in Vienna, which set the stage for future dialog to develop consensus recommendations for study design (see Chapter 12).

Research funds to support validation studies. As noted, we have set up a peer review process to evaluate applications that test the utility and validity of the ROME II criteria for functional GI disorders. To date we have awarded five grants, and expect to continue this process.

Establish an epidemiological database. We have begun the process of developing questionnaires to administer in international surveys in order to set up a database for future studies.

We are hopeful that this second edition will provide important information to help health professionals care for their patients with functional gastrointestinal disorders. Ultimately, we believe that our patients will benefit.

Douglas A. Drossman, M.D.,
and the Rome II Coordinating Committee
March 2000

Acknowledgments

On behalf of the Multinational Working Teams to Develop Diagnostic Criteria for Functional Gastrointestinal Disorders, the Coordinating Committee would like to thank our sponsors and supporters. From the pharmaceutical industry, the following sponsors merit special commendation: **Special Sustaining Sponsor:** Janssen Pharmaceutica, L. P.; **Full Sponsors:** AstraZeneca, Glaxo Wellcome, Novartis, Pfizer, Roberts Pharmaceuticals, SmithKline Beecham, and Solvay Pharmaceuticals; and **Partial Sponsors:** Procter and Gamble, Sanofi Winthrop, and TAP Holdings. In addition, the following professionals and organizations contributed generously of their time and expertise: the Food and Drug Administration (FDA); the Japan International Gastrointestinal Motility Society; the Functional Brain Gut Research Group; the International Foundation for Functional Gastrointestinal Disorders; the National Institute of Digestive Diseases and Kidney Disorders (NIDDK-NIH); Associazione per la NeUro-Gastroenterologia e la Motilità Gastrointestinale (ANEMGI), for support and sponsorship in Rome; and the 52 authors representing 13 countries who worked tirelessly to produce these documents. Finally, special thanks go to our reviewers, to Ms. Carlar Blackman for her creative intelligence and tireless effort to keep the numerous projects and activities underway; to George Degnon for his skills in coordinating our meetings and for his sound advice; Ms. Emanuela Crescini for her coordination of the meeting in Rome; to B. Williams & Associates for design and publication advice; and to Lou Ann Brower for genuine interest in producing the best in a final product.

Rome II

The Functional Gastrointestinal Disorders

Chapter 1

The Functional Gastrointestinal Disorders and the Rome II Process

Douglas A. Drossman

A Conceptual Change

Over the last few decades, and in particular, since publication of the previous edition of this book over five years ago, the functional gastrointestinal disorders (FGIDs) have become widely accepted as legitimate diagnostic entities worthy of clinical attention and scientific investigation. This has occurred, not because of their high prevalence in society [1–6] and gastroenterologic practice [7–9], but because of recent changes in the way these conditions are conceptualized. Despite the fact that these disorders, defined as a "variable combination of chronic or recurrent gastrointestinal symptoms not explained by structural or biochemical abnormalities"[10], have been present throughout history, the lack of identifiable pathology precluded their categorization (by Western biomedical standards) as bona fide diseases. The first published account of a functional gastrointestinal disorder was made over 180 years ago [11]. Since then, only occasional reports were published until the middle of this century, when their systematic investigation began [12–14].

However, over the last 25 years, scientific interest in understanding these disorders, and clinical attention toward caring for patients with these disorders has grown progressively (see Chapter 13). This change has been mirrored over the last few years by an impressive increase in the number of scientific publications, professional organizations and interest groups, grant applications, and pharmaceutical contracts.

The reasons for the increased attention to these disorders may be related to their legitimization as diagnostic entities. In part, the use of newer investigative techniques in gastrointestinal physiology (e.g., barostat, ambulatory monitoring, PET/fMRI studies), epidemiology (e.g., population studies, factor analysis), and clinical assessment (e.g., symptom-based criteria) have led to new knowledge about these disorders. But, in addition, this new interest follows important changes in how clinicians and investigators conceptualize the functional disorders, and human illness in general [15].

The prevailing assumption in Western medicine has been that medical illness is based on the identification of histopathologic disease [15,16]. The Biomedical Model presumes that identifiable abnormalities in the structure and function of organs and tissues, or its biochemical associations—disease—have a linear and causal relationship to the person's perception of ill health—illness. This concept has been supported and exemplified through the rapid growth over the last century of information on gastrointestinal histopathology, its endoscopic and radiological correlates, and most recently, their molecular determinants. But this presumption has also given us a distorted understanding of the true nature of gastrointestinal (and other) illness (i.e., the person's perception of ill health). Only about 10% of medical illnesses seen by physicians are explained by specific diseases [17], and gastroenterologists are all too familiar with the poor correlation between the morphologic findings on endoscopy and their patient's symptoms. Even persons with a structural ("organic") diagnosis such as inflammatory bowel disease [18] or cancer show considerable variation in the experience and behavior relating to their disease.

With regard to the functional gastrointestinal disorders, adherence to this bio-medical approach relegates them to being "non-entities," and this has produced more confusion than answers. It is unsettling to try to understand and treat the majority of patients in gastrointestinal practice with functional symptoms and no clear-cut structural, biochemical, or physiological basis. The initial enthusiasm (and hope) in the 1970s and early 1980s that these symptoms might be fully explained as a result of disordered motility was too simplistic, and it was not borne out by clinical experience or later investigations. Increased gut contractility is often not present when patients report pain, and when abnormal contractions are present, they may not be associated with symptoms. Even the counter-assumption, that functional gastrointestinal disorders must be psychiatric (due to high frequencies of psychiatric disturbances among patients) has been seriously challenged. Epidemiological studies have shown that persons with irritable bowel syndrome who do not seek health care are psychologically much like healthy subjects [19–21].

While some adherents to the biomedical approach might resolve this dilemma by rejecting those gastrointestinal complaints not currently understood in terms of disturbed physiology [22], most clinicians and clinical investigators seek a framework to understand, categorize and treat those common symptoms that patients bring to their physicians. These symptoms are real, though multi-determined, and they vary with cultural, social, interpersonal and psychological influences [15,16].

Possibly the publication in the late 1970s of the Systems or Biopsychosocial Model of illness [23,24] contributed to the acceptance of and interest in the research and clinical care of patients with functional gastrointestinal disorders (FGIDs). This model provided a conceptual basis for understanding and legitimizing these gastrointestinal symptoms not easily attributed to specific diseases, and has opened the way to multidisciplinary research that truly advances our understanding of these disorders. For example, imaging studies of the brain (PET, fMRI, evoked potentials) [25] and neurophysiologic studies of the brain-gut axis [26–28] are beginning to show that functional gastrointestinal symptoms result not from disturbances in the bowel per se, but from dysregulation in neuroenteric pathways that alter pain thresholds, motility, and behavior [15]. Finally, the Biopsychosocial Model provides the rationale for the use of psychopharmacological, behavioral, and psychological forms of treatment [29] for these conditions.

The Biopsychosocial Conceptualization

Figure 1 illustrates the proposed relationship between psychosocial and physiological factors with functional gastrointestinal symptoms and the clinical outcome. Early in life, genetics and environmental influences (e.g., family attitudes toward bowel training or illness in general, major loss or abuse history, or exposure to an infection) may affect one's psychosocial development (susceptibility to life stress, psychological state, coping skills, social support) and/or the development of gut dysfunction (abnormal motility or visceral hypersensitivity). In addition, the presence and nature of an FGID is determined by the interaction of psychosocial factors and altered physiology via the brain-gut axis. So, one individual afflicted with a bowel disorder but with no psychosocial disturbances and good coping and social support may not seek medical care. Another, having similar symptoms, but with coexistent psychosocial disturbance, high life stress, or poor social support, may see physicians frequently and have a generally poor outcome. It is also noted that the clinical outcome will, in turn, affect the severity of the disorder (double-sided arrow). The implication for the clinician and investigator is that psychosocial factors, while not etiologic, are relevant to understanding the patient's adjustment to a functional gastrointestinal disorder and to planning treatment. This psychosocial context, when linked with our growing understanding of the pathophysiology of the FGIDs as briefly described below,

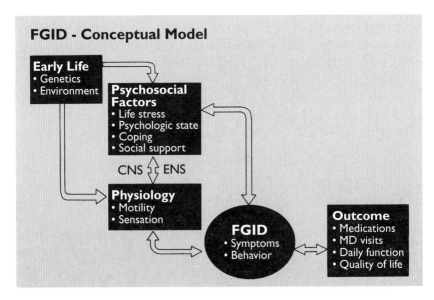

Figure 1. A biopsychosocial conceptualization of the pathogenesis and clinical expression of the functional GI disorders.

gives shape to rational bases for future research and the approach to patient care.

— Pathophysiological Observations on the Functional Gastrointestinal Disorders

In proposing the diagnostic groupings listed in Table 1, we recognize that despite differences in location and symptom features these groupings share common features with regard to their motor and sensory physiology, central nervous system relationships, and the approach to patient care. What follows are general observations and guidelines for these disorders.

Abnormal Motility

It is well recognized that many gastrointestinal symptoms such as vomiting, diarrhea, acute abdominal pain, and incontinence, among others, are generated by disturbed gastrointestinal motility. Furthermore, in healthy subjects, strong emotion or environmental stress can lead to increased motility in the esophagus [30], stomach [31], small intestine [32], and colon [33]. The functional gastrointestinal disorders are characterized by having an even greater motility response to stressors (psychological or physiological) when compared to normal subjects [34–36], and candidate electrical activity markers have been proposed that may facilitate these responses [34,37]. However, in these acute stress situations, the motor responses are only partially correlated with symptoms [34,38]. Thus, while abnormal motility plays an important role in understanding many of the functional gastrointestinal disorders and their symptoms, they are not sufficient to explain patient reports of chronic or recurrent abdominal pain.

Visceral Hypersensitivity

As anticipated from the previous section, many of the FGIDs associated with chronic or recurrent pain—e.g., functional chest pain of presumed esophageal origin (A3), functional dyspepsia (B1), irritable bowel syndrome (C1), functional abdominal pain syndrome (D1), and functional anorectal pain (F2)—usually is not well correlated with changes in gastrointestinal motility, and in some cases motility disturbances do not exist. One exception is Type I or II sphincter of Oddi dysfunction (E2), where sphincterotomy leads to reduction in bile duct pressures and reduced pain. The poor association of pain with gastrointestinal motility in most of these functional gastrointestinal disorders has led

Table 1. Functional Gastrointestinal Disorders

A. Esophageal Disorders

A1. Globus
A2. Rumination syndrome
A3. Functional Chest Pain of Presumed Esophageal Origin
A4. Functional Heartburn
A5. Functional Dysphagia
A6. Unspecified Functional Esophageal Disorder

B. Gastroduodenal Disorders

B1. Functional Dyspepsia
    B1a. Ulcer-like Dyspepsia
    B1b. Dysmotility-like Dyspepsia
    B1c. Unspecified (nonspecific) Dyspepsia
B2. Aerophagia
B3. Functional Vomiting

C. Bowel Disorders

C1. Irritable Bowel Syndrome
C2. Functional Abdominal Bloating
C3. Functional Constipation
C4. Functional Diarrhea
C5. Unspecified Functional Bowel Disorder

D. Functional Abdominal Pain

D1. Functional Abdominal Pain Syndrome
D2. Unspecified Functional Abdominal Pain

E. Functional Disorders of the Biliary Tract and the Pancreas

E1. Gallbladder Dysfunction
E2. Sphincter of Oddi Dysfunction

F. Anorectal Disorders

F1. Functional Fecal Incontinence
F2. Functional Anorectal Pain
    F2a. Levator Ani Syndrome
    F2b. Proctalgia Fugax
F3. Pelvic Floor Dyssynergia

G. Functional Pediatric Disorders

G1. Vomiting
    G1a. Infant regurgitation
    G1b. Infant rumination syndrome
    G1c. Cyclic vomiting syndrome
G2. Abdominal pain
    G2a. Functional dyspepsia
        G2a1. Ulcer-like dyspepsia
        G2a2. Dysmotility-like dyspepsia
        G2a3. Unspecified (nonspecific) dyspepsia
G2b. Irritable bowel syndrome
G2c. Functional abdominal pain
G2d. Abdominal migraine
G2e. Aerophagia
G3. Functional diarrhea
G4. Disorders of defecation
    G4a. Infant dyschezia
    G4b. Functional constipation
    G4c. Functional fecal retention
    G4d. Functional non-retentive fecal soiling

to studies that relate the pain to abnormalities in visceral sensation [40–43]. These patients have a lower pain threshold with balloon distension of the bowel (visceral hyperalgesia), or they have increased sensitivity even to normal intestinal function (e.g., allodynia), and there may be an increased or unusual area of somatic referral of visceral pain. Current studies are attempting to find whether visceral hypersensitivity the FGIDs relates to:

(1) altered receptor sensitivity at the viscus itself;
(2) increased excitability of the spinal cord dorsal horn neurons, or
(3) altered central modulation of sensation [38].

Another recent observation is that visceral hypersensitivity may be induced (stimulus hyperalgesia) in response to rectal or colonic distension in normals [44], and to a greater degree, in persons with IBS [45]. So it is possible that the pain of a functional gastrointestinal disorder may relate to sensitization resulting from chronic abnormal motor hyperactivity (e.g., discrete clustered contractions), gastrointestinal infection (e.g., *H. pylori* for functional dyspepsia and enteric infections for IBS), or trauma/injury to the viscera.

— Inflammation

Another area of recent interest relates to the possibility that increased inflammation in the enteric mucosa or neural plexi may contribute to symptom development [46]. This may occur by peripheral sensitization (see above) and/or hypermotility activated by induction of mucosal inflammatory cytokines [47]. This hypothesis follows clinical observations that about one-third of patients with IBS report that their symptoms began after an acute enteric infection, and conversely that one-third of patients presenting with an acute enteric infection will go on to develop IBS-like symptoms [48,49].

— Brain-Gut Interactions

To bring these observations together, basic and clinical investigators have emphasized a more integrative biopsychosocial understanding of these symptoms as being generated by a combination of intestinal motor, sensory, and CNS activity: the "brain-gut axis" [50]. In this conceptualization, higher neural centers are seen to modulate peripheral intestinal motor and sensory activity, and vice versa. So, extrinsic (vision, smell, etc.) or intrinsic (emotion, thought) information have, by the nature of their neural connections from higher centers, the capability to affect gastrointestinal sensation, motility, secretion, and inflammation. Conversely, viscerotopic effects (e.g., nociception) reciprocally affect central pain perception, mood, and behavior. For example, spontaneously induced contractions of the colon in rats lead to activation of the locus coeruleus in the pons, an area closely connected to pain and emotional centers in the brain [51]. Conversely, increased arousal or anxiety is associated with a decrease in the frequency of MMC activity of the small bowel [52].

Brain-gut interactions may also play a role in our understanding of post-infectious IBS. In a recent study of patients without prior bowel symptoms who were admitted for acute gastroenteritis, 23% developed IBS-like symptoms three months later. When comparing those who developed IBS symptoms with those who did not, the authors found:

(1) psychosocial difficulties (life stress and hypochondriasis) predicted who would go on to develop IBS symptoms;

(2) altered gut physiology (abnormal motility and visceral hypersensitivity) was present at three months in both groups, (i.e., with or without symptoms);

(3) increased inflammatory cells were present only in the group with IBS symptoms [49].

This suggests that while an acute infection leads to physiological disturbances in the gut (altered sensation and motility), it is the psychological distress that contributes to the experience of the symptoms. Furthermore, stress may perpetuate IBS symptoms by means of CNS facilitation of inflammation via disruption of the hypothalamic-pituitary-adrenal/cytokine stress pathway [18,53].

Now, after decades of studying the gastrointestinal physiology of the FGIDs, we have begun to use positron emission tomography (PET), functional magnetic resonance imaging (fMRI) and related imaging modalities to identify features of the brain physiology of these conditions [25]. These kinds of studies may help us to understand the role of the CNS in modulating visceral pain. It may also provide a marker for studying responses to psychological treatments or psycho-pharmacological agents. For example, the recent finding that depressed patients with active anterior cingulate gyrus activity on PET imaging were more likely to respond to antidepressants [54] suggests areas of new research on specifying the use of various treatments for patients with an FGID.

It is no longer rational to try to discriminate whether physiological or psychological factors produce pain or other bowel symptoms, dysmotility, or inflammation. Instead, the FGIDs appear to be understood in terms of dysregulation of brain-gut function, and the task is to determine the degree to which each is remediable.

A treatment approach that is consistent with the concept of brain-gut dysfunction is likely to focus on the neuropeptides and receptors that are present in both the enteric and central nervous systems. Putative agents include the enkephalins, Substance P, calcitonin gene-related polypeptide (CGRP), thyrotropin releasing hormone (TRH), 5 hydroxytryptamine (5-HT) and its congeners, and cholecystokinin (CCK), among others. These neuropeptides have integrated activities on gastrointestinal function and human behavior depending upon their location. Pharmacological treatment trials are underway in which the diverse but interconnected symptoms of pain, bowel dysfunction, and psychosocial distress so commonly associated with the FGIDs will be addressed. The information gained from these studies promise to increase our understanding of these conditions and to yield more effective treatment.

— Psychosocial Factors

As neurophysiologic investigation of the brain-gut axis continues to yield new findings as related to the clinical expression of the FGIDs, our understanding of the role of psychosocial factors remains important in our understanding of the individual patient. While psychosocial factors do not define these disorders, and are not required for diagnosis (see below), they are important modulators of the patient's experience and behavior, and ultimately, the clinical outcome. Research on the psychosocial aspects of patients with FGIDs yields three general observations:

1. *Psychological stress exacerbates gastrointestinal symptoms.* Psychological stress or one's emotional responses to stress can affect gastrointestinal function and produce symptoms in healthy subjects, but does so to a greater degree in patients with functional gastrointestinal disorders [55]. Identification of specific psychological stressors associated with exacerbation of symptoms or poor outcomes may help in planning treatment using psychological or psychopharmacological methods.

2. *Psychological disturbances modify the experience of illness and illness behaviors such as health care seeking.* Research showing that patients with FGIDs have greater psychological disturbance than otherwise healthy subjects and patients with medical disease [56–69] is based on data drawn from patients seen at referral centers. This overestimates the true association. Since we know that for IBS psychosocial factors relate to health care seeking more strongly than to the disorder per se [19,20,70], it is likely that psychosocial factors modulate the illness experience and illness behaviors such as health care seeking. Thus, major psychosocial trauma (e.g., sexual or physical abuse history) is more common in re-

ferral centers than in primary care, and is associated with a more severe disorder and a poorer clinical outcome, independent of the medical diagnosis [71–73]. In addition, psychosocial trauma may lower pain threshold and increase pain reporting tendency (response bias) [74].

3. *Having a functional gastrointestinal disorder may have psychosocial consequences.* Having a functional gastrointestinal disorder (or any chronic illness) has psychosocial consequences in terms of one's general well-being, daily functional status, concerns related to control over the symptoms, and the implications of the illness in terms of future functioning at work and at home. From a research standpoint, this can be understood in terms of the patient's health-related quality of life (HRQOL) [75]. This differs from disease assessment since the evaluation includes psychosocial (e.g., daily function, recreation, sexual function, etc.) as well as symptom- or disease-related factors. Furthermore, validation rests with the patient, rather than with physiologic or physician-based standards. Several new HRQOL instruments have been developed to evaluate patients with FGIDs (see Chapter 4).

Rationale for Symptom-Based Diagnostic Criteria

The classification system presented in this book is based on the premise that each category is determined by symptom clusters that "breed true" across clinical and population groups. This presumption provides a framework for identification and investigation of these disorders, which can be modified as new scientific data in the research areas discussed above emerges. In effect, patients fulfilling criteria for a particular diagnosis represent a group who are more similar to each other with regard to the underlying pathophysiology and choice of treatment than to those having other diagnoses. The assumption of clinical similarities within groups having these symptom clusters is not perfectly true, as the section below on qualifications will discuss. At the least, diagnostic categories reduce the difficulties that existed in previous studies where arbitrary selection criteria yielded mixed clinical populations and uncertain findings [76].

The rationale for classifying the functional gastrointestinal disorders into symptom-based subgroups has three bases [77].

— Site-Specific Differences

Patients with functional gastrointestinal disorders report a wide variety of symptoms affecting different regions of the gastrointestinal tract. These symptoms have in common disturbances in sensory and/or motor gastrointestinal function, which can overlap across anatomic regions. For example, epidemiological studies show that over one-third of patients with IBS have dyspeptic symptoms, and vice versa [78], thereby implicating an epidemiological and possibly neurophysiological link. However, there are other studies that support the assumption of specific syndromes [79–81]. We can conclude that the functional gastrointestinal disorders fall into distinct groups, albeit all related due to similar pathophysiological mechanisms [82].

The clinical value of separating the functional gastrointestinal symptoms into discrete conditions is that they can be reliably diagnosed and more specifically treated. Thus, globus (A1) resulting from a disturbance of upper esophageal sphincter function is distinct from gallbladder dyskinesia (E1) and levator ani syndrome (F2a). Each disorder, while possibly having similar underlying features (abnormal motility or decreased sensation threshold), displays a different clinical presentation.

The Rome II Multinational Working Teams have classified the functional gastrointestinal disorders into six subcategories based on anatomic region: Esophageal (A), Gastroduodenal (B), Bowel (C), Functional Abdominal Pain (D), Biliary (E), and Anorectal (F). Functional Abdominal Pain is separated from the functional bowel disorders because its pathophysiology may relate more to altered brain than to gut function. Also, within each subcategory site, there can be several disorders, each with specific clinical features that distinguish them. For example, irritable bowel syndrome (C1), functional constipation (C3), and functional diarrhea (C4) are all functional bowel disorders attributed to the colon and rectum. Irritable bowel syndrome is characterized by pain associated with change in bowel function, while functional diarrhea is defined in terms of loose stools and no pain, and functional constipation is understood as delayed transit and/or defecatory difficulties with or without pain. As a result, each condition has a different diagnostic and treatment approach.

— Epidemiologic Data

Further support of symptom-based criteria is based on epidemiological studies that show homology across various studies and populations. For example, the frequencies of bowel symptom patterns reported from England, France and China (see Chapter 7) are nearly identical. Similarly, the frequencies of functional constipation (3.0%) and diarrhea (1.6%) in the U.S. Householder Study [1] using Rome I Diagnostic Criteria are similar (3.0% and 1.2%, respectively) to data from the National Health Interview Survey, which used an entirely different assessment method [83].

These observations are also upheld by factor analysis, a method to identify groups of symptoms that aggregate into discrete clusters. For example, a factor analysis study using two community samples [84] identified an irritable bowel factor, and these symptoms were very similar to those developed from a clinical population of irritable bowel patients using discriminant function analysis (Manning criteria) [79]. The data from these and other well designed studies provide the basis to develop criteria for these disorders.

— Need for Diagnostic Standards in Clinical Care and Research

Since no physiological mechanisms define these disorders, physiologic assessment remains an investigative tool that is not easily applied to clinical settings. Because it is the symptoms that patients bring to physicians, it is important to categorize them for clinical practice. Symptom-based diagnostic criteria have achieved world wide acceptance, beginning with the American Psychiatric Association's Diagnostic and Statistical Manual of Mental Disorders (DSM-IIIR) [85], the American Rheumatologic Association's Primer [86], and most recently with the Rome I Criteria [87]. Their use has helped clinicians categorize these disorders in a way that simplifies the diagnostic and treatment approach, and it has probably reduced the ordering of unneeded diagnostic studies.

Another intended purpose of symptom-based criteria is to standardize the selection of patients for clinical trials. For example, in previous studies with irritable bowel syndrome, heterogeneous patient groups (e.g., combining those with predominant diarrhea with those having predominant constipation) increased the possibility that a medication (e.g., to control diarrhea) would not be found effective [76]. Symptom-based criteria allow patient groups to be selected based on the predominant symptom pattern, and this helps to evaluate the predicted effects of a particular treatment. For example, within psychiatry, there is evidence that panic disorder is clinically distinct from generalized anxiety, and is more closely linked to depression, even though anxiety is common to both. Therefore, anxiety and panic disorders are classified separately in DSM-IV. Furthermore, by being able to study these conditions separately, investigators found that patients with panic disorder respond better to antidepressants than patients with generalized anxiety.

The publication of the Rome I Criteria [87] has attracted the interest of clinical investigators, pharmaceutical companies, and federal regulatory agencies, and reaffirms the continued need for standardized diagnostic criteria for clinical research [88]. However, a process needs to be set up to modify these criteria as new scientific data emerges. The Multinational Working Teams have taken on that responsibility, organized as Rome II, and will continue to evaluate and seek to validate the Criteria.

— Qualifications for the Use of Symptom-Based Criteria

We recognize that there are important limitations and qualifications to the use of symptom-based criteria that need to be addressed [77].

Other Diseases May Coexist that Need To Be Excluded

The high frequency of the functional gastrointestinal disorders in epidemiological and clinical studies assures their coexistence with other diseases. In fact, IBS and inflammatory bowel disease (IBD) appear to have a greater than chance association [89], and IBD may even predispose to IBS [90]. Similarly, *H. pylori* needs to be excluded and/or treated among patients with functional dyspepsia. So, for research purposes, it is necessary to exclude other diseases before a functional gastrointestinal designation can be applied. But within clinical practice, the coexistence of functional and organic disorders is a reality that requires careful clinical judgment. For example, a patient with mild ulcerative proctitis who develops crampy abdominal pain and diarrhea might not require an increase in steroid medication since the symptoms are more likely related to the co-morbidity of IBS.

Symptoms May Overlap Across Functional Gastrointestinal Conditions

Due to presumably similar pathophysiological features, it is understandable that symptom patterns overlap across the FGIDs [1]. But for research purposes, it is important to separate these conditions in a consistent and reproducible manner. Therefore, the Criteria include statements that permit a hierarchical separation of disorders. By convention, if criteria are fulfilled for both IBS (C1) and functional dyspepsia (B1), then the diagnoses coexist. However if the individual fulfills criteria for IBS but has upper gastrointestinal pain that is relieved by defecation, then the subject is diagnosed to have IBS only. For certain categories we also include an unspecified designation (e.g., unspecified functional bowel disorder) to permit the inclusion of patients with functional gastrointestinal symptoms who do not meet more specific categories.

Symptoms Must be Present for at Least 12 Weeks Over the Previous Year

Short-lived functional gastrointestinal symptoms are of little clinical significance, and acute infectious disorders that can mimic a functional gastrointestinal disorder are common. Therefore, to make a diagnosis of a functional gastrointestinal disorder, we require that symptoms be present for at least 12 weeks out of the previous year. There are a few exceptions: Chronic Functional Abdominal Pain Syndrome (D1) requires a six month history to be consistent with the DSM psychiatric classification, while fecal incontinence (F1), and some of the pediatric and other anorectal functional gastrointestinal disorders require symptoms being present for only a few weeks to fulfill diagnostic criteria. The 12-week qualification is a change from the Rome I criteria which only required that symptoms be present in the previous three months. The reasons for this change are that FGIDs are conditions that have a waxing and waning course, and (particularly for epidemiological surveys) symptoms might not have been present in the previous three months, but may have existed prior to that time. The 12 weeks may not be consecutive, and within each week, symptoms are only required for 1/7 days.

In addition, we recognize the difficulty in translating the time requirement into a questionnaire. For some purposes, investigators may choose the last three months as the time requirement. This choice may be preferred for entry into clinical trials and for clinical surveys (see appendices B and C).

Correlation of Symptoms with Disturbed Motility Varies

Some functional gastrointestinal disorders are closely linked to disturbances in visceral or somatic muscle motor function. Examples include sphincter of Oddi dysfunction (E2) or functional incontinence (F1). However, for certain other functional gastrointestinal disorders, motility disturbances may be found which do not necessarily correlate with symptoms (e.g., discrete clustered contractions in irritable bowel syndrome [C1]). Finally, functional abdominal pain (D) is an example where the symptoms are closely linked to disturbances in central (CNS) activity rather than motility; it is an "abnormal perception of normal function," more than abnormal gastrointestinal function. These observations lend support to the pathophysiological heterogeneity of these disorders.

Diagnostic Categories Do Not Include Psychosocial Criteria

While it is commonly recognized that psychosocial factors can profoundly affect the onset, course and outcome of the FGIDs [29], they are not specific to the FGIDs. Also, psychosocial disturbances are not present to the same degree in patients with FGID who are not seeking health care [19,20]. For these reasons, psychosocial items are not included in the Criteria, though their role in influencing health status and outcome is emphasized (see Chapter 4).

Definitions and Criteria are Determined by Clinical Consensus

Because morphologic or physiologic standards to diagnose the functional gastrointestinal disorders do not exist, the proposed diagnostic criteria are derived from clinical investigation and are validated by the consensus of experts in the field (the Rome Working Team Committees and their consultants). We recognize that experienced clinicians and investigators may have different interpretations to any set of symptoms based on training, experience, and personal beliefs. The diagnosis of patients according to consensus criteria begins the process for future studies that will seek to validate and/or modify these criteria based on the scientific evidence. Using the Rome I consensus criteria as a starting point, all changes for the Rome II Criteria require evidence. Thus, any changes had to be based on existing scientific data, or on a rational recommendation that is agreed upon by the Working Team, the Coordinating Committee, and the reviewers. In addition, Rome II is supporting clinical studies designed to test the utility and validity of the new Criteria. The results from these and other studies will form the basis for future modifications of the Criteria.

Given these caveats, the formulation of symptom-based diagnostic criteria for the FGIDs is rational, practical and much needed. The process for developing these criteria is a rigorous one, and is outlined below.

The idea of using a consensus process was initiated by Professor Aldo Torsoli for the International Congress of Gastroenterology in Rome (*Roma '88*). Dr. Torsoli, the President of this Congress, proposed having working team committees address issues not easily resolved by usual scientific inquiry or review of the literature [91]. The committees were charged to formulate a consensus statement and to make clinical recommendations that would be published in the journal *Gastroenterology International*. The decision process was derived from the Delphi method [92], which fosters a team effort to produce consistency in opinion, or consensus (although not necessarily total agreement), for difficult questions not easily addressed. In effect, any member's opinion must be presented to the rest of the group in a convincing manner in order for it to be accepted as a consensus statement. Since the *Roma '88* meetings, numerous Working Teams have published articles in *Gastroenterology International*, and this led to the preparation and publication of a book [87]. In 1995, the Rome II Coordinating Committee took on the responsibility to carry these activities further. Several new committees were added including one that developed a new pediatric classification system. The Coordinating Committee then developed a rigorous three-year, ten-step process for the creation of these chapters.

(1) The Coordinating Committee identified individuals with international research and clinical expertise to chair each of the ten Working Teams. Each Chair was charged to develop a manuscript for this book and also for a supplement in the journal *GUT*.

(2) Upon acceptance, the chair, with consultation from the Coordinating Committee, identified a co-chair, and recruited an international panel of up to five additional members with similar clinical and investigative skills to take on the specific assignments necessary for creation of the manuscripts.

(3) Each Working Team then produced a document in response to their specific assignment. This was a synthesis of the literature including their expert opinion on the diagnostic approach, and the physiological, psychological, and treatment aspects for a particular functional disorder or scientific content area.

(4) The chair then incorporated all documents into a manuscript that was sent back to the entire Team for review.

(5) This process of modification and re-review by the Working Team was repeated two more times.

(6) The Working Team then met for three days in June, 1998, to revise the document, using the Delphi method [92]. This permitted a face-to-face meeting to achieve consensus on the Diagnostic Criteria and scientific content.

(7) Following the meeting, the chair sent the revised document to a minimum of six outside international experts, in addition to scientists in the pharmaceutical industry, for their review and commentary.

(8) The Working Team chairs then responded to the reviewers' comments, either by modifying the manuscripts as requested, or providing a written response that addressed the reviewers' concerns.

(9) The revised manuscripts and the commentaries by the reviewers and authors were then sent to the Coordinating Committee, which met in November, 1998, and again in February, 1999, to critically review these materials and to submit a critique back to the authors.

(10) Finally, when the document was completed, all members provided written approval and it was returned back to the Coordinating Committee for a final check on content and style before submitting it for publication.

Approach to Treatment

Given the evidence that physiologic and psychosocial factors interact to explain symptom severity and illness behavior, it is rational to consider both in planning treatment. This section presents general treatment guidelines for patients with FGIDs [93,94]. It is assumed that patients fulfill criteria for a FGID and that diagnostic studies have excluded other specifically treatable disorders. Detailed treatment recommendations specific for each disorder are found in later chapters.

— The Therapeutic Relationship

The basis for implementing a strong physician-patient relationship is supported by evidence that patients with functional gastrointestinal disorders have anywhere from a 30% to 80% placebo response rate regardless of treatment. To establish a therapeutic relationship, the physician must:

(1) obtain the history through a nondirective, nonjudgmental, patient-centered interview;
(2) conduct a careful examination and cost-efficient investigation;
(3) determine the patient's understanding of the illness and his or her concerns (*"What do you think is causing your symptoms?"*);
(4) provide a thorough explanation of the disorder;
(5) identify and respond realistically to the patient's expectations for improvement (*"How do you feel I can be helpful to you?"*);
(6) set consistent limits (*"I appreciate how bad the pain is, but narcotic medication is not indicated"*);
(7) involve the patient in the treatment (*"Let me suggest some treatments for you to consider"*); and
(8) establish a long-term relationship with a primary care provider [93].

Because the FGIDs are chronic, it is important to determine the immediate reasons for the patient's visit: (*"What led you to see me at this time?"*), and to evaluate the patient's verbal and nonverbal communication. Possible causes include:

(1) new exacerbating factors (dietary change, concurrent medical disorder, side effects of new medication);
(2) personal concern about a serious disease (recent family death);
(3) environmental stressors (e.g., major loss, abuse history);
(4) psychiatric co-morbidity (depression, anxiety);

(5) impairment in daily function (recent inability to work or socialize); or

(6) a "hidden agenda," such as narcotic or laxative abuse, pending disability, unconscious secondary gain, or somatic representation of psychosocial conflict.

Once the reasons for the visit are determined, treatment is based on the severity and nature of the symptoms, the physiologic and psychosocial determinants of the patient's illness behavior, and the degree of functional impairment. These factors can separate patients into mild, moderate, and severe categories.

— Patients with Mild Symptoms

Patients with mild or infrequent symptoms are usually seen in primary care practices and do not have major impairment in function or psychological disturbance. These patients may have concerns about the implications of their symptoms, but they do not make frequent physician visits, and usually maintain normal activity levels. Here, treatment is directed toward education, reassurance that no serious disease exists, and achievement of a healthier lifestyle.

1. Education. It is helpful to explain that functional gastrointestinal symptoms are very real, and the intestine is overly responsive to a variety of stimuli such as food, hormonal changes, medication, and stress. Pain resulting from spasm or stretching of the gut, from a sensitive gut, or both, can be experienced anywhere in the abdomen [95], and can be associated with changes in gastrointestinal function leading to symptoms (e.g., pain, nausea, vomiting, diarrhea, etc.). The physician should emphasize that both physiologic and psychological factors interact to produce symptoms.

2. Reassurance. The physician should elicit patient worries and concerns and provide appropriate reassurance. While this can be an effective therapeutic intervention, if it is communicated in a perfunctory manner and before necessary tests are completed, the patient will reject it.

3. Diet and medication. Offending dietary substances (e.g., lactose, caffeine, fatty foods, alcohol, etc.) and medications that adversely cause symptoms should be identified and possibly eliminated. Sometimes a food diary is helpful.

— Patients with Moderate Symptoms

A smaller proportion of patients, usually seen in primary or secondary care, report moderate symptoms and have intermittent disruptions in activity, for example, missing social functions, work, or school. They may identify a close relationship between symptoms and inciting events such as dietary indiscretion, travel, or distressing experiences. They may be more psychologically distressed than patients with mild symptoms. For this group, additional treatment options are recommended.

1. *Symptom monitoring.* The patient can keep a symptom diary for one to two weeks to record the time, severity, and presence of associated factors [96]. This may help to identify inciting factors, such as dietary indiscretions or specific stressors not previously considered. The physician can then review possible dietary, lifestyle, or behavioral modifications with the patient. This encourages the patient's participation in treatment, and as symptoms improve, increases his or her sense of control over the illness.

2. *Pharmacotherapy directed at specific symptoms.* Medication can be considered for symptom episodes that are distressing or that impair daily function. The choice of medication will depend on the predominant symptom and is outlined in later chapters of this book. In general, prescription medications should be considered as ancillary to dietary or lifestyle modifications for chronic symptoms, but can be used during periods of acute symptom exacerbation.

3. *Psychological treatments.* Psychological treatments may be considered for motivated patients with moderate to severe gastrointestinal symptoms [97] and for patients with pain symptoms [98,99]. It is more helpful if the patient can associate symptoms with stressors [100]. These treatments, which include cognitive-behavioral therapy, relaxation, hypnosis, psychotherapy, and combination treatments, help to reduce anxiety levels, encourage health promoting behaviors, give the patient greater responsibility and control in the treatment, and improve pain tolerance [94]. See Chapter 4 for more details.

— Patients with Severe Symptoms

Only a small proportion of patients with FGIDs (e.g., with chronic functional abdominal pain [D]) has severe and refractory symptoms. These patients also have a high frequency of associated psychosocial difficulties, including diagnoses of anxiety, depression or somatization, personality disturbance, and chronically impaired daily functioning. There may be a history of major loss or abuse, poor social networks or coping skills and "catastrophizing" behaviors. These patients may see gastroenterology consultants frequently and hold unrealistic expectations to be "cured." They may deny a role for psychosocial factors in the illness and may be unresponsive to psychological treatment or to pharmacological agents directed at the gut.

1. The physician's approach. These patients need an ongoing relationship with a physician (gastroenterologist or primary care physician) who provides psychosocial support through repeated brief visits. In general, the physician should: (a) perform diagnostic and therapeutic measures based on objective findings rather than in response to patient demands; (b) set realistic treatment goals, such as improved quality of life rather than complete pain relief or cure; (c) shift the responsibility for treatment to the patient by giving therapeutic options, and (d) change the focus of care from treatment of disease to adjustment to chronic illness.

2. Antidepressant treatment. The tricyclic antidepressants (e.g., amitriptyline, imipramine, doxepin), and more recently, the serotonin reuptake inhibitors (e.g., fluoxetine, sertraline, paroxetine) have a role in controlling pain via central analgesia [101], as well as relief of associated depressive symptoms. Antidepressants should be considered for unremitting pain and impaired daily functioning, coexistent symptoms of major or atypical depression, or panic attacks. Even without depressive symptoms, these agents may help when the pain is dominant and consuming. A poor clinical response may be due to insufficient dose or failure to adjust the dosage based on therapeutic response or side effects [102]. Treatment should be instituted for at least three to four weeks. If effective, it can be continued for three to twelve months and then tapered. Benzodiazepine-type anxiolytics usually are not indicated.

3. Pain treatment center referral. Pain treatment centers provide a multidisciplinary team approach toward rehabilitation of patients who have become seriously disabled. One controlled study [103] showed that patients with chronic pelvic pain who underwent an interdisciplinary pain management program had decreased pain scores, decreased anxiety and depression, and improved psychosocial functioning six months after treatment.

Concluding Comment

As we enter the new millennium, it seems likely that that many of the methods and techniques currently in use for understanding and treating patients with functional gastrointestinal disorders, will be modified or replaced concurrent with our changing understanding of these disorders. And if we look back over the last 20 years in the field, the changes have been remarkable: an explosion in diagnostic instrumentation, now involving the brain and gut; improved research methods to assess clinical symptoms and outcomes; and most importantly, a shift from dualistic and reductionistic views on diagnosis and treatment to a more integrated and comprehensive biopsychosocial understanding. While it is likely that potent new treatments will follow our growing pathophysiologic knowledge of these disorders, it is unlikely that they will replace some of the fundamental clinical principles: active listening, careful decision-making, an effective patient-physician relationship, and a patient-centered biopsychosocial plan of care.

We believe that the development and work of the Rome Working Teams over the last ten years have contributed to this progress in a number of ways. Rome Criteria reinforce an appreciation of the utility of symptom-based diagnosis. These Criteria give researchers the opportunity to select subjects in a standard fashion for clinical research. Clinicians are now provided with a database of information on the epidemiology, pathophysiology, and diagnostic and treatment approaches for these conditions. Finally, the Rome Working Teams contributed in major ways to the legitimization of these disorders as worthy of future investigation. In representing the Rome Working Teams, we invite your continuing interest and support.

References

1. Drossman DA, Li Z, Andruzzi E, et al. U.S. Householder survey of functional gastrointestinal disorders: prevalence, sociodemography and health impact. Dig Dis Sci 1993;38:1569–80.

2. Sandler R. Epidemiology of irritable bowel syndrome in the United States. Gastroenterology 1990;99(suppl 2):409–15.

3. Talley NJ, Zinsmeister AR, Schleck CD, et al. Dyspepsia and dyspepsia subgroups: a population-based study. Gastroenterology 1992;102:1259–68.

4. Thompson WG, Heaton KW. Functional bowel disorders in apparently healthy people. Gastroenterology 1980;79:283–88.

5. Bommelaer G, Rouch M, Dapoigny M, et al. Epidemiology of functional bowel disorders in apparently healthy people. Gastroenterol Clin Biol 1986;10:7–12.

6. Bi-zhen W, Qi-Ying P. Functional bowel disorders in apparently healthy Chinese people. Chinese J Epidiol 1988;9:345–49.

7. Switz DM. What the gastroenterologist does all day: a survey of a state society's practice. Gastroenterology 1976;70:1048–50.

8. Ferguson A, Sircus W, Eastwood MA. Frequency of "functional" gastrointestinal disorders. Lancet 1977;2:613–14.

9. Mitchell CM, Drossman DA. Survey of the AGA membership relating to patients with functional gastrointestinal disorders. Gastroenterology 1987;92:1282–84.

10. Drossman DA, Thompson WG, Talley NJ, et al. Identification of subgroups of functional bowel disorders. Gastroenterol Internat 1990;3:159–72.

11. Powell R. On certain painful afflictions of the intestinal canal. Med Trans Roy Coll Phys 1818;6:106–17.

12. Almy TP, Tulin M. Alterations in colonic function in man under stress: experimental production of changes simulating the "irritable colon". Gastroenterology 1947;8:616–26.

13. Almy TP. Experimental studies on the irritable colon. Am J Med 1951;10:60–67.

14. Chaudhary NA, Truelove SC. The irritable colon syndrome: a study of the clinical features, predisposing causes, and prognosis in 130 cases. Quart J Med 1962; 31:307–22.

15. Drossman DA. Presidential address: gastrointestinal illness and biopsychosocial model. Psychosomat Med 1998;60:258–67.

16. Drossman DA. Psychosocial mechanisms in GI illness. In: Kirsner JB, Editor. The Growth of Gastroenterologic Knowledge in the 20th Century. Philadelphia:Lea & Febiger;1993;419–32.

17. Kroenke K, Mangelsdorff AD. Common symptoms in ambulatory care: incidence, evaluation, therapy, and outcome. Am J Med 1989;86:262–66.

18. Drossman DA. Psychosocial factors in ulcerative colitis and Crohn's disease. In: Kirsner JB, Editor. Inflammatory Bowel Disease. Ed. 5. Philadelphia:W.B. Saunders Company; 1999.

19. Drossman DA, McKee DC, Sandler RS, et al. Psychosocial factors in the irritable

bowel syndrome: a multivariate study of patients and nonpatients with irritable bowel syndrome. Gastroenterology 1988;95:701–708.

20. Whitehead WE, Bosmajian L, Zonderman AB, et al. Symptoms of psychologic distress associated with irritable bowel syndrome: comparison of community and medical clinic samples. Gastroenterology 1988;95:709–14.

21. Smith RC, Greenbaum DS, Vancouver JB, et al. Psychosocial factors are associated with health care seeking rather than diagnosis in irritable bowel syndrome. Gastroenterology 1990;98:293–301.

22. Christensen J. Heraclides or the physician. Gastroenterol Internat 1990;3:45–48.

23. Engel GL. The need for a new medical model: a challenge for biomedicine. Science 1977;196:129–36.

24. Engel GL. The clinical application of the Biopsychosocial model. Am J Psychiatry 1980;137:535–44.

25. Aziz Q, Thompson DG. Brain-gut axis in health and disease. Gastroenterology 1998;114:559–78.

26. Accarino AM, Azpiroz F, Malagelada JR. Attention and distraction: effects on gut perception. Gastroenterology 1997;113:415–22.

27. Collins SM, Assche GV, Hogaboam C. Alterations in enteric nerve and smooth-muscle function in inflammatory bowel diseases. Inflam Bowel Dis 1997;3:38–48.

28. Clauw DJ, Chrousos GP. Chronic pain and fatigue syndromes: overlapping clinical and neuroendocrine features and potential pathogenic mechanisms. Neuroimmunomodulation 1997;4:134–53.

29. Drossman DA, Creed FH, Olden KW, et al. Psychosocial aspects of the functional gastrointestinal disorders. Gut 1999;45(suppl 11):25–30.

30. Young LD, Richter JE, Anderson KO, et al. The effects of psychological and environmental stressors on peristaltic esophageal contractions in healthy volunteers. Psychophysiology 1987;24:132–41.

31. Wolf S, Wolff HG. Human Gastric Function. New York:Oxford University Press; 1943.

32. Kellow JE, Langeluddecke PM, Eckersley GM, et al. Effects of acute psychologic stress on small-intestinal motility in health and the irritable bowel syndrome. Scand J Gastroenterol 1992;27:53–58.

33. Almy TP, Kern F Jr, Tulin M. Alteration in colonic function in man under stress: II. Experimental production of sigmoid spasm in healthy persons. Gastroenterology 1949;12:425–36.

34. Kumar D, Wingate DL. The irritable bowel syndrome: a paroxysmal motor disorder. Lancet 1985;2:973–77.

35. Narducci F, Snape WJ, Battle WM, et al. Increased colonic motility during exposure to a stressful situation. Dig Dis Sci 1985;30:40–44.

36. Welgan P, Meshkinpour H, Beeler M. Effect of anger on colon motor and myoelectric activity in irritable bowel syndrome. Gastroenterology 1988;94:1150–56.

37. Kellow JE, Phillips SF, Miller LJ, et al. Dysmotility of the small intestine in irritable bowel syndrome. Gut 1988;29:1236–43.

38. Drossman DA, Whitehead WE, Camilleri M. Irritable bowel syndrome: a technical review for practice guideline development. Gastroenterology 1997;112:2120–37.

39. Geenen JE, Hogan WJ, et al. The efficacy of endoscopic sphincterotomy after cholecystectomy in patients with sphincter-of-Oddi dysfunction. New Engl J Med 1989;320:82–87.

40. Richter JE, Barish CF, Castell DO. Abnormal sensory perception in patients with esophageal chest pain. Gastroenterology 1986;91:845–52.

41. Mearin F, Cucala M, Azpiroz F, et al. The origin of symptoms on the brain-gut axis in functional dyspepsia. Gastroenterology 1991;101:999–1006.

42. Whitehead WE, Holtkotter B, Enck P, et al. Tolerance for rectosigmoid distention in irritable bowel syndrome. Gastroenterology 1990;98:1187–92.

43. Clouse RE, Lustman PJ, McCord GS, et al. Clinical correlates of abnormal sensitivity to intraesophageal balloon distention. Dig Dis Sci 1991;36:1040–45.

44. Ness TJ, Metcalf AM, Gebhart GF. A psychophysiological study in humans using phasic colonic distension as a noxious visceral stimulus. Pain 1990;43:377–86.

45. Munakata J, Naliboff B, Harraf F, et al. Repetitive sigmoid stimulation induces rectal hyperalgesia in patients with irritable bowel syndrome. Gastroenterology 1997;112:55–63.

46. Collins SM. Is the irritable gut an inflamed gut? Scand J Gastroenterol 1992; 27(suppl 192):102–105.

47. Collins SM. The immunomodulation of enteric neuromuscular function: implications for motility and inflammatory disorders. Gastroenterology 1996;111: 1683–99.

48. McKendrick W, Read NW. Irritable bowel syndrome—post salmonella infection. J Infection 1994;29:1–4.

49. Gwee KA, Leong YL, Graham C, et al. The role of psychological and biological factors in post-infective gut dysfunction. Gut 1999;44:400–406.

50. Mayer EA, Raybould HE. Role of visceral afferent mechanisms in functional bowel disorders. Gastroenterology 1990;99:1688–1704.

51. Svensson TH. Peripheral, autonomic regulation of locus coeruleus noradrenergic neurons in brain: putative implications for psychiatry and psychopharmacology. Psychopharmacology 1987;92:1–7.

52. Valori RM, Kumar D, Wingate DL. Effects of different types of stress and/or "prokinetic" drugs on the control of the fasting motor complex in humans. Gastroenterology 1986;90:1890–1900.

53. Drossman DA. Mind over matter in the postinfective irritable bowel. Gut 1999; 44:306–307.

54. Mayberg HS, Brannan SK, Mahurin RK, et al. Cingulate function in depression: a potential predictor of treatment response. Neuroreport 1997;8:1057–61.

55. Whitehead WE, Crowell MD, Robinson JC, et al. Effects of stressful life events on bowel symptoms: subjects with irritable bowel syndrome compared to subjects without bowel dysfunction. Gut 1992;33:825–30.

56. Young SJ, Alpers DH, Norland CC, et al. Psychiatric illness and the irritable bowel syndrome: practical implications for the primary physician. Gastroenterology 1976;70:162–66.

57. Palmer RL, Crisp AH, Sonehill E, et al. Psychological characteristics of patients with the irritable bowel syndrome. Postgrad Med J 1974;50:416–19.

58. Magni G, DiMario F, Bernasconi G, et al. DSM-III diagnoses associated with dyspepsia of unknown cause. Am J Psychiatry 1987;144:1222–23.

59. Walker EA, Roy-Byrne PP, Katon WJ, et al. Psychiatric illness and irritable bowel syndrome: a comparison with inflammatory bowel disease. Am J Psychiatry 1990;147:1656–61.

60. Craig TKJ, Brown GW. Goal frustration and life events in the aetiology of painful gastrointestinal disorder. J Psychosomat Res 1984;28:411–21.

61. Whitehead WE, Winget C, Fedoravicius AS, et al. Learned illness behavior in patients with irritable bowel syndrome and peptic ulcer. Dig Dis Sci 1982;27:202–208.

62. Drossman DA, Leserman J, Nachman G, et al. Sexual and physical abuse in women with functional or organic gastrointestinal disorders. Ann Intern Med 1990;113:828–33.

63. Nyren O, Adami HO, Gustavsson S, et al. Excess sick-listing in nonulcer dyspepsia. J Clin Gastroenterol 1986;8:339–45.

64. Sloth H, Jorgensen LS. Predictors for the course of chronic non-organic upper abdominal pain. Scand J Gastroenterol 1989;24:440–44.

65. Sloth H, Jorgensen LS. Chronic non-organic upper abdominal pain: diagnostic safety and prognosis of gastrointestinal and non-intestinal symptoms: a 5- to 7-year follow-up study. Scand J Gastroenterol 1988;23:1275–80.

66. Talley NJ, Jones M, Piper DW. Psychosocial and childhood factors in essential dyspepsia. Scand J Gastroenterol 1988;23:341–46.

67. Bradley LA, Richter JE, Pulliam TJ, et al. The relationship between stress and symptoms of gastroesophageal reflux: the influence of psychological factors. Am J Gastroenterol 1993;88:11–19.

68. Clouse RE, Lustman PJ. Psychiatric illness and contraction abnormalities of the esophagus. New Engl J Med 1983;309:1337–42.

69. Wilson JA, Deary IJ, Maran AG. Is globus hystericus? Brit J Psychiatry 1988;153:335–39.

70. Sandler RS, Drossman DA, Nathan HP, et al. Symptom complaints and health care seeking behavior in subjects with bowel dysfunction. Gastroenterology 1984;87:314–18.

71. Drossman DA. Sexual and physical abuse and gastrointestinal illness. Scand J Gastroenterol 1995;208(suppl):90–96.

72. Drossman DA, Li Z, Leserman J, et al. Health status by gastrointestinal diagnosis and abuse history. Gastroenterology 1996;110:999–1007.

73. Longstreth GF, Wolde-Tsadik G. Irritable bowel-type symptoms in HMO examinees: prevalence, demographics, and clinical correlates. Dig Dis Sci 1993;38:1581–89.

74. Scarinci IC, Haile JM, Bradley LA, et al. Pain perception and psychosocial correlates of sexual/physical abuse among patients with gastrointestinal disorders. Gastroenterology 1992;102:A509.

75. Guyatt GH, Feeny DH, Patrick DL. Measuring health-related quality of life. Ann Intern Med 1993;118:622–29.

76. Klein KB. Controlled treatment trials in the irritable bowel syndrome: a critique. Gastroenterology 1988;95:232–41.

77. Drossman DA. Do the Rome Criteria stand up? In: Goebell H, Holtmann G, Talley NJ, Editors. Functional Dyspepsia and Irritable Bowel Syndrome: Concepts and Controversies (Falk Symposium 99). Dordrecht: Kluwer Academic Publishers; 1998:11–18.

78. Agreus L, Svardsudd K, Nyren O, et al. Irritable bowel syndrome and dyspepsia in the general population: overlap and lack of stability over time. Gastroenterology 1995;109:671–80.

79. Manning AP, Thompson WG, Heaton KW, et al. Towards positive diagnosis of the irritable bowel. Brit Med J 1978;2:653–54.

80. Whitehead WE. Functional bowel disorders: are they independent diagnoses? In: Corazziari E, Editor. NeUroGastroenterology. Berlin:Walter de Gruyter;1996: 65–74.

81. Whitehead WE, Li Z, Drossman DA, et al. Factor analysis of GI symptoms supports Rome criteria for functional GI disorders. Gastroenterology 1994;106:A589.

82. Whitehead WE, Gibbs NA, Li Z, et al. Is functional dyspepsia just a subset of the irritable bowel syndrome? Baillieres Clin Gastroenterol. 1998;12:443–61.

83. LeClere FB, Moss AJ, Everhart JE, et al. Prevalence of major digestive disorders and bowel symptoms, 1989. Advance data from vital and health statistics: no. 212. Hyattsville, Maryland:National Center for Health Statistics;1992.

84. Whitehead WE, Crowell MD, Bosmajian L, et al. Existence of irritable bowel syndrome supported by factor analysis of symptoms in two community samples. Gastroenterology 1990;98:336–40.

85. American Psychiatric Association. Diagnostic and Statistical Manual of Mental Disorders—DSM-IV. Washington, DC:American Psychiatric Association; 1994.

86. Schumaker HR, Klippel JH, Robinson DR. Primer on the Rheumatic Diseases. Atlanta, Georgia:Arthritis Foundation;1988.

87. Drossman DA, Richter JE, Talley NJ, et al. The Functional Gastrointestinal Disorders: Diagnosis, Pathophysiology and Treatment. McLean,VA:Degnon Associates;1994.

88. Camilleri M. What's in a name? Roll on Rome II. Gastroenterology 1998;114: 237–37.

89. Bayless TM. Inflammatory bowel disease and irritable bowel syndrome. Med Clin North Am 1990;49:21–28.

90. Isgar B, Harman M, Kaye MD, et al. Symptoms of irritable bowel syndrome in ulcerative colitis in remission. Gut 1983;24:190–92.

91. Torsoli A, Corazziari E. The WTR's, the Delphic Oracle and the Roman Conclaves. Gastroenterol Internat 1991;4:44.

92. Milholland AV, Wheeler SG, Heieck JJ. Medical assessment by a delphi group opinion technic. New Engl J Med 1973;298:1272–75.

93. Drossman DA, Thompson WG. The irritable bowel syndrome: review and a graduated, multicomponent treatment approach. Ann Intern Med 1992;116: 1009–1016.

94. Drossman DA. Diagnosing and treating patients with refractory functional gastrointestinal disorders. Ann Intern Med 1995;123:688–97.

95. Swarbrick ET, Hegarty JE, Bat L, et al. Site of pain from the irritable bowel syndrome. Lancet 1980;2:443–46.

96. Shimberg EF. Relief from IBS. New York:M. Evans;1988.

97. Whitehead WE. Behavioral medicine approaches to gastrointestinal disorders. J Consult Clin Psych 1992;60:605–12.

98. Keefe FJ, Dunsmore J, Burnett R. Behavioral and cognitive-behavioral approaches to chronic pain: recent advances and future directions. J Consult Clin Psychol 1992;60:528–36.

99. Linssen ACG, Spinhoven P. Multimodal treatment programmes for chronic pain: a quantitative analsis of existing research data. J Psychosomat Res 1992; 36:275–86.

100. Guthrie E, Creed F, Dawson D, et al. A randomised controlled trial of psychotherapy in patients with refractory irritable bowel syndrome. Brit J Psychiatry 1993;163:315–21.

101. Onghena P, Houdenhove BV. Antidepressant-induced analgesia in chronic nonmalignant pain: a meta-analysis of 39 placebo-controlled studies. Pain 1992; 49:205–19.

102. Cakkues AL, Popkin MK. Antidepressant treatment of medical-surgical inpatients by nonpsychiatric physicians. Arch Gen Psychiatry 1987;44:157–60.

103. Kames LD, Rapkin AJ, Naliboff BD, et al. Effectiveness of an interdisciplinary pain management program for the treatment of chronic pelvic pain. Pain 1990;41(1): 41–46.

Chapter 2

Fundamentals of Neurogastroenterology: Basic Science

Jackie D. Wood *and*

David H. Alpers, Co-Chairs,

with Paul L. R. Andrews

General Principles of Enteric Nervous Control

Neural networks for control of digestive functions are positioned in the brain, spinal cord, prevertebral sympathetic ganglia, and in the walls of the specialized organs that make up the digestive system. Control involves an integrated hierarchy of neural centers. Starting at the level of the gut, Figure 1 diagrams four levels of integrative organization. Level 1 is the enteric nervous system (ENS), which has local circuitry for integrative functions independent of extrinsic nervous connections. The second level of integration occurs in the prevertebral sympathetic ganglia where peripheral reflex pathways are influenced by preganglionic sympathetic fibers from the spinal cord. Levels 3 and 4 are within the central nervous system (CNS). At the third level, sympathetic and parasympathetic outflow to the gut is determined in part by reflexes with sensory fibers that travel with autonomic nerves. The fourth level includes higher brain centers that supply descending signals that are integrated with incoming sensory signals at level 3. The neural networks at Level 1 within the walls of the gut integrate contraction of the muscle coats, transport across the mucosal lining, and intramural blood flow into organized patterns of behavior. These networks form the ENS, which is considered to be one of the three subdivisions of the autonomic nervous system together with sympathetic and parasympathetic divisions.

Outflow in motor neurons of the ENS may either contract or relax the muscles. Absorption from the lumen and secretion into the lumen are also controlled by the ENS. Neural activity controls intramural blood flow and the distribution of flow within the muscle layers and mucosa. Malfunctions of neural control are becoming increasingly recognized as underlying factors in functional gastrointestinal disorders (FGIDs).

The musculature, mucosal epithelium, and blood and lymphatic vasculature are the effector systems of the digestive tract. Moment-to-moment behavior of any of the specialized compartments of the gut reflects the integrated activity of these three systems. The ENS coordinates activity of each system to achieve organized behavior of the whole organ. This is accomplished by timing of excitatory and inhibitory inputs to each effector system individually. This kind of integration occurs in the intestine where mucosal secretion and muscle activity are coordinated in a timed sequence during propulsion of the luminal contents [1,2].

The ENS is like a minibrain with a library of programs for different patterns of gut behavior. Emesis is an example of a program stored in the library. During emesis, propulsion in the upper small intestine is reversed for rapid movement of the contents toward the open pylorus and relaxed stomach. This program is downloaded from the library either by commands from the brain or by local sensory detection of noxious substances in the lumen [3].

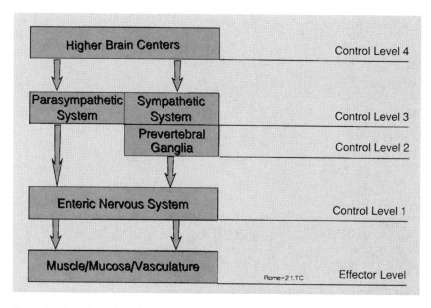

Figure I. Neural control of the gut is hierarchic with four basic levels of integrative organization. Level 1 is the ENS which behaves like a local "minibrain." The second level of integrative organization is in the prevertebral sympathetic ganglia. The third and fourth levels are within the CNS. Sympathetic and parasympathetic signals to the digestive tract originate at level three and represent the final common pathways for outflow of information from the central nervous to the gut. The fourth level includes higher brain centers that provide input for integrative functions at level three.

The heuristic model for the ENS (fig. 2) is the same as for the CNS. Like the CNS, the ENS functions with three categories of neurons identified as sensory, inter- and motor neurons.

Sensory neurons have receptor regions specialized for detecting changes in stimulus energy. Elsewhere in the body, sensory receptors are classified according to the kinds of energy they detect. These include photo-, thermo-, chemo-, and mechanoreceptors, each of which, except for photoreceptors, are found in the gut. The receptor regions transform changes in stimulus energy into signals coded by action potentials that subsequently are transmitted along sensory nerve fibers to other points in the nervous system.

Interneurons are connected by synapses into networks that process sensory information and control the behavior of motor neurons. Multiple connections among many interneurons form "logic" circuits that decipher action potential

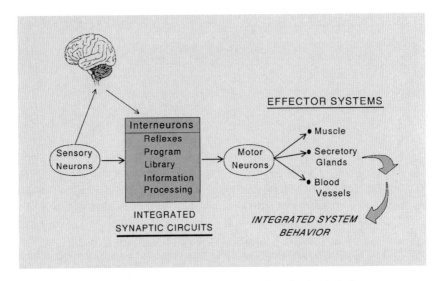

Figure 2. The conceptual model for the ENS is the same as for the CNS. Sensory neurons, interneurons, and motor neurons are connected synaptically for flow of information from sensory neurons to interneuronal integrative networks to motor neurons to effector systems. The ENS organizes and coordinates the activity of each effector system into meaningful behavior of the integrated organ. Bi-directional communication occurs between the CNS and ENS.

codes from sensory neurons and signals from elsewhere in the nervous system. These are recognized as integrative or reflex circuits because they organize reflex responses to sensory inputs.

Motor neurons are the final common pathways for transmission of control signals to the effector systems. In the digestive tract, motor signals may initiate, sustain, or suppress the behavior of the effector.

Innervation of the Digestive Tract

The digestive tract is innervated by the autonomic nervous system and by sensory nerves projecting to the spinal cord (splanchnic and sacral afferents) and brain stem (vagal afferents). Neuronal cell somas of the autonomic innervation are found in the brain stem and in ganglia located both outside and within the walls of the digestive tract. Cell bodies of extrinsic sensory nerve fibers are either in the nodose ganglia of the vagi or in dorsal root ganglia of the spinal cord.

The sympathetic, parasympathetic. and enteric divisions of the autonomic nervous system makeup the autonomic innervation. Sympathetic and parasympathetic pathways transmit signals between the CNS and the gut. This is the extrinsic component of innervation. Neurons of the enteric division form the local intramural control networks and are the intrinsic components of innervation. The parasympathetic and sympathetic subdivisions are identified by the positions of the ganglia containing the cell bodies of the postganglionic neurons and by the point of outflow from the CNS. Comprehensive autonomic innervation of the digestive tract consists of interconnections between the brain, the spinal cord, and the ENS (fig. 1).

— Parasympathetic Nervous System

The parasympathetic division of the autonomic innervation is subdivided anatomically into cranial and sacral divisions due to neuroanatomic organization in which neurons that send fibers to the gut are located both in the brain stem and in the sacral region of the spinal cord. Projections to the digestive tract from these regions of the CNS are preganglionic efferents. Neuronal cell bodies of the cranial division reside in the medulla oblongata and project in the vagal nerves. Cell bodies of the sacral division are located in the sacral region of the spinal cord and project in the pelvic nerves to the large intestine. Efferent fibers in the pelvic nerves make synaptic contact with neurons in ganglia located on the serosal surface of the colon and in ganglia of the ENS deeper within the large intestinal wall. Efferent vagal fibers form synapses with neurons of the ENS in esophagus, stomach, the small intestine, and colon, as well as the gallbladder and pancreas.

— Sympathetic Nervous System

The sympathetic division of the autonomic innervation is positioned in thoracic and lumbar regions of the spinal cord. Efferent sympathetic fibers leave the spinal cord in the ventral roots to make their first synaptic connections with neurons in prevertebral sympathetic ganglia located in the abdomen. The prevertebral ganglia are the coeliac, the superior mesenteric, and the inferior mesenteric ganglia. Cell bodies in the prevertebral ganglia project to the digestive tract where they form synapses with neurons of the ENS in addition to innervating the blood vessels, mucosa, and specialized regions of the musculature.

— Enteric Nervous System

Cell bodies of neurons of the ENS division of the autonomic nervous system are in ganglia within the walls of the digestive tract. The system consists of ganglia and interganglionic fiber tracts that form ganglionated plexuses. The ganglionated plexuses are continuous around the circumference of the gastrointestinal tract and along its length. The myenteric and submucous plexuses are the prominent ganglionated plexuses of the ENS (fig. 3).

The myenteric plexus, known also as Auerbach's plexus, is the major plexus of the ENS. It is located between the longitudinal and circular muscle layers of most all regions of the gastrointestinal tract. It is a two-dimensional array of neurons, ganglia, and interganglionic fiber tracts situated in close apposition to the longitudinal muscle. This organization is assumed to be an adaptation for sustaining function of the neural circuits as the nervous system is subjected to the mechanical forces and deformations that occur during contraction of the muscle or expansion and stretching of the wall as the lumen fills. Most of the motor neurons that innervate the circular and longitudinal muscle coats are found in the myenteric plexus [4–6].

The submucous plexus is a ganglionated plexus situated throughout the submucosal space between the mucosa and circular muscle coat (fig. 3). It is most prominent as a ganglionated network in the small and large intestine. No ganglionated submucous plexus exists in the esophagus, and ganglia are sparse in the submucosal space of the stomach. In larger mammals (e.g., pig, humans), the submucous plexus consists of an inner submucous network (Meissner's plexus) located at the serosal side of the muscularis mucosae and an outer plexus (Schabadasch's plexus) adjacent to the luminal side of the circular muscle coat. In human small and large bowel, a third intermediate plexus lies between the Meissner's and Schabadasch's plexus [7].

Motor innervation of the intestinal crypts and villi originates in the submucous plexus. Neurons in submucosal ganglia send fibers to the myenteric plexus and also receive synaptic input from axons projecting from the myenteric plexus [8,9]. The interconnections link the two networks into a functionally integrated nervous system.

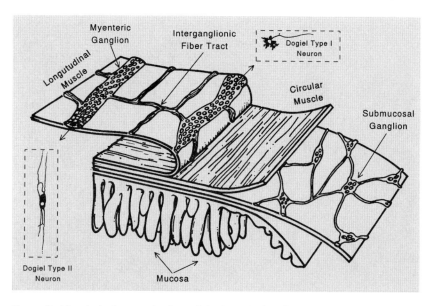

Figure 3. Morphologic organization of the intestinal wall showing the two principal ganglionated plexuses of the ENS, the primary muscles, the mucosa and shapes of two main types of neurons found in ganglia of the ENS.

Structure, function, and neurochemistry of enteric ganglia differ significantly from other autonomic ganglia. Unlike other autonomic ganglia, where function is mainly as relay-distribution centers for signals transmitted from the CNS, enteric ganglia are interconnected to form a nervous system with mechanisms for integration and processing of information like those found in the brain and spinal cord. On this basis, the ENS is sometimes referred to as "the brain-in-the-gut."

Many properties of the ENS resemble the CNS. Examples are:

(1) *Complex Integrative Functions*—Like the brain, the ENS executes complex integrative functions that control single effector systems and coordinate the behavior of a variety of different systems.

(2) *Sensory neurons*—Sensory neurons transmit information to the neural circuits of the ENS for processing same as in the CNS.

(3) *Interneurons*—Interneurons are synaptically connected into information processing circuits in both the ENS and CNS, but generally not in other autonomic ganglia.

(4) *Motor Neurons*—Enteric motor neurons are the final common pathways for flow of information from interneuronal processing circuits to the

effector systems. Their function is analogous to that of motor neurons from the spinal cord to the skeletal muscles.

(5) *Glial Elements*—The supporting cells of the ENS are like glial cells in the brain, but unlike the Schwann cells found associated with other autonomic ganglia. Enteric glial elements structurally and chemically resemble astroglia of the brain.

(6) *Synaptic Neuropil*—A synaptic neuropil is present in both enteric ganglia and the CNS. Neuropils are tangled meshworks of fine nonmyelinated nerve fibers that are segregated in parts of the ganglia away from the cell bodies that give rise to the fibers. This is consequential because in all integrative nervous systems, most of the information processing occurs in microcircuits within a synaptic neuropil.

(7) *Multiple Synaptic Mechanisms*—As in the brain, the neural circuits of the ENS have several different mechanisms of synaptic transmission involved in the handling of information.

(8) *Multiple Neurotransmitters*—Most of the neurotransmitters found in the brain and spinal cord are also involved in synaptic transmission in the ENS.

(9) *Absence of Connective Tissue*—Collagen, which forms part of the connective tissue for the structural support of autonomic ganglia, is absent from the interior of enteric ganglia, as in the CNS.

(10) *Small Extracellular Space*—Unlike other autonomic ganglia, extracellular space is reduced by close packing of glial elements.

(11) *Isolation from Blood Vessels*—No blood vessels enter enteric ganglia of the intestine and a blood-ganglion barrier analogous to the blood-brain barrier is inserted between the vasculature and the synaptic circuits of the ganglia.

Enteric Interneurons

Interneurons together with sensory neurons and motor neurons make-up the three primary classes of enteric neurons. Enteric interneurons are synaptically interconnected into integrated circuits that process sensory information and direct the activity of motor neurons to the musculature, secretory epithelium, and blood vasculature. Animal studies suggest that enteric interneurons have individualized properties including specific morphology, directionality of projections, length of axonal projections, electrical and synaptic behavior, and neurotransmitter codes [10].

Multiple synaptic connections contact the cell bodies of interneurons and their axons and dendrites in the ganglionic neuropil. Synaptic connections are made between axons and cell bodies, between axons and dendrites, and from axon to axon. Whereas the bulk of information processing in integrative nervous systems occurs in the synaptic neuropil, only the cell bodies of enteric neurons are presently accessible for electrophysiologic study of electrical and synaptic behavior. As in the brain, the interneuronal microcircuits account for the higher functions that are required for integrated control and coordination of behavior of effector systems within the complete organ.

Enteric Motor Neurons

Motor neurons innervate the effector systems. The motor neuron pool of the ENS contains both excitatory and inhibitory neurons. Excitatory motor neurons release neurotransmitters that stimulate cells of effector systems. Inhibitory motor neurons release neurotransmitters that suppress the activity of the effector cells.

Excitatory Motor Neurons

Excitatory motor neurons release neurotransmitters that evoke muscle contractions and mucosal secretion. Mechanisms of excitation-secretion coupling in the mucosal epithelium of specialized compartments (e.g., stomach and intestine) and excitation-contraction coupling in the smooth musculature are well understood, but beyond the scope of this chapter.

Acetylcholine and substance P are the principal neurotransmitters released from excitatory motor neurons to evoke contraction of the muscles [11–13]. Acetylcholine and vasoactive intestinal peptide are excitatory neurotransmitters that evoke secretion from intestinal crypts [14–16]. The receptors for acetylcholine at the neuroeffector junctions are the muscarinic receptor subtype. Receptors for substance P at neuromuscular junctions are the NK-1 subtype. Axons of excitatory motor neurons to the intestinal circular muscle generally project in the orad direction and excitatory motor axons to the longitudinal muscle coat project in the aboral direction [5]. Axons of excitatory gastric motor neurons generally project in the oral direction to both the musculature and mucosa [17,18]. Cell bodies of intestinal secretomotor neurons send their axons in the aboral direction [19,20].

Inhibitory Motor Neurons

Inhibitory motor neurons release neurotransmitters that suppress contractile activity of the muscles. Inhibitory neurotransmitters activate receptors on the muscle cell membranes to produce inhibitory junction potentials. Inhibitory junction potentials are hyperpolarizing potentials that move the membrane potential away from the threshold for discharge of action potentials and thereby reduce the excitability of the muscle.

Early evidence implicated a purine nucleotide, possibly ATP, as the inhibitory transmitter released by enteric inhibitory motor neurons. Consequently, for the gut, the term "purinergic neuron" temporarily became synonymous with inhibitory motor neuron [21]. The evidence for ATP as the inhibitory transmitter is now combined with evidence for vasoactive intestinal peptide (VIP), pituitary adenylate cyclase activating peptide (PACAP), and nitric oxide as inhibitory transmitters [22–26]. Enteric neurons with vasoactive intestinal peptide and/or nitric oxide synthase innervate the circular muscle of the stomach, intestines, gall bladder, and the various sphincters. Moreover, they can be measured after release into the external milieu when inhibitory motor neurons are active in functional motor behavior of the intestine [22–23].

The functional significance of inhibitory motor neurons is related to the specialized physiology of the musculature. The intestinal musculature behaves as a self-excitable electrical syncytium. This implies that action potentials and slow waves spread from muscle fiber to muscle fiber in three dimensions. The action potentials trigger phasic contractions as they spread. A non-neural pacemaker system of electrical slow waves accounts for the self-excitable characteristic of the electrical syncytium. In this construct, the electrical slow waves are an extrinsic factor to which the circular muscle responds.

Consideration of the functional characteristics of the musculature raises the question of why the circular muscle fails to respond with action potentials and contractions to all slow wave cycles? The question also arises as to why action potentials and contractions do not spread in the syncytium throughout the entire length of intestine each time they occur. Answers to the these questions lie in the functional significance of enteric inhibitory motor neurons.

The circular muscle can only respond to an electrical slow wave when the inhibitory motor neurons in a segment of intestine are switched off by input from other neurons in the control circuits. Likewise, action potentials and associated contractions can propagate only into disinhibited regions of the musculature. This means that inhibitory neurons determine when the ongoing slow waves initiate a contraction, as well as the distance and direction of propagation once the contraction has begun.

Inhibitory motor neurons to the circular muscle discharge continuously, with action potentials and contractions in the muscle occur only when the inhibitory neurons are switched off by input from interneurons in the control circuits. In sphincters, the inhibitory neurons are normally quiescent and are switched to an active state with timing appropriate for coordination of the opening of the sphincter with physiological events in adjacent regions. When this occurs, the inhibitory neurotransmitter relaxes ongoing muscle contraction in the sphincteric muscle and prevents excitation-contraction in the adjacent muscle from spreading into and closing the sphincter. In nonsphincteric circular muscle, the state of activity of inhibitory motor neurons determines the length of a contracting segment by controlling the distance of spread of action potentials within the three-dimensional electrical geometry of the syncytium. Contraction can occur in segments in which ongoing inhibition has been switched off, while adjacent segments with continuing inhibitory activity cannot contract. The boundaries of the contracted segment reflect the transition zone from inactive to active inhibitory motor neurons. The directional sequence in which the inhibitory motor neurons are switched off establishes the direction of propagation of the contraction. Normally, they are switched off in the aboral direction, resulting in contractile activity that propagates in the aboral direction. In the abnormal conditions of vomiting, the inhibitory motor neurons must be switched off in the reverse sequence to account for small intestinal propulsion that travels toward the stomach [3].

Observations of the continuous patterned discharge of action potentials in some of the myenteric neurons of dog, cat, guinea pig, and rabbit small intestine were early evidence for the continuous neuronal inhibition of the circular muscle [27]. The continuous release of inhibitory neurotransmitters (VIP and nitric oxide) can be detected in the dog small intestine [28–29]. Spontaneously occurring inhibitory junction potentials that may reflect an ongoing release of the inhibitory neurotransmitter can sometimes be recorded from the muscle. Nevertheless, in most preparations in vitro, the ongoing inhibitory activity is manifest in the muscle as a steady hyperpolarization and decreased input resistance, both of which reduce the probability that the electrical current of the slow waves will depolarize the muscle to spike threshold. The steady inhibitory hyperpolarization probably reflects smoothing of many inhibitory junction potentials due to:

(1) the release of transmitter from multiple sites during asynchronous discharge of different nerve fibers;
(2) long diffusion distances associated with neurotransmitter release; and
(3) the syncytial properties of the muscle

As a general rule, any treatment or condition that ablates the intrinsic inhibitory neurons results in tonic contracture and "achalasia" of the intestinal circular muscle. Several circumstances that involve functional ablation of the intrinsic inhibitory neurons are associated with conversion from a hypo-irritable condition of the circular muscle to a hyper-irritable state. These are

(1) local anesthetic drugs [15];
(2) long periods of cold storage [15];
(3) hypoxic vascular perfusion of an intestinal segment [30];

(4)   surgical ablation [31];

(5)   congenital absence, as in the piebald mouse and Hirschsprung's disease [32].

All evidence suggests that some of the intrinsic inhibitory neurons are tonically active, and that blockade or ablation of these neurons releases the circular muscle from the inhibitory influence. The behavior of the muscle in these cases is tonic contracture and disorganized phasic contractile activity reminiscent of fibrillation.

Enteric Reflexes

Reflexes are a form of neurally-mediated behavior of effector systems that occurs in response to stimulation of sensory neurons. Reflex behavior is described as stereotypical in nature. For example, the response in the wall of the intestine to distension or mucosal stroking is reflex contraction of the circular muscle coat above the site of stimulation and inhibition of the circular muscle below the site. This pattern of behavior is reproduced each time mechano-receptors are activated by stretch of the wall or deformation of the mucosa. This behavioral pattern, like that of all reflexes, mirrors the output of a set of fixed "hardwired" connections within the interneuronal circuitry.

Enteric Pattern Generators

Pattern generators are neural networks that generate rhythmic or repetitive behavior in effector systems. They are formed by interneuronal synaptic connections that are preprogrammed to produce an adaptive pattern of effector behavior. Pattern-generating circuitry consists of motor programs that signal the motor neurons for the control of repetitive cyclical behaviors such as the cyclical patterns of intestinal motility observed in the fasting state. The sequence of events in stereotyped repetitions of motor outflow to the effector system is determined by the program circuit. Programmed motor behavior, unlike reflex behavior, does not require sensory input to start the program, and feedback information from sensory neurons is unnecessary for the sequencing of the steps in the program. For many of the behaviors generated by programmed motor circuits (e.g., chewing, swallowing, breathing), the entire sequence of the motor program may be initiated by input signals from a single neuron called a command neuron. Cyclic patterns of secretory and contractile behavior seen in the large intestine in response to histamine release from enteric mast cells is an example of the output of pattern-generating circuitry in the ENS [1,2].

Central Command Signals

The parasympathetic nerves have long been recognized as the major pathway for the transmission of control signals from the brain to the digestive tract; whereas, the general neurophysiological mechanisms underlying the effects of vagal nerve stimulation on the upper gut and sacral nerves on the lower bowel have been clarified only recently. New awareness of the independent integrative properties of the ENS has led to revision of earlier concepts of mechanisms of vagal influence.

Earlier concepts of parasympathetic innervation presumed that ganglia of the digestive tract were the same as parasympathetic ganglia in other visceral systems. In other systems, parasympathetic ganglia are like sympathetic ganglia, except the ganglia of the parasympathetic system are either within the walls of the organ or in much closer apposition than ganglia of the sympathetic innervation. In these systems, the ganglia generally have a relay-distribution function. Earlier concepts supposed that the parasympathetic innervation of the gut was similar. Efferent vagal fibers were believed to form synapses directly with ganglion cells that innervated the cells of the effector systems. This concept, illustrated in Figure 4 for vagal nerves, is inconsistent with current evidence and should be abandoned.

The earlier concept placed the "computer" entirely within the CNS, whereas current concepts place "microprocessor" circuits within the wall of the gut in close proximity to the effector systems. A number of neurons equal to that of the spinal cord is present in the ENS. The number of neurons required for program control of the digestive processes would greatly expand the CNS if situated there. Rather than having the neural control circuits exclusively within the CNS and transmitting every byte of control information over long transmission lines, vertebrate animals have evolved with most of the circuits for automatic feedback control located in close proximity to the effector systems.

Figure 4 illustrates the current concept of CNS involvement in gut function using the vagus as the example. Local integrative circuits of the ENS are organized for many program operations independent of input from the CNS. Subsets of neural circuits are preprogrammed for control of distinct patterns of behavior in each effector system and for the coordination of activity of multiple systems. Enteric motor neurons are the final common transmission pathways for the variety of different programs and reflex circuits required for ordered gut function.

Rather than controlling individual motor neurons, messages transmitted by parasympathetic efferent fibers are command signals for the activation of expanded blocks of integrated circuits positioned in the gut wall. This explains the

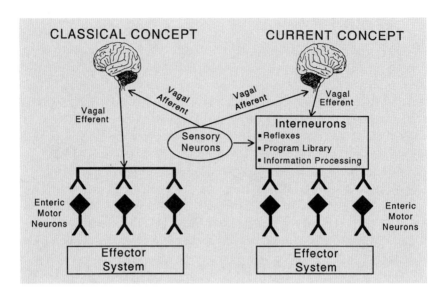

CLASSICAL CONCEPT

CURRENT CONCEPT

Vagal Efferent

Vagal Afferent

Vagal Afferent

Vagal Efferent

Sensory Neurons

Interneurons
• Reflexes
• Program Library
• Information Processing

Enteric Motor Neurons

Enteric Motor Neurons

Effector System

Effector System

Figure 4. Classical outmoded concept and current concept of relations between the brain and the digestive tract. The classical concept viewed vagal preganglionic fibers as synapsing directly with enteric motor neurons as illustrated on the left side of the diagram. In the current concept, vagal efferent fibers transmit command signals from the brain to the integrative and motor program circuitry of the ENS as shown on the right side of the diagram.

strong influence of a small number of efferent fibers (approx. 10% of vagal fibers are efferent) on motility and other effector systems over extended regions of the stomach or intestine. In this respect, the ENS is analogous to a micro-computer with its own independent software; whereas, the brain is like a larger mainframe that receives information from and issues commands to the enteric computer.

Pathophysiology: Disinhibitory Motor Disease

The physiology of neuromuscular relations in the intestine predicts that spasticity and achalasia will accompany any condition where inhibitory motor neurons are destroyed. Without inhibitory control, the self-excitable syncytium of non-sphincteric regions will contract continuously and behave as an obstruction. This happens because the muscle is freed to respond to the pacemaker with contractions that propagate without any amplitude, distance, or directional control. Contractions spreading in the uncontrolled syncytium collide randomly resulting in fibrillation-like behavior in the affected intestinal segment.

Loss or malfunction of inhibitory motor neurons is the pathophysiologic basis of disinhibitory motor disease. It underlies several forms of chronic intestinal pseudo-obstruction and sphincteric achalasia (Table 1). Neuropathic degeneration is a progressive disease that in its earlier stages may be manifest as symptoms that may be confused with IBS.

— FGID and Chronic Intestinal Pseudo-obstruction

Both myopathic and neuropathic forms of chronic intestinal pseudo-obstruction are recognized. Degenerative changes in the musculature underlie the myopathic form, whereas neuropathic forms arise from degenerative changes in the ENS. Failure of propulsive motility in the affected length of bowel reflects loss of the neural microcircuits that program and control the repertoire of motility patterns required for the necessary functions of that region of bowel. Pseudo-obstruction occurs in part because contractile behavior of the circular muscle is hyperactive but disorganized in the denervated regions [33]. Manometrically determined hyperactivity is a diagnostic sign of the neuropathic form of chronic small bowel pseudo-obstruction in humans. The hyperactive and disorganized contractile behavior reflects the absence of inhibitory nervous control of the muscles that are self-excitable (autogenic) when released from the braking action

Table 1. Disinhibitory Motor Disease

(1) Pseudo-obstruction	(2) Achalasia Lower Esophageal Sphincter
(a) Chagas Disease	(3) Biliary Dyskinesia
(b) Paraneoplastic Syndrome	(Sphincter of Oddi Achalasia)
(c) Hirschsprungs Disease	
(d) Idiopathic	

imposed by inhibitory motor neurons. Chronic pseudo-obstruction is therefore symptomatic of the advanced stage of a progressive enteric neuropathy. Retrospective review of patients' records suggest that some FGID-like symptoms can be an expression of early stages of the neuropathy [34,35].

Degenerative noninflammatory and inflammatory enteric neuropathies are two forms of the disease that culminate in pseudo-obstruction. Non-inflammatory neuropathies can be either familial or sporadic [36]. The mode of inheritance may be autosomal recessive or dominant. In the former, the neuropathologic findings include a marked reduction in the number of neurons in both myenteric and submucous plexuses, and the presence of round, eosinophilic intranuclear inclusions in about 30% of the residual neurons. Histochemical and ultrastructural analysis reveals the inclusions not to be viral particles, but rather proteinaceous material forming filaments [37,38]. Members of two families have been described with intestinal pseudo-obstruction associated with the autosomal dominant form of enteric neuropathy [39,40]. The numbers of enteric neurons were decreased in these patients, with no alterations being found in the CNS or parts of the autonomic nervous system outside the gut.

Degenerative inflammatory enteric neuropathies are characterized by a dense inflammatory infiltrate confined to enteric ganglia. Paraneoplastic syndrome, Chagas disease and idiopathic degenerative disease are recognizable forms of pseudo-obstruction related to inflammatory neuropathies.

Paraneoplastic syndrome is a form of pseudo-obstruction where commonality of antigens between small-cell carcinoma of the lungs and enteric neurons leads to immune attack resulting in loss of neurons [41]. The majority of patients with symptoms of pseudo-obstruction in combination with small-cell lung carcinoma have immunoglobulin-G autoantibodies that react with enteric neurons [42]. The antibodies react with a variety molecules expressed on the nuclear membrane of neurons, including Hu and Ri proteins, and with cytoplasmic antigens (Yo protein) of the Purkinje cells in the cerebellum [43–46]. Immunostaining with sera from paraneoplastic patients shows a characteristic pattern of staining in enteric neurons [43]. The detection of anti-enteric neuronal antibodies is a means to a specific diagnosis; nevertheless, the mechanisms by which the antibodies damage the neurons is unresolved.

The association of enteric neuronal loss and symptoms of pseudo-obstruction in Chagas' disease also reflects autoimmune attack on the neurons that mimics the situation in achalasia and paraneoplastic syndrome. *Trypanosoma cruzi*, the blood-borne parasite that causes Chagas' disease, has antigenic epitopes similar to antigens of enteric neurons [47]. This activates the immune system to assault the gut neurons coincident with the attack on the parasite.

Idiopathic inflammatory degenerative neuropathy occurs unrelated to neoplasms, infectious conditions or other known diseases [34,35,48]. De Giorgio et al. [34] and Smith et al. [35] described two small groups of patients with early complaints of symptoms similar to FGID that progressively worsened and were later diagnosed as idiopathic degenerative inflammatory neuropathy based on full-thickness biopsies taken during exploratory laparotomy that revealed chronic intestinal pseudo-obstruction. Each patient had inflammatory infiltrates localized to the myenteric plexus. Sera from the two cases reported by Smith et al. [35] had circulating antibodies against enteric neurons similar to those found in secondary inflammatory neuropathies (i.e., anti-Hu), but with different immunolabeling patterns characterized by prominent cytoplasmic rather than nuclear staining.

Recognition of the complex functions of the ENS leads to the conclusion that early neuropathic changes are expected to be manifest as functional symptoms that worsen with progressive neuronal loss. In diagnostic motility studies (e.g., manometry), degenerative loss of enteric neurons is reflected by hypermotility and spasticity [33] because inhibitory motor neurons are included in the missing neuronal population.

Higher Brain Centers

Final common pathways for output from higher centers to the gut exit the brain in efferent vagal fibers and descending pathways in the spinal cord that connect to sympathetic preganglionic neurons in the thoraco-lumbar region and parasympathetic preganglionic neurons in the sacral region. Several higher brain regions transmit to these outflow centers. Frontal regions of the cerebral cortex, bed nucleus of the stria terminalis, paraventricular nucleus of the hypothalamus, and the central nucleus of the amygdala project to the vagal outflow center in the medulla oblongata. These areas of the brain share information with the limbic regions where emotional responses to sensory input from the outside world as well as signals of volitional origin are processed.

Vagal afferent fibers from the upper gastrointestinal tract form synapses in the nucleus tractus solitarius (NTS, fig. 5). They are thought to mediate non-noxious physiologic sensations (e.g., distension, satiety, and nausea). The NTS is the relay station for transfer of vagal afferent information from the proximal gut to higher brain centers. There are direct projections from the NTS to the autonomic nuclei in the dorsal motor nucleus of the vagus and the nucleus ambiguus. Information is relayed from the NTS to the motor nuclei involved in chewing and swallowing and to more rostral brain stem regions that are connected to more rostral centers. There are also longer projections that terminate in higher centers such as frontal regions of the cerebral cortex, thalamus, hypothalamus and limbic and insular cortical areas involved in neuroendocrine function. Information relayed by the NTS influences the outflow of both volitional and non-volitional signals from higher brain centers.

Linked interactions between higher brain centers, emotional state, and gastrointestinal disorders are well recognized. Abdominal pain, diarrhea, nausea, and emesis can all be manifestations of emotional or traumatic stress. Moreover, emotional stress can disrupt normal behavior leading to altered food intake, changes in physical activity, treatment seeking, or any combination of these. The same symptoms following stress can occur in psychiatrically normal individuals, as well as in those with psychiatric illness. Findings that antidepressant medications relieve some functional bowel symptoms is evidence of disorder in the higher brain centers that influence the outflow of commands to the gut. Nevertheless, the effect is not evident for all antidepressants and is not necessarily related to effects on mood [49]. The stress-related symptoms and behavioral changes (i.e., sleep disturbances, muscle tension, pain, altered diet, abnormal illness behavior) associated with FGIDs probably reflect subtle malfunctions in the brain circuits responsible for interactions of higher cognitive functions and central centers that determine outputs to the gastrointestinal tract, and not to psychiatric illness alone.

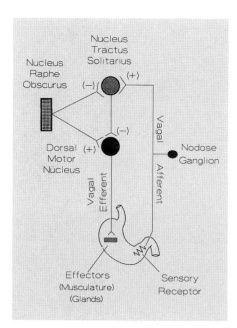

Figure 5. Vago-vagal reflex circuits are made-up of vagal afferent neurons, second-order interneurons in the NTS and vagal efferent neurons. Vago-vagal reflex circuits are influenced by other regions of the brain. A vago-vagal reflex circuit in which increased sensory activity suppresses the excitatory outflow in gastric vagal efferent fibers is illustrated. Inputs to the circuit from the nucleus raphe obscurus overrides inhibition of the sensory input and increases excitatory outflow in the vagal efferent. This involves inhibition of the second-order neuron in the NTS with simultaneous excitation of the vagal efferent in the dorsal motor nucleus.

Malfunctions may occur in the circuitry of any of the CNS centers. For example, thyrotropin-releasing hormone (TRH) is a neurotransmitter released in the dorsal vagal complex by neurons that have their cell bodies in the nucleus raphe obscurus (fig. 5). Abnormal levels of TRH in the dorsal vagal complex produced by experimental injection or presumably by hyperactivity in the TRH neurons results in gastric erosions that duplicate stress-induced pathology. Synaptic projections into the dorsal vagal complex from the nucleus raphe obscurus also release 5-hydroxytryptamine (5-HT). Actions of TRH on vagal motor neurons are greatly potentiated by 5-HT [50]. This suggests that abnormal firing in the serotonergic neurons from the midbrain raphe system could also lead to pathologic changes reflecting hypersecretion of acid in the stomach. All of the pathologic signals emerging from the higher brain circuits to the stomach are transmitted by the vagal nerves.

— Vago-Vagal Reflexes

Vagal integrative centers in the brain are more directly involved in the control of the specialized digestive functions of the esophagus, stomach, and the functional cluster of duodenum, gall bladder, and pancreas than in the distal small bowel and large intestine. The circuits in the dorsal vagal complex and their interactions with higher centers are responsible for the rapid and more precise control required for adjustments to rapidly changing conditions in the upper digestive tract during anticipation, ingestion, and digestion of meals of varied composition.

A reflex circuit known as the vago-vagal reflex underlies moment-to-moment adjustments required for optimal digestive function in the upper digestive tract (fig. 5). The afferent side of the reflex arc consists of vagal afferent neurons connected with a variety of sensory receptors specialized for detection and signaling of mechanical parameters such as muscle tension and mucosal brushing, or luminal chemical parameters such as pH, osmolarity, and glucose concentration. The afferent neurons are synaptically connected with neurons in the dorsal motor nucleus of the vagus (DMV) and in the NTS. The NTS, which lies directly above the DMV, makes synaptic connections with the neuronal pool in the DMV. A synaptic neuropil formed by processes from neurons in both nuclei tightly link the two into an integrative center, which together with the area postrema and nucleus ambiguus, form the dorsal vagal complex. The dorsal vagal neurons are second or third order neurons representing the efferent arm of the reflex circuit. They are the final common pathways out of the brain to the enteric circuits innervating the effector systems.

Efferent vagal fibers form synapses with neurons in the ENS to activate circuits which ultimately drive outflow of signals in motor neurons to the effector systems. When the effector system is the musculature, its innervation consists of both inhibitory and excitatory motor neurons that participate in reciprocal control. If the effector systems are gastric glands or digestive glands of the duodenal cluster unit, the secretomotor neurons are excitatory and stimulate secretory behavior.

The circuits for CNS control of the upper gastrointestinal tract are organized much like those dedicated to control of skeletal muscle movements where fundamental reflex circuits are located in the spinal cord. Inputs to the spinal reflex circuits from higher order integrative centers in the brain (e.g., motor cortex and basal ganglia) complete the neural organization of skeletal muscle motor control. Memory, processing of incoming information from outside the body, and integration of proprioceptive information are ongoing functions of higher brain centers responsible for intelligent organization of the outflow to the skeletal muscles by way of the basic spinal reflex circuit. The basic connections of the vago-vagal reflex circuit are like somatic motor reflexes, in being "fine tuned" from moment to moment by input from higher integrative centers in the brain.

The dorsal vagal complex has extensive connections for information sharing with both forebrain and brainstem centers. Afferent information into the NTS and the area postrema is relayed to several rostral centers. The same rostral centers reciprocate by projecting higher order information in descending connections to the vago-vagal reflex circuits. These interactions account for the effects of emotional state and external stimuli from the environment on functions of the digestive tract.

Synaptic transmission in the microcircuits of the dorsal vagal complex involves a varied array of neurotransmitters. These include acetylcholine, biogenic amines, amino acids, and peptides most of which are identified as neurotransmitters elsewhere in the brain and in the ENS. Glutamate, which is universally excitatory in brain microcircuits, has the same action in dorsal vagal circuits. Likewise, gamma-amino butyric acid, which is universally inhibitory in the brain, also acts as an inhibitory transmitter in the dorsal vagal complex. Of the brain-gut peptides, TRH, corticotropin-releasing factor (CRF), bombesin, calcitonin gene-related peptide, substance P, oxytocin, arginine vasopressin, somatostatin, and opioids are among the peptides that influence gastrointestinal signal transmission along both vagal and spinal transmission pathways. For TRH, CRF and oxytocin, this represents function as neurotransmitters in addition to well known roles as hormones released into the hypothalamic-hypophyseal portal blood vessels to regulate pituitary function.

Muscle Physiology (Relevant to Neural Control)

Gastrointestinal motility is the organized application of forces of muscle contraction that results in physiologically significant movement of intraluminal contents [51]. The ENS organizes motor behavior by transmitting control signals to the muscles. Mechanisms for interpretation of the signals are incorporated in the muscle cell membranes and mainly involve membrane excitability. The biophysical processes in the smooth muscle cell membranes have evolved in parallel with the nervous system. This accounts for the functional compatibility that is apparent as the two systems work in cooperative tandem. In order to understand normal and disordered motor function, basic knowledge of enteric neurophysiology and smooth muscle physiology must be integrated.

— Electrical Syncytial Properties of Smooth Muscles

Action potentials generated by the sarcoplasmic membrane trigger contractions of the circular muscle coat in all regions of the digestive tract. When intramural enteric nerves are blocked experimentally with anesthetics, action potentials and the associated contractions still spread in three dimensions throughout the bulk of circular muscle [52,53]. This occurs because the muscle fibers are electrically connected for action potentials to cross the fiber boundaries and travel from muscle fiber to muscle fiber in three-dimensions. Low resistance electrical junctions (i.e., gap junctions) account for electrical coupling from fiber to fiber [54,55].

Phasic contractions are evoked in the muscle as each action potential propagates from fiber to fiber. Phasic contractions are transient twitch-like contractions and differ from tonic contractions where tension is maintained for prolonged periods. When action potentials propagate through the muscle repeatedly at sufficiently high frequency, the twitch-like contractions can summate to give the appearance of a tonic contraction.

— Electrical Slow Waves in Gastrointestinal Musculature

Electrical slow waves have been the focus of investigative interest for much of the twentieth century [56] because of their importance as pacemakers that trigger action potentials and coincident contractions in the musculature (fig. 6). The muscle fiber membranes possess all the voltage-activated ionic channels necessary for generation of action potentials. Electrical slow waves depolarize the membranes of the muscle fibers to the threshold for the opening of voltage-activated calcium channels that carry the inward current for generation of action potentials [57]. As with action potentials in other excitable membranes, the repolarization phase of smooth muscle action potentials results from outwardly directed ionic current in voltage- and/or calcium-activated potassium channels [58].

Electrical slow waves are seen as rhythmic cycles of depolarization and repolarization when recorded with electrodes on the serosal surfaces of the gut (fig. 6). They are omnipresent in the gastric antrum and intestine of most species. Electrical slow waves are autogenic events that do not require the nervous system [52,53]. Current evidence suggests that a network of specialized cells called *Interstitial Cells of Cajal* (ICCs) generate the slow waves [59,60]. In small animals (e.g., mice), networks of ICCs located between the longitudinal and circular muscle layers are thought to produce slow waves and transmit them to the circular muscle through low resistance electrical junctions that connect the ICCs to the muscle fibers. In larger animals with thicker circular muscle coats (e.g., dogs and humans) slow wave generation occurs also in ICCs in a specialized network located at the mucosal side of the circular muscle as well as in the interspace between longitudinal and circular muscle coats [61–63].

Action potentials are not associated with every intestinal slow wave, and the frequency of phasic contractions may therefore not be the same as that of the

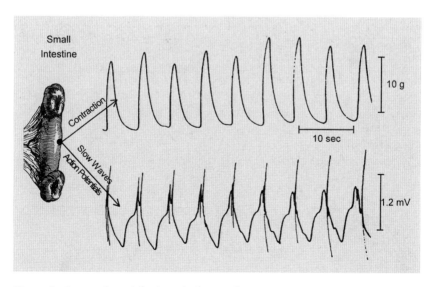

Figure 6. Contraction of the intestinal musculature is triggered by action potentials. Muscle action potentials are triggered by electrical slow waves and appear at or near the slow wave's crest.

slow waves. Nervous mechanisms determine when slow waves evoke action potentials and associated contractions.

Some action potentials and associated contractions are independent of slow waves. Both the small and the large intestine can show propagated action potentials and powerful propulsive contractions not associated with slow waves. In these cases, action potential discharge occurs continuously over more than one slow wave cycle and is often so intense that slow waves are obliterated on the electrical records. This kind of motor activity called power propulsion may travel in the oral or aboral direction to accomplish rapid propulsion over long stretches of intestine. Power propulsion in the oral direction is part of the emetic motility program in the upper small intestine [3]. It is triggered to travel in the aboral direction in response to noxious stimulation such as enterotoxins, parasitic antigens or radiation toxicity in the small and large intestine and is associated with secretion of large amounts of water and electrolytes into the lumen. This is neurally programed behavior that is an adaptation for the rapid expulsion of noxious agents from the intestinal lumen [2,3,64–68]. Operation of the program in the large intestine is accompanied by symptoms of abdominal pain and diarrhea in animals and humans [69].

— Muscle Pathophysiology

Abnormalities of muscle function underlie a subset of gastrointestinal motility disorders that include altered gastric emptying and myopathic forms of chronic intestinal pseudo-obstruction. Electrical dysrhythmia in the gastric antrum is a muscle dysfunction associated with disordered gastric emptying, nausea, and vomiting and epigastric discomfort and pain. Tachygastria and bradygastria are contrasting antral dysrhythmias in which the frequency of occurrence of electrical slow waves is significantly higher than the normal 3 cycles per minute in the former and significantly reduced below the 3-cycle norm in the latter. Gastric slow wave dysrhythmias are common in women in early pregnancy and are also documented in a subgroup of anorexia nervosa patients [70,71].

Diseases involving the small intestinal musculature include collagen-related diseases (e.g., scleroderma and lupus) and a group of diseases with smooth muscle degeneration known as familial and childhood visceral myopathies [72,73]. The latter are myopathic forms of chronic intestinal pseudo-obstruction that are characterized by hypomotility in manometric studies of small bowel motility. Hypomotility in myopathic forms of intestinal pseudo-obstruction contrasts with manometric patterns of hypermotility that characterize the neuropathic form of chronic pseudo-obstruction. Early symptoms of either form may be confused as a FGID.

Relevance of ICCs for disordered muscle function is not yet clear. Interstitial cells of Cajal are depleted in the aganglionic constricted terminal segment of the large intestine in Hirschsprung's disease, and this is associated with abnormality of slow wave generation [74]. A similar condition of the ICCs and slow wave behavior is found in patients with infantile hypertrophic pyloric stenosis [75]. Both diseases are associated with neuropathic alterations of the ENS in the affected regions of gut. This raises the question of whether the alterations in the networks of ICCs are primary or secondary to aganglionosis.

Sensory Neurophysiology

Sensory neurons belong to the third category of enteric neurons (fig. 2). They function in concert with the other two categories (i.e., interneurons and motor neurons).

Sensory afferent fibers of neuronal cell bodies in nodose and dorsal root ganglia transmit information from the gastrointestinal tract and gallbladder to the CNS for processing. These fibers transmit a steady stream of information to the local processing circuits in the ENS and to prevertebral sympathetic ganglia and the CNS. The gut has mechano-, chemo- and thermoreceptors. Mechano-receptors sense mechanical events in the mucosa, musculature, serosal surface, and mesentery. They supply both the enteric minibrain and the CNS with information on stretch-related tension and muscle length in the wall and on the movement of luminal contents as they brush the mucosal surface. Mesenteric receptors code for gross movements of the organ. Chemoreceptors generate information on the concentration of nutrients, osmolarity, and pH in the luminal contents. Recording of sensory information exiting the gut in afferent fibers reveals that most receptors are multimodal in that they respond to both mechanical and chemical stimuli. Thermoreceptors supply the brain with deep-body temperature data used in regulation and perhaps sensations of temperature change in the lumen. Presence in the gastrointestinal tract of pain receptors (nociceptors) equivalent to those connected with C-fibers and A-delta fibers elsewhere in the body is likely, but not unequivocally confirmed except for the gallbladder [76].

The biophysical principles of sensory function in the gastrointestinal tract are like those found elsewhere in the body. Each sensory neuron has at least one neurite with a generator region that converts a change in stimulus energy into an action potential code. The frequency of action potential discharge is a code for transmission of information on intensity of the stimulus to central processing circuits.

Sensory information on the mechanical state of the musculature and distension of the visceral wall is coded by mechanoreceptors. Whether the neuronal cell bodies of intramuscular and mucosal mechanoreceptors belong to dorsal root ganglia, enteric ganglia, or both, is uncertain [77,78]. Stretch sensitive mechanoreceptors have pathophysiologic importance because a consistent finding in patients diagnosed with the irritable bowel syndrome (IBS) is abnormally high sensitivity to stretch that translates into pain [79,80]. The heightened sensitivity to distension and conscious awareness of the GI-tract experienced by IBS patients is a generalized phenomenon throughout the gut, including the esophagus [81]. The mechanism is unclear. However, three general explanations are apparent:

(1) hypersignals from sensitized mechanoreceptors may be accurately decoded by the brain as hyperdistension;

(2) malfunctioning brain circuits may be misinterpreting accurate information;

(3) combined sensing and central processing malfunction could be in effect.

Hyposensory perception, particularly in the recto-sigmoid region, is at the opposite extreme of gastrointestinal sensory abnormality. Sensory suppression in this region of the gut, either in the pathway for recto-anal stretch reflexes or in the transmission pathway from the recto-sigmoid to conscious perception of distension, can be an underlying factor in the pathogenesis of chronic constipation and associated symptoms [82]. Hyperglycemia is another pathologic disturbance that can lead to sensory neuropathy and suppressed sensations of recto-sigmoid fullness [83].

Mounting evidence suggests that sensory transduction of chemical information related to nutrient concentrations in the small bowel involves enteroendocrine peptides and amines (e.g., cholecystokinin and 5-HT) and a mechanism akin to sensory function in taste buds [84]. Mucosal enteroendocrine cells appear to "taste" the lumen and release cholecystokinin in direct proportion to the concentration of products of protein digestion and lipids. The amount of cholecystokinin release is a transform of the nutrient concentration, which in turn, acts to evoke concentration-dependent action potential discharge in vagal afferent neurons, and probably a subpopulation of enteric neurons. The vagal sensory fibers branch in the wall of the stomach and upper small bowel for simultaneous transmission to both the big brain and the enteric minibrain [85]. The spike frequency transmitted by each sensory neuron becomes a transform of the stimulus strength for simultaneous decoding in the brain and enteric processing circuitry. The neuronal receptors for cholecystokinin belong to the CCK-A subtype [86,87].

Vagal sensory mechanisms involving cholecystokinin are implicated in the complex nervous functions involved in the sensations of satiety and control of food intake [86]. Disordered vagal sensory mechanisms are also suspect in the poorly understood pathophysiology of functional dyspepsia [88].

Action potential discharge in vagal sensory nerve terminals and the mucosal terminals of a unique population of intrinsic enteric neurons can be initiated by the action of 5-HT released from mucosal enterochromaffin cells [88,89]. The 5-HT receptors at the vagal afferent terminals belong to the 5-HT$_3$ subtype. Identification of these receptors is relevant to anti-emetic efficacy of 5-HT$_3$ receptor antagonists described later in the chapter.

— Mechanoreceptors

Low- and high-threshold receptors are involved in coding of mechano-sensory information from the gastrointestinal and biliary tracts. Low-threshold splanchnic afferents respond to innocuous levels of distension; high-threshold afferents respond to distending pressures only when the pressure is greater than a set threshold. High-threshold afferent fibers are predominantly unmyelinated C-fibers. Low-threshold afferents are myelinated fibers of the A-delta class. Low-threshold mechanoreceptors are presumed to be the afferent component of normal autonomic regulatory reflexes. It is unknown for certain if activity in low-threshold pathways reach the level of conscious perception; nevertheless, it is likely that some nonpainful sensations such as fullness or the presence of gas are derived from this kind of activity. High-threshold afferents are thought to be the sensory analogs of sharp-localized pain in organs such as the gallbladder where pain is the only consciously perceived sensation [90]. Combined involvement of both low- and high-threshold fibers in nociperception cannot be excluded. Cervero and Jänig [76] suggested for organs such as the urinary bladder and colon, where distension can evoke sensations ranging from mild fullness to intense pain, that activation of differing proportions of low- and high-threshold mechano-receptors account for the range of sensations. Acute visceral pain could emerge from activation of high-threshold nociceptive fibers; whereas, chronic forms of visceral pain could be attributed to sensitization of both types of mechanoreceptors by conditions such as inflammation or ischemia. Application of acetic acid or other irritants to the large intestinal mucosa in animals lowers the threshold and sensitizes both the high- and low-threshold distension sensitive afferents. This is peculiar to the large intestine and not found for cutaneous afferents (J.N. Sengupta, personal communication). Involvement of another class of splanchnic afferents termed "silent nociceptors" is also suspect in chronic pain.

The term "silent nociceptor" refers to afferents that do not respond to the strongest of distending stimuli. These normally silent receptors appear to become sensitized by inflammatory mediators. Spontaneous action potential discharge and responses to normally innocuous mechanical distension can be recorded in the previously unresponsive afferents after the bowel is inflamed by experimentally applied irritants or inflammatory substances.

— Sensory Pathways

Nociceptive afferents form synapses with spinothalamic neurons in spinal laminae I and V-VII after entering the dorsal horn and crossing to the contralateral side. Synaptic convergence of afferent fibers from cutaneous regions and visceral organs onto common populations of spinothalamic neurons accounts for the component of visceral pain often described as referred pain. Referral of gallbladder pain to the right upper abdominal quadrant and right shoulder is an example of this phenomenon.

Axons of spinothalamic neuronal cell bodies in the gray matter of the dorsal horn form the spinothalamic tracts in the anterolateral regions of the spinal white matter and are responsible for direct transmission of ascending sensory information to thalamic relay nuclei and on into the cerebral cortex (fig. 7). This is known as the specific thalamo-cortical projection pathway because the sensory information crosses only two synapses (one in the contralateral spinal cord and one in the thalamus) before reaching processing centers in the cortex. Afferent information from the viscera may also reach the cortex by way of spinoreticular, spinomesencephalic, and spinosolitary tracts, and by way of the dorsal columns. The spinoreticular, spinomesencephalic and spinosolitary tracts are known as nonspecific thalamo-cortical projections because the sensory information first crosses synapses in the brain stem and then the thalamus before reaching the cortex (fig. 7). Recent evidence suggests that some nociceptive neurons of laminae III and IV project their axons in the dorsal columns along with the axon collaterals of large diameter-myelinated primary afferent fibers to synapses in the cuneate and gracile nuclei in the medulla oblongata [91,92].

Integration of somatic and visceral input from spatially diverse regions of the body occurs in the synaptic processing centers of the spinothalamic pathways, including visceral inputs from both vagal and dorsal root afferents. From the thalamic integrative centers, sensory information is projected to higher centers in the insular cortex, primary somatosensory cortex, and the prelimbic, limbic, and infralimbic areas of the medial prefrontal cortex.

— Central Processing Revealed by Brain Imaging

Modern advances in brain imagining have begun to illuminate sites in the cerebral cortex where processing of sensory information from the digestive tract takes place. Four techniques have been used [93]:

(1) positron emission spectroscopy (PET), including single proton emission computerized tomography (SPECT);
(2) cortical evoked potentials (CEPs);
(3) magnetoencephalography (MEG); and
(4) functional magnetic resonance imaging (fMRI)

PET and SPECT both use radiotracer molecules to measure physiological processes (e.g., blood flow) and biochemical mechanisms (e.g., glucose uptake

Figure 7. The antero-lateral spinothalamic pathway relays sensory information on pain to the contralateral side of the brain. Information in the pathway is projected to the brain-stem reticular formation, midbrain tectum, ventral posterior lateral nucleus, specific regions of the thalamus and the primary and secondary somatosensory cortex and posterior parietal cortex.

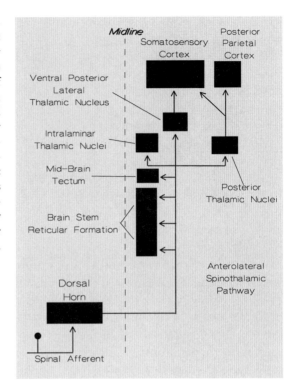

and receptor binding) and depend on manufacture of radio-isotopes of interest and imaging of the manufactured tracer over time in the brain by detectors of gamma radiation [93]. Although studies of this nature in patients with FGID are in an early stage, reasonable documentation for the practicality of the method and reproducibility of changes found in studies of depression and mood disorders is currently available [93]. Because FGIDs are frequently associated with depression [94–96], results with neuroimaging in functional bowel patients will require controls for the changes seen in depression and other psychiatric disorders. PET has now been used to map regions of the cortex in which activity (monitored as increased regional blood flow) is increased by painful distension of the esophagus and by anticipation of painful rectal distension in patients with IBS [97–99].

CEPs are the electrically manifested cerebral responses to sensory stimuli, and are recorded by electrode placements on the scalp. CEP recording requires relatively inexpensive technology, but is influenced by environmental and psychologic variables of importance in FGID patients [99]. CEPs are elicited by both electrical stimulation and balloon distension in the esophagus. Transcranial magnetic stimulation identifies corticofugal pathways from cortex to esophagus in humans [99]. The significance of these kinds of investigation for patients with nonulcer dyspepsia or noncardiac chest pain is unclear; nevertheless, they show that afferent information from the esophagus is integrated at multiple levels of cerebral organization.

MEG measures time-variant magnetic fields generated by current flow in the brain microcircuits [99]. MEG has been used mainly to assess esophageal afferent pathways. The cortical representation of the upper esophagus is unilateral and that of the distal esophagus is bilateral. The primary somatosensory cortex is activated more consistently after proximal esophageal stimulation; whereas, after distal stimulation the secondary somatosensory cortex shows activation. Because vagal afferents seem not to project to the primary somatosensory cortex, activation of this area during esophageal distension suggests that spinal afferents are involved in nonpainful sensations arising from the esophagus. The insular cortex receives vagal as well as spinal afferent input and has connections with the limbic cortex that may be involved with autonomic responses to visceral sensations. MEG has not yet been applied to investigation of hypersensitivity of the esophagus to distension in IBS patients.

fMRI exploits the diamagnetic properties of oxyhemoglobin to provide an enhanced signal and measure increased blood flow without an increase in oxygen consumption. As with MEG, these methods have not been used to evaluate esophageal hypersensitivity in IBS patients.

— Abnormal Central Processing in FGID

Irritable Bowel Syndrome

In healthy subjects, either painful distension by a balloon in the recto-sigmoid region or anticipation of painful distension is associated with increased activity in the anterior cingulate cortex [98]. In IBS patients, activation of the anterior cingulate cortex does not occur. Instead, the left prefrontal cortex becomes activated, as if a shift had occurred and anomalous processing was taking place in this part of the brain.

The cingulate cortex is thought to be an integrative center for both emotional experience and specific representation for pain, which may account for linkage of pain and emotional state. This cortical region is formed around the rostrum of the corpus callosum and has projections into the motor regions of the cortex. The "affect" areas of the cingulate cortex has extensive connections with the amygdala and periaqueductal gray matter and with autonomic nuclei in the brain stem [100].

The cingulate cortex integrates autonomic and endocrine functions and is involved in recall of emotional experiences. Cognition appears to reside in the caudal portion of the anterior cingulate cortex together with circuits delegated to premotor functions and processing of nociceptive information.

PET scans show that rectal hypersensitivity induced in IBS patients by repetitive stimulation of the sigmoid colon [101,102] is associated with increased activity in thalamic regions. Differing autonomic responses to painful rectal stimuli that are suggestive of anomalous processing of visceral afferent information are also found in IBS patients [103]. These studies are generally suggestive that anomalous central processing of visceral afferent information is occurring in FGIDs; nevertheless, association between the abnormalities detected in the brain images and the cognitive sensations experienced by the irritable bowel patients remain unclear.

Non-Cardiac Chest Pain

Regions of the cerebral cortex involved in processing of information evoked by balloon distension in the esophagus have also been imaged effectively by PET [97]. Nonpainful distension produces bilateral activation along the postcentral gyrus, in the insular cortex and the frontal and parietal operculum overlaying the insular cortex. Painful distension in right-handed persons evokes stronger activation of the same cortical regions together with expansion of activation to basal areas of the right anterior insular cortex and the anterior cingulate gyri. Suppression of activity in the right prefrontal cortex occurs during both painful and nonpainful distension. Aziz and Thompson [99] interpreted these findings to suggest that sensory-discriminative aspects of esophageal distension are processed together with somatic sensations in the primary somatosensory cortex, and the affective-motivational aspects of sensation are integrated in the anterior cingulate cortex. They interpreted suppression in the prefrontal cortex, where cognitive-evaluative aspects of sensation are thought to occur, as indicative of the employment of strategies by the subjects to cope with the sensations arising from the esophagus.

— Central Modulation of Nociception

Stimulation of low-threshold myelinated primary afferent fibers (A_{alpha} and A_{beta} fibers) suppresses the response of dorsal horn neurons to inputs from unmyelinated (C-fibers) nociceptive afferents. Blockade of conduction in the large myelinated afferents enhances responses of dorsal horn neurons to inputs from the unmyelinated afferents. Firing of neurons in the dorsal horns therefore reflects a balance between inputs in nociceptor fibers and myelinated afferents that are not directly involved in pain transmission [104]. These observations underlie the "spinal gating" concept of pain transmission (fig. 8). Both fast-conducting myelinated afferents (e.g., skin tactile receptors) and slow-conducting nociceptive C-fibers form synapses with spinothalamic neurons that project afferent information to the brain. Both also have collaterals that form synapses on inhibitory interneurons to the same spinothalamic neurons. Synaptic input to the inhibitory interneurons from large myelinated afferents is excitatory, whereas input from the non-myelinated afferents is inhibitory. The finding that stimulation of large diameter myelinated afferents inhibit the neurons that signal pain has led to the successful practice of stimulating axons in the dorsal columns and peripheral nerves transcutaneously as a therapy for pain. This may also underlie efficacy of some forms of acupuncture.

The gating theory implies that pain perception at the spinal level is determined by amounts of activity in both nociceptive and non-nociceptive sensory afferents. At supraspinal levels of neural organization, nociceptive signals can be modulated at successive synaptic relays as they ascend the brain.

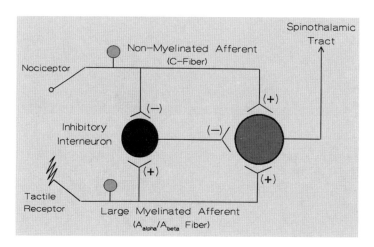

Figure 8. The gate control hypothesis for modulation of transmission of pain involves four kinds of neurons. Inhibitory interneurons are spontaneously active and normally suppress transmission of nociceptive information by spinothalamic neurons. The inhibitory interneurons are excited by input from large-diameter, fast-conducting (A_{alpha}/A_{beta}) myelinated afferents and inhibited by activity in nociceptive C-fibers. Activity in the large-diameter tactile afferents thereby reduces the intensity of pain signals to the brain.

Important pain modulatory pathways that descend to the spinal cord from centers in the brain also exist [104]. In animal models, stimulation of the gray matter surrounding the third ventricle, cerebral aqueduct, and fourth ventricle produces analgesia. In human neurosurgical therapy, stimulating electrodes placed in the periventricular gray region, the ventrobasal complex of the thalamus, or the internal capsule effectively suppress the perception of pain. The patients in these cases continue to experience sensations of touch, pressure, and temperature in the bodily areas where pain is suppressed. A descending inhibitory pathway that terminates on nociceptive neurons in the spinal cord accounts for the analgesic effects of stimulation in the brain. The pathway includes neurons in the periventricular and periaqueductal gray matter in the midbrain that send excitatory projections to the rostroventral medulla. The rostroventral medulla is a region that includes the nucleus raphe magnus and the adjacent nucleus reticularis paragigantocellularis. Serotonergic neurons from the rostroventral medulla project down the cord to form inhibitory synapses on neurons in laminae I, II, and V of the dorsal horn, where nociceptive afferent neurons terminate. Stimulation in the rostroventral medullary region inhibits dorsal horn neurons including spinothalamic neurons that respond to noxious stimulation. Additional descending fiber systems originate in the medulla and pons to supply inhibitory input to nociceptive dorsal horn neurons.

Pain is suppressed by administration of morphine into the same brain regions where electrical stimulation produces analgesia. Application of the opioid antagonist, naloxone, in these same regions blocks morphine action. Morphine and naloxone have similar actions when injected into the spinal cord. This suggests that opiates act on descending pain modulatory pathways as well as on the processing circuitry at the spinal level.

Opioid substances bind to receptors for three classes of endogenous opioid peptides that include the enkephalins, proopiomelanocortin family, and the dynorphin family. Each of the endogenous opioid peptides is expressed from one of three genes that code for large precursor proteins. Post-translational processing of proopiomelanocortin gives rise to beta-endorphin, melanocyte-stimulating hormone, and adrenocorticotropic hormone. Proenkephalin gives rise to met-enkephalin, leu-enkephalin, and a variety of short peptide fragments that also have potent analgesic properties. Prodynorphin gives rise to dynorphin.

The supraspinal analgesic actions of opiates are mediated partially by descending monoaminergic projections to the spinal cord. Neurons that form the descending modulatory pathway from the rostroventral medulla use 5-HT as a neurotransmitter and a descending projection from the pontine region releases norepinephrine in the dorsal horn. The analgesic action of opiates is lost following lesioning of these neurons. Injection of 5-HT or norepinephrine into the

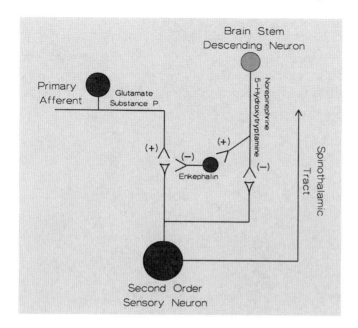

Figure 9. Descending projections from supraspinal centers suppress transmission of nociceptive signals at the level of the spinal cord. Nociceptive primary afferents form synapses with second-order spinothalamic neurons. Enkephalin-containing interneurons inhibit excitatory transmission from the nociceptive afferents to the spino-thalamic projection neurons. Descending projections from brain stem neurons release norepinephrine or 5-HT to both excite enkepha-linergic inhibitory interneurons and inhibit spinothalamic projection neurons.

spinal cord produces analgesia and application of 5-HT antagonists in the cord suppresses the analgesic action of centrally applied opiates. Figure 9 shows putative synaptic interactions among nociceptive afferents, second order neurons in the dorsal horn, and descending modulatory pathways.

Integration of Visceral and Somatic Information

The "spinal gating" concept of nociceptive transmission applies for non-visceral sensory areas of the body innervated by A_{alpha} and A_{beta} myelinated afferents. The digestive and other viscera are not innervated by large diameter, myelinated afferents and this raises the question of whether equivalent synaptic gating modulates central processing of visceral nociceptive information.

Large diameter myelinated afferents from skin or muscle proprioceptors project in the dorsal columns of the spinal cord to form their first synapse in the nucleus gracilis or nucleus cuneatus in the medulla. Evidence suggests that the gracilis and cuneatus nuclei are also centers where visceral input is processed prior to relaying the information on to the ventro posterolateral nucleus of the thalamus. The visceral input involves synaptic connections with dorsal column neurons [91].

A large proportion of neurons in the dorsal column nuclei respond both to mild (non-painful) stimulation of the skin and visceral distension [105], and lesions in these nuclei reduce thalamic responses to both colorectal distension and innocuous cutaneous stimulation [106]. This suggests that the dorsal column nuclei mediate transfer of both noxious visceral and innocuous cutaneous information to the ventro posterolateral thalamic nucleus. There is no effect of lesions of gracilis or cuneatus nuclei or the dorsal columns on thalamic responses to noxious mechanical cutaneous stimuli [92]. This input is carried by spinothalamic sensory pathways other than the dorsal columns. The convergence of information from the viscera and skin in the nucleus gracilis and cuneatus is reminiscent of the convergence of inputs from large diameter, myelinated afferents and non-myelinated C-fibers in the spinal dorsal horn–spinothalamic pathway. Nevertheless, whether filtering of visceral nociceptive information analogous to "spinal-gating" of pain information occurs in the dorsal column nuclei remains as an open question.

— Genesis of Nonpainful Sensations

Pain is a cardinal symptom of FGID; nevertheless, other sensations including bloating, abdominal distension, early satiety, incomplete evacuation and nausea may also be symptoms [107]. Prolonged activation of the pathways responsible for these may lead to permanent reconfiguration of central neural circuits, which include alterations in c-fos activation, reflexes, cognitive perception, and overt behavior. The functional neuroanatomy and neurophysiology underlying these sensations is unclear mainly due to lack of appropriate animal models. Humans can describe sensations experienced in response to a defined stimulus; whereas in animal studies, if a similar stimulus activates an identified population of afferents, it can only be assumed that the particular sensation in humans is mediated by the same afferents. Little is known about abdominal sensory physiology in humans. Electrical recordings from the isolated posterior vagal nerve in humans does reveal a prominent group of fibers with conduction velocities characteristic of unmyelinated afferents found in animals [108]. Lesion studies would appear to be a useful approach to identification of peripheral afferents responsible for specific sensations. Nevertheless, these are definitive only if a sensation is abolished. In such cases, it is necessary to rule out interruption of efferent nerves in the mixed population that may evoke the sensation (e.g., by stimulating acid secretion or muscle spasm). Splanchnic afferents appear to be involved in the sensation of nausea, because nausea can be evoked by gastric distension in patients with bilateral vagotomy and pyloroplasty [109]. This suggests that stimulation of splanchnic afferents can evoke the sensation, but does not exclude vagal involvement in the intact subject. Vagal stimulation has long been implicated as a factor in nausea [110]. In contrast to vagal afferents, stimulation of greater splanchnic nerves does not evoke an emetic response in animal models.

Vagal afferents continuously transmit gastrointestinal information to the brainstem with little reaching the level of consciousness. Failure to reach conscious awareness does not mean the information is not processed at higher levels of central organization. In FGID, some symptomatology may be related to signals reaching consciousness that would normally be filtered by processing in lower levels of the brain. Aside from primary sensory abnormalities, there is a possibility for inappropriate secondary sensory signals to be experienced as discomfort. In this case, inappropriate efferent signals evoke abnormal activity of the musculature or secretory glands that is subsequently detected by primary afferents and transmitted to the brain where it is interpreted as a disagreeable sensation. There is also the possibility that sensations originating from inappropriate activity in higher brain circuitry are projected to the digestive tract.

Nausea and Vomiting

Nausea and vomiting are common symptoms of FGIDs. Nausea and vomiting are both viewed as components of a protective mechanism against accidentally ingested toxins [111]. Nausea is responsible for the genesis of an aversive response either by taste, sight or smell such that the animal avoids the toxin on future occasions. Vomiting expels the toxin from the upper gastrointestinal tract, whereas diarrhea and power propulsion fulfill a similar function in the lower gut (fig. 10). Nausea immediately reduces food consumption thereby reducing further intake of a contaminant. Probably more importantly, nausea induces an aversive response linking the sensation to recently ingested food that contained the toxin. In humans, nausea can be more aversive than pain. Effects of inappropriate induction of nausea in the clinic are seen in patients undergoing anti-cancer chemotherapy who may experience reduced food intake, anticipatory emetic responses, and aversion to further courses of therapy. Aside from its

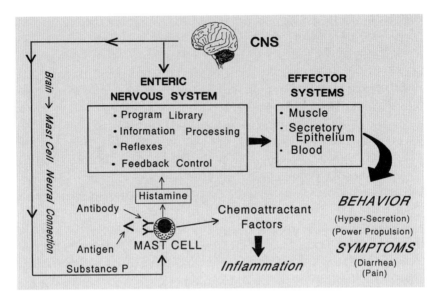

Figure 10. Conceptual model for enteric neuro-immuno physiology. The ENS is a mini-brain located in close apposition to the gastrointestinal effectors it controls. Enteric mast cells are in position to detect foreign antigens and signal their presence to the ENS. Stimulated mast cells release several paracrine mediators simultaneously. Some of the mediators signal the ENS while others act as attractant factors for polymorphonuclear leukocytes responsible for acute inflammatory responses. The ENS responds to the mast cell signal by initiating a program of coordinated secretion and propulsive motility that expels the source of antigenic stimulation from the bowel. Symptoms of abdominal pain and diarrhea result from operation of the neural program. Neural inputs to mast cells from the brain stimulates simultaneous release of chemoattractant factors for inflammatory cells and chemical signals to the ENS with effects that mimic antigenic stimulation.

adaptive advantage in evolution, some animals including humans, experience nausea and vomiting as a symptom in response to an extended range of drugs, therapies, disease processes and altered mental states.

The somatic motor acts of retching and vomiting are preceded by changes mediated by the autonomic nervous system. These include salivation, tachycardia, cutaneous vasoconstriction, sweating, relaxation of the proximal stomach, and retrograde propulsive contractions in the upper small bowel. Relaxation of the proximal stomach is mediated by activity in vagal efferent fibers that leads to activation of enteric inhibitory motor neurons [3,112]. Proximal gastric relaxation reduces emptying of potentially contaminated contents, places the stomach in an advantageous position for mechanical compression, and accommodates the small bowel contents returned by retrograde propulsion in the small bowel. No evidence suggests that the pre-emetic gastric relaxation or retrograde propulsive contractions are responsible for the sensation of nausea.

After emptying of the small bowel into the relaxed stomach, the emetic reflex progresses from predominantly autonomic to somatic nervous control. Retching often precedes vomiting. Retching differs from vomiting in that the peri-esophageal fibers of the diaphragm do not relax. The function of retching is unclear. Vomiting can occur without prior retching. Retching may provide for sensory "sampling" of gastric contents for fluidity optimal for expulsion and may also be a "wind-up" function for a central motor program. Factors that determine the number of retches preceding a vomit are unknown. In animal models, vagal afferents appear to be involved because the number of retches are inversely related to the gastric volume. The predominant force for expulsion is compression of the stomach by intense contraction of the abdominal musculature and diaphragm. This occurs coincident with relaxation of the lower esophageal sphincter, shortening of the esophagus and inhibition of motor neurons in the spinal phrenic nucleus that innervate the peri-esophageal (crural) fibers of the diaphragm [112,113].

"Vomiting center" is a convenient shorthand term for description of the brainstem structures that contain the neural program for organization of autonomic and somatic motor outflow in generation of the emetic response. Input to the vomiting center from vagal afferents, the area postrema, vestibular system, and higher brain structures can induce nausea and trigger the emetic pattern generator in humans. Stimulation of rostral brain regions (e.g., amygdala) can evoke nausea and vomiting [114].

Both abdominal and cardiac vagal afferents can trigger vomiting. Whereas the cardiac afferents may be involved in emesis associated with myocardial infarction, abdominal afferents are more relevant for FGID. Vagal afferents innervate virtually every region of the digestive tract including the liver. The relative ease with which emesis can be evoked by stimulation in varied regions is unknown. The stomach and small intestine are commonly assumed to be the most sensitive sites, as expected from the protective function of emesis. In view of this, it might be argued that the presence of nausea or vomiting signals activity originating in the proximal gut. Nausea is readily induced by distension of the stomach [115], but rarely by distension in the sigmoid colon [101]. Nausea and other sensations of discomfort to overdistension of the stomach may reflect excessive activation of the muscle mechanoreceptors normally involved in gastric vago-vagal reflexes.

Vomiting can also be evoked by stimulation of vagal afferents that innervate the mucosal regions of the stomach and small bowel. Paracrine signaling from mucosal enteroendocrine cells to vagal afferent terminals is believed to be the mechanism of mucosal sensory transduction, with a major involvement of 5-HT and cholecystokinin as paracrine mediators. Mucosal enterochromaffin cells are implicated in the mechanisms by which treatments with cytotoxic drugs and radiation lead to nausea and vomiting. These treatments can lead to generation of free radicals in the enterochromaffin cells leading to influx of calcium that in turn triggers exocytotic release of 5-HT. This can lead to elevated input into the NTS as the released 5-HT stimulates 5-HT_3 receptors located on the vagal afferent terminals [11]. 5-HT_3 receptor antagonists abolish the effects of cytotoxic drugs and radiation in animal models, but are less efficacious in humans. This suggests involvement of additional mechanisms in humans.

The area postrema is an access route to the vomiting center apart from vagal afferents. It is recognized as a circumventricular region located at the caudal extremity of the floor of the fourth cerebral ventricle. It is not isolated by the blood-brain barrier and sends projections to the NTS. Lesion studies and the area postrema's sensitivity to systemically circulating agents such as apomorphine and morphine underlie its identification as "the chemoreceptor trigger zone for emesis" [116]. Some emetic agents (e.g., opiates) may act on dendrites that project into the area postrema from neuronal cell bodies in the NTS [116]. The open blood-brain barrier in the region of the area postrema may also provide access for circulating endocrine signals, as evidenced by blockade of the emetic response to systemic injection of the gut hormone peptide PYY after ablation of the area postrema [117].

The vomiting center should be an ideal target for antiemetic drug therapy because a drug acting there could potentially block both retching and vomiting irrespective of the initial trigger. Several classes of agents that may work in this way have been identified in animal studies. These include 5-HT_{A1} receptor agonists [118], opiate receptor agonists [119], the capsaicin analog resiniferatoxin [120], and neurokinin receptor antagonists [121]. Neurokinin antagonists block retching and vomiting induced by activation of vagal afferents with electrical stimulation, intragastric irritants, cisplatin, and radiation. They also block retching and vomiting evoked by stimulation of the area postrema with apomorphine or loperamide and stimulation of the vestibular system with motion. Early results from clinical trials suggest that the neurokinin antagonists block the sensation of nausea as well as retching and vomiting. This suggests action at a site before divergence of the pathways responsible for the sensation of nausea and the motor behavior of emesis. The most likely site of action is the NTS [121]. Observations that a non-peptide neurokinin-1 receptor antagonist can block the emetic response to abdominal vagal afferent stimulation raises the possibility that this class of drugs may have potential for modifying other nonpainful sensations arising from the upper digestive tract [121].

The primary pathways involved in induction of nausea are the same as those for vomiting; nevertheless, much less is known about the neural mechanisms of nausea. Whereas retching and vomiting are mediated entirely by circuitry of the vomiting center in the brain stem, the sensation of nausea must involve processing in more rostral circuitry. The cerebral origins of the sensation are not known precisely. Magnetic Source Imaging in humans implicates activation in the inferior frontal gyrus for nausea induced by vestibular stimulation and oral administration of ipecac [122]. Electrical stimulation in relatively discrete sites in the cerebral hemispheres are capable of inducing nausea [114].

Elevation of plasma vasopressin and gastric antral dysrhythmia are two physiologic changes consistently associated with nausea in humans. These occur in nausea evoked by illusory self-motion, motion, apomorphine, pregnancy, or chemotherapy. Vasopressin can be massively elevated to greater than fifty times maximal antidiuretic levels. Although both are reliable indicators of nausea, in neither case is it clear whether the elevated vasopressin and gastric dysrhythmia are causal of nausea or consequential links to a general response to stress [123]. In a study of mild nausea induced by illusory self-motion (subject seated inside a vertically-striped rotating drum), neither elevated vasopressin nor gastric dysrhythmia were more likely to occur in nauseated subjects than in subjects that did not experience nausea [124]. This suggests that elevated vasopressin and alterations in gastric electric activity are more likely reflections of complex responses to the stress of nausea. A positive correlation between vasopressin levels and levels of anxiety reported by the subjects is consistent with this.

Sensations of Urgency and Incomplete Stool Evacuation

The sensory physiology underlying nonpainful sensations of urgency and incomplete stool evacuation involves mechanosensory detection at the level of the distal large intestine, transmission in spinal pathways to the brain, and central processing of the information. Low-threshold mechanoreceptors present in the sigmoid colon and rectum, and in the attached mesentery, are the most likely source of afferent information of nonpainful modality. Hirschsprung's disease patients can discriminate between gas and feces after recovery from surgical resection of the terminal large intestine, suggesting that mechanoreceptors in the musculature of the pelvic floor may be responsible for some of the sensations generally referred to the recto-sigmoid and anal regions [125].

Information from mechanoreceptors in the distal bowel is transmitted to the lumbar spinal cord by afferent fibers in the lumbar splanchnic and colonic nerves, and to the sacral spinal cord by afferents in the pelvic nerves. Afferents in the lumbar splanchnic and colonic nerves are accompanied by sympathetic fibers projecting to the intestine and those in the pelvic nerves by parasympathetic efferents. Nevertheless, reference to the sensory fibers in the mixed nerves as "sympathetic" or "parasympathetic" afferents is incorrect. Information from Golgi tendon organs and intrafusal muscle fibers in the pelvic floor musculature is transmitted by primary spinal afferents occupying the pudendal nerves.

How sensory information is processed centrally to produce the nonpainful sensations associated with the distal gut and anus is not understood. Sensory detection is an ongoing process that provides a steady stream of information on the state of the lower bowel to the CNS. However, like the upper gut, most of the information is processed without being consciously perceived. In the absence of means for understanding central mechanisms, most hypotheses are focused on alterations of sensory detection in the periphery.

Normal adults require signaling at the level of consciousness for appreciation of the need to defecate. This dictates voluntary aspects of the process while autonomic reflexes are initiated without conscious awareness. Central processing at the level of consciousness may also elect to postpone defecation. When this happens, the urge to defecate subsides but eventually returns as stimulation by fecal presence persists. The mechanisms by which the sensation of urgency temporarily subsides include receptor adaptation, accommodation in the recto-sigmoid region, and spinal or cerebral gating of the afferent signals. Disordered function at any of these levels could underlie exaggerated sensations of urgency. Sensitization of the mechanoreceptors in the recto-sigmoid region could generate an exaggerated signal such that small fecal volumes entering the region are interpreted centrally as larger volumes. A decrease in rectal tone due to a defective accommodation reflex might drive a higher level of activity along afferent pathways to the CNS or heightened sensations of urgency could arrive from errors in the central processing of normal information from the recto-sigmoid and pelvic floor regions.

Sensations of successful evacuation or incomplete evacuation are also derived from central processing of afferent information arising from the recto-sigmoid and pelvic floor. A population of these afferents respond intensely and preferentially to innocuous proximo-distal shearing stimuli applied to the mucosa of the recto-sigmoid region [126]. Silence in the afferents could be interpreted as a signal that a stool has been completely evacuated and that normal nondefecatory functions can resume. A feeling of incomplete evacuation could result from peripheral or central sensitization of these afferents such that a small volume of residual stool or viscous mucus would be misinterpreted as incomplete evacuation.

The enteric immune system is colonized by populations of immune/inflammatory cells that are constantly changing in response to luminal conditions and during pathophysiologic states. In its position in the colon, the mucosal immune system encounters one of the most contaminated of bodily interfaces with the outside world. The system is exposed daily to dietary antigens, bacteria, viruses, and toxins. Physical and chemical barriers at the epithelial interface do not exclude the large antigenic load in its entirety, causing the mucosal immune system to be chronically challenged.

Observations in antigen sensitized animals suggest direct communication between the immune system and the ENS that may be normal or become pathologic [2,64,127–131]. The communication results in adaptive behavior of the bowel in response to circumstances within the lumen that are threatening to the functional integrity of the whole animal. Communication is chemical in nature (paracrine) and incorporates specialized sensing functions of the immune cells for specific antigens together with the capacity of the ENS for intelligent interpretation of the signals. Flow of information in immuno-neural integration starts with immune detection and signal transfer to the ENS. The enteric minibrain interprets the signal and responds by calling up from its library of stored programs, a specific program of coordinated mucosal secretion and propulsive motility that functions to clear the antigenic threat from the intestinal lumen. Side effects of the program are symptoms of abdominal pain and diarrhea.

The enteric immune system becomes sensitized by foreign antigens in the form of foodstuffs, toxins, and invading organisms. Once the system is sensitized, a second exposure to the same antigen triggers predictable integrated behavior of the intestinal effector systems [3,129–132]. Neurally coordinated activity of the musculature, secretory epithelium, and blood vasculature results in organized behavior of the whole intestine that rapidly expels the antigenic threat. Recognition of an antigen by the sensitized immuno-neuro apparatus leads to activation of a specialized propulsive motor program that is integrated with copious secretion of water, electrolytes and mucus into the intestinal lumen [27,127,129–134]. Detection by the enteric immune system and signal transmission to the enteric minibrain initiates the defensive behavior, which is analogous to emetic defense in the upper GI tract (fig. 10). The neurally organized pattern of muscle behavior that occurs in response to an offending antigen in the sensitized intestine is called power propulsion [13]. This specialized form of propulsive motility forcefully and rapidly propels any material in the lumen over long distances and effectively empties the lumen. Its occurrence is associated with cramping lower abdominal pain and diarrhea [69,135,136].

Power propulsion is one of the neural programs contained in the library of programs stored in the enteric minibrain. Output of the program reproduces the same stereotyped motor behavior in response to radiation exposure, mucosal contact with noxious stimulants or antigenic detection by the sensitized enteric immune system [137]. Whether functional bowel symptoms sometimes reflect paradoxical output of the program is unresolved. The neural program for power propulsion incorporates connections between myenteric and submucous plexuses that coordinate mucosal secretion with the motor behavior. The program is organized to stimulate copious secretion that flushes the mucosa and suspends the offensive material in solution in the receiving segment ahead of the powerful propulsive contractions, which in turn, empty the lumen. The overall benefit is rapid excretion of material recognized by the immune system as threatening.

— Immunoneural Communication

Several kinds of immune/inflammatory cells including lymphocytes, macrophages, polymorphonuclear leukocytes, and mast cells are putative sources of paracrine signals to the ENS. Signaling between mast cells and the neural elements of the local microcircuits is the best understood.

Intestinal mast cells proliferate during exposure to threatening invaders, such as the parasitic nematode *Trichinella spiralis*. Following an initial exposure to the nematode, immunoglobulins specific for *T. spiralis* antigens are bound to receptors on the mast cells where they confer memory for recognition of the sensitizing antigens. Binding and cross-linking of the antigens with the antibodies triggers degranulation of the mast cells. Degranulation releases a variety of paracrine messengers which may include serotonin, histamine, prostaglandins, leukotrienes, platelet-activating factor, and cytokines (fig. 10). Among these, histamine is implicated as a significant messenger in communication between the enteric immune system and the ENS in animal models.

Applications of histamine, to simulate degranulation of mast cells in guinea-pig colon, evokes rhythmic bursts of chloride secretion coordinated with contraction of the musculature. Neural blockade or application of histamine H_2 receptor antagonists stops the cyclic behavior. Several days after sensitization to either *T. spiralis* or milk protein, re-exposure to the parasite or food antigen evokes a pattern of cyclical secretory behavior like that seen during exposure to histamine [131–138].

Electrophysiologic recordings in neurons of the submucous plexus during histamine application show cyclical discharge of action potentials in the same pattern as the cyclical changes in mucosal secretory behavior [139]. Antigen exposure evokes similar responses in neurons of the sensitized intestine [140,141]. Both the action of histamine and the effects of antigen on neuronal behavior are mediated by histamine H_2 receptors.

The patterned discharge of action potentials by the neurons is the neural correlate of the secretory and contractile responses that are linked during exposure to histamine. It reflects activity of a neural pattern generator that sequentially activates and inactivates secretomotor neurons to drive periodic bursts of water and electrolyte secretion that undoubtedly lead to neurogenic diarrhea in the intact animal. The combination of evidence suggests that recognition of sensitizing antigens by intestinal mast cells leads to release of histamine, which signals activation of a neuronal pattern generator from the library of programs stored in the local neural network.

— Brain-Mast Cell Interaction

Enteric mast cells appear to be involved in other defense mechanisms that are separated from antigen sensing and local signaling to the ENS. An hypothesis that mast cells are relay nodes for transmission of selective information from the brain to the ENS is plausible and of sufficient significance to justify attention. Evidence from ultrastructural and light microscopic studies suggest that enteric mast cells are innervated by projections from the CNS [127,142,143]. Functional evidence supporting the brain to mast cell connection is found in reports of Pavlovian conditioning of mast cell degranulation in the gastrointestinal tract [144]. Release of mast cell protease into the systemic circulation is a marker for degranulation of enteric mucosal mast cells. This can be demonstrated as a conditioned response in rats to either light or auditory stimuli and in humans as a conditioned response to stress [145]. The findings support a brain to enteric mast cell connection.

Findings that stimulation of neurons in the brain stem by TRH evokes degranulation of mucosal mast cells in the rat small intestine is additional evidence for brain-mast cell interactions [146]. In the upper gastrointestinal tract of the rat, intracerebroventricular injection of TRH evokes the same kinds of gastric inflammation and erosions as cold-restraint stress. In the large bowel, restraint stress exacerbates nociceptive responses and these effects are associated with increased release of histamine [147]. Intracerebroventricular injection of corticotropin releasing factor (CRF) mimics the responses to stress. Intracerebroventricular injection of a CRF antagonist or pretreatment with mast cell stabilizing drugs suppressed stress-induced responses.

Mast cell degranulation may release mediators that sensitize "silent" nociceptors in the large intestine. In animal models, degranulation of intestinal mast cells results in a reduced threshold for pain responses to balloon distension [148]. Treatment with mast cell stabilizing drugs prevents lowering of the pain threshold.

— Brain-Mast Cell Connection: Implications for FGID

The brain-to-mast-cell connection has clinical relevance for FGIDs. It implies a mechanism linking central psycho-emotional status to irritable states of the digestive tract. The irritable state of the bowel (abdominal discomfort and diarrhea), known to result from degranulation of intestinal mast cells and release of signals to the ENS, is expected to occur irrespective of the mode of stimulation of the mast cells (see fig. 10). Degranulation and release of mediators evoked by neural input will have the same effect on motility and secretory behavior as degranulation triggered by antigen detection. This may explain the similarity of bowel symptoms between those associated with noxious insults in the lumen and those associated with psychogenic stress in susceptible individuals.

The immunoneurophysiologic evidence reinforces the hypotheses that moment-to-moment behavior of the gut, whether it be normal or pathologic, is determined primarily by integrative functions of the ENS. The enteric minibrain processes signals derived from local sensory receptors, the CNS, and immune/inflammatory cells (e.g., mast cells). Enteric mast cells utilize the capacity of the immune system for detection of new antigens and long-term memory that permits recognition of the antigen if it ever reappears in the gut lumen. Should the antigen reappear, the mast cells signal its presence to the enteric minibrain. The minibrain interprets the mast cell signal as a threat and calls up from its program library secretory and propulsive motor behavior organized for quick and effective eradication of the threat. Operation of the program protects the integrity of the bowel, but at the expense of the side effects of abdominal distress and diarrhea. The same symptomatology is expected to result from activation of neural pathways that link psychologic states in the brain to the mast cells in the gut. The immunoneurophysiology in this respect is suggestive of mechanisms with susceptibility to malfunctions that could result in symptoms resembling FGIDs.

Modern methods of PET and single proton emission computerized tomography (SPECT) imaging have been used to follow localized changes in cerebral blood flow or glucose metabolism and thereby mapping of the brain areas involved in cognitive processing in normal subjects and patients with psychiatric disorders [93,149,150]. In unipolar depression found in both patients 60 years of age and older and those with familial depression, blood flow and glucose metabolism in the ventral prefrontal cortex increases during emotional agitation when compared with normal subjects. This region of the brain is involved in language, attention, memory, motor planning, and emotional expression, and the prefrontal cortex is thought to modify long-lasting effects centered in the amygdala. The amygdala, on the other hand, may mediate largely negative emotional associations and thoughts that are integrative functions counteracted by the integrative processes in the prefrontal cortex. The ventrolateral, orbital and subgenual prefrontal areas are all heavily connected with limbic structures (e.g., the amygdala), which have been implicated as sites of emotional arousal and which also have connections with the dorsal vagal complex.

On the one hand, the multiple connections of the dorsolateral prefrontal cortex and the types of cognitive tasks that are processed there raises doubts as to whether core emotional features of depression can be attributed to this brain region. On the other hand, this area is clearly important as suggested by the decreased neural activity seen in PET scans of the amygdala, the ventral prefrontal cortex, and the medial thalamus in response to antidepressant drugs. The magnitude of the blood flow decreases in these regions correlates negatively with subjective ratings of thought and emotion. These changes are normalized when the depression is resolved in some, but not all, studies.

Patients with bipolar depression or secondary depression do not show identical abnormalities in the ventrolateral and lateral orbital portions of the prefrontal cortex. Cerebrovascular lesions associated with bipolar mood disorders involve the right ventral prefrontal cortex, right striatum, right thalamus, or right basotemporal cortex including the amygdala, in contrast with involvement of the left prefrontal cortex and caudate in unipolar depression. These findings have led to the hypothesis that mood disorders may arise from a variety of structural/functional lesions at multiple sites in the limbic-thalamic-cortical circuits [146]. The amygdala and mediodorsal nucleus of the thalamus may interact with the prefrontal cortex in this circumstance. A second part of the hypothesis states that different lesions could produce different phenotypes. Because many of the FGIDs are associated with unipolar and not bipolar depression, such selectivity would predict that the abnormalities found on PET or SPECT scans will not be identical with those found in all forms of depression. In view of the fact that brain imaging has identified abnormalities associated with psychiatric disorders, there will be need to repeat the same studies in well-defined groups of patients with FGIDs in order to start the process of understanding the relationships in brain dysfunction in the two groups of disorders.

— Neuroendocrine Abnormalities

The relevance of changes in CNS blood flow or glucose metabolism for depression and FGIDs can be made only by analogy, as studies with depressed FGID patients have yet to be performed. Nevertheless, hyperactivity of the hypothalamic-pituitary-adrenocortical system (HPA) occurs in both depression and chronic stress, which are conditions strongly associated with FGIDs. Evidence for increased central drive to the HPA axis in depressive illness includes increased levels of corticotropin releasing factor (CRF) in the cerebrospinal spinal fluid and increased expression of CRF in cells in the paraventricular nucleus of the hypothalamus observed in post-mortem examination and adrenal hypertrophy found on CT scan, MRI or post-mortem examination [151]. Moreover, increased serum or urinary cortisol has been reported following provoking life events or in patients with chronic psychosocial difficulties [149, 150]. During successful (but not unsuccessful) treatment of depression, serum cortisol and cerebrospinal fluid levels of CRF normalize, although these changes could be secondary to other changes in the CNS [152].

Directions for the Future

— Neurogastroenterology

Many lines of evidence implicate dysfunction in the nervous system as a significant factor underlying symptomatology in patient complaints and behavior that fit criteria for FGID. This justifies future attention to the neural factors underlying development of symptomatology in patient complaints and behavior that fit criteria for FGID and also justifies accelerated expansion of current interest in the subspeciality of neurogastroenterology. Neurogastroenterology encompasses the investigative sciences dealing with functions, malfunctions, and malformations in the brain and spinal cord and the sympathetic, parasympathetic, and enteric divisions of the autonomic innervation of the digestive tract. Psychologic and psychiatric relations to FGID are significant components of the neurgastroenterologic domain. Acceptance of "neurogastroenterology" as the name for the subspeciality of gastroenterology where the bulk of future progress in understanding FGID is expected will undoubtedly escalate in the future. This should signal its acceptance as a bona fide field of gastroenterologic research and clinical practice [153,154].

— Central Nervous System

The CNS is key to understanding conscious perception of real gastrointestinal pain, genesis of non-painful sensations, the emotional consequences of real pain perception, and psychologic origins of projection of discomfort to the bowel. Spinal pathways and gating mechanisms for nociceptive and non-nociceptive sensations of gastrointestinal origin are poorly explored areas amenable to investigation, with potential for understanding and treatment for disordered sensory aspects of FGID. Advances in understanding the basic neurophysiology of nausea and vomiting is expected to focus on origins in the CNS. Targeting of basic mechanisms of nausea and vomiting for pharmacotherapy with agents such as the non-peptide NK-1 receptor antagonists holds future promise. Nevertheless, future research should not ignore evidence that the peripheral nervous system, especially vagal afferents, is of equal importance in the basic physiology and pharmacology of nausea and vomiting.

New technologies for imaging or otherwise detecting activity in the functioning brain have strong potential for better understanding of how malfunctions of central processing are related to symptoms in FGID patients. These approaches will be necessary for distinguishing peripheral sensitization of sensory detection from abnormalities of central processing as underlying neuropathology in the hypersensitivity to gut pain in IBS patients. They offer promise for improved insight into abnormality of processing in the brain nuclei involved in cognitive perception of gut sensations, integration into emotional consciousness, and psychogenic aspects of behavioral phenotype.

— Enteric Nervous System

Consideration that the ENS is an independent integrative nervous system with most of the neurophysiologic complexities found in the CNS stimulates the premonition that FGID symptoms may originate there as well. Lack of understanding of how subtle malfunctions may occur in the synaptic microcircuits of the ENS is the basis of "functional" as the description for some forms of disordered gastrointestinal motility. This is reminiscent of neurologic disorders, such as Parkinsonian tremors, ballisms, and choreas, that were classified as "functional" prior to understanding of neurotransmission in microcircuits of somatic motor centers in the brain. Parkinson's disease is a classic example of a functional somatic motor disorder that was ultimately explained as malfunction of dopaminergic neurotransmission in localized brain centers. Like the status of understanding of somatic motor control centers in the brain a half-century ago, now as we enter the twenty-first century, the ENS remains a virtual "black box" that must be opened scientifically in order to acquire real understanding of FGIDs.

Acquisition of new knowledge of the neurobiology of the enteric minibrain will require application of the same methodologies that unified functional concepts for the CNS. Electrophysiologic and synaptic behavior of individual enteric neurons, identification of neurotransmitters, identification of how specific neuronal types are wired into synaptic circuits and the emergent properties of microcircuits in the programing of motor and secretory behavior are areas open to innovative investigation. Further investigation of enteric sensory physiology and the influence of inflammation and noxious insult holds promise for understanding why the digestive tract is sensitized to distension in patients afflicted with functional dyspepsia or noncardiac chest pain.

— Enteric Neuroimmune Interactions

Interactions of the enteric immune system and the ENS is an area where progress can be expected in understanding FGIDs. Enteric mast cells may be a key cell type responsible for signaling the ENS to program behavior that results in FGID-like symptoms and for initiating inflammatory cascades that generate chemical mediators (e.g., cytokines) currently known to have potent actions on enteric neurons. Other immune cells (e.g., lymphocytes and macrophages) that have been largely ignored in this respect will also require more focused attention. Evidence that activation of enteric mast cells can occur by central nervous input as well as local insults requires further exploration to determine if a brain-mast cell connection underlies gut reactions to stress.

Cases where autoimmune attack is targeted to enteric neurons requires future investigative scrutiny because current evidence suggests that FGID-like symptoms may signal the onset of the immunologic event that culminates in symptoms of chronic pseudo-obstruction. This appears to be true for explained forms of neuropathic autoimmunity (paraneoplastic syndrome and Chagas' disease) and the idiopathic form. Future directions should include attention to development of tests for enteric neuropathic autoimmunity that can be applied in diagnostic workups during early indications of FGID.

— Musculature

The potential for disordered function of the gastrointestinal, esophageal, and biliary tract musculature to contribute to FGID-like symptoms in subgroups of patients requires targeted consideration. Genetic and acquired myopathies fall into this area. Efforts focused on development of deeper insight into the basic physiology of the pacemaker system (ICCs) of the gastrointestinal musculature and the pathophysiologic basis of disease in this system are justified as added lines of investigation relevant to FGIDs.

References

1. Cooke HJ, Wang YZ, Rogers RC. Coordination of Cl⁻ secretion and contraction by a histamine H(2)-receptor agonist in guinea pig distal colon. Am J Physiol 1993; 265:G973–G978.
2. Wood JD: Neuro-immunophysiolgy of colon function. Pharmacology 1993;47 (suppl 1):7–13.
3. Lang IM, Sarna SK. Motor and myoelectric activity associated with vomiting, regurgitation, and nausea. In: Wood JD, editor. Handbook of Physiology: The Gastrointestinal System: Motility and Circulation. 1. Bethesda, Maryland: American Physiological Society, 1989; p 1179–98.
4. Brookes SJH, Steele PA, Costa M. Identification and immunohistochemistry of cholinergic and non-cholinergic circular muscle motor neurons in the guinea-pig small intestine. Neuroscience 1991;42:863–78.
5. Brookes SJH, Song ZM, Steele PA, et al. Identification of motor neurons to the longitudinal muscle of the guinea pig ileum. Gastroenterology 1992;103:961–73.
6. Brookes SJH, Chen BN, Hodgson WM, et al. Characterization of excitatory and inhibitory motor neurons to the guinea pig lower esophageal sphincter. Gastroenterology 1996;111:108–17.
7. Timmermans JP, Adriaensen D, Cornelissen W, et al. Structural organization and neuropeptide distribution in the mammalian ENS, with special attention to those components involved in mucosal reflexes. Comp Biochem Physiol 1997;118:331–40.
8. Song ZM, Brookes SJH, Costa M. Identification of myenteric neurons which project to the mucosa of the guinea-pig small intestine. Neurosci Let 1991;129:294–98.
9. Song ZM, Brookes SJH, Costa M. All calbindin-immunoreactive myenteric neurons project to the mucosa of the guinea-pig small intestine. Neurosci Let 1994; 180:219–22.
10. Brookes SJH, Meedeniby ACB, Jobling P, et al. Orally projecting interneurones in the guinea-pig small intestine. J Physiol 1997;505.2:473–91.
11. Daniel EE, Parrish MB, Watson EG, et al. The tachykinin receptors inducing contractile responses of canine ileum circular muscle. Am J Physiol 1995;31:G161–G170.
12. Hellstrom PM, Murthy KS, Grider JR, et al. Coexistence of three tachykinin receptors coupled to Ca^{++} signaling pathways in intestinal muscle cells. J Pharmacol Exp Ther 1994;270:236–43.
13. Mao YK, Wang YF, Daniel EE. Characterization of neurokinin type 1 receptor in canine small intestinal muscle. Peptides 1996;17:839–43.
14. Cooke HJ. Neurobiology of the intestinal mucosa. Gastroenterology 1986;90: 1057–81.
15. Cooke HJ. Complexities of nervous control of the intestinal epithelium. Gastroenterology 1988;94:1087–1096.
16. Cooke HJ. Role of the "little brain" in the gut in water and electrolyte homeostasis. FASEB 1989;J 3:127–38.

17. Reiche D, Schemann M. Ascending choline acetyltransferase and descending nitric oxide synthase immunoreactive neurones of the myenteric plexus project to the mucosa of the guinea pig gastric corpus. Neurosci Let 1998;241:61–64.
18. Schemann M, Schaaf C. Differential projection of cholinergic and nitroxidergic neurons in the myenteric plexus of guinea pig stomach. Am J Physiol 1995;32: G186–95.
19. Neunlist M, Frieling T, Rupprecht C, et al. Polarized enteric submucosal circuits involved in secretory responses of the guinea-pig proximal colon. J Physiol (Lond) 1998;506:539–50.
20. Neunlist M, Schemann M. Projections and neurochemical coding of myenteric neurons innervating the mucosa of the guinea pig proximal colon. Cell Tissue Res 1997;287:119–25.
21. Burnstock G. Purinergic neurons. Pharmacol Rev 1972;34:509–81.
22. Grider JR, Cable MB, Said SI. Vasoactive intestinal peptide as a neural mediator of gastric relaxation. Am J Physiol 1985;248:G73–G78.
23. Grider JR, Makhlouf GM. Colonic peristaltic reflex: identification of vasoactive intestinal peptide as mediator of descending relaxation. Am J Physiol 1986;251: G40–G45.
24. Jin JG, Murthy KS, Grider JR, et al. Stoichiometry of neurally induced VIP release, NO formation, and relaxation in rabbit and rat gastric muscle. Am J Physiol 1996;34:G357–69.
25. Murthy KS, Grider JR, Jin JG, et al. Interplay of VIP and nitric oxide in the regulation of neuromuscular activity in the gut. Arch Internat Pharmacodyn Ther 1995;329:27–38.
26. Murthy KS, Makhlouf GM. Vasoactive intestinal peptide pituitary adenylate cyclase-activating peptide-dependent activation of membrane-bound NO synthase in smooth muscle mediated by pertussis toxin-sensitive G(i1-2). J Biol Chem 1994;269:15977–80.
27. Wood JD. Electrical and synaptic behavior of enteric neurons. In: Wood JD, editor. Handbook of Physiology: The Gastrointestinal System: Motility and Circulation. Bethesda, Maryland:American Physiological Society;1989:p 465–17.
28. Manaka H, Manaka Y, Kostolanska F, et al. Release of VIP and substance-P from isolated perfused canine ileum. Am J Physiol 1989;257:G182–90.
29. Vergara P, Woskowska Z, Cipris S, et al. Somatostatin excites canine ileum ex vivo: Role for nitric oxide? Am J Physiol 1995;32:G12–G21.
30. Hukuhara T, Kotania S, Sato G. Effect of destruction of intramural ganglion cells on colon motility: possible genesis of congenital megacolon. Japan J Physiol 1961; 11:635–40.
31. Schiller WR, Suriyapa C, Mutchler JHW, et al. Surgical alteration of intestinal motility. Am J Surg 1973;125:122–28.
32. Wood JD. Electrical activity of the intestine of mice with hereditary megacolon and absence of myenteric ganglion cells. Am J Dig Dis 1973;18:477–88.

33. Stanghellini V, Camilleri M, Malagelada JR. Chronic idiopathic intestinal pseudo-obstruction: clinical and intestinal manometric findings. Gut 1987;23:824–28.

34. De Giorgio R, Bassotti G, Stanghellini V, et al. Clinical, morpho-functional and immunological features of idiopathic myenteric ganglionitis. Gastroenterology 1996;110:A655.

35. Smith VV, Gregson N, Foggensteiner L. Acquired intestinal aganglionosis and circulating autoantibodies without neoplasia or other neural involvement. Gastroenterology 1997;112:1366–71.

36. Camilleri M, Phillips SF. Disorders of small intestinal motility. Gastroenterol Clin N Am 1989;18:405–24.

37. Palo J, Haltia M, Carpenter S, et al. Neurofilament subunit-related proteins in neuronal intranuclear inclusion. Ann Neurol 1984;15:316–21.

38. Monoz-Garcia D, Ludwin SK. Adult-onset neuronal intranuclear hyaline inclusion disease. Neurology 1986;36:785–90.

39. Roy AD, Bharucha H, Nevin NC, et al. Idiopathic intestinal pseudo-obstruction: a familial visceral neuropathy. Clin Gen 1980;18:292–97.

40. Mayer EA, Schuffler MD, Rotter JI, et al. Familial visceral neuropathy with autosomal dominant transmission. Gastroenterology 1986;91:1528–35.

41. Schuffler MD, Baird HW, Fleming CR. Intestinal pseudo-obstruction as the presenting manifestation of small cell carcinoma of the lung: a paraneoplastic neuropathy of the gastrointestinal tract. Ann Intern Med 1983;98:129–34.

42. Lennon VA, San DF, Fusk MF, et al. Enteric neuronal autoantibodies in pseudo-obstruction with small-cell lung carcinoma. Gastroenterology 1991;100:137–42.

43. Altermatt HJ, Rodriguez M, Scheithauer BW. Paraneoplastic anti-Purkinje and type 1 antineuronal nuclear autoantibodies bind selectively to central, peripheral autonomic nervous system cells. Lab Invest 65:412–20,1991.

44. Rosenblum MK: Paraneoplastic and autoimmunologic injury of the nervous system: the anti-hu syndrome. Brain Pathol 1993;3:199–212.

45. Jean WC, Dalmau J, Ho A, et al. Analysis of the IgG subclass distribution and inflammatory infiltrates in patients with anti-hu-associated paraneoplastic encephalomyelitis. Neurology 1994;44:144–47.

46. Heidenreich F, Schober R, Brinck U, et al. Multiple paraneoplastic syndromes in a patient with antibodies to neuronal nucleoproteins (anti-Hu). J Neurol 1995; 242:210–16.

47. Wood JN, Hudson L, Jessel TM, et al. A monoclonal antibody defining antigenic determinants on subpopulations of mammalian neurones and Trypanosoma cruzi parasites. Nature (Lond) 1982;296:34–37.

48. Krishnamurthy S, Shuffler M.D. Pathology of neuromuscular disorders of the small intestine and colon. Gastroenterology 1997;93:610–39.

49. Magni G. The use of antidepressants in the treatment of chronic pain: a review of the current evidence. Drugs 1991;42:730–48.

50. McCann MJ, Hermann GE, Rogers RC. Nucleus raphe obscurus (nRO) influences vagal control of gastric motility in rats. Brain Res 1989;486:181–84.

51. Wood JD. Gastrointestinal Motility. In: Rhoades RA, Tanner GA , editors. Medical Physiology. Boston: Little Brown; 1995: p 505–29.

52. Prosser CL, Sperelakis N. Transmission in ganglion-free circular muscle from cat intestine. Am J Physiol 1956;187:536–45.

53. Wood JD. Excitation of intestinal muscle by atropine, tetrodotoxin and xylocaine. Am J Physiol 1972;222:118–25.

54. Dewey MM, Barr L. Intracellular connection between smooth muscle cells: the nexus. Science 1962;137:670–72.

55. Gabella G. Structure of muscles and nerves in the gastrointestinal tract. In: Johnson LR, editor. Physiology of the Gastrointestinal Tract. New York: Raven Press; 1981: p 197–241.

56. Szurszewski JH. The enigmatic electrical slow wave. Gastroenterology 1997;113: 1785–87.

57. Sanders KM. Colonic electrical activity: concerto for two pacemakers. News Physiol Sci 1989;4:176–81.

58. Carl A, Bayguinov O, Shuttleworth CWR, et al. Role of Ca^{2+}-activated K^+ channels in electrical activity of longitudinal and circular muscle layers of canine colon. Am J Physiol 1995;37:C619–27.

59. Sanders KM. A case for interstitial cells of Cajal as pacemakers and mediators of neurotransmission in the gastrointestinal tract. Gastroenterology 1996;111:492–515.

60. Rumessen JJ, Thuneberg L. Pacemaker cells in the gastrointestinal tract: Interstitial cells of Cajal. Scand J Gastroenterol 1996;31:82–94.

61. Thuneberg L. Interstitial cells of Cajal: intestinal pacemaker cells? In: Beck F, Hild W, van Limbrorgh J, et al., editors. Advances in Anatomy, Embryology and Cell Biology. Berlin: Springer-Verlag;1982: p 1–130.

62. Barajas-Lopez C, Berezin I, Daniel EE, et al. Pacemaker activity recorded in interstitial cells of Cajal of the gastrointestinal tract. Am J Physiol 1989;257:C830–35.

63. Langton P, Ward SM, Carl A, et al. Spontaneous electrical avtivity of interstitial cells of Cajal isolated from canine proximal colon. Proc Nat Acad Sci (USA) 1989; 86:7280–84.

64. Castro GA. Gut immunophysiology; regulatory pathways within a common mucosal immune system. News Physiol Sci 1989;4:59–64A.

65. Castro GA. Parasite infections and gastrointestinal motility. In: Wood JD, editor. Handbook of Physiology: The Gastrointestinal System: Motility and Circulation. Bethesda: American Physiological Society;1989:p 1133–52.

66. Castro GA. Immunophysiology of enteric parasitism. Parasitol Today 1989;5: 11–19,1989.

67. Mathias JR, Clench MH. Alterations of small intestine motility by bacteria and their enterotoxins. In: Wood JD, editor. Handbook of Physiology: The Gastrointestinal System: Motility and Circulation. Bethesda: American Physiological Society;1989: p 1153–77.

68. Andrews PLR, Davis CJ, Bingham S, et al. The abdominal visceral innervation and

the emetic reflex pathways, pharmacology, and plasticity. Can J Physiol Pharmacol 1990;68:325–345.

69. Phillips SF: Motility disorders of the colon. In Yamada T, editor. Textbook of Gastroenterology, 2nd Ed. Philadelphia: J. B. Lippincott,1995: p 1856–75.

70. Koch KL, Stern RM, Vasey MW, et al. Gastric dysrhythmias and nausea of pregnancy. Dig Dis Sci 1990;35:961–68.

71. Abel TL, Malagelada JR, Lucas AR, et al. Gastric electromechanical and neurohormonal function in anorexia nervosa. Gastroenterology 1987;93:958–65.

72. Schuffler MD, Pope CE. Studies of idiopathic intestinal pseudoobstruction: II. Hereditary hollow visceral myopathy: family studies. Gastroenterology 1977;73: 339–44.

73. Anuras S, Mitros FA, Soper RT, et al. Chronic intestinal pseudoobstruction in young children. Gastroenterology 1986;91:62–70.

74. Vanderwinden JM, Liu H, Delaet MH. Study of the interstitial cells of Cajal in infantile hypertrophic pyloric stenosis. Gastroenterology 1996;111:279–88.

75. Vanderwinden JM, Rumessen JJ, Liu H, et al. Interstitial cells of Cajal in human colon and in Hirschsprung's disease. Gastroenterology 1996;111:901–10.

76. Cervero F, Jänig W. Visceral nocireceptor: a new world order? Trends Neurosci 1992;15:374–78.

77. Wood JD. Physiology of the enteric nervous system. In: Johnson LR, editor. Physiology of the Gastrointestinal Tract. New York: Raven Press;1994:p423–82.

78. Furness JB, Kunze WAA, Bertrand PP, et al. Intrinsic primary afferent neurons of the intestine. Prog Neurobiol 1998;54:1–18.

79. Whitehead WE, Holtkotter B, Enck P, et al. Tolerance for rectosigmoid distention in iritable bowel syndrome. Gastroenterology 1990;98:1187–92.

80. Lembo T, Munakata J, Mertz H, et al. Evidence for the hypersensitivity of lumbar splanchnic afferents in irritable bowel syndrome. Gastroenterology 1994;107: 1686–96.

81. Richter JE, Barish CF, Castell DO. Abnormal sensory perception in patients with esophageal chest pain. Gastroenterology 1986;91:845–62.

82. Loening-Baucke V. Sensitivity of the sigmoid colon and rectum in children treated for chronic constipation. J Ped Gastroenterol Nutr 1984;3:454–59.

83. Chey WD, Kim M, Hasler WL, et al. Hyperglycemia alters perception of rectal distention and blunts the rectoanal inhibitory reflex in healthy volunteers. Gastroenterology 1995;108:1700–1708.

84. Fujita T. Taste cells in the gut and on the tongue: their common, paraneuronal features. Physiol Behav 1991;49:883–85.

85. Berthoud HR, Powley TL. Vagal afferent innervation of the rat fundic stomach: morphological characterization of the gastric tension receptor. J Com Neur 1992; 319:261–76.

86. Smith GP, Jerome C, Norgren R. Afferent axons in abdominal vagus mediate satiety effect of cholecystokinin in rats. Am J Physiol 1985;249:R638–41.

87. Davison JS, Clarke GD. Mechanical properties and sensitivity to CCK of vagal gastric slowly adapting mechanoreceptors. Am J Physiol 1988;255:G55–G61.

88. Talley NJ. 5-Hydroxytryptamine agonists and antagonists in the modulation of gastrointestinal motility and sensation: clinical implications. Aliment Pharmacol Therap 1992;6:273–89.

89. Bertrand PP, Kunze WAA, Bornstein JC, et al. Analysis of the responses of myenteric neurons in the small intestine to chemical stimulation of the mucosa. Am J Physiol 1997;36:G422–35.

90. Cervero F. Afferent activity evoked by natural stimulation of the biliary system in the ferret. Pain 1982;13:137–51.

91. Alchaer ED, Lawand NB, Westlund KN, et al. Pelvic visceral input into the nucleus gracilis is largely mediated by the postsynaptic dorsal column pathway. J Neurophysiol 1996B;76:2675–90.

92. Alchaer ED, Lawand NB, Westlund KN, et al. Visceral nociceptive input into the ventral posterolateral nucleus of the thalamus: a new function for the dorsal column pathway. J Neurophysiol 1996A;76:2661–74.

93. Drevets WC, Todd RD. Neuroimaging in psychiatry. In: Guze, editor. Adult Psychiatry. St Louis, MO: Mosby;1997: p 53–82.

94. Lydiard RB, Fossey MD, Marsh W, et al. Prevalence of psychiatric disorders in patients with irritable bowel syndrome. Psychosomatics 1993;34:229–34.

95. Young SJ, Alpers DH, Norland CC, et al. Psychiatric illness in irritable bowel syndrome: practical implications for the primary physician. Gastroenterology 1976;70:162–66.

96. Walker E.A., Roy-Byrne P.P., Katon W.J. Irritable bowel syndrome and psychiatric illness. Am J Psychiatry 1990;147:565–72.

97. Aziz Q, Andersson JLR, Valind S, et al. Identification of human brain loci processing esophageal sensation using positron emission tomography. Gastroenterology 1997; 113:50–59.

98. Silverman DHS, Munakata JA, Ennes H, et al. Regional cerebral activity in normal and pathological perception of visceral pain. Gastroenterology 1997;112:64–72.

99. Aziz Q, Thompson DG. Brain-gut axis in health and disease. Gastroenterology 1998;114:559–78.

100. Devinsky O, Morrell MJ, Vogt BA. Contributions of anterior cingulate cortex to behaviour. Brain 1995;118:279–306.

101. Ness TJ, Metcalf AM, Gebhart GF. A psychophysical study in humans using phasic colonic distension as a noxious visceral stimulus.1990; Pain 43:377–86.

102. Munakata J, Naliboff B, Harraf F, et al. Repetitive sigmoid stimulation induces rectal hyperalgesia in patients with irritable bowel syndrome. Gastroenterology 1997;112:55–63.

103. Mayer EA, Munakata J, Mertz H, et al. Visceral hyperalgesia and the irritable bowel syndrome. In: Gebhart G, editor. Visceral Pain: Progress in Pain Research and Management: 2. Seattle: IASP;1995: p 429–68.

104. Willis WD. The Pain System: The Neural Basis of Nociceptive Transmission in the Mammalian Nervous System. Basel: Karger;1985.

105. Berkley KJ, Hubscher CH. Are there separate central nervous system pathways for touch and pain? Nature Med 1995;1:766–73.

106. Al-Chaer ED, Westlund KN, Willis WD. Nucleus gracilis: integrator for visceral and somatic information. J Neurophysiol 1997;78:521–27

107. Whorwell PJ, McCallum M, Creed FH et al. Non-colonic features of irritable bowel syndrome. 1986;Gut 27:37–40.

108. Andrews PLR, Taylor TV. An electrophysiological study of the posterior abdominal vagus nerve in man. Clin Sci 1982;63:169–73.

109. Troncon LEA, Thompson DG, Ahuwalia NK et al. Relations between upper abdominal symptoms and gastric distension abnormalities in dysmotility like functional dyspepsia and after vagotomy. 1995;Gut 37:17–22.

110. Lewis T. Pain. New York;Macmillan:1992.

111. Andrews PLR, Davis CJ. The physiology of emesis induced by anti-cancer therapy. In: Reynolds DJ, Andrews PLR, Davis CJ, editors. Serotonin and the Scientific Basis of Anti-emetic Therapy. Oxford: Oxford Clinical Communications; 1995: p25–49.

112. Lang IM, Sarna SK, Dodds WJ. Pharyngeal, esophageal, and proximal gastric responses associated with vomiting. Am J Physiol 1993;265:G963–72.

113. Grelot L, Miller AD. Vomiting—its ins and outs. News Physiol Sci 1994;9:142–47.

114. Sem-Jacobsen CW. Depth Electrographic Stimulation of the Human Brain and Behavior. Springfield, Ill.:Thomas; 1968.

115. Khan MI, Read NW, Grundy D. Effect of varying the rate and pattern of gastric distension on its sensory perception and motor activity. Am J Physiol 1993;27: G824–27.

116. Reynolds DJM. Where do 5-HT3 receptor antagonists act as anti-emetics? Reynolds DJ, Andrews PLR, Davis CJ, editors. Serotonin and the scientific basis of anti-emetic therapy. Oxford: Oxford Clinical Communications;1995: p 111–26.

117. Harding RK, McDonald TJ. Identification and characterization of the emetic effects of peptide YY. Peptides 1989;10:21–24.

118. Lucot JB. 5–HT$_{1A}$ receptor agonists as anti-emetics. In: Reynolds DJ, Andrews PLR, Davis CJ, editors. Serotonin and the Scientific Basis of Anti-emetic Therapy. Oxford: Oxford Clinical Communications;1995: p 222–27.

119. Rudd JA, Naylor RJ. Opioid receptor involvement in emesis and anti-emesis. In: Reynolds DJ, Andrews PLR, Davis CJ, editors. Serotonin and the Scientific Basis of Anti-emetic Therapy. Oxford: Oxford Clinical Communications; 1995: p 208–21.

120. Andrews PLR, Bhandari P. Resinferatoxin, an ultrapotent capsaicin analogue, has anti-emetic properties in the ferret. Neuropharmacology 1993;32:799–806.

121. Watson JW, Gonsalves SF, Fossa AJ et al. The role of the NK1 receptor in emetic responses: the anti-emetic effects of CP-99,994 in the ferret and the dog. Br J Pharmacol 1995;115:84–94.

122. Miller AD, Rowley HA, Roberts TPL et al. Human cortical activity during vestibular- and drug-induced nausea detected using MSI. Ann NY Acad Sci 1996;781: 670–72.

123. Koch KL. A noxious trio: nausea, gastric dysrhythmias and vasopressin. Neurogastroenterol Motil 1997;9:141–42.

124. Kiernan BD, Soykan I, Lin Z et al. A new nausea model in humans produces mild nausea without electrogastrogram and vasopressin changes. Neurogastroenterol Motil 1997;9:257–63.

125. Holschneider AM, Boerner W, Buurman O, et al. Clinical and electromanometrical investigations of postoperative continence in Hirschsprung's disease. Zeit Kinderchir 1980;29:39–48.

126. Bahns E, Halsband U, Jänig W. Responses of sacral visceral afferents from the lower urinary tract, colon and anus to mechanical stimulation. Pflügers Arch 1987;410:296–303.

127. Stead RH, Tomioka M, Quinonez G, et al. Intestinal mucosal mast cells in normal and nematode-infected rat intestines are in intimate contact with peptidergic nerves. Proc Nat Acad Sci USA 1987;84:2975–79.

128. Perdue MH, Marshall J, Masson S. Ion transport abnormalities in inflamed rat jejunum: involvement of mast cells and nerves. Gastroenterology 1990;98:561–67.

129. Wood JD. Communication between minibrain in gut and enteric immune system. News Physiol Sci 1991;6:64–69.

130. Wood JD. Gastrointestinal neuroimmune interactions. In: Holle GE, Wood JD, editors. Advances in the Innervation of the Gastrointestinal Tract. Amsterdam: Elsevier Scientific Press; 1992; p 607–15.

131. Wang YZ, Palmer JM, Cooke HJ. Neuro-immune regulation of colonic secretion in guinea pigs. Am J Physiol 1991;260:G307–14.

132. Harari Y, Russell DA, Castro GA. Anaphylaxis mediated epithelial Cl secretion and parasite rejection in rat intestine. J Immunol 1987;128:1250–55.

133. Baird WW, Cutbert AW. Neuronal involvement in type 1 hypersensitivity reactions in gut epithelia. Brit J Pharmacol 1987;92:647–55.

134. Wang YZ, Cooke HJ. H_2 receptors mediate cyclical chloride secretion in guinea pig distal colon. Am J Physiol 1990;258:G887–93.

135. Cowles VE, Sarna SK. Effects of T. spiralis infection on intestinal motor activity in the fasted state. Am J Physiol 1990;259:G693–G701.

136. Cowles VE, Sarna SK. Trichinella spiralis infection alters small bowel motor activity in the fed state. Gastroenterology 1991;101:664–69.

137. Sarna SK, Otterson MF, Cowles VE. In vivo motor response to gut inflammation. In: Collins SM, Snape WJ, editors. Effects of Immune Cells and Inflammation on Smooth Muscle and Enteric Nerves. Boca Raton: CRC Press; 1991:p 181–95.

138. Sethi AK, Sarna SK. Colonic motor activity in acute colitis in conscious dogs. Gastroenterology 1991:100:954–63.

139. Frieling T, Cooke HJ, Wood JD. Histamine receptors on submucous neurons in the guinea-pig colon. Am J Physiol 1992;264:G74–80,1992.

140. Frieling T, Cooke HJ, Wood JD. Neuroimmune communication in the submucous plexus of guinea-pig colon after sensitization to milk antigen. Am J Physiol 1994A;267:G1087–93.

141. Frieling T, Palmer JM, Cooke HJ, et al. Neuroimmune communication in the submucous plexus of guinea pig colon after infection with Trichinella spiralis. Gastroenterology 1994B;107:1602–1609.

142. Williams R.M., Berthoud H.R., Stead R.H. Association between vagal afferent nerve fibers and mast cell in rat jejunal mucosa. Gastroenterology 1995;108:A941.

143. Gottwald T, Lhotak S, Stead RH. Effect of truncal vagotomy and capsaicin on mast cells and IgA-positive plasma cells in rat jejunal mucosa. Neurogastroenterol Motil 1997;9:25–33.

144. MacQueen G, Marchall J, Perdue M et al. Pavlovian conditioning of rat mucosal mast cells to secrete rat mast cell protease II. Science 1989;243:83–84.

145. Santos J, Saperas E, Nogueiras C et al. Release of mast cell mediators into the jejunum by cold pain stress in humans. Gastroenterology 1998;114:640–48.

146. Santos J, Esteban S, Mourelle M. Regulation of intestinal mast cells and luminal protein release by cerebral thyrotropin-releasing hormone in rats. Gastroenterology 1996;111:1465–73.

147. Gue M, Del Rio-Lacheze C, Eutamene H, et al. Stress-induced visceral hypersensitivity to rectal distension in rats: role of CRF and mast cells. Neurogastroenterol Motil 1997;9:271–79.

148. Coelho A, Fioramonti J, Bueno L. Mast cell degranulation induces delayed rectal allodynia in rats: role of histamine and 5-HT. Dig Dis Sci 1998;43:727–37.

149. Drevets WC, Raichle ME. Neuroanatomical circuits in depression: implications for treatment mechanisms. Psychopharmacol Bull 1992;28:261–74.

150. Dreverts WC, Vodeem TO, Price JL, et al. A functional anatomical study of unipolar depression. J Neurosci 1992;12:3628–41.

151. Demitrack MA. Neuroendocrine correlates of chronic fatigue syndrome: a brief review. J Psychiat Res 1997;31:69–82.

152. Dinan TG, Majeed T, Lavelle E et al. Blunted serotonin-mediated activation of the hypothalamic-pituitary axis in chronic fatigue syndrome. Psychoneuroendocrinology 1997;31:261–67.

153. Grundy D. The changing face of gastrointestinal motility. J Gastrointest Mot 5:231–32.

154. Krammer H-J, Enck P, Tack J. Neurogastroenterology from the basics to the clinics. Z Gastroenterol 1997;suppl 2:3–68.

Chapter 3

Principles of Applied Neurogastroenterology: Physiology/Motility-Sensation

John E. Kellow, Chair,

Michel Delvaux, Co-Chair, *with*

Fernando Azpiroz,

Michael Camilleri,

David G. Thompson,

and Eamonn M. M. Quigley

Summary

Many of the symptoms characteristic of the functional gastrointestinal disorders (FGIDs) are consistent with dysfunction of the motor and/or sensory apparatus of the digestive tract. The aspects of sensorimotor dysfunction most relevant to the FGIDs include: alterations in gut contractile activity, in myoelectrical activity, in tone and compliance, and in transit, as well as an enhanced sensitivity to distension, in each region of the gastrointestinal tract. Assessment of these phenomena involves a number of techniques, some well-established and others requiring further validation. Using such techniques, researchers have reported a wide range of alterations in sensory and motor function in the FGIDs. Little relationship has been established to date, however, between such dysfunction and symptoms, and so the clinical relevance of the former remains unclear. Moreover, the proportions of patients in the various symptom subgroups who display dysfunction require better characterization. Progress is occurring in several areas, especially in relation to functional dyspepsia and irritable bowel syndrome. Based on the data gathered to date, a number of recommendations for further progress can be made.

Introduction

Motility of the digestive tract encompasses the phenomena of myoelectrical activity, contractile activity, tone, compliance and transit; these vary according to the specific regions of the gut. Traditionally, many of the symptoms characteristic of the functional gastrointestinal disorders (FGIDs) have been regarded as consistent with alterations in one or more of these components, e.g., impaired gastric emptying and/or defective gastric accommodation underlying the postprandial symptoms in functional dyspepsia, and disordered colonic contractile activity and transit underlying the altered bowel habit in irritable bowel syndrome [1,2]. Such *dysmotility* has been documented repeatedly in FGID patients and most likely reflects dysfunction at one or more levels of the brain-gut axis. Moreover, evidence accumulated in the past decade suggests that patients with FGIDs also exhibit sensory afferent dysfunction, manifest as an altered *sensitivity*, selectively affecting the visceral territory [reviewed in 3–5].

This chapter provides (1) a general overview of the basic concepts, definitions, regional patterns, and techniques of assessment of digestive tract sensorimotor physiology in health; (2) a summary of the main sensorimotor alterations documented in the most common FGIDs; (3) discussion of the current clinical implications of such dysfunction; and (4) some recommendations for future research in this area.

Overview of Digestive Tract Sensorimotor Physiology

Motor and sensory functions of the gastrointestinal tract are mediated through neurotransmitters in the enteric nervous system and in the extrinsic nerves that connect the gastrointestinal tract to the central nervous system (fig. 1). The following discussion covers aspects of normal gut sensorimotor function at the level of the whole organ that are of relevance to the FGIDs. For both conceptual and historical reasons, motility and sensation, although clearly intimately related, are initially considered separately.

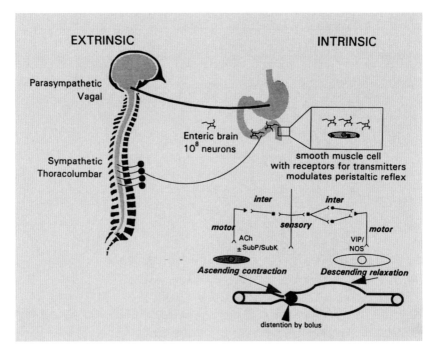

Figure 1. Extrinsic and intrinsic control of gastrointestinal motility. The extrinsic sympathetic and parasympathetic supply to the gut modulates the function of the enteric brain located in ganglionated plexi along the gastrointestinal tract. Transmitters released from the enteric neurons, which are the intrinsic neural control of the gut, modulate the peristaltic relex. The major transmitters in the peristaltic reflex are shown on the right, acetylcholine and substance P are the predominant excitatory neurotransmitters, and VIP and nitric oxide are the predominant inhibitory neurotransmitters. ACh=acetylcholine; SubP=substance P; SubK=substance K; VIP=vasoactive intestinal polypeptide; NOS=nitric oxide synthase. (With permission, The Annual Review of Medicine, Vol 50, to be published and copyrighted in 1999, by Annual Reviews.)

— Basic Concepts and Definitions

Motility

Contractile Activity and Tone

Gastrointestinal contractions may be classified on the basis of their duration; contractions may be of short duration (phasic contractions), or may be more sustained (tone). In the small intestine, a phasic contraction is usually defined as a contraction, the duration of which does not exceed the span of a slow wave cycle; however, some longer lasting motor events are also considered phasic, e.g., "prolonged propagated" contractions. A more prolonged state of contraction, referred to as "tone," may be clearly recognized in some regions such as the proximal stomach (accommodation response to a meal) and the colon (response to feeding). Phasic contractions may be superimposed on this tone; the luminal-occluding properties of phasic contractions thus depend, to some extent, on tone. Tone may also be a feature of sphincteric regions.

The spatial organization of contractions differs at all levels of the gastrointestinal tract. The *stomach* and *small intestine* present different patterns of contractility during fasting and postprandial states (discussed further below) [6]. The *colon* displays several forms of contractility: irregular contractions and high amplitude propagated contractions are associated with electrical activities called short and long spike bursts [7]. The *rectum* demonstrates irregular contractions and periodic rectal motor activity.

Compliance and Related Phenomena

Compliance refers to the capability of a region of the gut to adapt to an imposed intraluminal distension. It is expressed as the ratio dV/dP and is obtained from the pressure-volume curve (fig. 2). In man, compliance reflects the contributions of several factors, including the capacity (diameter) of the organ, the elastic properties and muscular activity of the gut wall, and the elasticity of surrounding organs. It can also be influenced by factors outside the wall such as ascites, organomegaly, or abdominal masses. Although compliance has sometimes been expressed as the pressure/volume ratio at one distension step, it is more accurately expressed as the entire pressure/volume curve. Compliance can differ markedly within an organ; for example the descending colon is less compliant than the ascending colon, while the sigmoid colon is less compliant than the transverse colon. The interpretation of compliance measurements remains controversial, however, because compliance is also influenced by the type of distension and—when phasic distension is applied—by the number of distension steps. Therefore, compliance should be compared between studies only when it has been measured in a similar way. Measurement of compliance has been applied to elucidate the mechanisms of rectal urgency in conditions such as ulcerative colitis [8] and scleroderma [9], both of which are associated with decreased rectal compliance.

A phenomenon related to compliance is wall tension. This reflects the force acting on the gut wall and results from the interaction between intraluminal content and the reaction of the muscular and elastic properties of the wall. Gut sensation depends at least in part on wall tension; in the whole gut segment, tension is operationally defined by Laplace's law (T = PR/2 for a sphere; T = PR for a cylinder, where T refers to wall tension; P, intraluminal pressure; and R, radius). Assessment of wall tension may therefore be important in the interpretation of results of sensation tests.

Transit

While flow reflects the local movements of intraluminal content, transit refers to the time taken for food or other material to traverse a specified region of the gastrointestinal tract. In clinical terms, transit is an extremely important aspect of motility, as it represents the net interaction of a number of the other parameters discussed above. Transit depends on the physical nature of the meal (e.g., solid vs. liquid emptying from the stomach), the composition of the meal (e.g., fat content or osmolality of the liquid phase); whether the marker used to measure transit is inert or part of the meal; the relation of marker ingestion to the interdigestive motility state in the small intestine; and the state of cleansing of the colon. Summaries of transit measurements commonly employed include the half time for emptying (t1/2) (e.g., stomach, colon) (fig. 3), the amount emptied from the stomach at 2 and 4 hours, and the mean colonic transit time.

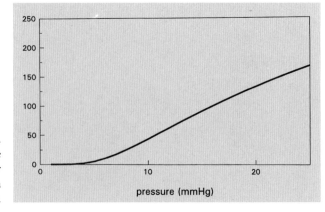

Figure 2. Compliance curve (dV/dP) drawn for human colon in a healthy subject.

pressure (mmHg)

Sensation

The bowel has no specialized sensory end organs, other than naked nerve endings and enteroendocrine cells within the wall, and Pacinian corpuscles in the mesentery [4]. Specialized sensory functions include the sensation of chemical, noxious, thermal, and mechanical stimuli; in recent years, the importance of visceral sensation has been increasingly appreciated, as the magnitude of the sensory traffic emanating from the gut has become evident (see Chapter 2 for more details). When compared to the field of motility, however, there remains a surprising lack of information regarding many key areas, such as receptors, afferent pathways, modulatory mechanisms, and normal perceptions. In brief, visceral afferent input is conveyed to the central nervous system by rapidly conducting myelinated A-delta fibers, and slower, nonmyelinated C fibers. These nerve fibers reach the central nervous system via either the vagus nerve (which consists of 60% afferent fibers at the level of the diaphragm), or spinal afferents. Spinal afferents have their cell bodies in the dorsal root ganglia, and constitute the first in a chain of three neurons conveying gut afferent input to conscious perception. The second order neuron is the dorsal horn neuron in the spinal

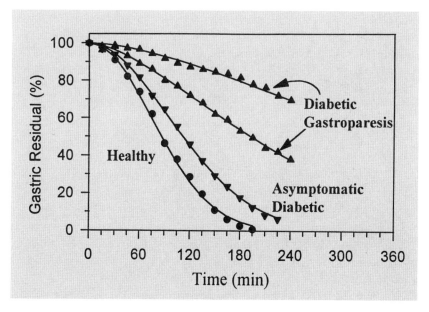

Figure 3. Gastric emptying of solids measured using scintigraphy. Note the delay in gastric emptying t1/2 in a symptomatic diabetic patient compared with an asymptomatic patient and a healthy subject.

cord, which sends information along the lateral spinothalamic or spinoreticular tracts. In addition, there is a midline dorsal column nociceptive pathway conveying pain sensation from abdominal and pelvic viscera to brainstem centers. The third order neurons project from the latter to cortical or subcortical centers, which convey the specific sensation (somewhat localized to the gut area), and the associated symptoms such as affective responses, appetite changes, or autonomic features. It is thought that pain results when sensory fibers are inflamed or stimulated more intensely. Sensations have a diffuse nature, unless the parietal peritoneum is stimulated, with resultant stimulation of somatic afferents. The dorsal horn neuron to which visceral fibers project also receives input from somatic nerves.

It is well established that conscious perception is elicited via spinal afferents. The vagus may exert a modulatory role on spinal afferent input and perception, but there is no firm evidence supporting vagal afferents directly eliciting perception. Visceral sensations are modulated by several factors [4]. *First*, a synapse between the en passant neuron of the spinal afferent and ganglion cells in the prevertebral ganglia mediates intestino-intestinal reflex responses; these responses may alter gut smooth muscle tone and increase or decrease the activation of nerve endings within the bowel wall or mesentery. *Second*, somatic afferents project on the same dorsal horn neurons in the spinal cord that synapse with visceral afferents; this common viscerosomatic projection results in referred pain (or somatic projection of the visceral stimulus) and may also control the ascending or central input of visceral stimuli by changing the excitability of the dorsal horn neuron. There is wide overlap of projections of somatic and visceral afferents over many spinal laminae; this probably accounts for the poor localization of visceral sensations. The dorsal horn neuron functions as a "gate" that controls central projections. Physical methods such as transcutaneous electrical nerve stimulation (TENS) or acupuncture can alter perception of visceral sensations by providing a competing stimulus to the same dorsal horn neuron. *Third*, descending noradrenergic and serotonergic pathways arising in the brainstem project to the dorsal horn neurons and modulate the latter's responses to gut stimuli. *Fourth*, the reticular formation and thalamic projections to cardiovascular or respiratory (autonomic) nuclei, satiety (hypothalamic), and emotional (limbic system) centers induce the changes in affect, appetite, pulse, respiratory rate, and blood pressure that may occur in response to visceral sensations.

Most stimuli in the gut are not consciously perceived. Sensitivity is an ambiguous term that has been used to refer to both conscious perception and to activity in sensory afferent pathways, whether related to perception or to reflex responses. In this chapter we will focus on the mechanisms that lead to the subjective experience of *conscious perception*. Several other terms, however, borrowed from the field of somatic sensitivity, have been applied to studies of the FGIDs. *Hypersensitivity* is the excessive sensation of afferent stimuli. *Hyperalgesia* is where a painful stimulus leads to a behavioral, perceptual or neurophysiologically-induced sensation greater in intensity and duration than normal. *Allodynia* reflects the painful sensation of a previously painless stimulus. Although these terms have led to a resurgence of interest in the anatomy and function of sensory pathways in the gastrointestinal tract, their appropriateness to the field of visceral sensitivity in the FGIDs remains to be established.

— Regional Patterns of Motility

In the various regions of the gastrointestinal tract, muscle layers of the gut wall and their innervation are adapted and organized to subserve the motor functions of that region. Along the gastrointestinal tract, the gut interacts with the central nervous system through either somatic or autonomic neurons, and communication between various parts of the gut is facilitated by the transmission of myogenic and neurogenic signals longitudinally along the gut, as well as by reflex arcs transmitted through autonomic neurons.

Stomach and Small Intestine

The main functions of gastric motility are to accommodate and store the ingested meal, to grind or *triturate* solid particles, and then to empty the meal in a regulated fashion into the duodenum [10–12]. Small intestinal motility mixes the meal with intestinal secretions, propels digesta in an aboral direction, and keeps the intestine clean (regardless of the delivery of food). Sphincters at the lower esophageal, pyloric, and ileocecal regions regulate transit across these regions and prevent orad reflux. Along the length of the gut, patterns of motor activity during fasting and after food differ fundamentally.

Fasting Gastrointestinal Motility

In the fasted state, motor activity is highly organized into a distinct and cyclically recurring sequence of events known as the migrating motor complex (MMC) [6]. The MMC consists of three distinct phases of motor activity that occur in sequence and migrate slowly along the length of the small intestine. Each sequence begins with a period of motor quiescence (phase 1), is followed by a period of apparently random and irregular contractions (phase 2), and culminates in a burst of uninterrupted regular phasic contractions (phase 3 or activity front) (fig. 4). The maximum frequency of contraction in the small intestine (12–14 cycles per minute) occurs during phase 3 of the MMC. Individual cycles last between one and two hours, originate in the stomach, or most frequently, the duodenum or proximal small intestine, and migrate aborally; the velocity of propagation slows as the activity front progresses distally. Cyclical motor activity has also been identified in the gallbladder and sphincter of Oddi [13].

During gastric phase 3 activity, basal tone in the lower esophageal sphincter is increased and exhibits superimposed phasic contractions, thereby preventing reflux of gastric contents during this time of intense phasic contractile activity. Tone increases in the proximal stomach, and superimposed phasic waves can be identified. True rhythmic activity occurs only in the distal antrum where contractions at 3 cycles per minute, the maximum rate of contraction in the stomach, may be seen at the end of phase 3. As phase 3 progresses, antro-pyloro-duodenal coordination increases and high amplitude contractions propagate through the antrum across the pylorus into the proximal duodenum where they may be associated with brief clusters of phasic contractions. In this way, the motor patterns of the proximal duodenum can be differentiated from the remainder of the duodenum, the jejunum, and most of the ileum. The distal ileum also demonstrates

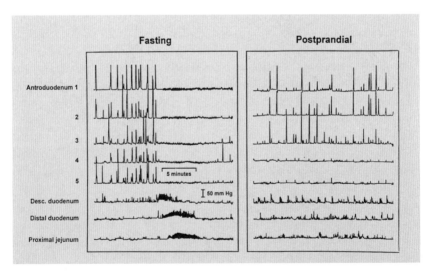

Figure 4. Example of fasting and postprandial motility in a healthy subject. Note the activity front (phase 3 of the migrating motor complex) during fasting (left panel) and the sustained but irregular contractile phasic pressure activity postprandially. (With permission, The Annual Review of Medicine, Vol 50, to be published and copyrighted in 1999, by Annual Reviews.)

regional specialization. Phase 3 of the MMC usually fades out in the distal ileum, and few complexes reach the ileocecal sphincter (ICS). Instead, irregular activity and clustered contractions predominate. On occasion, a high amplitude wave sweeps through the region and across the ICS into the cecum. This "giant migrating" or "prolonged propagating" contraction is thought to clear the ileum of refluxed colonic material. Tone is not a prominent or consistent feature at the ileocecal sphincter, and it is thought that the transport of ileal contents into the colon and the prevention of colo-ileal reflux result mostly from coordinated ileal phasic contractions rather than to fluctuations in ICS tone [14].

Postprandial Gastrointestinal Motility

If food is ingested, the cyclical pattern is abolished, or at least suppressed, and replaced in the stomach by regular antral contractions, and in the small bowel, by irregular, random contractions which may be sustained for 2.5 to 8 hours, depending on the size and nature of the meal (fig. 4). Thereafter, the fasted pattern resumes, or recurs, when a substantial part of the meal has emptied from the small bowel.

On arrival of a swallow sequence at the esophago-gastric junction, the gastric fundus undergoes receptive relaxation, partly mediated by the vagus nerve. As the meal enters the stomach, tone and phasic contractions in the proximal stomach are inhibited leading to accommodation. An important component of the normal response to a meal, and of the gastric emptying process, is the ability of the antro-pyloric region to discriminate solids by size and to retain solid particles greater than 2 mm in diameter. The antro-pyloric mill grinds ("triturates") larger particles; when the size of the solids is reduced to 2 mm or less, they are emptied with the liquid phase. While trituration proceeds, solid emptying does not occur, giving rise to the lag phase, the duration of which is directly related to the size and consistency of the solid component of the meal. After a typical solid/liquid meal, the lag phase lasts approximately 60 minutes; once the particles are triturated, the emptying phase occurs and typically proceeds in a linear fashion. The content of the meal, however, exerts a profound effect on motility and emptying—thus liquids, digestible solids, and relatively large undigested solids clearly empty at different rates.

Trituration is a function of the coordinated shearing forces that are set up within the stomach. These include high amplitude waves that originate in the proximal antrum and are propagated to the pylorus. As these contractions traverse the mid-antrum, the pylorus is open and duodenal contractions are inhibited, permitting trans-pyloric flow of liquids and suspended or liquefied solid particles. On reaching the distal antrum, the terminal contraction closes the pylorus promoting retropulsion of particles that are too large to have exited through the pylorus. In this manner, solid food particles continue to move into, through and out of the antrum, until they are small enough to exit the pylorus. All parameters of duodenal motility that are related to antral and pyloric contractions and contribute to gastric emptying can be considered as antro-pyloro-duodenal coordination. Antro-pyloro-duodenal coordination is suppressed during the lag phase and isolated pyloric contractile waves are prominent, perhaps serving to maintain the solid particles in the stomach until trituration has occurred. Once emptying begins, the incidence of antro-pyloro-duodenal coordination again increases and that of isolated pyloric waves diminishes. Gastric emptying of liquids and solids suspended in the liquid phase is ultimately dependent on the interplay between the propulsive force generated by tonic contractions of the proximal stomach and the resistance presented by the antrum, pylorus, and duodenum. The tonic contractions may contribute to the second shearing force, as content is propelled aborally, and this may manifest as a common cavity wave or contractions that can be detected in the body and antrum of the stomach. Indigestible solids are not emptied during this postprandial stage but during phase 3 MMC activity when they are swept out of the stomach. A number of factors, both physiological and pathophysiological, are known to influence the gastric emptying rate of a meal (Table 1).

The postprandial motor response in the small intestine features intense but apparently uncoordinated motor activity. More detailed studies suggest, however, that there may be considerable organization within this activity. Although contractions propagating over long distances are suppressed in the postprandial period, more localized contractile events are common and serve to advance the meal slowly in a cauded direction and to promote mixing and digestion. As MMC activity is less evident in the terminal ileum, the transition from the fasted to the fed state is also less readily defined in this region, and a clear differentiation in the terminal ileum between fasting and postprandial motor activity may prove difficult.

In the small intestine, the generation and propagation of the MMC appear to be independent of extrinsic nerves and are intrinsic to the gut; the ability to switch from the fasted to the fed state, however, is largely dependent on the vagus [15]. In the stomach the motor response to feeding is, in large part, mediated through the vagus. While the integration of the gastric component with the small bowel MMC remains incompletely understood, it appears that both extrinsic nerves (especially the vagus) and hormonal factors (in particular motilin) are involved. Thus, phase 3 activity that begins in the stomach is associated with a rise in the serum motilin level and exogenously administered motilin induces this same activity. However, other activity fronts that begin in the proximal jejunum occur without a rise in serum motilin [16,17].

Table 1. Some Factors Modulating Gastric Emptying and Colonic Transit

Modulating Factor	Effect on Emptying Rate/Transit
A. Gastric Emptying	
I Meal factors	
Volume	Rate proportional to volume
Acidity	Slows
Osmolality	Hypertonic meals empty more slowly
Nutrient density	Rate inversely proportional to nutrient density
Fat	Slows
Certain amino acids (e.g., L-tryptophan)	Slow
II Other factors	
Ileal fat	Slows (ileal brake)
Rectal/colonic distension	Slows
III Extrinsic neural control	
Vagotomy	Accelerates liquid emptying
	Slows solid emptying
IV Hormonal control	
CCK	Slows
Gastrin	Accelerates
B. Colonic Transit	
I Meal factors	
Fiber	Accelerates
Fat	Slows
Osmotic agents	Accelerates
(e.g., disaccharide intolerance)	
II Neurohormonal control	
Vagal, Sacral parasympathetic	Accelerates
Sympathetic	Slows

Colon and Anorectum

The motor functions of the colon include propulsion and accommodation or storage [7]. Propulsion is achieved by a number of motor events, which include individual contractions, contractile bursts, and high amplitude, rapidly-propagated contractions, i.e., pressure events that sweep through the colon to propel contents from the ascending or transverse colon to the sigmoid colon or rectum. These high amplitude propagated contractions have been correlated to some extent with large volume movements of the intraluminal content of the colon that were initially recognized on barium studies as "mass movements" [18]. Studies performed with simultaneous monitoring of content movements and motility confirmed this association of mass movements with propulsion of the content over long distances [19]. They correspond to the migrating long spike bursts described on electromyographic recordings [20]. Prolonged recordings of colonic motility have shown that these high amplitude propagated contractions occur more often in the morning and during the postprandial period [21,22]. The other motor events may propel contents over short distances in either an orad or an aboral direction, and their primary function appears to be to facilitate mixing. A number of factors influence the rate of colonic transit (Table 1). Periodic or cyclical motor activity has not been identified in the human colon but is evident in the rectum—the rectal motor complex (RMC). Although the RMC is also more prominent during sleep, it does not appear to be synchronized with the small intestinal MMC and its precise function and regulation remain unclear.

Accommodation and storage are essential functions of the colon, as fluids, electrolytes, and some products of carbohydrate and fat digestion are salvaged by bacterial metabolism; the mechanisms of such salvage remain unclear. Accommodation and storage are at least partly mediated by colonic tone. Fluctuations in tone also facilitate distribution of material in the colon, and alter thresholds for perception of luminal distension. Tone demonstrates considerable diurnal variation, increasing slowly following a meal, relaxing during sleep and increasing dramatically upon waking (fig. 5) [23]; these variables also influence phasic activity similarly.

The anorectum serves two important functions, namely, defecation and continence. Defecation is achieved through the integration of a series of motor events and involves both striated and smooth muscle. When colonic contents reach the rectum, a sensation of rectal fullness is generated by rectal afferents, probably arising from activation of stretch receptors in the mesentery or pelvic floor muscles. In response to this, a "sampling" reflex, also known as the rectoanal inhibitory or rectosphincteric reflex, is generated and leads to internal anal sphincter relaxation and external sphincter contractions. At this stage, the individual can decide to postpone or, if it is considered socially acceptable, proceed with defecation. To facilitate the process, the puborectalis muscle and external anal sphincter relax, thereby straightening the rectoanal angle and opening the anal canal. The propulsive force for defecation is then generated by contractions of the diaphragm and the muscles of the abdominal wall, which now propel the rectal contents through the open sphincter. The internal anal sphincter is a continuation of the smooth muscle of the rectum and is under sympathetic control. It provides approximately 80% of normal resting anal tone. The external anal sphincter and pelvic floor muscles are striated muscles, innervated, respectively,

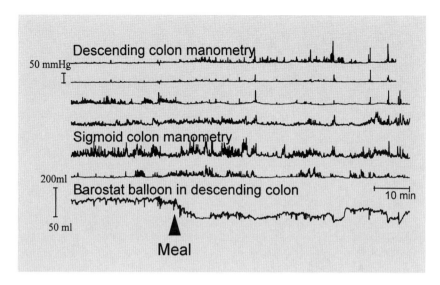

Figure 5. Colonic motility measured by means of manometry and barostatically-controlled balloon in a healthy subject. Note the postprandial increase in phasic pressure activity in the descending colon, and the reduction in balloon volume signifying an increase in colonic tone.

by sacral roots 3 and 4 and the pudendal nerve. The anorectum represents, therefore, the other site of convergence of the somatic and autonomic nervous systems and is susceptible to disorders of both striated and smooth muscle, as well as to diseases of the central, peripheral, and autonomic nervous systems (see Chapter 9).

— ## Current Techniques to Evaluate Sensorimotor Physiology

Motility

Techniques applicable to the measurement of gastrointestinal motor function can be grouped under five main headings: transit, wall motion, intraluminal manometry, myoelectric recordings, and assessment of tone. Although a critical appraisal of the indications and pros and cons of these techniques is beyond the scope of this review, some of their applications in the stomach, small bowel, colon, and anorectum are discussed briefly below, and summarized in Table 2. Techniques used in the esophagus are discussed in Chapter 5.

Table 2. Measurement of Gastrointestinal Motility

Recording Techniques	Main Applications
I Transit	
radio-opaque markers and X-ray*	gastric emptying, colonic transit
hydrogen breath tests	orocecal transit
scintigraphy*	gastric emptying
	small bowel & colonic transit
	dynamics of defecation
radio-labeled C-substrate breath tests	gastric emptying
	orocecal transit
magnetic resonance imaging	gastric emptying
pharmacologic markers	
acetaminophen	gastric emptying of liquids
sulfasalazine	orocecal transit time
intraluminal impedance	bolus transport
II Wall motion	
ultrasonography	gastric antro-pyloric contractions
	gastric compartment volumes (areas)
scintigraphy	gastric antral contractions
magnetic resonance imaging	gastric contractions
III Intraluminal phasic pressure	
water-perfused manometry*	phasic contractions at all levels
solid-state transducers	of the digestive tract
impedance transducers	
IV Myoelectrical activity	
electrogastrography	gastric-surface electrical recordings
intraluminal electromyographic	gastric, small intestinal and colonic
recordings	electrical activity
needle electromyography	anal sphincter & pelvic floor muscle
	activity
V Tone, compliance & wall tension	
barostat	gastric, small bowel, colorectal tone
	and compliance
tensostat	tension

* most widely available methods

Stomach

Scintigraphy

Scintigraphic techniques are the most commonly used for the assessment of gastric motor function [24]. Various types of meals and isotopes can be used, the important principle being that the isotope should remain totally bound with the meal during emptying. To assess solid phase emptying ^{99m}Tc-labeled scrambled egg is commonly used; this isotope should not leach into the liquid phase. Similarly, a liquid marker such as Indium-DTPA-labeled water should not be adsorbed into the solid phase. To achieve standardized results, meals should always be consumed in the same position; correction for movement of the meal in three dimensions within the stomach can be made by using anterior and posterior cameras and calculating a geometric mean. Because of variations in test substance, method of scanning and of calculations, each laboratory should establish its own range of normal values from a control population of adequate size and age- and gender-distribution. Scintigraphic studies are sensitive and specific for the demonstration of gastric stasis, the sensitivity of the emptying study being related to the nature of the test material. Indigestible solid-phase meals may provide the most useful clinical information.

Recently, ^{13}C octanoic acid and ^{13}C acetate breath tests have been developed to measure solid and liquid emptying [25]. In several studies, the ^{13}C octanoic acid breath test has demonstrated reproducibility comparable to standard scintigraphy; as it employs the stable isotope ^{13}C, no radiation is involved, and this approach has the greatest potential to become an office-based test of gastric emptying.

Ultrasonography

This noninvasive method, most suited to study gastric wall movements and volume configurations, can provide a detailed but short-term evaluation of antropyloric function. Thus, novel two-dimensional and sophisticated three-dimensional methods can yield information regarding relationships between antral volume, pyloric patency, transpyloric flow and antral and duodenal contractions [26,27]. More widespread clinical application of ultrasonography is limited by the short observation time feasible, and by the paucity of data from studies in disease states. Other limitations include the inability to visualize the upper body and fundus, the need for frequent acquisition, and the time required for quantitative analysis.

Electrogastrography (EGG)

Until recently, technical problems limited the usefulness of this relatively simple and noninvasive technique. Using sophisticated electronic equipment, several laboratories have reported the consistent and reliable recording of gastric electric activity from surface electrodes. Because of interference from a multitude of artifacts, as well as competing biological signals, the raw EGG signal is difficult to decipher and its analysis depends on such computer–based methods as application of fast Fourier transformation and running spectral analysis. Two parameters appear most predictive of motor function: slow wave frequency and the power ratio. The gastric slow wave can be readily and reliably recorded in fasting conditions and following meal ingestion, and this technique can detect abnormal frequencies (bradygastria and tachygastria) in response to environmental and pharmacological manipulation, as well as in disease states. The change in power related to meal ingestion, or power ratio, appears to correlate with gastric emptying; recent studies suggest that this phenomenon reflects a real increase in the electrical signal rather than an artifact related to alterations in the spatial relationship between the surface electrode(s) and the gastric antrum. Though noninvasive and, therefore, most attractive for clinical use, the clinical role of EGG remains to be established [28–32].

Magnetic Resonance Imaging
Echo-planar magnetic resonance imaging has been employed to assess gastric emptying and to evaluate regional gastric motor function [33,34]. There is now considerable evidence to indicate that this noninvasive, though expensive, technique provides detailed information on gastric function and appears to be particularly valuable in the assessment of regional gastric emptying, including the intragastric distribution of the meal [35]. Most recently, MRI technology has been applied to the assessment of gastric contractility [36]. Given the relatively limited access to this technique in clinical practice, and the expense involved, it seems unlikely that it will ever achieve widespread use as a clinical modality for the assessment of gastric emptying.

Barostat
Conventional techniques to measure phasic contractile activity fail to measure tone; the barostat was developed to overcome this deficiency. This instrument, primarily used for research purposes, controls intraluminal pressure in a segment of the gut (e.g., stomach, colon) by a feedback regulation of air volume within an intraluminal bag [37]. Isobaric volume changes reflect variations in gut tone: when the gut relaxes, the volume increases, and vice versa. This isobaric approach applies a low tension on the gut wall and measures muscular activity by the changes in muscle length.

However, the barostat has limitations and potential technical pitfalls that require proper attention. Important technical aspects include the use of an oversized bag, carefully deflated at the beginning of the experiment, and a separate channel in the connecting tube for direct pressure monitoring within the bag. Subjects should be positioned so that the air within the bag is located in the upper part of the abdominal cavity, otherwise overlying viscera will obscure the responses. The operating pressure in the barostat is individually adjusted 1–2 mmHg above intra-abdominal pressure. Intra-abdominal pressure may be approximately determined by increasing the pressure slowly, until the barostat captures volume variations associated with respiration [37,38]. It is important to emphasize that this minimal distending pressure, which equilibrates intra-abdominal pressure, is unrelated to gastric tone. Likewise, the barostat volume recording does not reflect the absolute level of tone; comparisons of baseline volume levels between subjects are meaningless, because they depend on the operating pressure, which is difficult to standardize precisely. Small differences in the setting of the operating pressure with respect to the intra-abdominal pressure level may condition marked differences in the intragastric air volume. Hence, at a constant pressure level the barostat only measures changes in tone. With this setting, the barostat is ideally suited to measure reflex motor responses as changes in air volume, particularly when the effects are relatively brief and reversible. Basal tone can be evaluated by measuring intragastric volume after complete inhibition of tone, for instance after administration of glucagon at the end of the experiment, and using this volume as a reference level for previous measurements.

Small Intestine
Measurement of Intestinal Transit
For many years, the sole technique for the assessment of intestinal motor function was the radiological observation of the passage of barium through the gut. Though fundamental to the definition of anatomic abnormalities, this technique was insensitive, subjective, and extremely difficult to quantify. Another technique, hydrogen breath testing, relies on the fact that carbohydrates which pass through the small intestine undigested and unabsorbed undergo fermentation by the colonic bacterial flora upon arrival at the cecum. The hydrogen gas produced is absorbed across the colonic mucosa, enters into the splanchnic circulation, and is exhaled in the breath. Therefore, the time from ingestion of a nonabsorbable carbohydrate to the onset of rise in breath hydrogen provides an index of the mouth-to-cecum transit time. Using either natural carbohydrate sources such as potatoes, rice, or beans, or artificial compounds such as lactulose, exhaled breath hydrogen analysis has been widely employed as an estimate of intestinal transit, and can be used in clinical practice. It should be remembered, however, that the transit time measured includes not only small intestinal tran-

sit, but also gastric emptying. Moreover, this test only provides information in regard to the arrival of the head of the meal and its interpretation is difficult if small intestinal bacterial overgrowth is present [39].

Scintigraphic techniques have also been employed to measure small intestinal transit. This has proved more problematic than the measurement of gastric emptying due to the disassociation of some isotopes from food during digestion, overlap both between individual loops of intestine and between the intestine and other organs, and difficulties in defining the arrival of the meal in the cecum or right colon. There is thus a lower reproducibility and accuracy in measurements of small bowel transit time than in measurements from other regions of the digestive tract. For these reasons, it is not usually employed in clinical practice. One recently described technique involves the use of Indium 111-labeled cation exchange resin pellets (amberlite) and can provide, in a single study, an accurate measure of gastric emptying, small bowel transit, and colonic filling [40].

Antroduodenal and Small Intestinal Manometry

The direct measurement of pressure activity in the antrum, duodenum, and small intestine is a technique which remains confined to specialized laboratories [5,24]. In most institutions, a multi-lumen perfused catheter assembly is employed, the assembly is customized according to the site in the intestine in which recordings are to be obtained, and stationery recordings obtained. Thus, for antro-duodenal recordings, the assembly should include an array of closely-spaced sensors to straddle the pylorus, as well as recording sites in the duodenum and proximal jejunum; for small intestinal recordings, several more widely-spaced recording sites may be more appropriate. These assemblies are placed under fluoroscopic guidance and recordings typically performed for several hours during fasting and following the ingestion of a standardized liquid/solid meal. Recordings are analyzed for the various parameters of the MMC, for the presence and nature of the motor response to the meal, and for abnormal patterns [24]. Such stationary recordings are well suited to evaluation of postprandial motility.

Ambulatory systems have been developed which combine solid-state miniaturized strain gauges, data loggers similar to those employed for 24-hour pH recordings, and appropriate computer software. Such systems permit prolonged (typically 24 hours) ambulatory recordings of motor activity from antrum, duodenum, jejunum, or ileum, and can be performed in the patient's home environment [41,42]. Ambulatory recordings are thus most suitable for evaluation of the MMC, the response to a number of meals can be assessed, and diurnal variations in gastrointestinal motor activity can be evaluated [43]. Nocturnal recordings are particularly useful for studying dysmotility of enteric origin.

Intraluminal Electromyographic Recordings

Electromyographic recordings from surgically-implanted serosal electrodes in a variety of animal models have been crucial to the description of interdigestive and postprandial motor patterns and have provided insights into a number of pathological states. Recordings from implanted electrodes have been performed to a limited extent in man. In these instances, serosal electrodes have been placed at the time of laparotomy for another procedure, and recordings performed for a limited time postoperatively. This approach has been adapted to permit electrode placement at the time of laparotomy and to enable correlation of short-term EMG recordings with full-thickness biopsy findings [44]. Efforts have also been made to obtain EMG recordings from electrodes mounted on a catheter and placed in the intestinal lumen [45]. In the small intestine, the information provided by such EMG recordings is to some extent equivalent to manometry, although reliable recordings require careful monitoring, and consequently the technique is not in general use.

Colon

Scintigraphy, manometry and barostat techniques, when used in the colon, employ similar principles as those for recordings in the stomach. Scintigraphy with images at 4, 24, and 48 hours provides an accurate estimate of colonic transit, and can identify accelerated or delayed colonic transit. Colonic manometry and barostat measurements can be used to detect colonic inertia, a condition in which slow transit constipation is associated with a lack of response to meal ingestion [46,47], or to cholinergic stimulation [46] or bisacodyl [48].

Radio-opaque Markers

Although in specialized laboratories and in clinical research studies, scintigraphy, manometry and the barostat have been applied to the investigation of colonic motor function, the radio-opaque marker technique remains the most widely employed clinical test of colonic motor function. While protocols vary, the essential component of this test is the definition of transit, through the colon, of orally-ingested radio-opaque markers. If transit is delayed, and the pattern of marker distribution is one of retention of markers throughout the colon, the diagnosis of colonic inertia is suggested. On the other hand, if markers are retained in the rectum or rectosigmoid region but have moved in a normal fashion through the remainder of the colon, "outlet" or defecatory dysfunction should be suspected.

Anorectum

A variety of techniques have been applied specifically to the assessment of anal sphincter and pelvic floor function [49]. These are discussed in more detail in Chapter 9 and include endorectal ultrasound, anorectal manometry, defecography (using either radiographic or scintigraphic technique), balloon expulsion tests, electromyography, and tests of rectal tone, compliance and sensation. Anorectal manometry aims to define resting anal sphincter tone (which primarily reflects the function of the internal anal sphincter and sympathetic innervation), the sphincter pressure during the squeeze maneuver (a reflection of external sphincter contraction and parasympathetic innvervation), the integrity of the rectoanal inhibitory or rectosphincteric reflex, and rectal sensation. However, the methods for evaluation of anorectal function to date have not been standardized.

Defecography provides a dynamic evaluation of the function of the pelvic floor during a variety of maneuvers, including attempted evacuation. It may also help to identify such anatomical features as prolapse and rectoceles, which are relevant if they fill preferentially and fail to empty during attempted defecation. More commonly, defecography and allied techniques, such as balloon expulsion, are used to detect ineffective or obstructed defecation, such as that associated with failure of relaxation of the puborectalis, leading to obstructed defecation. An important objective in the clinical assessment of patients with incontinence is to define localized and potentially surgically correctable defects in the anal sphincter. Focal defects that may have been detected on EMG in the past are most clearly delineated by endorectal ultrasound.

Sensation

Stimulation techniques
The processes of digestion involve numerous stimuli within the gastrointestinal tract. These physiological stimuli induce specific reflexes to accomplish the digestive function, and normally the whole process evolves in an unperceived fashion. Studies on visceral sensitivity in healthy subjects therefore require probing stimuli which induce perception, and this can be achieved using a number of different types of stimulation. A summary of stimulation techniques and the measurement of the responses is shown in Table 3.

Gastrointestinal Distension
Distension of the gut can be performed by means of a distending device—a balloon or similar tool—mounted over a tube. High-compliance latex balloons made with condoms have relatively low intrinsic pressures, and compliance can be calculated with a reasonably small error. Flaccid bags with negligible intrinsic pressure require no corrections and may be preferable. However, the bag has to be oversized, because if the capacity of the bag is attained during a distension, the function of the gut is not reliably recorded.

Table 3 Assessment of Gastrointestinal Sensation

Stimulus	Type	Gastrointestinal distension, transmucosal electrical nerve stimulation, thermal stimulation
	Intensity	Pressure, volume
Responses	Perception	Quality, threshold, intensity (scores & scales), location, duration, affectivity (pleasantness—unpleasantness)
	Objective responses	
	Reflex responses	Gastrointestinal, e.g., gastric accommodation during distension or with intraluminal lipid, e.g., intestino-intestinal reflexes (excitatory and inhibitory reflexes) General—autonomic parameters
	Central responses	Cortical evoked potentials—EEG, MEG Measurement of cerebral blood flow— PET, SPECT, FMRI

Abbreviations: EEG=electroencephalogram; MEG=magneto-encephalography; PET=positron emission tomography; SPECT=single photon emission computerized tomography; FMRI=functional magnetic resonance imaging.

Most studies use air to produce gut distension because its resistance to flow through small tubes is relatively low. Furthermore, air does not pose the problem of hydrostatic pressure differences along the connecting line. However, air is compressible, and hence, the actual distending volume depends on the pressure within the distending device. In a conventional balloon inflated with a syringe this compression is negligible. However, the barostat and other devices have large pumps which may be deformable, and thus air compression requires careful corrections before interpreting distension data. Location of the balloon relative to other viscera should be controlled by changing body position, otherwise viscera lying on top of the distending balloon will artificially increase the intraballoon pressure and confound the responses. It has been reported that perception of gut distension depends on the rate and the pattern of distension. However, the effects of dynamic distension are difficult to interpret, because distension also involves work related to visceral displacements within the abdominal cavity.

Distensions can be simply produced by manual inflation using a syringe, or with more sophisticated methods, for instance, the barostat (see earlier) which applies fixed intraluminal pressures [37] or the tensostat, which applies fixed tension levels to the gut wall [50]. The barostat is an electronic pressure clamp that adapts the volume of air within a distending bag to maintain the desired intrabag pressure. By analogy, the tensostat is a computerized distension system, that, based on intrabag pressure and volume, calculates wall tension and drives an air pump to maintain the desired tension level. Recent studies suggest that perception of gut distension relies on stimulation of tension receptors, while intraluminal volume and wall stretch seem not to be determinants [50–53]. Hence, the tensostat probably allows a better standardization of distending stimuli, regardless of the capacity and compliance of the organ tested. Recently a method for studying intestinal gas dynamics has been described. This method measures both gas tolerance and transit, and hence, provides an integrated evaluation of the sensory and reflex responses to intraluminal gas loads [54].

Other Stimuli

(i) Transmucosal electrical nerve stimulation. Testing somatic sensitivity involves a variety of stimuli, each activating a specific pathway. For instance, "A beta" low threshold mechanoreceptors, which produce a faint tactile sensation at levels near the detection threshold, can be assessed by cotton wisps. At detection, electrical stimulation activates the same pathways, but directly stimulates afferent axons independently of the receptors [55]. By analogy to transcutaneous electrical nerve stimulation, transmucosal electrical nerve stimulation can be used as an alternative test of visceral sensitivity. Electrical stimulation may be produced via intraluminal electrodes mounted over a tube [56].

(ii) Thermal stimulation. Nonpainful thermal stimuli provide important information in somatosensory testing. Thinly myelinated "A delta" fibers mediate sensation of cool, and "C-fibers" mediate warmth sensation. Hence, warmth and cool detection can be used to evaluate these specific pathways [55]. The responses to visceral thermostimulation are not as well characterized, but thermal stimulation may be also applicable in the gut, for instance, using intraluminal water-filled bags [57].

Factors that Modify the Sensory Responses to Gut Stimuli
Many factors, both local and extraintestinal, can modify visceral perception and therefore require attention in testing sensitivity. For instance, perception of gut distension depends on gut compliance [58,59], while a recent study has shown that tone is a factor which influences the perception of rectal balloon distension [60]. Furthermore, perception may be modified by previous or simultaneous stimuli [61], as well as the speed of distension [62] and the length of the gut stimulated [61]. Perception is also influenced by extrinsic mechanisms, including

somato-visceral interactions [63], sympathetic arousal [64] and cognitive-affective phenomena (see below) [65,66].

Measurement of the Responses

Gut stimuli may induce conscious perception, reflex responses, and central responses, and each of these may be evaluated in the laboratory. Distending stimuli in particular may also be applied to measure gut compliance, that is the local response to distension.

Measurement of Conscious Perception

There is no "gold standard" to measure visceral perception. A variety of techniques used to measure somatic pain can be adapted to test visceral sensitivity. The use of rating scales and questionnaires allows evaluation of the intensity of perception and other characteristics, such as the type and location of the sensation. Other methods include paradigms for threshold detection. However, somatic and visceral sensitivity bear significant differences that are still not well defined and may limit interpretation of results when using "borrowed" methodology. For instance, in contrast to somatic sensations, non-painful visceral sensations are abnormal, and interestingly, these are frequently the main complaint in patients with FGIDs. While most techniques used to test somatic sensitivity deal with pain, this may not be the ideal reference point in the assessment of visceral perception. In fact, other authors incorporate rating scales for gas, urgency, distension, satiety, and nausea, apart from pain, when assessing sensation in response to isobaric graded distensions. Further details are contained in a recent publication in which the detailed procedures and protocols for the evaluation of visceral sensitivity, using barostat technology, are discussed [67].

Early studies showed that slow distension of the stomach produces a sensation of fullness; this is replaced by pain when intragastric pressure is increased beyond a given intensity threshold [68], and referral is to the epigastric and periumbilical regions [69]. Mechanical distension of the small bowel is usually perceived as a diffuse pressure sensation or a fullness in the epigastrium [70]; in the jejunum distensions can also be perceived as colicky [71]. The intensity of perception is stimulus related, although the character of the sensations can be similar across a range of distensions between the threshold for perception and the threshold for discomfort. Distension of the descending or sigmoid colon evokes diffuse abdominal distress described variously as cramping, gas-like and/or elevated intra-abdominal pressure [2]. Sensations produced by distension of the sigmoid colon are referred to the lower abdomen, lower back and perineum and are graded with increasing pressure in the balloon or barostat bag [72]. Both sensory and affective components of the sensation in this latter study were found to increase over the course of ten consecutive stimuli, together with an increase in the area of the referred sensation. Some data suggest that it may be important to evaluate the affective component or hedonic dimension of the sensory experience (pleasantness–unpleasantness), but such data on visceral perception are scarce [55].

Measurement of Gut Compliance and Related Phenomena

As defined earlier, compliance is the pressure-volume relationship within the gut. Basically, compliance may be evaluated using any distending system: at different levels of distension both parameters are correlated. The most appropriate way of expressing compliance is the pressure/volume plot, because compliance may vary at different levels of distension. There is no basis to suspect that compliance measurements may be different using distensions at fixed volumes, at fixed pressure by the barostat, or even at fixed tension levels by the tensostat. On the other hand, distension of the gut may elicit reflexes, such as the propulsive peristaltic reflex or an accommodative relaxation. Since compliance depends in part on the muscular activity of the organ under study, these reflexes may modify compliance. However, the precise effects of local reflexes on compliance at different levels of distension and at different sites in the gastrointestinal tract cannot be ascertained, and remain to be characterized.

Recently, probes consisting of a series of ring electrodes have been used to measure the cross-sectional diameter of a tubular hollow viscus such as the esophagus, duodenum, ureter, and rectum [73–77]. Such impedance planimetry measurements can thus monitor the reductions of the luminal cross-sectional diameter as a result of a contraction, as well as detect the increase in diameter during the process of flow over the sensors. These careful measurements may also permit a thorough evaluation of dimensions, which will increase the fidelity of measurements of wall elastic properties and wall tension. More work needs to be completed in this field, and the potential of studying asymmetrical hollow organs such as the stomach requires further validation. Incorporation of a distension balloon in the device also facilitates measurement of the sensory thresholds, while carefully monitoring the physical properties of the wall of the viscus.

Evaluation of Reflex Responses

Gut stimuli which induce perception may also induce reflex responses. These types of reflex responses have been well characterized in experimental animals because they have been used as an indirect index of nociception. However, responses in healthy humans differ from those in acute experiments in anesthetized animals, largely because the magnitude of the stimuli applied in conscious subjects is much smaller. As discussed earlier, manometry and electro-myography are well-established methods to measure phasic motor activity of the gut in humans. However, since phasic activity is intermittent, it may be difficult to assess responses to brief stimuli, especially since most reflexes induced by distension are inhibitory. The barostat is therefore useful in this setting to measure changes in gut tone.

In the small bowel, distension of the distal jejunum triggers retrograde reflexes that induce a small and inconstant relaxation in the proximal jejunum at a short distance (5 cm), but a prominent relaxation at a long distance (40 cm). Further, the distal jejunum does not respond to distension of the proximal jejunum, whereas the proximal jejunum responds to both antegrade and retrograde reflexes, with distending stimuli inducing similar relaxation responses at orad and caudad sites. The reflex responses to gut distension are heterogeneous; indeed, some data indicate that perception and reflex responses are dissociable and probably mediated by different mechanisms [39,78].

In the colon, important reflexes include ascending inhibitory reflexes such as the rectocolonic and colonogastric inhibitory reflexes [79]. Thus, irritation of the rectal mucosa by glycerol results in a left colonic reflex marked by a relaxation with superimposed powerful contractions perceived by the subjects [80], while distension of the rectum may impair gastric motility [81] and small intestinal motility [82]. Also, voluntary suppression of defecation for one week results in delayed gastric emptying [83]. Descending excitatory reflexes include the gastrocolonic and ileocolonic reflexes [84,85]. Such reflexes illustrate the complex relationships existing between the various segments of the digestive tract, and thus the potential for stimuli generating abnormal sensorimotor function in multiple areas of the gut.

The RIII reflex is a polysynaptic reflex that is elicited by electrical stimulation of a sensory nerve, via a cutaneous electrode. This stimulation results in a response that is measured at the level of a flexor muscle in the ipsilateral limb. The threshold and amplitude of the RIII reflex are closely related to those of the concomitant cutaneous sensations evoked by electrical stimulation [86]. This experimental setup allows an evaluation of somatic perception. Recent work [87] has also shown that this RIII reflex can be inhibited by visceral sensations reaching the level of pain. Thus, inhibition of this RIII reflex could be used as a technique to evaluate visceral sensations, and the interaction between somatic and visceral sensitivity.

Measurement of Central Responses: Detection of Afferent Signals within the Brain
In the last five years a number of techniques have been developed which allow the detection and location of signals within the CNS from the gastrointestinal tract

(reviewed in detail in [88]). Nevertheless, it cannot be ascertained whether the signals really derive from peripheral afferents or from central reflex pathways. The use of such techniques is currently largely restricted to research activity; it is possible that simplified versions of these measures may, however, find a role in clinical practice.

(i) Cortical Evoked Potentials (CEP). This technique is a development of the standard techniques used in clinical neurophysiology for the detection of visual and auditory evoked potentials. The technique involves the repeated, high frequency stimulation of an area of the gastrointestinal tract at a precisely defined interval and the coordinated recording of EEG activity from the brain's surface within a time period of interest. Using averaged signals, extraneous brain activity is reduced in amplitude whilst the electrical responses of interest become more prominent. Sophisticated mapping equipment and recording from multiple electrodes attached to the surface of the scalp enables identification of the sites on the somatosensory cortex activated by the upper and lower gut, and the latencies of the pathways can be determined. This provides an estimate of nerve conduction velocities but has little significance in the central processing of visceral signals.

(ii) Magnetoencephalography (MEG). This technique is a sophisticated development of electroencephalography (see above), involving the use of highly sensitive magnetometers placed over the scalp to detect minute changes in magnetic field induced by cortical afferent nerve activity. This technique has a major advantage over EEG in that the magnetic field is not dispersed by overlying tissue (e.g., skull); therefore the source of the magnetic signal can be accurately localized. With this technique it is now possible to identify the locus for specified gut areas on the primary somatosensory cortex within 2 to 3 millimeters resolution. EEG and MEG detect surface projection to the cerebral cortex and cannot be used to assess deeper structures, e.g., thalamus, limbic system.

(iii) Cerebral Blood Flow
   Positron Emission Tomography (PET). This technique, the current "gold standard" for identifying brain activation, involves the use of a sophisticated detecting apparatus capable of recognizing the passage of positrons emitted from the brain. Radio-labeled water produced in a cyclotron is injected intravenously and circulates around the body, its concentration within the brain depending upon blood flow. By comparing the areas of blood flow between stimulated and unstimulated conditions, those areas that are activated by gut stimulation can be identified. The current state of the art equipment is capable

of identifying areas of cerebral activation within 2–3 millimeters resolution. Statistically-based mapping routines permit a "subtraction" assay to demonstrate focal increases in blood flow over baseline (surrounding structures). Unlike electrical and magnetic studies, however, the temporal resolution of the technique is relatively low, so that identification of sequences of activation in response to a specific gut stimulus is not possible. Because FGIDs are frequently associated with depression [89], results of neuroimaging in such patients require controls for the changes observed in depression and other psychiatric disorders [90,91]. The interpretation of the functional significance of differences in CNS blood flow, however, remains difficult.

Single Photon Emission Computerized Tomography (SPECT). SPECT is an adaptation of measured cerebral blood flow using gamma-emitting isotopes. It requires sham and active stimulation studies for comparisons of flow, and since the gamma-emitter (typically ^{99m}TC) has a halflife measured in hours, it needs repeat studies separated by at least one day to resolve focal increases in blood flow over background. It is possible that the availability of a larger number of appropriate radioligands for SPECT will lead to increased application of neuroimaging to investigate aspects of brain function in a variety of disorders, including the FGIDs.

(iv) Functional Magnetic Resonance Imaging (FMRI). This is the newest technique available for studying the processing of gut signals. The technique uses standard magnetic resonance imaging equipment but employs sophisticated data processing to identify areas of regional variation in blood flow induced by gut stimulation. When areas of the brain are activated by neuronal stimulation, the ratio of oxygenated to de-oxygenated hemoglobin flowing through the brain is altered and a change in the magnetic signal emitted from that brain area occurs. This technique has a spatial resolution which approaches that of PET, but greater temporal resolution, and has the major advantage of freedom from radiation exposure so that it can be employed repeatedly both in healthy subjects and in patients. With the further developments of the technique, it should be possible to study whether patients with FGID have an aberrant processing of gut signals by the CNS to explain their apparent "hypersensitivity."

Thus, in summary, different stimulation techniques currently employed in research laboratories can be applied for the assessment of visceral sensation. Conscious perception is modulated by a net of mechanisms at different levels of the afferent pathways. Hence, sensitivity studies require proper control of these factors which may modify perception. By analogy to somatosensory testing, a combination of techniques may in future conceivably allow a precise characterization of sensory dysfunctions in clinical practice.

Alterations in Digestive Tract Sensorimotor Physiology in Selected Functional Gastrointestinal Disorders

Each of the techniques of measurement discussed in the previous section has been applied to patients with FGIDs. The techniques most utilized, however, have been scintigraphy, manometry, electrogastrography, ultrasonography, and increasingly, barostat studies for assessing gut tone and sensitivity. The disorders of functional dyspepsia (FD) and irritable bowel syndrome (IBS) will be used to highlight the use of these techniques; where available, data from the subgroups of functional diarrhea and functional constipation are also presented. It should be noted that many of these studies were performed prior to the current classification of the specific symptom subgroups; this is particularly relevant given the symptom overlap between FD and IBS. The use of the current classification, however, should not restrict further attempts at relating specific symptoms to sensorimotor dysfunction, e.g., stool form, urgency etc. It also should be emphasized that in many studies a "normal range" (e.g., mean ± 2SD, or 95% confidence limits) was not formally established, leading to difficulties in interpreting the significance of the work.

— Functional Dyspepsia

Motility

It is now established that gastrointestinal dysmotility is present in a portion of patients with FD, and may be an important factor in symptom generation. Most studies have evaluated the stomach and small bowel.

Stomach

A wide range of techniques has been used to study gastric motor function in FD. Examples of these are shown in Table 4. The frequently demonstrated postprandial gastric antral hypomotility [108] is consistent with the scintigraphic studies showing delayed gastric emptying. It is possible, however, that excessive postprandial antral distension in FD impedes the lumen-occlusive nature of normal antral contractions producing a false impression of antral hypomotility on manometric recordings. "Pylorospasm," and impaired antroduodenal coordination, are other entities that have been postulated to play a role in FD [109,110], but have received little attention. Myoelectric dysrhythmias may be an electrophysiological marker predictive for gastric stasis [111]—such dysrhythmias may inhibit the development of normal postprandial peristalsis thereby producing gastroparesis; alternatively, normal gastric slow waves may fail to link to, or couple with, abnormal circular muscle activity, resulting in electro-mechanical dissociation and gastroparesis [28,95].

Table 4. Alterations in Gastric Motility in Functional Dyspepsia

Measurement Technique	Reference	Major Findings
Myoelectric activity	You et al. [92] Geldof et al. [93] Koch et al. [94] Chen et al [95]	Alterations in gastric slow waves (tachygastria, bradygastria) in patients with chronic idiopathic nausea and vomiting and FD
Contractile activity	Malagelada [96]	Reduced number and/or amplitude of gastric antral pressure waves in 25–40% of a heterogeneous group of patients, including FD
	Pieramico et al. [97]	No difference in postprandial antral motility index between *H. pylori* positive and negative FD patients
	Testoni et al. [98]	Decreased frequency of gastric phase 3 MMC in *H. pylori* chronic gastritis
	Qvist et al. [99]	No difference between *H. pylori* positive and negative FD patients in phase 3 MMC; alterations in antroduodenal motor activity normalized after *H. pylori* eradication
Gastric emptying	Jian et al. [100] Waldron et al. [101] Stanghellini et al. [102] Caballero-Plasencia et al. [103]	Scintigraphic delay in gastric emptying in 30–75% of patients
Regional gastric motor dysfunction	Scott et al. [104] Troncon et al. [105]	Altered intragastric distribution of food (scintigraphy, ultrasonography) in FD
	Bolondi et al. [27] Hausken et al. [106]	Demonstration of a wide gastric antrum in FD (ultrasonography)
	Ahluwalia et al. [107]	Impaired antral emptying in FD (ultrasonography)
	Gilja et al. [108]	Impaired proximal gastric accommodation in FD (ultrasonography)
	Coffin et al.[63]	Impaired duodenogastric reflex

Abbreviations: FD=functional dyspepsia.

Small Intestine

Small intestinal dysmotility, with or without associated gastric dysmotility, has been described in patients with FD. Both conventional stationary [112,113] and ambulatory antroduodenal and duodenojejunal [114] manometric techniques have been employed. Motor abnormalities have included absence or reduced incidence of MMC cycles [112,113,115], aberrant propagation of phase 3 of the MMC [113,115], longer duration of phase 2 activity [115], a higher prevalence of burst activity [112,115,116], and an abnormal postprandial motor response [116].

Sensation

The symptoms of FD cannot be entirely explained on the basis of disturbed upper gut motility or secretion; in many patients motility [104,117,118], as well as gastric secretion [119], are normal.

Stomach

Studies demonstrating an enhanced perception of gastric distension in FD are summarized in Table 5. This phenomenon has now assumed a central role in the putative mechanisms of symptom generation in FD patients, and appears the area most likely to yield the most definitive information on the pathogenesis of this disorder. Moreover, both the cold pressor test and transcutaneous electrical nerve stimulation have shown these complementary studies of somatic sensitivity to be normal in FD patients [63,126], supporting the concept of selective visceral hypersensitivity. There is conflicting data regarding gastric compliance during fasting in FD. Thus, Bradette et al. [120] and Mearin et al. [122] found no difference in compliance, although in the former study the data are not clearly shown. Lemann et al. [121] demonstrated a small, but not statistically significant, increase in compliance. In the two studies that found reduced compliance, one [124] did not employ state-of-the-art technology, while the difference in compliance was not statistically significant in the other [64].

As is evident from the foregoing, gastric sensitivity has been evaluated most often using distending stimuli [127]. One study, however, has reported increased sensitivity of the gastric mucosa to acid and duodenal contents in patients with FD [128]; other potential types of stimulation outlined earlier (transmucosal electrical nerve stimulation, thermal stimulation) have not been explored.

Small Intestine

Whether sensory dysfunction extends beyond the stomach in patients with FD is controversial. For example, increased gastric but normal duodenal sensitivity was shown in a specific subset of FD patients predominantly com-

Table 5. Alterations in Gastric Sensation to Distension in Functional Dyspepsia

Reference	Major Findings
Bradette et al. [120] Lemann et al. [121] Mearin et al. [122] Coffin et al. [63] Mertz et al. [123] Troncon et al. [124]	Heightened perception of gastric distension; gastric compliance overall normal
Klatt et al. [125]	Pain threshold in normal range in approx. 50% of FD patients

Abbreviations: FD=functional dyspepsia.

plaining of postcibal bloating [62]. However, other studies have reported an increased perception of small intestinal distension in patients with FD [128,129].

— Irritable Bowel Syndrome

Motility

The extensive literature on gastrointestinal motility in IBS patients has accrued over more than three decades. The more sophisticated measurement techniques developed over the last 10 years, however, have enabled better characterization of altered motor patterns in IBS.

Colon and Rectum

Most studies utilizing the more invasive measurement techniques in IBS, particularly the earlier studies, have been undertaken examining the colon (especially the distal colon) and rectum, because of their greater accessibility. Some examples of relevant studies of colorectal dysmotility in IBS and related disorders are summarized in Table 6.

Small Intestine and Other Regions of the Gut

The small intestine in IBS has been explored in relatively few studies. However, a range of subtle alterations in small bowel interdigestive motor activity has been documented, including alterations in the periodicity of interdigestive cycles, small differences in phase 3 duration and propagation velocity, and phase 2 contractile patterns [147–150]. The finding of an increased prevalence of phase 2 clustered contractions in some IBS patients (both predominant consti-

Table 6. Alterations in Colorectal Motility in Irritable Bowel Syndrome, Functional Diarrhea, and Functional Constipation

Measurement Technique	Reference	Major Findings
Myoelectric activity	Chaudhary and Truelove [130]	Increased phasic contractions post-prandially in those with prominent gastrocolonic reflex more common in IBS
	Snape et al. [131]	3 cycles/minute electrical activity
	Bueno et al. [20]	Increased long spike bursts in diarrhea; irregular short spike burst activity in constipation
	Latimer et al. [160]	Myoelectric activity similar in IBS and "psychologic" controls
	Welgan et al. [132]	No increase in 3 cycles/minute activity in IBS
Contractile activity and tone	Connell et al. [133]	Increased colonic contractions in constipation, reduced contractions in diarrhea
	Misiewicz et al. [134]	Lower rectosigmoid motility index in IBS-diarrhea than controls, fasting and postprandially
	Whitehead et al. [135]	Increased rectosigmoid response to distension in IBS-diarrhea > IBS-constipation > controls
	Bazzocchi et al. [136]	Increase in higher amplitude (>35mmHg) contractions in functional diarrhea
	Vassallo et al. [137]	Fasting and postprandial colonic (descending) tone normal
	Bradette et al. [138]	No significant abnormality in colonic tone in IBS
	Crowell & Musial [139]	Impaired adaptive relaxation of the rectum in IBS in response to chronic distension
	Choi et al. [140]	Increased HAPC's in functional diarrhea
Compliance	Whitehead et al. [135]	Rectal compliance normal
	Bradette et al. [138]	Colonic compliance normal
Transit	Cann et al. [141]	Accelerated and delayed whole gut transit in IBS-diarrhea and IBS-constipation respectively
	Vassallo et al. [142]	More rapid emptying of right hemi colon in IBS-diarrhea than controls, related to stool weight

Table 6. *(cont'd)*

Measurement Technique	Reference	Major Findings
	Bazzochi et al. [143] Stivland et al. [144] van der Sijp et al. [145]	Delayed colonic transit in severe idiopathic constipation

Abbreviations: HAPC=high amplitude propagating contraction.
Modified from Drossman et al. [146], with permission.

pation and predominant diarrhea)—most prominent when patients were studied using ambulant technology in their home and/or work environment, with a relatively unstructured experimental protocol—[149,151] has not been confirmed in some other studies of small bowel manometry in IBS that have used different protocols [152–54]. Schmidt et al. [150], however, documented longer periods of clustered contractions in IBS than in controls, and the same authors have recently shown, by applying sophisticated analysis techniques from nonlinear dynamics, that phase 2 motor activity of the small intestine is more random in IBS than in health [154]. In postprandial jejunal motor recordings in IBS patients, no major alterations have been observed; some patients have a shorter duration of the fed pattern and a higher amplitude and frequency of contractions than healthy subjects, but the initial response of the small intestine to food appears intact [149,155,156]. Small bowel transit time has been variably reported as rapid [141] or normal [157] in IBS patients with predominant diarrhea. Gastric emptying may be delayed in some IBS patients [157], and small bowel dysmotility appears to be more prevalent in such patients [158]. In contrast, gastric emptying may be more rapid than usual in patients with functional diarrhea [159], and antral hypomotility may be present in patients with slow-transit constipation [46].

In summary, the following general conclusions can be reached regarding gastrointestinal motility in IBS [146]: (1) the motor patterns recorded from the colon and small intestine in patients with IBS are quantitatively similar to those seen in healthy controls; (2) there is no consensus on the patterns of motility associated with the symptoms of diarrhea and constipation; (3) some patients with diarrhea-predominant IBS have accelerated transit in the small bowel and/or colon [141,142]; (4) some patients with constipation-predominant IBS have slowed or delayed transit [141,143]; (5) the more recent studies [132,160] do not support the earlier claims [131,161] that IBS is characterized by three cycles per minute colonic myoelectric activity; and (6) IBS patients display increased motor activity in response to environmental or enteric stimuli, such as psychological stress [151,162,163], meals [155,164,165], balloon inflation [135,166] and cholecystokinin [67,155,167].

Sensation

It has been shown repeatedly that a proportion of patients with IBS display an increased conscious perception to painful distensions in the small bowel and colon, and in some studies, an increased perception of apparently normal motor events in the gut. An increased or unusual area of somatic referral of visceral pain may also be present [4].

Colon and Rectum

Patients with IBS perceive colonic distension at lower volumes than healthy subjects [168,169]. Such hypersensitivity to distension has been well documented in both the distal colon and more proximal colonic segments in IBS patients [138,166,170]. Table 7 summarizes a selection of studies investigating colorectal sensation in IBS. Although reports of pain from balloon distension studies can be influenced by response bias [179,181], the low thresholds for balloon distension occur even when controlling for neuroticism [166]. Furthermore, patients with IBS have normal [166] or even increased, thresholds [180] for painful stimulation of somatic neuroreceptors. It is unclear whether the novel reports of alterations in cerebral blood flow in IBS patients [178,181] provide mechanistically important insights; such descriptive observations require validation in large patient groups. Reflex responses in the colon and rectum to gut stimulation have received little attention to date in IBS.

Small Intestine and Other Regions of the Gut

Visceral hypersensitivity in patients with IBS may also affect different levels of the small bowel [56,173,183–85]. Using TENS applied via intraluminal electrodes. researchers showed that the small bowel in patients with IBS exhibits a selective hypersensitivity to mechanical, but not to electrical, stimuli. Such increased sensitivity to mechanical stimuli was not due to a reduced compliance of the gut wall [56], and response bias could be reasonably excluded because TENS in these patients induced normal perception, even though both electrical and mechanical stimuli produced a similar character of sensation. It is not merely experimental distension of the small bowel that reveals an enhanced visceral sensitivity, as some IBS patients display an increased awareness of the passage of the phase 3 MMC [182]. Other physiological stimuli such as feeding and nonperceived rectal distension also appear to modulate jejunal perception to distension to a different extent in IBS patients when compared to healthy subjects [184].

Whether the ileum [155,171] exhibits greater or lesser hypersensitivity than the jejunum in IBS is not established. Patients with IBS display a distorted referral pattern of gut sensations, and perceive intestinal distensions more diffusely over the abdomen than healthy controls [168,169,171,185]. Interestingly, it has been shown that normally perceived electrical stimuli also have an expanded referral area [56]. Visceral and somatic afferents converge onto the same sensory neurons in the spinal cord, and sensitization of these neurons by noxious visceral input produces an expansion of their somatic receptive fields [4,186]. Perhaps not surprisingly, the sensory dysfunction in IBS seems to affect the entire gut, including the stomach and the esophagus [177,187–89].

Table 7. Alterations in Colorectal Sensation to Distension in Irritable Bowel Syndrome

Reference	Major Findings
Conscious perception	
Ritchie [170]	↓sigmoid threshold for pain
Whitehead [135]	↓threshold for pain in rectum
Moriatry and Dawson [171]	unusual somatic referral pattern
Whitehead [166]	↓threshold for pain in colon
Prior et al. [172], Sun et al. [62]	↓threshold for gas, urgency, and pain in IBS diarrhea
Hammer et al. [175]	↓rectal sensory threshold
Bradette et al. [138]	↓threshold for discomfort in left colon
Hasler et al. [174]	↓threshold for rectal sensation, modified with somatostatin analog
Lembo et al. [175]	↓threshold for discomfort, unusual somatic referral patterns, threshold modified with topical lidocaine
Mertz et al. [176]	↓threshold for perception (hyperalgesia) with normal threshold in rectum; unusual somatic referral pattern
Zighelboim et al.[177]	thresholds in rectum not different in IBS patients and controls
Cerebral blood flow	
Silverman et al. [178]	Increased dorsolateral prefrontal cortex blood flow anticipation of rectal pain

Modified from Drosman et al. [146], with permission.

Clinical Implications of Sensorimotor Dysfunction in the Functional Gastrointestinal Disorders

Documentation of sensorimotor dysfunction in at least some patients with FGID gives rise to four main questions relevant to clinical practice. These are (i) what are the possible mechanisms of such dysfunction?; (ii) what are the relationships between sensorimotor dysfunction and symptoms?; (iii) what is the role of current tests of sensorimotor function in helping to establish a diagnosis of FGID?; and (iv) can treatment of specific types of sensorimotor dysfunction lead to clinical improvement? Only limited data are currently available in each of these areas.

— Putative Origins of Sensorimotor Dysfunction in the FGID

Alterations in gut motor activity in the FGIDs may arise from a number of putative mechanisms. These include: (i) enteric mechanisms such as motor dysfunction associated with minor degrees of inflammation and consequent changes in neurotransmitter release [190–92]; (ii) local reflex mechanisms, occurring in response to specific nutrients such as lipid [193] or to mechanical distension [63]; (iii) extrinsic neural mechanisms such as abnormalities in extrinsic autonomic innervation [194]; and (iv) central mechanisms, whereby higher neural centers (e.g., in response to psychosocial stimuli) modulate peripheral intestinal motor activity [195]. Similar mechanisms have been advanced to account for the enhancement of visceral sensation in the FGID [4,196]. These include: (i) altered receptor sensitivity at the viscus itself, occurring through recruitment of silent nociceptors or peripheral sensitization in response to ischemia or inflammation; (ii) increased excitability of the spinal cord dorsal horn neurons, where repeated distension of the intestine produces central (spinal) hyperalgesia with enhanced intensity and expanded somatic referral of the visceral stimulus; and (iii) altered central modulation of sensation involving psychological influences on the interpretation of these sensations, or altered central regulation of ascending signals from the dorsal horn neurons in the spinal cord. Because the mechanisms of central interpretation of afferent signals are not known, it is not clear whether psychological or neurophysiological mechanisms work singly or in concert in the conscious perception of incoming signals.

— Enteric Triggers of Sensorimotor Dysfunction

In IBS, the fact that patients are hypersensitive to mechanical, but not electrical, stimuli implies that the structure primarily responsible for the hypersensitivity may be the mechanical receptor in the gut wall. Further recent studies indicate that tension applied to the gut wall may be the trigger for sensations resulting in hypersensitivity in IBS patients [197,198]; tension may stimulate specific "in series" mechanoreceptors in the gut wall. Lembo et al. [175], however, by comparing the sensations triggered with different distending protocols in IBS patients, spinal cord patients, and controls, have concluded that the primary abnormality may be at the level of the spinal afferents.

In recent years, considerable interest has been generated regarding the relationship between the enteric nervous system and the immune system, especially in relation to the FGIDs [191,192]. In IBS, a further stimulus has been recent epidemiologic evidence [199,200] confirming earlier work [130] that symptoms may commence and persist after an episode of acute infective diarrhea (although life event stress also appears to be implicated). Studies in animals and in man have suggested that a minimal inflammatory process may be able to induce hypersensitivity of afferent nerve pathways, e.g., an increase in rectal sensitivity has been reported in patients following salmonella gastroenteritis [201]. In rodents, findings of potential relevance are that intestinal inflammation provoked by instillation of chemical irritants can induce hypersensitivity to distension [202], and that transient mucosal inflammation alters enteric neuromuscular function which persists after recovery from the infection and mucosal restitution [203]. A special role has been recognized for mast cells in the interconnection of neurological and immunological processes [204,205]. In particular, Khan and Collins [206] have shown that IL1 mRNA was expressed more in IBS patients mast cells than in controls. It remains unclear, however, whether there is a distinct and more prolonged physiological motor response to an initial inflammatory state in the human colon. In FD, it is logical to suggest that mucosal inflammation may also play a role in some patients [207], particularly given the high prevalence of *Helicobacter pylori*. Studies of the role of *Helicobacter pylori* in FD have, however, to date not supported this hypothesis [125,208,209], although recent preliminary data [210] suggest that *Helicobacter*-positive FD may be associated with postprandial hypersensitivity.

Although there is some clinical evidence to incriminate "food intolerance" in the pathogenesis of IBS [211,212], little substantive evidence exists to link the phenomenon to dysmotility or visceral hypersensitivity. In animal studies, however, it has been demonstrated that intestinal anaphylaxis can result in motility changes mediated via visceral afferents [213]. In these experiments, changes in c-fos expression in some nuclei of the thalamus suggested that motility abnormalities were triggered by long reflexes arising from the damaged gut and reaching the central nervous system. Also, recent studies have shown that colonic antigen challenge of sensitized rats results in local mast cell activation and modulation of both local colonic and remote jejunal myoelectrical activity [214]. In man, it appears that, using experiments with cold pain stress, the central nervous system is also capable of modulating intestinal mast cell activity; interestingly, there was a greater release of mast cell mediators in food-allergic patients than in healthy subjects [215]. In FD, attention is now also being paid to particular meal components, e.g., higher fat meals appear to provoke more symptoms [216], and duodenal lipid infusion specifically enhances gastric hypersensitivity to distension [217].

— Central Triggers of Sensorimotor Dysfunction

In FD, it has been proposed that abnormal proximal gastric accommodation may be due to an underlying vagal defect [124]; both FD and postvagotomy patients have a similar impairment of gastric accommodation. Other studies have supported such a concept [128,218,219]. Moreover, barostat studies in diabetic patients emphasize the importance of vagal control in normal adaptive relaxation of the stomach [220,221]. On the other hand, studies of vection-induced nausea and gastric dysrhythmias [222,223] raise the possibility of central neurohumoral dysfunction in the pathogenesis of FD. Thus, motion sickness-susceptible and resistant individuals differed in their central release of vasopressin, rather than displaying a peripheral resistance to its effects. In IBS, Smart et al. [224] documented abnormal vagal function, while Aggerwal et al. [194] demonstrated vagal dysfunction to be specifically associated with a constipation-predominant subgroup of patients, whereas patients with diarrhea-predominant symptoms had evidence of sympathetic adrenergic dysfunction.

Important factors also influencing sensorimotor dysfunction include psychological stress and other cognitive aspects (see Chapter 4, and review article by Whitehead and Palsson [225]). In FD, Haug et al. [219] have suggested that reduced vagal activity could be a mediating mechanism by which psychologic factors influence gastrointestinal sensorimotor physiology and evoke dyspepsia. Indeed, Bennett et al. [226] have documented a correlation in FD between delayed gastric emptying and psychological factors, especially suppression of anger. In IBS the effects on small bowel motility of acute psychological stress—produced in a laboratory situation—were shown to be, in most cases, not significantly different from controls; these findings contrast with those produced by mental stressors of longer duration, where a pattern similar to clustered contractions was provoked, suggesting that stress of a more chronic nature evokes a different type of response from that of acute stress [151]. Psychological stress may hasten mouth-to-cecum transit in diarrhea-predominant IBS, but slow transit time in constipation-dependent IBS [141]. In a recent study in IBS [183], the psychosocial profiles associated with three different and increasing levels of sensory and/or motor dysfunction displayed a similar pattern of increasing severity and intensity of psychosocial disturbance. Relevant to this area is the finding that perception of small intestinal distensions was higher during attention than during distraction, and the area of somatic projection was greater during attention [65].

In the colon, the motor response to psychologic stress in IBS has been reported as either similar to [160] or higher than [132] in control subjects. Erckenbrecht et al. [227] demonstrated that a psychological stress (dichotomous listening) applied during or before rectal distension induced hypersensitivity to the distension; this effect was maintained for at least one hour after the end of the stressful period. More recent preliminary studies, however, have shown contradictory results; a short psychological stress (5 minutes) had virtually no measurable effect on pressures triggering rectal sensations in IBS patients with rectal hypersensitivity or in healthy volunteers [228]. However, in this study, the "distraction" effect was much more marked in healthy controls than in patients—in the latter group, the pressure that triggered rectal discomfort increased by only 15% compared to baseline, while it increased by 60% in controls. Ford et al. [67] have observed that stress (dichotomous listening) provokes a moderate increase in the intensity of sensations recorded by healthy subjects for a given painful stimulus, at the level of the sigmoid, but not the transverse, colon. The sensation of gas (bloating) was also increased during the period over which the psychological stress was applied. Active relaxation had no effect on the intensity of pain and had little effect on gas sensation, which was less intense at the highest distension step, both in the transverse and sigmoid colons. There was no effect of stress or relaxation on the compliance of the colon. In a recent study in healthy subjects [229], mental stress induced a clear distracting effect during the time it was applied, while the intensity of reported symptoms, at least for the painful sensations, was increased. In addition, stress induced significant changes in compliance of the rectum. Hypervigilance is also a factor that influences symptom reporting by IBS patients during rectal distension testing [230]. There were differences between IBS patients and controls when one technique of testing (ascending method of limits) was used, but not when another (tracking) was used in the same subjects. In studies of altered cerebral perfusion (thalamic and cortical areas) induced by rectal distension in IBS patients, differences between patients and controls appear due to an anticipation phenomenon observed in the patients [178]. Further studies in IBS [181], however, suggest that rectal hypersensitivity induced by repetitive distension of the sigmoid colon may be due to an aberrant thalamic response to pain.

— Relationships between Sensorimotor Dysfunction and Symptoms

Studies have generally shown a disappointing lack of correlation between sensorimotor dysfunction and symptoms in the FGIDs. Ideally, a number of criteria should be satisfied to define a causal relationship between the two, namely,

   (i)   a consistent association between symptoms and the sensorimotor disorder;
   (ii) a correlation in time and severity between symptoms and the sensorimotor disorder;
   (iii) an improvement in the sensorimotor disorder associated with clinical improvement; and
   (iv) the production of symptoms by experimental induction of the sensorimotor disorder.

None of these criteria have been shown to date to be fulfilled reliably in the FGIDs, and so the clinical relevance of sensorimotor dysfunction in such patients remains unclear. Moreover, it needs to be borne in mind that dysmotility per se could lead to distension of an organ and symptoms usually considered as related to visceral hypersensitivity.

Recent studies have addressed the issue of symptoms and sensorimotor dysfunction in more detail, and when more sophisticated techniques are used, some potentially important correlations have emerged. In FD, in the largest and most comprehensive study to date, Stanghellini et al. [102] evaluated 343 patients, of whom one third had delayed gastric emptying. Factors that predicted gastric stasis included female gender and low body weight; symptoms were generally unhelpful, although severe postprandial fullness and vomiting were consistently predictive of gastroparesis. Preliminary results of studies in another large group of FD patients have confirmed that those with delayed gastric emptying, as determined by the octanoic acid breath test, are more likely to suffer from postprandial fullness, and also nausea and vomiting. Also, Fock et al. [231], measuring gastric emptying of indigestible solids, have shown that gastroparesis is associated with the subgroup of dysmotility-like FD, while Hausken et al. [106], and subsequently Hveem et al. [232], have shown a relationship between antral widening and the degree of abdominal discomfort occurring soon after eating. The relationship between symptoms and ultrasonographic assessments of gastric motor function in FD was also examined using glyceryl trinitrate (GTN), an exogenous donor of NO [233]. In a double-blind, placebo-controlled, cross-over design, concomitant improvement of postprandial proximal gastric accommodation, and of epigastric pain, nausea, and total symptom scores, was demonstrated in response to GTN. Distal antrum measures, however, were not significantly altered by GTN, suggesting that in FD, defective accommodation of the proximal stomach may be more directly related to symptom generation than dysmotility of the antrum. Recent preliminary studies also support this concept. Thus, in patients with FD, the stomach accommodated less in the postprandial period than in healthy controls, and this was not related to vagal efferent dysfunction [210]. Moreover, Tack et al. [209] have shown that impaired accommodation to a meal is present in 40% of patients with FD. Impaired gastric accommodation was not associated with hypersensitivity to distension, presence of *H. pylori*, or delayed gastric emptying. The symptom of early satiety was independently associated with impaired gastric accommodation, and weight loss, occurring secondarily to early satiety, was more prevalent in patients with impaired accommodation. Administration of the 5-HTIP receptor agonist sumatriptan was able to restore gastric accommodation in patients with impaired postprandial gastric relaxation, and improve early satiety in a double-blind, placebo-controlled, cross-over design [209]. In another study, with a larger number of FD patients, those patients with hypersensitivity to gastric distension were more likely to suffer from epigastric pain, belching, and weight loss, but such visceral hypersensitivity was not associated with gastric motor abnormalities or with *H. pylori* infection [234]. It is plausible that gastric hyporeflexia is an important factor in the reduced tolerance of FD patients to intragastric volume increase, thereby contributing to the generation of clinical symptoms in the absence of major motor dysfunction. The magnitude of the normal proximal gastric relaxation is regulated by nutrient-dependent enterogastric reflexes, and as the relaxatory input decreases, the proximal stomach gradually transfers intragastric content into the antrum [235]. A gastric hyporeactivity to enterogastric reflexes would predictably result in defective accommodation of the proximal stomach and antral "overload." In turn, impaired meal accommodation would potentiate the hypersensitivity to distension, because the stomach tolerates smaller volumes when not properly relaxed [58].

In IBS, studies examining the inter-relationships between motility and sensation have enabled some correlation with symptoms. Whitehead et al. [166]

demonstrated that rectal hypersensitivity is associated with motor hyperactivity in response to gut stimuli; both hypersensitivity and hyperreactivity could contribute to the perception of rectal tenesmus and fecal urgency in IBS. There is some evidence that postprandial symptoms in IBS may be associated with alterations in the colonic response to feeding [132,137]. In the small bowel, the most striking finding in IBS patients has been that of episodes of cramping abdominal pain directly related to the usually nonperceived, intermittent, large amplitude peristaltic waves in the terminal ileum [155], supporting the concept of visceral hypersensitivity. These peristaltic waves are more frequent in the postprandial period. Also, IBS patients with jejunal hypersensitivity displayed a higher prevalence of postprandial dysmotility than those without jejunal hypersensitivity [183]; this finding may be relevant to the prominent postprandial symptoms experienced by some IBS patients. In contrast, in the group with normal jejunal sensitivity, there was a higher prevalence of fasting dysmotility. Recent studies using a new methodology to evaluate intestinal gas dynamics further substantiate the role of combined sensory and motor disturbances in symptom production. These studies have shown that "gas" symptoms in IBS patients may be related either to impaired intestinal handling of gas leading to retention and gut distension, to gut hypersensitivity with poor gas tolerance, or to both [54].

— Tests of Sensorimotor Function in the Diagnosis of the FGIDs

Although each of the techniques to assess motility can provide important information regarding one or more motor functions of the digestive tract, none has enabled characterization of definitively "abnormal" motor patterns in FGID patients. In patients with severe motility-like FD, for example, despite the use of prolonged recordings and advanced computer-aided analysis, and the demonstration of motor alterations, it was not possible to identify a *specific* small intestinal motor pattern which enabled discrimination between patients and those with other disorders, or even with healthy individuals [114]. Thus, although several different types of motor dysfunction have been more frequently observed in various patient groups, such alterations may be encountered in healthy subjects, or else they are not demonstrable in a significant number of patients. Moreover, the possibility that physiological disturbance may be transient is an important confounding factor. The specificity and the sensitivity of the tests is therefore low, and consequently the clinical utility of the "investigation" is limited. Also, more widespread use of many of these procedures in clinical practice is limited because they are often either time consuming and relatively expensive (e.g., gastric emptying and colonic transit measurements by isotopic methods), or invasive (e.g., intestinal manometry, colonic recordings by endoluminal probes, barostat recordings). Notwithstanding these considerations, and the inherent variability in motor parameters due to factors such as posture, determination of intra-abdominal pressure, etc., a recent study has established, in 35 healthy subjects, the lower range of normal (mean minus 2 SD) for gastric accommodation. This, calculated as the mean increase in intraballoon volume during 60 minutes after the meal compared to 30 minutes before the meal at minimal distending pressure + 2, was 64 ml [209].

As with motility, based on the data outlined earlier, it is clear that the currently available tests to assess gut sensation do not enable a positive diagnosis of these syndromes. In FD, although patients with significant symptoms after meals exhibit discomfort at lower levels of gastric distension than healthy controls, the differences are relatively small. Similarly, in IBS, although it has been reported that patients may have significant discomfort during sigmoidoscopy, when specifically tested these patients may exhibit normal thresholds to rectal balloon distension [4]. Also, there appears to be little specificity of the responses to distension tests for the FGID subgroups, or to the organ considered most relevant in the pathophysiology of the syndrome, i.e., the stomach for FD, or the colon and rectum for IBS. In IBS, it is not yet possible to define abnormal values, e.g., the rectal pressure which can characterize "hypersensitive" patients, due to the lack of large studies in healthy subjects. Based on those studies which have included control subjects, a limit of approximately 28 mmHg for the pain threshold discriminating between IBS patients (who display a threshold lower or equal to 28 mmHg) and controls (usually approximately 32 mmHg or above) during rectal distension, could be proposed [138,177,178,236–38], but these distinctions may not be reliable as sensory thresholds are clearly influenced by a number of factors discussed earlier, including the intensity of symptoms at the time of study [176]. In the case of gastric distension in FD, data from large numbers of patients and controls are currently not available, although Tack et al. [240] in 35 healthy subjects, has reported that the lower range of normal (mean minus 2 SD) for the distending pressure inducing discomfort is 7.1 mmHg above minimal distending pressure. It should be emphasized that these results from one study require confirmation in other laboratories.

Despite the foregoing, several of the techniques are well standardized and interpretable in the clinical context; these include radio-opaque marker transit, anorectal manometry, scintigraphic gastric emptying assessment, and antroduodenal manometry. An important role for such tests in clinical practice is to enable identification of disturbances that clearly indicate the likely presence of another specific disorder, such as the low amplitude contractions (postprandial intestinal contractions < 10 mmHg at manometry) suggestive of an infiltrative disorder of gastrointestinal smooth muscle, or other severe enteric myopathic disorder which would exclude the diagnosis of FGID [24]. On the other hand, normal fasting and postprandial small bowel motor patterns are a strong indication of normal enteric neurotransmitter function.

If such clearly abnormal findings are not identified, what then is the clinical relevance of other alterations in sensorimotor function in a patient with FGID? Currently, alterations in transit, and to a lesser extent manometric alterations, provide objective demonstration of dysfunction and invite trials of specific drug therapies to attempt to correct the dysfunction. In the case of other tests, particularly those that assess perception, or reflex responses such as gastric accommodation or the colonic response to feeding, further research to evaluate their specificity and predictive value is required. The expectation is that more precise identification of such physiological alterations will facilitate the recognition of further patient subgroups deserving a directed therapeutic approach.

— Pharmacotherapy of the Sensorimotor Dysfunction in the FGIDs

Modulation of sensorimotor function can be accomplished by different types of interventions aimed at different levels of the brain-gut axis. For the purposes of this review, only pharmacotherapy will be discussed; the use of interventions such as biofeedback therapy for fecal incontinence and pelvic floor dyssynergia [237,238], and hypnosis to reduce hypersensitivity to rectal distension and to decrease contractile activity, especially in IBS [172,239], are considered in other chapters.

Motility

A range of medications is available to potentially restore some of the alterations in motor function identified in the FGIDs. Most evidence for the efficacy of such medications is available for those which improve disordered gut transit, such as delayed gastric emptying, and delayed or accelerated colonic and/or small bowel transit, and to a lesser extent altered contractile activity such as antral hypomotility or an exaggerated colonic motor response to feeding. Little evidence is available for modulation of other components of dysmotility such as alterations in tone or compliance, although a recent study has demonstrated that cisapride is able to enhance gastric accommodation to a meal in

Table 8 Examples of Pharmacological Modulation of Motor Dysfunction in FD and IBS

Agent	Mechanisms of action	Effects on sensorimotor function	Efficacy in FGIDs
Cisapride	$5HT_4$ agonism enhances acetylcholine release; in addition $5HT_3$ antagonism	Accelerates gastric emptying, small and large bowel transit; enhances gastric accommodation in health; lowered threshold to gastric distension	May improve symptoms in FD, especially in patients with gastroparesis; may improve symptoms in IBS-constipation
Domperidone	Dopamine antagonist	Accelerates gastric emptying	May improve symptoms in FD
Erythromycin	Motilin agonist	Accelerates gastric emptying; induces gastric phase 3 activity; causes contraction of the gastric fundus.	Not known
Loperamide	Binds to mu and delta opioid receptors in gastrointestinal tract	Retards small and large bowel transit; enhances intestinal water & ion absorption; increases rectal sphincter tone	Improves stool frequency/consistency in IBS-diarrhea
Ondansetron	$5HT_3$ receptor antagonist	May accelerate gastric emptying; prolongs colonic transit	May improve stool consistency in IBS-diarrhea
Mebeverine	Smooth muscle relaxant	Reduces postprandial sigmoid motility; alters small bowel motility	May improve abdominal pain in IBS
Dicyclomine	Anticholinergic	Reduces postprandial sigmoid motility	May improve abdominal pain in IBS
Octreotide	Somatostatin analog	Induces phase 3 MMC-like activity in small bowel; retards small bowel transit; decreases visceral perception in colon.	May increase rectal threshold in IBS

healthy subjects [240]. Some examples of agents which can modify motor function of the gut and which have been studied in the FGIDs, are shown in Table 8. Further details are available in a number of recent general reviews [1,241,242] and summaries of the effects of individual agents or classes of agent 243–248].

Several other classes of drugs are currently under evaluation; these include drugs inhibiting contractile activity in the gut such as the selective muscarinic antagonists (for example, darifenacin), MK2-antagonists, beta 3-adrenoreceptor agonists, and gut selective calcium channel blockers (for example, pinaverium bromide). Medications such as these may theoretically enable a reduction of contractile activity in the gut without significant effects on other systems. Other agents with potential for stimulation of motor activity and transit include loxiglumide, acting via blockade of CCKA-receptors, and 5-HT$_4$ agonists; these latter agents display prokinetic effects in the mid and distal gut, and may prove useful for disorders such as IBS and functional constipation. Drugs under evaluation to induce a relaxation of the proximal stomach include sumatriptan [209], clonidine [52] and buspirone [249].

Sensation

The demonstration of altered visceral perception in patients with FGIDs has led to a focus of attention on substances that may influence sensation by acting at peripheral, spinal, supraspinal, or even several levels of brain-gut interaction. These substances have been considered in detail by Bueno et al. [250]. Most of these compounds have undergone only limited, if any, testing in humans and in the FGIDs.

The specific 5-HT$_3$ receptor antagonists such as ondansetron and granisetron, and the somatostatin analog octreotide, referred to earlier, may have some peripheral visceral antinociceptive actions, and they represent promising classes of agents acting in peripheral sites [251]. The kappa-opioid receptor angonist fedotozine is another drug which can affect sensory thresholds to gastric and colonic distension in man, and which has been shown to improve symptoms in FD [252] and IBS [253].

Compounds modulating visceral sensitivity by acting centrally (as well as peripherally) include the tricyclic antidepressants in low dose, and adrenoreceptor agonists such as clonidine. The serotonin reuptake inhibitors have not been the subject of a systematic study in FD or IBS. Tricyclic antidepressants have been shown to be superior to placebo for improving the symptoms of abdominal pain, nausea and diarrhea in IBS [254,255] and in FD [256], but their precise site or sites of action remain unclear.

Further work is needed in many areas to address the clinical relevance of sensorimotor dysfunction in the FGID: in particular, advances in the four main areas discussed earlier are of crucial importance. *First*, a greater understanding of enteric neural control and modulation, and of the mechanisms for dysfunction, will depend, to a large extent, on continuing advances in the basic science arena, e.g., the electrophysiology of individual enteric neurons, identification of neurotransmitters, receptor subtypes and their interrelationships, the integration of specific neurons into the programs of motor and secretory activity, and the interactions between the enteric immune system and nervous system. Human physiological studies addressing more specific hypotheses can then be undertaken. Relevant to the latter is further characterization of the interactions between the enteric nervous system and its local environment, such as the luminal content, hormonal fluctuations, presence of inflammation, etc. For example, the effects of *Helicobacter pylori* eradication on sensorimotor function of the gastroduodenum in FD, and the effects on neuronal plasticity remain to be established. Also, more reliable identification of postinfective IBS patients will lead to exploration of potentially important alterations in local reflex activity and neuroimmune interactions in the small and large bowel. Alterations of CNS control are clearly of major importance, given the evidence to date, and the role of autonomic dysfunction in the FGID warrants further attention, especially evaluation of abdominal autonomic function using more specific tests. The *interaction* between central trigger factors, including psychological factors, and peripheral trigger factors needs greater exploration, at both the basic and whole organ level. More precise characterization of these interactions may enable better definition of the proportions of patients with dysmotility, hypersensitivity, combined dysfunction, or no demonstrable physiological alterations. This is important as the efficacy and approach to therapy is likely to be different in these various subgroups. It should be stated that, despite the accumulating evidence discussed earlier in support of visceral hypersensitivity, further definitive studies are required to confirm this phenomenon as a major pathogenic factor in the genesis of symptoms in the functional gastrointestinal disorders.

Second, to determine relationships between symptom subgroups, individual symptoms and sensorimotor dysfunction, the patient populations under study require strict definition. Even minor variations in inclusion/exclusion criteria between studies of pathophysiological mechanisms, may of themselves, lead to major discrepancies in findings. For example, the relevance of the predominant alteration of bowel habit in IBS, such as diarrhea, constipation, and associated changes in stool form and consistency, and also the presence or absence of concomitant dyspeptic symptoms in the context of sensorimotor dysfunction, remain to be established. Cross-correlation of physiological dysfunction with symptoms may only be possible if the particular symptoms experienced by the patient at the time of investigation are evaluated. The severity and extent of such symptoms may then facilitate further studies assessing the natural history of sensorimotor dysfunction and its relationship to the natural history of symptoms, i.e., why patients display a range from individual syndromes with minor intermittent and transient symptoms originating in a single gut region, to more extensive and constant symptomatology involving multiple overlapping syndromes with symptoms referred from multiple (more generalized) gut foci.

Third, it is clear that new approaches and methods are required to study sensorimotor dysfunction in man, in order to overcome the considerable limitations of the current techniques. The specificity and predictive value of testing can only be improved with the development of novel, validated, technologies. Thus, more sophisticated techniques to assess compliance, wall tension, and accommodation, and to assess more precisely the flow of luminal content and gas, are required. New techniques for brain imaging and spinal monitoring are required to attempt to discriminate between patients with FGID who display gut hypersensitivity due to sensitization of primary visceral afferents and/or the spinal cord, from patients who have aberrant brain processing of sensations. At the same time as the development of more sophisticated technology, such tests, together with existing techniques, need standardization to enable the completion of multicenter studies and facilitate comparability of data between centers. In this regard also, the development of minimally or noninvasive techniques of investigation, which can function as true surrogate markers of sensorimotor dysfunction, and which can be repeated in patients after various therapeutic maneuvers, is important.

Fourth, the main challenge for pharmacological research on FGID over the next decade will be the development of new drugs to relieve specific sensorimotor dysfunctions and hopefully, to thus relieve specific symptoms. As discussed earlier, much effort to date has been applied largely to developing drugs with either an inhibitory or excitatory effect on digestive tract motor function. On the other hand, the increasing interest in visceral afferent pathways has resulted in the identification of a number of neurotransmitters involved in the processing of information from the gut to the brain (acting either centrally, peripherally or both) and which may affect sensitivity [250]. It is important to note, however, that almost all of these neurotransmitters act on both the afferent and the efferent pathways, so caution is necessary in defining the mechanisms of drug action. In FD, the targets for restoring normal sensitivity and improving postprandial symptoms are most likely to be facilitation of accommodation and reduction of afferent hypersensitivity; the latter is clearly a more difficult task than the former.

In the investigation of new drugs to modulate visceral sensitivity, assessment of compliance, tone and wall tension are important areas. For example, somato-statin has been shown on several occasions to significantly increase sensory thresholds in IBS patients, with values returning to those observed in control subjects. The action of such drugs, however, could also be an indirect one to an effect on gut motor activity, either by stimulation or most likely by inhibition. For example, after the first report by Prior and Read [257] that granisetron, a selective 5-HT$_3$ antagonist, markedly increased sensory thresholds to rectal distension, other studies failed to observe such an effect with other similar compounds [173]. It was subsequently shown that 5-HT$_3$ antagonists may act on visceral sensitivity by modifying compliance or tone rather by an action on sensory afferents. Thus, another 5-HT$_3$ antagonist, ondansetron, reduces postprandial colonic tone in humans, and the novel agent, alosetron, increases compliance of the human colon and increases significantly the volumes measured at sensory thresholds during colonic distension, while not affecting pressure thresholds [258]. Sensory testing may need to correct for changes in wall tension to more thoroughly appraise the effects of pharmacological agents on afferent function. Of course, only when documentation of correction of abnormal, or restoration of normal, sensorimotor function can be reliably achieved, will it be possible to determine whether such correction is related to improved clinical outcomes in the FGIDs. Moreover, whether such correction can be achieved wholly via pharmacologic approaches, or whether additional or separate cognitive or similar strategies are required, remains to be established. Assuming progress can be made in each of the above areas, and against the backdrop of the recent substantial gains, a cautious optimism in regard to the future of neurogastro-enterology studies in the FGIDs seems justified.

References

1. Malagelada JR. Functional dyspepsia: insights on mechanisms and management strategies. Gastroenterol Clin North Am 1996;25:103–12.
2. Phillips SF: Motility disorders of the colon. In: Yamada T, editor. Textbook of Gastroenterology. 2nd Ed. Philadelphia: JB Lippincott;1995;1856–75.
3. Mayer EA, Raybould HE. Role of visceral afferent mechanisms in functional bowel disorders. Gastroenterology 1990;99:1688–1704.
4. Mayer EA, Gebhart GF. Basic and clinical aspects of visceral hyperalgesia. Gastroenterology 1994;107:271–293.
5. Camilleri M, Saslow SB, Bharucha AB. Gastrointestinal sensation: mechanisms and relation to functional gastrointestinal disorders. Gastroenterol Clin North Am 1996;25:247–58.
6. Quigley EMM. Gastric and small intestinal motility in health and disease. Gastroenterol Clin North Am 1996;25:113–45.
7. Sarna SK. Physiology and pathophysiology of colonic motor activity (part one of two). Dig Dis Sci 1991;36:827–62.
8. Rao SSC, Read NW, Davison PA, et al. Anorectal sensitivity and responses to rectal distension in patients with ulcerative colitis. Gastroenterology 1987;93:1270–75.
9. Leighton JA, Valdovinos MA, Pemberton JH, et al. Anorectal dysfunction and rectal prolapse in progressive systemic sclerosis. Dis Colon Rectum 1993;36:182–85.
10. Malagelada JR, Azpiroz F. Determinants of gastric emptying and transit in the small intestine. In: Handbook of Physiology. 2nd Edition. The Gastrointestinal System, Volume 1, Part 2, Bethesda, MD:American Physiological Society;1989: 909–38.
11. Meyer, JH, et al. Effect of size and density on gastric emptying of indigestible solids. Gastroenterology 1985;89:805–13.
12. Minami H, McCallum RW. The physiology and pathophysiology of gastric emptying in humans. Gastroenterology 1984;86:1592–1610.
13. Toouli J. Biliary tract. In: Kumar D, Wingate D, editors. An Illustrated Guide to Gastrointestinal Motility. 2nd Ed. London: Churchill Livingstone;1993:393–409.
14. Phillips SF, Quigley EMM, Kumar D, et al. Motility of the ileocolonic junction. Gut 1988;29:390–406.
15. Weisbrodt NW. The regulation of gastrointestinal motility. In: Motility Disorders of the Gastrointestinal Tract. Anuras S, editor. New York: Raven Press Ltd.; 1992:27–48.
16. Bormans V, Peeters TL, Janssens J, et al. In man, only activity fronts that originate in the stomach correlate with motilin peaks. Scand J Gastroenterol 1987;22:781–84.
17. Tack J, Janssens J, Vantrappen G, et al. Effect of erythromycin on gastric motility in controls and in diabetic gastroparesis. Gastroenterology 1992;103:72–79.
18. Holzknecht G. Die normale Peristaltik des Colons. Munch Med Wochenschr; 1909;56:2401–2403.
19. Holdstock DJ, Misiewicz JJ, Smith T, et al. Propulsion (mass movement) in the human colon and its relationship to meals and somatic activity. Gut 1970;11:91–99.

20. Bueno L, Fioramonti J, Ruckebusch Y, et al. Evaluation of colonic myoelectrical activity in health and functional disorders. Gut 1980;21:480–85.

21. Frexinos J, Bueno L, Fioramonti J. Diurnal changes in myoelectric spiking activity of the human colon. Gastroenterology 1985;88:1104–10.

22. Narducci F, Bassotti G, Gaburri M, et al. Twenty-four hour manometric recording of colonic motor activity in healthy man. Gut 1987;28:17–25.

23. Steadman CJ, Phillips SF, Camilleri M, et al. Variations of muscle tone in the human colon. Gastroenterology 1991;101:373–81.

24. Camilleri M, Hasler WL, Parkman HP, et al. Measurement of gastroduodenal motility in the gastrointestinal laboratory. Gastroenterology 1998;115:747–62.

25. Ghoos YF, Maes BD, Geypeus BJ et al. Measurement of gastric emptying rate of solids by means of a carbon-labelled octanoic acid breath test. Gastroenterology 1993;104:1640–47.

26. Berstad A, Hausken T, Gilja OH, et al. Volume measurement of gastric antrum by 3-D ultrasonography and flow measurements through the pylorus by duplex technique. Dig Dis Sci 1994;39:97–108.

27. Bolondi L, Bortolotti M, Santi V et al. Measurement of gastric emptying time by real-time ultrasonography. Gastroenterology 1985;89:752–59.

28. Chen JDZ, Schirmer BD, McCallum RW. Serosal and cutaneous recordings of gastric myoelectrical activity in patients with gastroparesis. Am J Physiol 1994;266: G90–98.

29. Mintchev MP, Kingma YJ, Bowes KL. Accuracy of cutaneous recordings of gastric electrical activity. Gastroenterology 1993;104:1273–80.

30. Sun WM, Smout A, Malbert C, et al. Relationship between surface electrogastrography and antropyloric pressures. Am J Physiol 1995;268:G424–G430.

31. Pfaffenbach B, Adamek RJ, Kuhn K, et al. Electrogastrography in healthy subjects: evaluation of normal values, influence of age and gender. Dig Dis Sci 1995;40: 1445–50.

32. Liang J, Chen JDZ. What can be measured from surface electrogastrography: computer simulations. Dig Dis Sci 1997;42:1331–93.

33. Evans DF, Lamont G, Stehling MK et al. Prolonged monitoring of the upper gastrointestinal tract using echo planar magnetic resonance imaging. Gut 1993; 34:848–52.

34. Schwizer W, Fraser R, Borovicka J, et al. Measurement of proximal and distal gastric motility with magnetic resonance imaging. Am J Physiol 1996;271:G217–G222.

35. Boulby P, Gowland P, Adams V, et al. Use of echo planar imaging to demonstrate the effect of posture on the intragastric distribution and emptying of an oil-water meal. Neurogastroenterol Motil 1997;9(1):41–47.

36. Kunz P, Crelier GR, Schwizer W, et al. Gastric emptying and motility: assessment with MR imaging-preliminary observations. Radiology 1998;207:33–40.

37. Azpiroz F, Malagelada JR. Gastric tone measured by an electronic barostat in health and postsurgical gastroparesis. Gastroenterology 1987;92:934–43.

38. Azpiroz F, Malagelada JR. Perception and reflex relaxation of the stomach in response to gut distention. Gastroenterology 1990;98:1193–98.

39. Strocchi A, Levitt MD. Breath hydrogen measurement of small bowel transit time. In: Schuster MM, editor. Atlas of Gastrointestinal Motility in Health and Disease. Baltimore, MD:Williams and Wilkins;1993:76–84.

40. Charles F, Camilleri M, Phillips SF, et al. Scintigraphy of the whole gut: clinical evaluation of transit disorders. Mayo Clin Proc 1995;70:113–18.

41. Evans PR, Bak Y-T, Kellow JE. Ambulant small bowel manometry in health: comparison of consecutive 24-h recording periods. J Ambul Monitoring 1996;9:193–202.

42. Holland R, Gallagher MD, Quigley EMM. An evaluation of an ambulatory manometry system in assessment of antroduodenal motor activity. Dig Dis Sci 1996;41:1531–37.

43. Quigley EMM, Deprez PH, Hellstrom P, et al. Ambulatory intestinal manometry: a consensus report on its clinical role. Dig Dis Sci 1997;92:2395–2400.

44. Familoni BO, Abell TL, Voeller G. Measurement of gastric and small bowel electrical activity at laparoscopy. J Laparoendoscopic Surg 1994;4:325–32.

45. Staumont G, Delvaux M, Fioramonti J, et al. Differences between jejunal myoelectrical activity after a meal during phase 2 of migrating motor complexes in healthy humans. Dig Dis Sci 1992;37:1554–61.

46. Bassotti G, Stanghellini V, Chiarioni G, et al. Upper gastrointestinal motor activity in patients with slow–transit constipation: further evidence for an enteric neuropathy. Dig Dis Sci 1996;41:1999–2005.

47. O'Brien MD, Camilleri M, van der Ohe M et al. Motility and tone of the left colon in constipation: a role in clinical practice? Am J Gastroentol 1996;91:2532–38.

48. Kamm MA, Lennard-Jones JE, Thompson DG et al. Dynamic scanning defines a colonic defect in severe idiopathic constipation. Gut 1988;29:1085–92.

49. Bartolo DCC, Kamm MA, Kuijpers H, et al. Working party report: defecation disorders. Am J Gastroenterol 1994; 89:s154–s159.

50. Bassotti G, Botti C, Erbella CS, et al. Colonic mass movements in diarrhea-predominant IBS patients. Gastroenterology 1990;98:A326.

51. Distrutti E, Azpiroz F, Soldevilla A, et al. Perception of rectal distention depends on wall tension but not on expansion. Gastroenterology 1996;110:A657.

52. Thumshirn M, Burton OD, Zinsmeister AR, et al. Modulation of gastric sensory and motor functions by nitrergic and a2-adrenergic agonists. Gastroenterology 1997;112:A837.

53. Piessevaux H, Tack J. Coulie B, et al. Perception of phasic tension changes in the proximal stomach in man. Gastroenterology 1998;114:G3375.

54. Serra J, Azpiroz F, Malagelada J-R. Intestinal gas dynamics and tolerance in humans. Gastroenterology 1998;115:542–50.

55. Gracely RH. Studies of pain in normal man. In: Wall PD, Melzack R, editors. Textbook of Pain, 3rd Ed. Edinburgh: Churchill Livingstone;1994:315–36.

56. Accarino AM, Azpiroz F, Malagelada J-R. Selective dysfunction of mechanosensitive intestinal afferents in the irritable bowel syndrome. Gastroenterology 1995; 108:636–43.

57. Villanova N, Azpiroz F, Malagelada J-R. Perception and gut reflexes induced by stimulation of gastrointestinal thermoreceptors in humans. J Physiol (London) 1997;502(1):215–22.

58. Notivol R, Coffin B, Azpiroz F, et al. Gastric tone determines the sensitivity of the stomach to distention. Gastroenterology 1995;108;330–36.

59. Tack J, Coulie B, Janssens J. 5-HT$_1$ activation has a major impact on gastrointestinal functions in man. Gastroenterology 1996;110:A1123.

60. Malcolm A, Phillips SF, Camilleri M, et al. Pharmacological modulation of rectal tone alters perception of distention in humans. Am J Gastroenterology 1997;92: 2073–79.

61. Serra J, Azpiroz F, Malagelada J-R. Perception and reflex responses to intestinal distension are modified by simultaneous or previous stimulation. Gastroenterology 1995;109:1742–49.

62. Sun WM, Read NW, Prior A, et al. Sensory and motor responses to rectal distention vary according to rate and pattern of balloon inflation. Gastroenterology 1990;99:1008–15.

63. Coffin B, Azpiroz F, Malagelada J-R. Somatic stimulation reduces perception of gut distension. Gastroenterology 1994;107:1636–42.

64. Iovino P, Azpiroz F, Domingo E, et al. The sympathetic nervous system modulates perception and reflex responses to gut distension in humans. Gastroenterology 1995;108:680–86.

65. Accarino, AM, Azpiroz F, Malagelada J-R. Attention and distraction: effects on gut perception. Gastroenterology 1997;113:415–22.

66. Ford MJ, Camilleri M, Zinsmeister AR, et al. Psychosensory modulation of colonic sensation in the human transverse and sigmoid colon. Gastroenterology 1995;109;1772–80.

67. Whitehead WE, Delvaux M. Standardization of procedures for testing smooth muscle tone and sensory thresholds in the gastrointestinal tract. Dig Dis Sci 1997;42:223–41.

68. Hurst AF: The sensibility of the alimentary canal in health and diseases. Lancet 1:1051–56;1911.

69. Bloomfield AL, Polland WS. Experimental referred pain from the gastrointestinal tract: part II: stomach, duodenum and colon. J Clin Invest 1931;10:453–73.

70. Rouillon JM, Azpiroz F, Malagelada J-R. Sensorial and intestino-intestinal reflex pathways in the human jejunum. Gastroenterology 1991;101:1606–12.

71. Bentley FH, Smithwick RH. Visceral pain produced by balloon distension of the jejunum. Lancet 1940:1(2);389–91.

72. Ness TJ, Metcalf AM, Gebhart GF. A psychophysical study in humans using phasic colonic distension as a noxious visceral stimulus. Pain 1990;43:377–86.

73. Gregersen A, Orvar IC, Christensen J. Biomechanical properties of duodenal wall and duodenal tone during phase I and phase II of the MMC. Am JPhysiol 1992;263:G795–G801.

74. Dall FH, Jorgensen CS, Hou D, et al. Biomechanical wall properties of the human rectum: a study with impedance planimetry. Gut 1993;34:1581–86.

75. Rao SSC, Hayek B, Summers RW. Impedance planimetry: an integrated approach for assessing sensory, active and passive isomechanical properties of the human oesophagus. Am J Gastroenterol 1995: 90;431–38.

76. Rao SSC, Gregerson H, Hayek B et al. Unexplained chest pain: the hypersensitive, hyperative, and poorly compliant oesophagus. Ann Intern Med 1996;124:950–58.

77. Patel RS, Rao SSC. Biomechanical and sensory parameters of the human esophagus at four levels. Am J Physiol 1998:275;G187–G191.

78. Rouillon JM, Azpiroz F, Malagelada J. Reflex changes in intestinal tone: relationship to perception. Am J Physiol 1991; 261: G280–G286.

79. Youmans WM, Meak WJ. Reflex and humoral gastrointestinal inhibition in unanesthetized dogs during rectal stimulation. Am J Physiol 1937;120:750–55.

80. Louvel D, Delvaux M, Staumont G, et al. Intracolonic injection of glycerol: a model for abdominal pain in Irritable Bowel Syndrome. Gastroenterology 1996; 110:351–361.

81. Youle MS, Read NW. Effect of painless rectal distention on gastrointestinal transit of solid meal. Dig Dis Sci 1984;29:902–906.

82. Kellow JE, Gill RC, Wingate DL. Modulation of human upper gastrointestinal motility by rectal distention in humans. Gut 1987;28:864–68.

83. Tjeerdsma HC, Smout AJP, Akkermans LMA. Voluntary suppression of defecation delays gastric emptying. Dig.Dis.Sci. 1983; 38: 832–36.

84. Toouli J. Biliary tract. In: Kumar D, Wingate D, editors. An Illustrated Guide to Gastrointestinal Motility. 2nd Edition. London: Churchill Livingstone;1993:393–409.

85. Wiley J, Tatum D, Kennalt et al. Participation of gastric mechanoreceptors and intestinal chemoreceptors in the gastro-colonic response. Gastroenterology 1988;94: 1144–49.

86. Willer JC. Comparative study of perceived pain and nociceptive flexion reflex in man. Pain 1977;3:69–80.

87. Bouhassira D, Sabate JM, Coffin B, et al. Effects of rectal distensions on nociceptive flexion reflexes in humans. Am J Physiol 1998;275:G410–G417.

88. Aziz Q, Thompson DG. Brain-gut axis in health and disease. Gastroenterology 1998;114:559–78.

89. Lydiard RB, Fossey MD, Marsh W, et al. Prevalence of psychiatric disorders in patients with irritable bowel syndrome. Psychosomatics 1993;34:229–34.

90. Utydenhoef P, Portelance P, Jacquy J, et al. Regional cerebral blood flow and lateralised hemispheric dysfunction in depression. Brit J Psychiatry 1983;143:128–32.

91. Ebert K, Feistel H, Barocka A. Effects of sleep deprivation on the limbic system and the frontal lobes in affective disorders: a study with TC-99m-HMPAO SPECT. Psychiatry Res 1991;40:247–51.

92. You Ch, Lee KY, Chey WY, et al. Electrogastrographic study of patients with unexplained nausea, bloating and vomiting. Gastroenterology 1980;79:311–14.

93. Geldof H, van der Schee EJ, van Blankenstein M, et al. Electrogastrographic study of gastric myoelectrical activity in patients with unexplained nausea and vomiting. Gut 1986;27:799–808.

94. Koch KL, Medina M, Bingaman S, et al. Gastric dysrhythmias and visceral sensations in patients with functional dyspepsia. Gastroenterology 1991;101: 999–1006.

95. Chen JDZ, Lin ZY, Pan J, Mccallum RW. Abnormal gastric myoelectrical activity and delayed gastric emptying in patients with symptoms suggestive of gastroparesis. Dig Dis Sci 1996;41:1538–45.

96. Malagelada JR, Stanghellini V. Manometric evaluation of functional upper gut symptoms. Gastroenterology 1985;88:1223–31.

97. Pieramico O, Ditschuneit H, Malfertheirner D. Gastrointestinal motility in patients with non-ulcer dyspepsia: a role for helicobacter pylori infection? Am J Gastroenterol 1993;88:364–68.

98. Testoni PA, Bagnolo F, Masci E, et al. Different interdigestive antroduodenal motility patterns in chronic antral gastritis with and without Helicobacter pylori infection. Dig Dis Sci 1993;38:2255–61.

99. Qvist N, Ramussen L, Axelsson CK. Helicobacter pylori associated gastritis and dyspepsia: the influence of migrating motor complexes. Scand J Gastroenterol 1994;29:133–37.

100. Jian R, Ducorot F, Ruskone A, Chaucsade S, et al. Symptomatic, radionuclide and therapeutic assessment of chronic idiopathic dyspepsia: a double-blind placeo-controlled evaluation of cisapride. Dig Dis Sci 1989;34:657–64.

101. Waldron B, Cullen PT, Kumar R, et al. Evidence for hypomotility in non-ulcer dyspepsia. Gut 1991;32:246–51.

102. Stanghellini V, Tosetti C, Patermico A, et al. Risk indicators of delayed gastric emptying of solids in patients with functional dyspepsia. Gastroenterology 1996;110:1036–42.

103. Caballero-Plasencia AM, Muros Navarro MC, Martin-Ruiz JL, et al. Dyspeptic symptoms and gastric emptying of solids in patients with functional dyspepsia: role of Helicobacter pylori infection. Scand J Gastroenterol 1995;30:45–51.

104. Scott AM, Kellow JE, Shuter B, et al. Intragastric distribution and gastric emptying of solids and liquids in functional dyspepsia: lack of influence of symptom subgroups and H.pylori-associated gastritis. Dig Dis Sci 1993;38:2247–54.

105. Troncon LE, Bennett RJ, Ahuwalia NK, et al. Abnormal intragastric distribution of food during gastric emptying in functional dyspepsia patients. Gut 1994; 35:327–32.

106. Hausken T, Berstad A. Wide gastric antrum in patients with non-ulcer dyspepsia: effect of cisapride. Scand J Gastroenterol 1992;27:427–32.

107. Ahluwaha NK, Thompson DG, Mantora H, et al. Evaluation of gastric antral motor performance in patients with dysmotility-like dyspepsia using real-time high resolution ultrasound. Neurogastroenterol Motil 1996;8:332–38.

108. Gilja OH, Hausken T, Wilhelmsen I, et al. Impaired accommodation of proximal stomach to a meal in functional dyspepsia. Dig Dis Sci 1996;41:689–96.

109. Mearin F, Malagelada J-R. Upper gut motility and perception in functional dyspepsia. Eur J Gastroenterol Hepatol 1992;4:615–21.

110. Bost R, Hostein J. Valenti M, et al. Is there an abnormal fasting duodenal reflux in nonulcer dyspepsia? Dig Dis Sci 1990;67:193–99.

111. Abell TL, Camilleri M, Hench VS, et al. Gastric electromechanical function and gastric emptying in diabetic gastroparesis. Eur J Gastroenterol Hepatol 1991; 3:163–67.

112. Stanghellini V, Ghidni C, Maccarini MR, et al. Fasting and postprandial gastrointestinal motility in ulcer and non-ulcer dyspepsia. Gut 1992;33:184–90.

113. Bassotti G, Pelli MA, Morelli A. Duodenojejunal motor activity in patients with chronic dyspeptic symptoms. J. Clin Gastroenterol 1990;12:17–21.

114. Wilmer A, Van Cutsem E, Andrioti A, et al. Ambulatory gastro-jejunal manometry in severe motility-like dyspepsia: lack of correlation between dysmotility, symptoms and gastric emptying. Gut 1998;42:235–42.

115. Jebbink HJA, van Berge-Henegouwen GP, Akkermans LMA, et al. Small intestinal motor abnormalities in patients with functional dyspepsia demonstrated by ambulatory manometry. Gut 1996;38:694–700.

116. Jebbink HJA, van Berge-Henegouwen GP, Akkermans LMA, et al. Antroduodenal manometry: 24-hour ambulatory monitoring versus short-term stationary manometry in patients with functional dyspepsia. Eur J Gastroenterol Hepatol 1995;7:109–16.

117. Camilleri M, Malagelada J-R, Kao PC, et al. Gastric and autonomic responses to stress in functional dyspepsia. Dig Dis Sci 1986;31:1169–77.

118. Tucci A, Corinaldesi R, Stanghellini V, et al. Helicobacter pylori infection and gastric function in patients with chronic idiopathic dyspepsia. Gastrenterology 1992;103:768–74.

119. Collen MJ. Loebenberg MJ. Basal gastric acid secretion in nonulcer dyspepsia with or without duodenitis. Dig Dis Sci 1989;34:246–50.

120. Bradette M, Pare P, Douville P, et al. Visceral perception in health and functional dyspepsia: crossover study of gastric distention with placebo and domperidone. Dig Dis Sci 1991;36:52–58.

121. Lemann M, Dederding JP, Flourie B, et al. Abnormal perception of visceral pain in response to gastric distention in chronic idiopathic dyspepsia. The irritable stomach. Dig Dis Sci 1991;36:1249–54.

122. Mearin F, Cucala M, Azpiroz F, et al. The origin of symptoms on the brain gut axis in functional dyspepsia. Gastroenterology 1991;101:999–1006.

123. Mertz H, Kodner A, Hirsh T, et al. Gastric balloon distention as a diagnostic test for non-ulcer dyspepsia. Gastroenterology 1994;106:A539.

124. Troncon LE, Thompson DG, Ahuwalia NK, et al. Relations between upper abdominal symptoms and gastric distention abnormalities in dysmotility like functional dyspepsia and after vagotomy. Gut 1995;37:17–22.

125. Klatt S, Pieramico O, Guethner C, et al. Gastric hypersensitivity in nonulcer dyspepsia: an inconsistent finding. Dig Dis Sci 1997;92:720–23.

126. Camilleri M, Malagelada J-R, Kao PC, et al. Gastric and autonomic responses to stress in functional dyspepsia. Dig Dis Sci 1986;31:1169–77.

127. George AA, Tsuchiyose M, Dooley CP. Sensitivity of the gastric mucosa to acid and duodenal contents in patients with non-ulcer dyspepsia. Gastroenterology 1991;101:3–6.

128. Greydanus MP, Vassallo M, Camilleri M, et al. Neurohormonal factors in functional dyspepsia: insights on pathophysiological mechanisms. Gastroenterology 1991;100:1311–18.

129. Holtmann G, Talley NJ, Goebell H. Assocation between H.pylori duodenal mechanosensory thresholds and small intestinal motility in chronic unexplained dyspepsia. Dig Dis Sci 1996;41:1285–91.

130. Chaudhary NA, Truelove SC. The irritable colon syndrome: a study of the clinical features, predisposing causes, and prognosis in 130 cases. Quart J Med 1962; 31:307–22.

131. Snape WJ, Carlson GM, Cohen S. Colonic myoelectric activity in the irritable bowel syndrome. Gastroenterolgoy 1976;70:326–30.

132. Welgan P, Meshkinpour H, Hoehler F. The effect of stress on colon motor and electrical activity in irritable bowel syndrome. Psychosom Med 1985;47:139–49.

133. Connell AM, Jones FA, Rowlands EN. Motility of the pelvic colon: IV. abdominal pain associated with colonic hypermotility after meals. Gut 1965;6:105–12.

134. Misiewicz JJ, Connell AM, Pontes FA. Comparison of the effect of meals and prostigmine on the proximal and distal colon in patients with and without diarrhea. Gut 1966;7:468–73.

135. Whitehead WE, Engel BT, Schuster MM. Irritable bowel syndrome: physiological and psychological differences between diarrhea-predominant and constipation-predominant patients. Dig Dis Sci 1980;25:6:404–13.

136. Bazzocchi G, Ellis J, Villanueva-Meyer J, et al. Effect of eating on colonic motility and transit in patients with functional diarrhea. Gastroenterology 1991; 101:1298–1306.

137. Vassallo MJ, Camilleri M, Phillips SF, et al. Colonic tone and motility in patients with irritable bowel syndrome. Mayo Clin Proc 1992;67:725–31.

138. Bradette M, Delvaux M, Staumont G, et al. Evaluation of colonic sensory thresholds in IBS patients using a barostat: definition of optimal conditions and comparisons with healthy subjects. Dig Dis Sci 1994;39:449–57.

139. Crowell MD, Musial F. Rectal adaptation for distention is impaired in the irritable bowel syndrome. Am J Gastroenterol 1994;89:1689.

140. Choi MG, Camilleri M, O'Brien MD, et al. A pilot study of motility and tone of the left colon in patients with diarrhea due to functional disorders and dysautonomia. Am J Gastroenterol 1997;92:297–302.

141. Cann PA, Read NW, Brown C, et al. Irritable bowel syndrome: relationship of disorders in the transit of a single solid meal to symptom patterns. Gut 1983; 24:405–11.

142. Vassallo M, Camilleri M, Phillips SF, et al. Transit through the proximal colon influences stool weight in the irritable bowel syndrome. Gastroenterology 1992; 102:102–108.

143. Bazzocchi G, Ellis J, Villanueva-Meyer J, et al. Postprandial colonic transit and motor activity in chronic constipation. Gastroenterology 1990;98:686–93.

144. Stivland T, Camilleri M, Vassallo M, et al. Scintigraphic measurement of regional gut transit in idiopathic constipation. Gastroenterology 1991;101:107–15.

145. van der Sijp JRM, Kamm MA, Nightingale JMD, et al. Radioisotope determination of regional colonic transit in severe constipation: comparison with radiopaque markers. Gut 1993;34:402–8.

146. Drossman DA, Whitehead WE, Camilleri M. Irritable Bowel Syndrome: a technical review for practice guideline development. Gastroenterology 1997;112: 2120–37.

147. Horowitz L, Farrer JT. Intraluminal small intestinal pressures in normal patients and in patients with functional gastrointestinal disorders. Gastroenterology 1962;42:455–64.

148. Kellow JE, Phillips SF. Altered small bowel motility in irritable bowel syndrome is correlated with symptoms. Gastroenterology 1987;92:1885–93.

149. Kellow JE, Gill RC, Wingate DL. Prolonged ambulant recordings of small bowel motility demonstrate abnormalities in the irritable bowel syndrome. Gastroenterology 1990;98:1208–18.

150. Schmidt T, Hackelsberger N, Widmer R et al. Ambulatory 24-hr jejunal motility in diarrhea-predominant irritable bowel syndrome. Scand J Gastroenterol 1996;31:581–89.

151. Kumar D, Wingate DL. The irritable bowel syndrome: a paroxysmal motor disorder. Lancet 1985; (ii): 973–77.

152. Kingham JCG, Brown R, Colson R et al. Jejunal motility in patients with functional abdominal pain. Gut 1984;25:375–80.

153. Gorard DA, Libby GW, Farthing MJG. Ambulatory small intestinal motility in 'diarrhea' predominant irritable bowel syndrome Gut 1994;35:203–10.

154. Wackerbauer R, Schmidt T, Widmer R et al. Discrimination of irritable bowel syndrome by non-linear analysis of 24-h jejunal motility. Neurogastroenterol Motil 1998;10:331–37.

155. Kellow JE, Phillips SF, Miller IJ, et al. Dysmotility of the small intestine in irritable bowel syndrome. Gut 1988;29:1236–43.

156. Small PK, Loudon MA, Hau CM, et al. Large-scale ambulatory study of postprandial jejunal motility in irritable bowel syndrome. Scand J Gastroenterol 1997;32:39–47.

157. Nielsen OH, Gjonip T, Christensen FN. Gastric emptying rate and small bowel transit time in patients with irritable bowel syndrome determined with 99MTC-labelled pellets and scintigraphy. Dig Dis Sci 1986;31:1287–91.

158. Evans PR, Bak Y-T, Shuter B, et al. Gastroparesis and small bowel dysmotility in irritable bowel syndrome. Dig Dis Sci. 1997;42:2087–2093.

159. Charles F, Phillips SF, Camilleri M, et al. Rapid gastric emptying in patients with functional diarrhea. Mayo Clin Proc 1997;72:323–28.

160. Latimer PR, Sarna SK, Campbell D, et al. Colonic motor and myoelectrical ac-

tivity: a comparative study of normal patients, psychoneurotic patients and patients with irritable bowel syndrome (IBS). Gastroenterology 1981;80:893–901.

161. Taylor I, Duthie DL, Smallwood R. The effect of stimulation on the myoelectrical activity of the rectosigmoid of man. Gut 1974;15:599–607.

162. Almy TP, Kern FJ, Tulin M. Alteration in colonic function in man under stress. II. experimental production of sigmoid spasm in healthy persons. Gastroenterology 1949;12:425–36.

163. Fukudo S, Suzuki J. Colonic motility, autonomic function, and gastrointestinal hormones under psychological stress on IBS. Tohoku J Exp Med 1987;151: 373–85.

164. Sullivan MA, Cohen S, Snape WJ. Colonic myoelectrical activity in irritable bowel syndrome: effect of eating and anticholinergics. New Engl J Med 1978; 298:878–83.

165. Rogers J, Henry MM, Misiewicz JJ. Increased segmental activity and intraluminal pressures in the sigmoid colon of patients with the irritable bowel syndrome. Gut 1989;30:634–41.

166. Whitehead WE, Holtkotter B, Enck P, et al. Tolerance for rectosigmoid distention in irritable bowel syndrome. Gastroenterology 1990;98:1187–92.

167. Harvey RF, Read AE. Effect of cholecystokinin on colon motility and symptoms in patients with the irritable bowel syndrome. Lancet 1973;1:1–3.

168. Evans PR, Dowsett JF, Bak Y-T , et al. Abnormal sphincter of Oddi response to cholecystokinin in postcholecystectomy syndrome patients with irritable bowel syndrome. Dig Dis Sci 1995;40:1149–56.

169. Swarbrick ET, Hegarty JE, Bat L, et al. Site of pain from the irritable bowel. Lancet 1980;2:443–46.

170. Ritchie J. Pain from distention of the pelvic colon by inflating a balloon in the irritable bowel syndrome. Gut 1973;14:123–32.

171. Moriarty KJ, Dawson AM. Functional abdominal pain: further evidence that whole gut is affected. Brit Med J 1982;284:1670–72.

172. Prior A, Colgan SM, Whorwell PJ. Changes in rectal sensitivity after hypnotherapy in patients with irritable bowel syndrome. Gut 1990;31:896–98.

173. Hammer J, Phillips SF, Talley NJ, et al. Effect of a 5-HT_3 antagonist (ondansetron) on rectal contractility and compliance in health and the irritable bowel syndrome. Aliment Pharmacol Ther 1993;7:543–51.

174. Hasler WL, Soudah HC, Owyang C. Somatostatin analog inhibits afferent response to rectal distention in diarrhea-predominant irritable bowel patients. J Pharmacol Exp Ther 1994;268:1206–11.

175. Lembo T, Munakata J, Mertz H, et al. Evidence for the hypersensitivity of the lumbar splanchnic afferents in irritable bowel syndrome. Gastroenterology 1994; 107:1686–96.

176. Mertz H, Naliboff B, Munakata J, et al. Altered rectal perception is a biological marker of patients with irritable bowel syndrome. Gastroenterology 1995;109: 40–52.

177. Zighelboim J, Talley NJ, Phillips SF, et al. Visceral perception in irritable bowel syndrome Dig Dis Sci 1995;40:819–27.

178. Silvermann DHS, Munakata JA, Ennes H, et al. Regional cerebral activity in normal and pathological perception of visceral pain. Gastroenterology 1997; 112: 64–72.

179. Scarinci IC, McDonald-Haile J, Bradley LA, et al. Altered pain perception and psychosocial features among women with gastrointestinal disorders and history of abuse: a preliminary model. Am J Med 1994;97;108–18.

180. Cook IJ, Vaan Eeden A, Collins SM. Patients with irritable bowel syndrome have greater pain tolerance than normal subjects. Gastroenterology 1987;93:727–33.

181. Munakata J, Silvermann DHS, Hoh CK, et al. Rectosigmoid sensitization correlates with thalamic response to rectal pain: an O-15-water PET study of normal subjects and IBS patients (abstr) Gastroenterology 1996;(Suppl.):A720.

182. Kellow JE, Eckerskey GM, Jones MP. Enhanced perception of physiological intestinal motility in the irritable bowel syndrome. Gastroenterology 1991;101: 1621–27.

183. Evans PR, Bennet EJ, Bak Y-T, et al. Jejunal sensorimotor dysfunction in irritable bowel syndrome: clinical and psychosocial features. Gastroenterology 1996;110: 393–404.

184. Evans PR, Kellow JE. Physiological modulation of jejunal sensitivity in health and in the irritable bowel syndrome. Am J Gastroenterol 1998;93:2191–96.

185. Kingham JCG, Dawson AM. Origin of chronic right upper quadrant pain. Gut 1985;26:783–88.

186. Cervero F, Laird JMA, Pozo MA. Selective changes of receptive field properties of spinal nociceptive neurones induced by noxious visceral stimulation in the cat. Pain 1992;51:335–42.

187. Trimble KC, Farouk R, Pryde A, et al. Heightened visceral sensataions in functional gastrointestinal disease is not site-specific: evidence for a generalized disorder of gut sensitivity. Dig Dis Sci 1995;40:1607.

188. Francis CY, Houghton LA, Whorwell PJ, et al. Enhanced sensitivity of the whole gut in patients with irritable bowel syndrome. Gastroenterology 1995;108:A601.

189. Constantini M, Sturniolo GC, Zaninitto G, et al. Altered oesophageal pain threshold in irritable bowel syndrome. Dig Dis Sci 1993;38:206–12.

190. Dykhuizen RS, Masson J, McKnight G et al. Plasma nitrate concentration in infective gastroenteritis and inflammatory bowel disease. Gut 1996;39:393–95.

191. Collins SM, Hurst SM, Main C, et al. Effect of inflammation of enteric nerves: cytokine-induced changes in neurotransmitter content and release. Ann NY Acad Sci 1992;664:415–24.

192. Collins SM. Is the irritable gut an inflamed gut? Scand J Gastroenterol 1992;27 (Suppl)192:102–105.

193. McLaughlin JT, Troncon LEA, Barlow J, et al. Evidence for a lipid specific effect in nutrient inducted human proximal gastric relaxation. Gut 1998;43:248–51.

194. Aggarwal A, Cutts TF, Abell TL, et al. Prominent symptoms in irritable bowel syn-

drome correlate with specific autonomic nervous system abnormalities. Gastroenterology 1996;110:393–404.

195. Valori RM, Kumar D, Wingate DL. Effects of different types of stress and of "prokinetic" drugs on the control of the fasting motor complex in humans. Gastroenterology 1986;90:1890–1900.

196. Sengupta JN,Gebhart GF. Gastrointestinal afferents and sensation. In: Johnson, LR, editor. Physiology of the Gastrointestinal Tract. Vol. 1, 3rd ed. New York: Raven;1994:483–519.

197. Distrutti E, Soldevilla A, Azpiroz F,et al. Gastric mechanoreceptors' response characterized by a computerized tensostat in humans. Gastroenterology 1996; 110:A657.

198. Lagier E, Delvaux M, Metivier S, et al. Colonic tone influences thresholds of sensory perception to luminal distention in IBS patients. Gastroenterology 1996; 110:A700.

199. Gwee KA, Graham JC, McKendrick NW, et al. Psychometric scores and persistence of irritable bowel after infectious diarrhoea. Lancet 1996;347;150–53.

200. Neal KR, Hebdon J, Spiller R. Prevalence of gastrointestinal symptoms six months after bacterial gastroenteritis and risk factors for development of the irritable bowel syndrome. Brit Med J 1997;314:779–82.

201. Bergin AJ, Donnelly, TC, McKendrick MW, et al. Changes in anorectal function in persistent bowel disturbance following salmonella gastroenteritis. Eur J Gastroenterol Hepatol 1993;5:617–20.

202. Morteau O, Hachet T, Caussette M, et al. Experimental colitis alters visceromotor response to colorectal distention in awake rats. Dig Dis Sci 1994;39:1239–48.

203. Barbara G, Vallance BA, Collins Stephen M. Persistent intestinal neuromuscular dysfunction after acute nematode infection in mice. Gastroenterology 1997;113: 1224–32.

204. Weston AP, Biddle WL, Bhatia PS, et al. Terminal ileal mucosal mast cells in irritable bowel syndrome. Dig Dis Sci 1993;38:1590–95.

205. Collins SM. The immunomodulation of enteric neuromuscular function: implications for motility and inflammatory disorders. Gastroenterology 1996;111: 1683–99

206. Khan I, Collins SM. Is there an inflammatory basis for a subset of patients presenting with diarrhea in the irritable bowel syndrome. Gastroenterology 1994; 106:A523.

207. Collins JS, Hamilton PW, Watt PC, et al. Quantitative histological study of mucosal inflammatory cell densities in endoscopic duodenal biopsy specimens from dyspeptic patients using computer-linked image analysis. Gut 1990;31: 858–61.

208. Mearin F, Ribot X, Balboa A, et al. Does Helicobacter pylori infection increase gastric sensitivity in functional dyspepsia. Gut 1995;37:47–51.

209. Tack J, Piesservau H, Coulie B, et al. Role of impaired gastric accommodation to a meal in functional dyspepsia. Gastroenterology (in press).

210. Thumshirn M, Saslow SB, Camilleri M, et al. Postcibal gastric sensory and motor dysfunctions in non-ulcer dyspepsia: what are the roles of Helicobacter pylori infection and vagal function? Gastroenterology 1998;114:A847.

211. Jones A, Shorthouse M, McLaughlan P, et al. Food intolerance: a major factor in the pathogenesis of the irritable bowel syndrome. Lancet 1982;2:1115–17.

212. Finn R, Smith MA, Youngs GR, et al. Immunological hypersensitivity to environmental antigens in the irritable bowel syndrome. Brit J Clin Pract 1987;41: 1041–43.

213. Castex N, Fioramonti J, Fargeas MJ, et al. c-fos expression in specific rat brain nuclei after intestinal anaphylaxis: involvement of 5-HT$_3$ receptors and vagal afferent fibers. Brain Res 1995;688:149–60.

214. Oliver MR, Tan DTM, Kirk DR et al. Colonic and jejunal motor disturbances after colonic antigen challenge of sensitized rat. Gastroenterology 1997;112:1996–2005.

215. Santos J, Saperas E, Nogueiras C et al. Release of mast cell mediators into the jejunum by cold pain stress in humans. Gastroenterology 1998;114:640–48.

216. Houghton LA, Mangall YF, Dwivedi A, et al. Sensitivity to nutrients in patients with non-ulcer dyspepsia. Eur J Gastroenterol Hepatol 1993;5:109–113.

217. Barbera R, Feinle C, Read NW. Abnormal sensitivity to duodenal lipid infusion in patients with functional dyspepsia. Eur J Gastroenterol Hepatol 1995;7: 1051–58.

218. Hausken T, Svebak S, Wilhelmsen I, et al. Low vagal tone and antral dysmotility in patients with functional dyspepsia. Psychosomat Med 1993;55;12–22.

219. Haug TT, Svebak S, Hausken T, et al. Low vagal activity as mediating mechanism for the relationship between personality factors and gastric symptoms in functional dyspepsia. Psychosomat Med 1994;56:181–86.

220. Undeland KA, Hausken T, Svebak S, et al. Wide gastric antrum and low vagal tone in patients with diabetes mellitus type I compared to patients with functional dyspepsia and healthy individuals. Dig Dis Sci 1996;41:9–16.

221. Undeland KA, Hausken T, Anderud S, et al. Lower postprandial gastric volume response in diabetic patients with vagal neuropathy. Neurogastroenterol Motil 1997;9:19–24

222. Muth ER, Stern RM, Koch KL. Effects of vection-induced motor sickness on gastric myoelectric activity and oral-caecal-transit time. Dig Dis Sci 1996;41: 330–34.

223. Kim MS, Chey WD, Owyang C, et al. Role of plasma vasopressin as a mediator of nausea and gastric slow wave dysrhythmias in motion sickness. Am J Physiol 1997;35:G853–G862.

224. Smart HL, Atkinson M. Abnormal vagal function in irritable bowel syndrome. Lancet 1987;2:475–78.

225. Whitehead WE, Palsson OS. Is rectal pain sensitivity a biological marker for irritable bowel syndrome: psychological influences on pain perception. Gastroenterology 1998;115:1263–71.

226. Bennett EJ, Kellow JE, Cowan H, et al. Suppression of anger and gastric emptying in patients with functional dyspepsia. Scand J Gastroenterol 1992;27:869–74.

227. Erckenbrecht J. Noise and intestinal motor alterations. In: Stress and Digestive Motility. Bueno L, Collins S, Junien JL, editors. London: John Libbey Eurotext; 1989:93–96.

228. Monnikes H, Heymann-Monnikes I, Arnold R. Patients with irritable bowel syndrome have alterations in the CNS-modulation of visceral afferent perception. Gut 1995;37:A168.

229. Metivier S, Delvaux M, Louvel D, et al. Influence of stress on sensory thresholds to rectal distention in healthy volunteers. Gastroenterology 1996;110:A717.

230. Naliboff BD, Munakata J, Fullerton S, et al. Evidence for two distinct perceptual alterations in irritable bowel syndrome. Gut 1997;41:505–12.

231. Fock KM, Khoo TK, Chia KS, et al. Helicobacter pylori infection and gastric emptying of indigestible solids in patients with dysmotility-like dyspepsia. Scand J Gastroenterol 1997;32:676–80.

232. Hveem K, Jones KL, Chatterton BE, et al. Scintigraphic measurement of gastric emptying and ultrasonographic assessment of antral area: relation to appetite. Gut 1996;38:816–21.

233. Gilja OH, Hausken T, Barg CJ, Berstad A. Effect of glyceryl trinitrate on gastric accommodation and symptoms in functional dyspepsia. Dig Dis Sci 1997;42: 2124–31.

234. Tack J, Piessevaux H, Coulie B, et al. Role of visceral hypersensitivity in patients with functional dyspepsia. Gastroenterology 1998;114;A301.

235. Moragas G, Azpiroz F, Pavia J, et al. Relations among intragastric pressure, postcibal perception and gastric emptying. Am J Physiol 1993;264:G1112–G1117.

236. Delvaux M, Louvel D, Lagier E, et al. Reproducibility of sensory thresholds triggered by rectal distention in healthy volunteers. Gastroenterology 1995;108: A590.

237. Enck P. Biofeedback training in disordered defecation: a critical review. Dig Dis Sci 1993;38:1953–60.

238. Whitehead WE, Thompson WG. Motility as a therapeutic modality. In: Schuster MM, editor. Atlas of Gastrointestinal Motility in Health and Disease. Baltimore, MD:Williams & Wilkins;1993:300–16.

239. Whorwell PJ. Hypnotherapy for selected gastrointestinal disorders. Dig Dis 1990;8:223–25.

240. Tack J, Broeckart D, Coulie B, et al. Influence of cisapride on gastric tone and on the perception of gastric distension. Alimen Pharmacol Ther 1998;12:761–66.

241. Farrugia G, Camilleri M, Whitehead WE. Therapeutic strategies for motility disorders. In: Camilleri M, editor. Gastrointestinal Motility in Clinical Practice. Philadelphia, PA: W. B. Saunders; Gastroenterology Clinics of North America 1996;25(1);225–46.

242. Pace F, Coremans G, Dapoigny M et al. Therapy of irritable bowel syndrome: an overview. Digestion 1995;56:433–42.

243. Wiseman LR, Fauld D. Cisapride: an updated review of its pharmacology and therapeutic efficacy as a prokinetic agent in gastrointestinal motility disorders. Drugs 1994;47:116–52.

244. Peeters TL. Erythromycin and other macrolides as prokinetic agents. Gastroenterology 1993;105:1886–99.

245. Owyang C. Octreotide in gastrointestinal motility disorders. Gut 1994;3(Suppl): s11–s14.

246. Poynard T, Naveau S, Mory B, et al. Meta-analysis of smooth muscle relaxants in the treatment of irritable bowel syndrome. Aliment Pharmacol Therap 1994;8: 499–510.

247. Awouters F, Megens A, Verlinden M, et al. Loperamide: survey of studies on mechanism of its antidiarrheal activity. Dig Dis Sci 1993;38:977–95.

248. Camilleri M, von der Ohe MR. Drugs effecting serotonin receptors. Baillieres Clin Gastroenterol 1994;8:301–19.

249. Coulie B, Tack J, Janssens J. Influence of buspirone-induced fundus relaxation on the perception of gastric distension in man. Gastroenterology 1997;112:A715.

250. Bueno L, Fioramonti J, Delvaux M, et al. Mediators and pharmacology of visceral sensitivity: From basic to clinical investigations. Gastroenterology 1997;112: 1714–43.

251. Bradette M, Delvaux M, Staumont G, et al. Octreotide increases thresholds of colonic visceral perception in IBS patients without modifying muscle tone. Dig Dis Sci 1994;39:1171–78.

252. Fraitag B, Homerin M, Hecketsweiler P. Double-blind dose response multicenter comparison of fedotozine and placebo in treatment of nonulcer dyspepsia. Dig Dis Sci 1994;39:1072–77.

253. Dapoigny M, Abitol JL, Geneve J et al. Fedotozine in irritable bowel syndrome: results of a 6 wk placebo-controlled multicenter therapeutic trial. Gut 1995;37: A159.

254. Clouse RE. Antidepressants for functional gastrointestinal syndromes. Dig Dis Sci 1994;39:2352–63.

255. Tanum L, Malt UF. A new pharmacologic treatment of functional gastrointestinal disorder: a double-blind placebo-controlled study with mianserin. Scand J Gastroenterol 1996;31:318–25.

256. Mertz H, Foss R, Kodner A, et al. Effect of amitriptyline on symptoms, sleep and visceral perception in patients with functional dyspepsia. Am J Gastroenterol 1998;93:160–65.

257. Prior A, Read NW. Reduction of rectal sensitivity and postprandial motility by granisetron, a 5-HT$_3$ receptor antagonist, in patients with irritable bowel syndrome. Aliment Pharmacol Ther 1993;7:175–80.

258. Delvaux M, Louvel D, Mamet JP, et al. Effect of alosetron on colonic sensitivity in patients with irritable bowel syndrome (IBS). Aliment Pharmacol Ther 1998; 12:849–55.

Chapter 4

Psychosocial Aspects of the Functional Gastrointestinal Disorders

Douglas A. Drossman, Chair,
Francis H. Creed, Co-Chair, *with*
Kevin W. Olden,
Jan Svedlund,
Brenda B. Toner,
and William E. Whitehead

Introduction

The functional gastrointestinal disorders (FGIDs) are the most frequent clinical conditions seen in gastroenterology practice [1,2], and they also comprise a major portion of primary care. Even for the majority of individuals who do not seek health care, these disorders are associated with significant work absenteeism [3], impaired health-related quality of life [3], and increased medical costs [4].

Furthermore, psychosocial factors are important in these disorders with regard to: (1) their effects on gut physiology; (2) their modulation of the symptom experience; (3) their influence on health behavior; (4) their impact on outcome; and (5) their influence on indications for behavioral interventions. For the majority of patients with milder symptoms who are most often seen in primary care, psychological stressors may not be prominent and psychological interventions are rarely needed. However, a smaller, but well recognized group of patients with refractory symptoms suffers considerable impairment in their health-related of life (HRQOL), and is more likely to have co-morbid psychological difficulties and/or pronounced health concerns that limit the effectiveness of traditional medical management. For example, they may frequently seek medical attention for "diagnosis and cure," and are at risk of receiving costly and unneeded diagnostic studies and treatments. It is this group of patients, with significant psychosocial difficulties contributing to their illness, that requires more sophisticated management strategies. Many of the data in this chapter relate to these patients seen at referral (tertiary) medical centers, but the concepts presented are relevant to all settings in gastroenterology practice.

In this chapter, a multinational panel of gastroenterologists, psychiatrists, psychologists, physiologists, and health service investigators provide historical, epidemiological, and clinical information on the relationship of psychosocial factors to gut physiology, symptom presentation, illness behavior, and outcome for patients with functional gastrointestinal disorders. In addition, we provide a comprehensive review of psychological and psychopharmacological treatment trials and make recommendations regarding future study design. A large number of the studies cited refer to irritable bowel syndrome (IBS) because it is over-represented in the studies done in the FGIDs. However, we have attempted to include studies of other FGIDs where possible.

Acknowledgments: The authors would like to thank Drs. Susan Levenstein, Rona Levy, Claus Buddeberg, Nick Diamant, Giovanni Fava, Marvin Schuster, and Gabriele Moser for their critical review of this manuscript, and Ms. Carlar Blackman and Sandy Hall for their valuable assistance in the preparation of this document.

We acknowledge that this document has been prepared by a working team of only North American and European investigators. It is important to recognize that these disorders occur within a larger social and cultural environment outside the individual, for example, within the social structures of class, race, and gender. Expression and meaning of the disorders themselves and the associated illness will vary across different cultural and social groups. Little data exist that address the social and cultural patterning of FGIDs.

Background Knowledge

— Historical Aspects

Our understanding of how psychosocial factors relate to the functional gastrointestinal disorders depends partly on the changing belief systems or explanatory ("folk") models of disease through the ages. Particularly when the psychological dimensions of a clinical problem are poorly understood, the research strategies for a particular disorder are strongly influenced by the prevailing climate of interest and success in the behavioral sciences [5]. For this reason, an historical review of the evolution of thought relating to the role of psychosocial factors in gastrointestinal illness is provided.

Antiquity Through the Late Nineteenth Century

Beliefs about the interaction between mind and body in Western civilization relate historically to two competing concepts: *dualism*, which separates, and *holism*, which unifies these two [5,6]. The most widely recognized proponent of dualism was the philosopher, Rene Descartes, who in 1637 proposed the separation of the thinking mind (*res cogitans*) from the body (*res extensa*) [7]. Consistent with dualism is the concept of psychogenesis: if mind and body are separate, then psychological processes (as an external factor) can cause (rather than be a part of) medical disease.

The concept of holism, from the Greek *holos*, or whole, was proposed by Plato, Aristotle, and Hippocrates in ancient Greece [7]. It postulates that mind and body are inseparable, so the study of medical disease must take into account the whole person rather than merely the diseased part. By the seventeenth century, these holistic ideas were overshadowed by the strong influence of Cartesian duality on Western medicine. Nevertheless, holistic theory was occasionally defended by authors such as Benjamin Rush [8], who sought to integrate psychological and medical knowledge in the diagnosis and treatment of medical illness. However, after Rush's death in 1813, psychiatry was separated from medical practice and was relegated to the asylums. In addition, Pasteur's discovery of microorganisms and Koch's development of the germ theory of disease further moved medicine in the direction of duality and biologic reductionism [9]. Only in recent years (for example, with tuberculosis and AIDS), have we learned that the social environment can influence susceptibility to disease and can affect its clinical expression.

With limited technology, research through the nineteenth century developed from natural observations, which were interpreted in terms of etiology. However, an important advance occurred in 1833 with William Beaumont's studies of

Alexis St. Martin, a soldier who developed a traumatic gastric fistula. Beaumont's studies systematically reported the association of emotions such as anger and fear on gastric mucosal morphology and motor function [10], and they are probably the first psychophysiological investigations of the human gastrointestinal tract.

Observational Studies—1900 to 1959

Studies of Gastrointestinal Function

Beaumont's work was the first in a series of studies of the effects of emotion on gastrointestinal function by Cannon [11], Pavlov [12], Selye [13], Wolf [14] and Engel [15]. Almy first reported increased sigmoid motility in response to stress in IBS patients as well as in healthy subjects, and later correlated specific mood states with the pattern of motility [16,17]. These studies provided scientific evidence that the gut is physiologically responsive to emotion and environmental (stressful) stimuli. However, no efforts were made to evaluate the reciprocal effects of changes in gut physiology on psychological functioning.

Psychosomatic Investigation of Gastrointestinal Disorders

At about the same time, Franz Alexander and coworkers [18] proposed that psychodynamic conflicts and specific personality features, in addition to a biologic predisposition (Factor X), contributed to the development of certain medical diseases. The proper environmental stimulus could activate the psychological conflict in a susceptible individual, and the biologically predisposed individual would, in turn, develop or experience an exacerbation of the disease. These studies were methodologically flawed due to small sample sizes, skewed sampling of psychiatric patients, poor experimental design, uncontrolled psychological assessment, and limited disease validation [19,20]. These studies also portrayed a more limited view of psychosocial theory since emotional factors were proposed as directly causative, rather than an enabling part of the illness. Furthermore, other contributing factors such as life stress, the social environment, illness behavior, and coping style were not considered. By the 1970s this theory became unpopular among patients and health professionals because of its stigmatizing features and as a result of advances in our understanding of the underlying pathophysiology of some "psychosomatic" diseases, including inflammatory bowel disease and peptic ulcer disease [19,21]

The Biomedical Era—1960–1979

With new medical technology, the "bad press" of psychoanalytically oriented psychosomatic research moved scientists into an era of biomedical (dualistic and reductionistic) research. The search for the etiology and pathophysiology of disease took precedence over the study of the patient. Psychosocial processes were considered important, but only as secondary phenomena.

Physiological Investigation of the Gastrointestinal Tract

By the early 1970s, using improved technology, gastrointestinal physiologists were developing and testing physiological systems to better evaluate the motor and electrical activity of the gastrointestinal system. Investigators were able to describe more specifically motility abnormalities in the gut of patients with functional gastrointestinal disorders, and such abnormalities were presumed to be etiologic for these symptoms. When patients with IBS were compared to normals, they had an enhanced motor response to various environmental stimuli such as psychological stress [16], peptide hormones [22], and fatty meals [23], and it was also occasionally observed that the increased motility was associated with symptoms of pain [24].

In the late 1970s interest focused on finding physiological markers (i.e., specific myoelectrical patterns for IBS and the other functional gastrointestinal disorders). One study described a possible IBS-specific pattern of myoelectrical activity in the gut [25] although this finding was not replicated in subsequent studies [26]. Despite the efforts toward physiological specificity, it soon became evident that the correlation between altered motility and painful symptoms was poor. It took another ten years before investigators began to consider alternative explanations for the symptoms of IBS.

Psychosocial Investigation of Gastrointestinal Disorders

Psychosocial investigation during this period remained out of the mainstream of medical research and was undertaken by psychologists and psychiatrists independent of the physiological studies. The work of these investigators laid the foundation for later multidisciplinary research by contributing new methods for evaluating, in a standardized way, the psychosocial dimensions of the functional gastrointestinal disorders (see below).

The Re-emergence of Holism—1980–1990s

Until the 1980s, with only a few exceptions in certain areas of research and clinical care, the biomedical model was dominant; it was believed that technologic advances would find the cause (and cure) of many gastrointestinal disorders. However, by the late 1980s this model lost ground due to a number of factors, including: (1) the available physiological data did not fully explain all the symptoms of many patients with functional gastrointestinal complaints; (2) social and political forces, as well as newer scientifically based methods of psychosocial assessment, shifted interest away from disease activity and toward the patient; and (3) advances in brain-gut physiology yielded findings that did not fit with a purely biomedical concept [27].

Beginning in 1977, Engel proposed the Biopsychosocial Model [28–30], a modern exposition of holistic (also called systems) theory. He proposed that illness and disease are the product of the interaction of biologic, psychological, and social subsystems operating at multiple levels. This model also provided a framework to integrate biologic and psychosocial data in medical care, and it contributed to later use of multidisciplinary research methodology.

Enhancements in Psychosocial Assessment Analysis

There were several improvements in psychosocial assessment and interpretation that helped to address growing evidence for the role of psychological factors in FGIDs [31–34].

Standardization of Psychiatric Diagnosis

The publication in 1972 of criteria for psychiatric disorders by Feighner et al. [35] heralded the use of standardized psychiatric criteria for psychiatric research. This led the American Psychiatric Association to develop their Diagnostic and Statistical Manual of Psychiatric Diagnosis, which is now in its fourth edition (DSM-IV) [36]. Using standardized psychiatric criteria, investigators confirmed that patients with IBS [37,38], esophageal motility disorders [39], and functional dyspepsia [40] have higher frequencies of psychiatric diagnoses (particularly in medical clinic patients) than those with other gastrointestinal problems, and the psychiatric diagnosis often antedated the onset of the bowel disorder [37].

Study of New Psychosocial Domains

Simple analyses found medical and psychiatric diagnoses, personality, and life stress insufficient to explain the illness experience. This led to the application of new standardized questionnaires [41] to assess psychological distress [42], social support [43], coping style [44], and functional status [45].

Epidemiological Psychosocial Assessment

The question as to whether psychosocial factors are linked to the functional gastrointestinal disorders was clarified through epidemiological techniques that first identified bowel patterns in the population [46,47] and later compared large samples of patients with IBS to others with IBS not seeing physicians. It was found that the psychological disturbances reported in IBS are not specific or intrinsic to the disorder, but do characterize the subset with IBS who see physicians [48,49].

Life Events Research

Meanwhile, psychiatric investigation shifted from case reports of psychody-namic processes to larger studies linking stressful life events with the incidence and prevalence of disease. This led to the use of standardized self-report ques-tionnaires measuring life changes first developed by Holmes and Rahe [50]. Al-though the results of these studies have been criticized due to the confounding effects of recall bias and illness behavior, they were the first to correlate the number of such life events with the likelihood of impaired health status.

The limitations of the Holmes and Rahe life events scale led to new ques-tionnaires [51] that evaluated not only the presence of a life event, but also its appraisal as positive or negative, and its intensity. Self-rating scales for assessing life events were further enhanced by the development of semi-structured re-search interviews and the categorization of events (entrances/losses; desirable/undesirable, etc.) [52,53]. Using the Life Event and Difficulties Schedule (LEDS) [54], Creed et al. found that while the frequency of life events was similar in pa-tients with functional and organic gastrointestinal illness, severe negative life events were more frequent in the functional gastrointestinal group, and these events preceded the onset of the gastrointestinal symptoms [55].

Illness Behavior

These epidemiological studies led to the awareness that IBS symptoms are com-mon and are not always perceived as an illness (i.e., no or adaptive illness be-havior) by the individual. Conversely, patients with IBS who are high health care utilizers may exhibit "maladaptive illness behaviors" [56].

Behavioral Medicine

The discipline of behavioral medicine evolved from studies showing that auto-nomic or other physiological functioning (e.g., gastrointestinal secretion and motility) could be modified through operant or classical conditioning [57], or through relaxation training [58]. Fordyce's early work demonstrated how the al-teration of environmental contingencies through operant conditioning would reduce the impact of chronic pain behaviors [59]. Conditioning experiences might also contribute to the development of a psychophysiological disorder such as IBS [27,60–62]. Behavioral interventions were proposed [63], for if gastrointestinal dysfunction is learned, then it may return to more normal function through learning techniques such as biofeedback. Early efforts to im-prove disordered gastrointestinal function [64,65] through biofeedback were generally unsuccessful for functional gastrointestinal disorders (the exception being treatment of fecal incontinence [66] and constipation [67]). For the func-tional gastrointestinal disorders, alternative techniques based on relaxation training and stress management were utilized.

Health Outcome Research

In understanding illness, health outcome research could be considered an application of the biopsychosocial (systems) model [68]. Possible medical and psychosocial explanatory variables are analyzed in a way that indicates their relative contribution and their interactions in predicting a selected outcome (e.g., health care visits, disease activity).

Newer Physiological Investigations Relating to Gastrointestinal Illness

Since the 1980s the focus of physiological research has shifted from etiology, i.e., a unidirectional relationship between psychosocial events (e.g., "stress") and gastrointestinal function, to increasing awareness of the reciprocal interaction of the physiological and psychosocial processes affecting illness via the brain-gut axis [27].

Psychoneuroimmunology and Psychoneuroendocrinology

Also new is the study of natural and experimentally induced stressors on cognitive and emotional centers, and their subsequent alteration of immune function, gut physiology, and disease susceptibility [69,70]. It is now clear that the central nervous system (CNS)—through the hypothalamic-pituitary (via corticotropic releasing hormone) and noradrenergic (via locus ceruleus) systems—coordinate both behavioral and immunological adaptation to stressful situations [71].

Psychophysiological Imaging

A new approach to understanding the physiology of brain-gut relationships in the FGIDs relates to the use of brain imaging techniques, including the use of cortical evoked potentials [72,73], Positron Emission Tomography (PET scanning) [74], and functional magnetic resonance imaging (fMRI) [75]. These modalities allow investigations of the effects of various gastrointestinal stimuli (e.g., visceral distension) on activating specific areas of the brain.

— A Biopsychosocial Conceptualization

The evolution of psychosocial and physiological investigation now provides a framework to understand more fully the relationships between psychosocial processes, gastrointestinal function, disease susceptibility, and clinical outcome. As shown in figure 1, the experience of symptoms and clinical outcomes can now be understood as the product of certain interacting subsystems. Early life factors, either

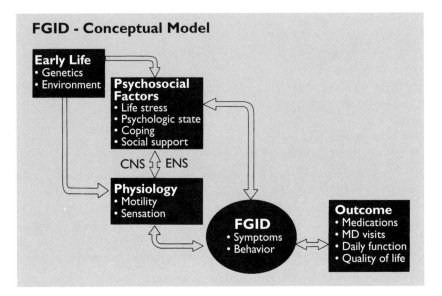

Figure 1. Biopsychosocial relationship between early life, psychosocial factors, physiology and pathology, symptom experience, and behavior and outcome.

biologic or behaviorally conditioned, will influence later psychosocial experiences, physiological functioning or susceptibility to developing a functional gastrointestinal disorder. This disorder, in turn, will be influenced by one's psychosocial milieu, leading to unique and varying effects on symptom expression and clinical outcome, as mediated through CNS/ENS (enteric nervous system) pathways.

— Psychophysiology

This section reviews the relationship between psychological distress and gastrointestinal symptoms as mediated by peripheral physiological events. Newly emerging data derived from Positron Emission Tomography (PET), Magnetic Resonance Imaging (MRI), and analysis of cortical evoked potentials is discussed Chapter 3. Three types of physiological events are considered in this section: smooth muscle contractions, striated muscle contractions, and pain in response to intraluminal distension. Additional information on the relationship of stress and gastrointestinal motility can be found elsewhere [76].

Smooth Muscle Contractions and Gastric Secretion

Esophagus

Motility disorders of the esophagus are expressed across a spectrum from occasional abnormal contractions in normal, asymptomatic individuals to the frequent, high amplitude, nonpropagated contractions that define diffuse esophageal spasm [77]. Twenty to 60% of patients with functional chest pain of esophageal origin have nonspecific esophageal motility disorders. There is a strong association between nonspecific esophageal motility disorder and psychiatric morbidity [39]. This association may reflect the effects of stress: laboratory studies suggest that loud noises [78] and experimental stress [79] can elicit increased contraction amplitude, but not tertiary contractions (i.e., non-propulsive contractions occurring independently of swallows), in normal subjects. Recently, patients with globus sensation and other pharyngoesophageal disorders have been reported to have a high frequency (over 60%) of psychiatric disorders [80].

Approximately 64% of people with symptoms of gastroesophageal reflux report that stress makes their symptoms worse [81]. Bradley and colleagues [82] investigated the effects of experimental stressors on reflux events and showed that patients with gastroesophageal reflux report increased symptoms of reflux when exposed to stressors, but the number of reflux events that actually occurred was unchanged. It is now believed that altered pain thresholds rather than abnormal esophageal motility contribute to functional chest pain [83,84] and functional gastroesophageal reflux [82].

Stomach

Psychological stress contributes to the development of peptic ulceration, possibly through interactions with other risk factors such as *Helicobacter pylori* infection and cigarette smoking [85]. Psychological stress may also affect the CNS control of acid secretion [86], or it may alter the immune response [87] thereby permitting the *Helicobacter* organism to flourish [88,89]. Gastric emptying of solids is delayed during experimentally induced stress [90], apparently through an inhibition of antral motility [91]. This may be relevant to the understanding of a subgroup of patients with functional dyspepsia [91].

Small Intestine

Three small bowel motor abnormalities have been described in patients with irritable bowel syndrome:

(1) *Discrete clustered contractions (DCC)* are brief bursts of contractions lasting about 10–15 seconds and occurring at intervals of 1–3 minutes. Patients

with irritable bowel syndrome are more likely than healthy controls to display this pattern [92,93] and may report abdominal pain in association with this motility pattern [92]. However, this finding is not specific to IBS [94].

(2) *Giant contractions* are said to occur if the contraction amplitude is greater than 75 mm Hg. These contractions are also seen in healthy subjects, but only in patients with IBS are they associated with reports of pain [95].

(3) *Hyper-reactivity* to stress or other provocative stimuli is also characteristic of IBS. Kellow and colleagues [95] have shown that inflation of a balloon in the terminal ileum elicits more contractions, and patients with IBS show a greater increase in activity than healthy controls. As described below, a similar pattern of hyper-reactivity is seen in the colon in patients with IBS. Since the contractions that are elicited are nonperistaltic, this motor hyper-reactivity to distension could contribute to symptoms of altered bowel habits by slowing the movement of chyme towards the colon.

Both experimentally induced and naturally occurring stressors disrupt the cyclic pattern of motility normally seen during fasting [96] as well as decrease the overall amount of contradictions [96–98]. Although patients with IBS show more discrete clustered contractions than healthy controls under resting conditions [92,93], this type of contractile activity is suppressed by experimental stress [97]. Cann and colleagues [99] reported that stress significantly speeded mouth-to-cecum transit time in diarrhea-predominant patients with IBS and significantly slowed transit time in constipation-predominant patients.

Colon

Patients with IBS have exaggerated motility in response to any type of stimulation. This hyper-reactivity occurs in response to psychological stress [17,100–103] as well as balloon distension [104,105], eating [106], and injection of cholecystokinin [22,107]. The contractions observed following experimental stressors and other provocative stimuli are principally nonperistaltic contractions, which could contribute to the symptoms of IBS by retarding the movement of gas and stool towards to rectum and anus. No specific pattern of motility has been identified that is unique to patients with IBS.

Smooth Muscle Tone

Some reports suggest that smooth muscle tone is increased in IBS [108]. Mental arithmetic stress has been shown to cause an immediate increase in smooth muscle tone in the rectum [109]. Eating also reliably alters smooth muscle tone in the colon and rectum [110,111].

Striated Muscle Contractions

The contribution of abnormal striated muscle contractions to functional gastrointestinal symptoms is limited to the pharyngoesophageal and
anorectal areas of the gastrointestinal tract, where these muscles participate in
swallowing and defecation.

Aerophagia

The excessive ingestion of air may underlie many cases of unexplained
upper and lower gastrointestinal symptoms [112–114]. The symptom most frequently reported by aerophagic patients is belching unrelated to meals, but they
also report bloating or abdominal distension, excessive flatus, a feeling of incomplete evacuation, and relief of abdominal pain with defecation or flatus.
The most common mechanism for aerophagia is excessively frequent swallowing. Every swallow carries 3–5 ml or more of air into the esophagus where
peristalsis may carry it into the stomach and small intestine. The frequency of
swallowing increases with stress or emotional arousal [114] and decreases with relaxation [115]. Thus, increased frequency of swallowing could mediate the effects
of stress on gastrointestinal symptoms, especially those related to bowel gas.

There is a small group of patients who have difficulty swallowing due to a fear
of choking or aspirating [116–118]. Such functional dysphagia appears to be due
to an inhibition and/or incoordination of the voluntary phase of swallowing.

Rumination Syndrome

This disorder is characterized by the frequent regurgitation, in the absence of nausea, of previously ingested food into the mouth where it is chewed
and then reswallowed or spit out [119]. Regurgitation involves a voluntary sequence of behaviors. It may be preceded by excessive air swallowing or by stimulating the palate with the tongue or fingers [120]. This is followed by descent of
the diaphragm and relaxation of the lower esophageal sphincter. The critical
event, however, is a brisk contraction of the abdominus rectus muscles to force
the contents of the stomach up the esophagus.

Rumination occurs frequently in mentally challenged and/or institutionalized
patients, especially children [121,122]. However, it may also occur in children
and adults of normal intelligence and has been seen as a component of an eating disorder. In children and mentally challenged adults, rumination often occurs
as a self-stimulatory behavior [123,124], but it may also develop as a means to gain
attention from adults [125,126]. Adult ruminators of normal intelligence often describe rumination as an idle pleasurable habit that is voluntary. Other adults first
present with a complaint of vomiting that usually occurs 10–30 minutes after eating. Gastrointestinal motility is normal in rumination [127].

Pelvic Floor Dyssynergia and Pelvic Floor Spasm

The symptoms which most people refer to when they call themselves constipated [128] are straining to defecate, a feeling of incomplete evacuation after defecation, and in a few people, digital facilitation of evacuation [67,128–131]. Preston and Lennard-Jones [132] were the first to describe the physiological basis for this type of constipation. During defecation, the puborectalis muscle (part of the pelvic floor) and external anal sphincter muscles should relax to open up the angle between the anus and the rectum and to allow the anal canal to dilate enough for stool to pass. In many patients with chronic constipation, however, the pelvic floor muscles fail to relax, or they may paradoxically contract during attempted defecation.

Chronically constipated patients are as a group more anxious and depressed than the general population [128,133–135]. This may be due to the tendency for anxious people to have tonically tense skeletal muscles [136]. Leroi and colleagues [137] have shown that a history of sexual abuse is commonly reported by women with pelvic floor dyssynergia. This history may predispose to increased pelvic floor tone.

Proctalgia Syndromes

Levator ani syndrome, which is characterized by chronic or recurring dull aching rectal pain, is also believed to be due to tense pelvic floor muscles [67]. It is distinguished from proctalgia fugax where the pain, presumably also related to pelvic floor spasm, is more short lived. The majority of patients with levator ani syndrome have increased tension in the pelvic floor muscles [138,139], and levator ani syndrome is often associated with constipation [138]. In an uncontrolled study, biofeedback training to teach relaxation of the pelvic floor muscles was associated with relief of rectal pain and with reductions in the severity of constipation [138].

Altered Perception of Intraluminal Distension

In recent years, investigators have reported that IBS, functional dyspepsia, and functional esophageal pain are associated with a lower threshold for reporting pain or other symptoms in response to intraluminal distension. This has led to speculation that altered visceral sensitivity is the pathophysiological mechanism common to all these disorders [140,141]. The evidence for and against this hypothesis is briefly summarized below.

Functional Esophageal Pain

Patients with functional esophageal pain are more likely to report pain at low volumes of esophageal balloon distension than are healthy controls [142,

143]. However, Bradley and Richter [144] reported a signal detection study which suggests that this increased sensitivity is due to response bias, i.e., a tendency to report pain at lower thresholds for psychological reasons unrelated to actual differences in receptor sensitivity. (See Whitehead, Delvaux, and colleagues [145] for further information on the distinction between perceptual sensitivity and perceptual response bias.)

Functional Dyspepsia

Several research teams have shown that patients with functional dyspepsia report bloating and discomfort or pain at a lower volume of intragastric balloon distension than healthy controls [146–150]. No studies published to date have distinguished perceptual sensitivity from perceptual response bias in patients with functional dyspepsia. However, in healthy subjects, distraction raises perception thresholds and increased attention (warning signal) lowers the threshold [151].

Irritable Bowel Syndrome

Ritchie [152] was the first to show that patients with IBS report pain at a lower volume of balloon distension in the sigmoid colon. This observation has been replicated by more than twenty subsequent studies. New observations that have extended Ritchie's original observations are as follows.

(1) Increased pain sensitivity in patients with IBS appears to be specific to the gastrointestinal tract, since these patients do not show lower thresholds for cutaneous pain [105,153–157].

(2) Although their cutaneous pain thresholds are normal, patients with IBS show increased sensitivity to intraluminal distension in the esophagus [158,159], stomach [157], and small intestine [98,155], as well as the colon, and they are more likely to notice the occurrence of the migrating motor complex in the duodenum than are healthy controls [160].

(3) Some studies [160,161] suggest that patients with IBS have increased sensitivity for nonpainful intensities of intraluminal distension, reporting sensations of flatus and urge to defecate at a lower volume of distension. However, other studies [108,162,163] failed to find lower thresholds for nonpainful sensations.

(4) Rectal distension activates a different part of the brain in patients with IBS as compared to healthy controls (lateral prefrontal cortex instead of anterior cingulate gyrus) [74].

(5) Stress [164] and a warning signal that increases attention to the distending stimulus [151] appear to lower the threshold at which pain is reported whereas relaxation [154,164] and distraction by another task [151] appear to raise the threshold for discomfort.

(6) When signal detection methodology is used to separate perceptual sensitivity from perceptual response bias, patients with IBS are not found to have increased perceptual sensitivity for intraluminal distension, although they do report pain at lower volumes of distension when tested using methods that confound perceptual sensitivity with response bias [108].

There is continuing controversy over whether the altered threshold to report pain in IBS represents a biological marker for IBS [163] or is due to perceptual response bias [165]. However, the increased sensitivity due to intraluminal distension could give rise to functional gastrointestinal symptoms since the predominant complaint relates to increased pain. Two groups have shown that changes in pain thresholds are correlated with changes in clinical symptoms of abdominal pain over a 3-month period of treatment [163,166].

— Brain-Gut Interactions

The above data support clinical observations that psychological and environmental stressors will affect intestinal motor and sensory activity (i.e., how symptoms are experienced). Furthermore, gastrointestinal symptoms have reciprocal effects on one's psychological state. The brain-gut axis is a theoretical model that describes the bi-directional neural pathways that link cognitive and emotional centers in the brain with the neuroendocrine centers, the enteric nervous system and the immune system [141,167]. For example, extrinsic (vision, smell, etc.) or enteroceptive (emotion, thought) information have, through their neural connections from higher centers, the capability to affect gastrointestinal sensation, motility, and secretion. Conversely, viscerotopic effects (e.g., nociception) reciprocally affect central pain perception, mood, and behavior [141].

Regulation of these anatomic connections occurs via brain-gut neurotransmitters including: vasoactive intestinal peptide (VIP), 5-hydroxytryptamine (5-HT), Substance P, calcitonin gene-related polypeptide (CGRP), cholecystokinin (CCK), and the enkephalins, among others. Since neurotransmitters are not site specific, they have varied influences on gastrointestinal, endocrine and immune function, as well as human behavior, depending on their location. As examples:

(1) The enkephalins can variably effect pain control [168], gastrointestinal motility [169], feeding activity [170], emotional behavior, and immunity [171];

(2) Administration of CCK increases gut motility and also elicits postprandial satiety in animals [172], and may influence conditions like bulimia nervosa [173];

(3) The 5-HT receptors, depending on the site of activity in brain and gut, are implicated in the functional gastrointestinal disorders [174–176], migraine headache [177], alcoholism, and disorders of mood [178];

(4) Lymphocytes, mast cells and macrophages contain receptors that respond to neurotransmitters and neuropeptides (e.g., endorphins, VIP), thereby providing the basis for stress and emotion to influence gastrointestinal inflammation and immune function [179,180], and contributing to the pathogenesis of visceral hyperalgesia [181];

(5) Finally, nitric oxide (NO) can increase the expression of proto-oncogenes (e.g., c-fos) involved in the transcriptional control of genes that encode production of certain neuropeptides (e.g., dynorphin), that lead to long-term changes in brain or gut function producing visceral sensitization [182].

Given these findings, a unifying hypothesis to explain the functional gastrointestinal disorders [27,183] is that they result from dysregulation of "brain-gut" and neuroenteric systems, much like anovulatory bleeding is a dysregulation of hypothalamic-pituitary-ovarian function rather than a disease of any of these structures. When compared to healthy subjects, patients with FGID have increased motor reactivity to various stressors including balloon distension, food, various peptides, and physical and psychological stressors [184,185], albeit with physiological variation in response between individuals, and for the same individual over time. Furthermore, patients with functional esophageal [186, 187], gastroduodenal [188], and bowel [105] disorders have decreased thresholds for gut pain in response to balloon distension and other stimuli (visceral hypersensitivity).

The role of the CNS in modulating motility is supported by evidence that:

(1) The motility disturbances in IBS disappear during sleep [92];
(2) MMC frequency decreases and propagating velocity increases progressively with alertness and arousal [92,189];
(3) Patients with IBS may have a different EEG sleep pattern than healthy subjects [190]; and
(4) Experimental stressors appear to have linked effects leading to simultaneous increases in EEG beta power activity and colonic motility that are significantly greater in patients with IBS [191].

The role of the CNS in modulating visceral perception [141] is supported by recent studies using PET, which differentiates patients with IBS from normals, based on regional cerebral perfusion. When evaluating the CNS response to rectal distension, or even the anticipation of rectal distension, patients with IBS, compared to controls, fail to activate the anterior cingulate cortex, an area of the limbic system associated with active opiate binding, but do activate the pre-frontal cortex, an area associated with hypervigilance and anxiety [74]. Therefore, patients with IBS may fail to use CNS down-regulating mechanisms in response to incoming or anticipated visceral pain. Instead, they may activate an area of the brain that amplifies pain perception.

The varied influence of environmental stress, personality, or thoughts and emotions on gut function effected through neurotransmitter release or receptor activity may explain the remarkable differences in symptoms that exist for patients having these disorders. For example, patients with IBS can have both constipation and diarrhea, or disturbed motility without pain, or even pain without dysmotility ("altered perception of normal function"). It also helps explain how psychosocial trauma (e.g., physical or sexual abuse history [192]) or poor coping style (e.g., "catastrophizing" [193]) profoundly affect symptom severity, daily function, and health outcome.

Based on these data, it is no longer reasonable to try to discriminate whether physiological or psychological factors cause pain or other bowel symptoms. Both are operative, and the task is to determine the degree to which each contributes and is remediable.

— Life Stress, Abuse History, and Other Psychological Factors

In this chapter the term "stress" will be used to describe environmental events ("stressful life events" or "stressors") or stressors such as loss of a close relative or childhood abuse [194]. Stress is also considered in the context of incongruity between the stressors and one's adaptation such as coping and calling on social supports. The term "stress" may also be used to indicate symptoms of anxiety and depression. These symptoms (e.g., of anxiety and depression) will be referred to as "psychological distress" (see section on Clinical Assessment, below, and Table 3) except when they are sufficiently marked to merit a psychiatric diagnosis (see Table 1); these are briefly described at the end of this chapter.

Accurate measurement of stressful life events and psychiatric disorder is essential for research purposes; otherwise inaccurate results may occur. However, the clinician may not choose to adopt these research tools in clinical practice since they are time-consuming and require specific training. Information relevant to clinical practice is provided in the section below on assessment.

Life Stress

Methodological Issues
Research Interview vs. Self-administered Questionnaire
The "gold standard" of life stress measurement has been the interview-based method set by the Life Events and Difficulties Schedule (LEDS) [54]. Interviewers with specific training use a semi-structured approach to elicit all possible stressful situations and to probe for details. The rating of severity is not made by the interviewer, who may have been influenced by the subject's psychological state or attitude to the event or its difficulty; it is made by an independent body of trained raters who are unaware of the respondent's attitude and who are blind to whether the subject belongs to the experimental or control group. Such a method can rarely be used because of the necessary research expertise and expense, but it has been used in five studies of gastrointestinal disorders [53,55, 195–197]. Self-administered questionnaires, on the other hand, are easy and inexpensive to administer. They can overcome any bias of an untrained interviewer and provide important subjective data. However, questionnaire data are influenced by personality traits which affect how a respondent reacts to stressful events and which may result in selective or distorted recall.

Timing of Events
Since most patients with functional gastrointestinal disorders have experienced their symptoms for several years prior to clinic attendance, it is difficult to know whether life stress precedes or follows illness onset. A stressful life event, (e.g., divorce) may be considered etiologic only if it occurred before the onset of a FGID. However, it may be important to determine whether stress exacerbates FGID, in addition to ascertaining whether stress preceded onset of the FGID; as this will affect the treatment strategy. Self-administered questionnaires cannot accurately date life events in relation to onset of symptoms because they cannot prompt respondents or check the accuracy of the replies [198,199], whereas trained interviewers can achieve an accurate record extending back over several years [200,201].

Type of Life Events
Measurement of life events does not simply include counting events in the months prior to onset of disorder. Account must be taken of the types of events. Those that are threatening to the individual are often of greatest significance.

In FGID, for example, the dissolution of intimate relationships is closely associated with onset [53]. Similarly, the development of peptic ulcer disease is *not* preceded by a general increase of life events [202], but is preceded by an increase in life events of high threat to the individual, especially those causing goal frustration [53].

Findings

One study of patients with IBS [203] used a self-administered questionnaire to record stressful life events every three months. The results were analyzed controlling for neuroticism (to allow for response bias). A significant relationship between symptom exacerbation and stressful situations over the preceding three months was found. Stressful life events also had a significant impact on health care visits and disability days. Craig and Creed [55] demonstrated a clear excess of severely stressful life events or chronic social difficulties (e.g., bereavement, marital separation, court appearance with threat of imprisonment) immediately before the onset of functional bowel disorders (60–66% of FGID patients had experienced severe life events compared to 25% of healthy controls). The level of stress in functional gastrointestinal disorder was similar to that occurring in patients who had taken a deliberate overdose of psychiatric medication.

From these data, we conclude that for patients in a gastrointestinal clinic, social stress plays an important part in explaining exacerbation of symptoms and treatment seeking.

Sexual and Physical Abuse

Recent studies have highlighted the high prevalence of sexual and physical abuse history in clinical settings and their affects on health outcome in gastrointestinal as well as several other medical and psychiatric conditions [204].

Methodological Issues

The measurement of sexual and physical abuse has not been studied in as much detail as stressful life events, and as yet, there is no agreement between researchers as to the optimal method of eliciting these data. Self-administered questionnaires preserve the anonymity of the respondent but still have no way of controlling for the effect of selective recall or selective disclosure.

Validity of Data

It is difficult to confirm whether a prior history of abuse has occurred. Verification from police records, family, or acquaintances grossly underestimates the true frequency of abuse; alternatively, within a referral clinical population, some have argued that patients who have co-morbid psychosocial difficulties may over-report certain experiences as abusive [205]. Furthermore, within psychiatric populations, the concept of "false memory syndrome" has been identified: a small percentage of patients in therapy may fabricate an abusive event in response to unintentional, but leading questions or suggestions by a psychotherapist. For research purposes, accuracy requires [204]:

(1) the evaluation must be confidential;
(2) an interview by a trained investigator in a supportive environment;
(3) the questions must not be coercive and should contain operational definitions (e.g., *"Has anyone ever touched your sex organs against your wishes?"* rather than *"Have you ever been abused?"*); and
(4) attention to the psychological profile of the patient must be considered.

In clinical practice, in contrast to research, the patient's disclosure of an abusive experience should be considered truthful, unless the data suggest otherwise [204]. The physician's belief in what the patient reports has implications for preserving the physician-patient relationship. Moreover, information on sexual and physical abuse has implications for patient management.

Types of Abuse
The varying criteria for defining abuse lead to wide ranges in the prevalence for this condition (from 6% to 62%) [206]. Because there can be several types of sexual or physical abuse (threat of abuse, exhibitionism, fondling or contact abuse, battering or physical abuse, and penetration or rape), it is relevant to determine which types of abuse lead to poorer health status. Among gastrointestinal patients, it has been found that rape (penetration), multiple experiences, and abuse experienced as life threatening are associated with poorer health status [207]. This has led to the development of an abuse severity score which for research purposes can be used to quantitate abuse severity (from 0 to 6) and predict adverse health outcome [208].

Findings
Prevalence
Studies suggest a strong epidemiological relationship between self-reported sexual and physical abuse history and functional gastrointestinal disorders [204]. In the first study [209] of 206 female gastrointestinal clinic attendees, rape or incest was reported by 31% of patients with functional gastrointestinal diagnoses compared to 18% for those with organic diagnoses. Forty-four percent of women reported any form of sexual or physical abuse but physicians were aware of this only in 17%; and 30% of the victims had not previously disclosed this history to anyone.

Later studies found similar high frequency rates (30–56%) from referral centers in the United States and Europe [210–213]. However, high frequencies of abuse (approaching 50%) are also reported by patients with chronic or recurrent painful functional conditions that are not gastrointestinal (e.g., pelvic pain, headaches, fibromyalgia) and certain behavioral disorders (e.g., bulimia nervosa, morbid obesity, substance abuse) [214,215]. Furthermore, the frequencies of abuse in primary care settings are lower (about one-half) [216]. Therefore, the association of abuse with FGID or any other chronic painful condition also depends on the clinical setting in which the patient is seen.

Consequences of Abuse on Health Status
Abusive Experiences Affect Health Status [204]. Gastrointestinal patients with abuse histories reported 70% more severe pain ($p<0.0001$); 40% greater psychological distress ($p<0.0001$); spent over two and one-half times more days in bed in the previous three months (11.9 vs. 4.5 days, $p<0.0007$); had almost twice as poor daily function ($p<0.0001$); saw physicians more often (8.7 vs. 6.7 visits over six months ($p<0.03$); and even underwent more surgical procedures (4.9 vs. 3.8 procedures, $p<0.04$) [192]. A diagnosis of functional gastrointestinal disorder has additional independent adverse effects on health status [192]. These findings also apply to patients with abuse histories seen in primary care settings, who report more non-gastrointestinal symptoms and operations than non-abused patients [216]. In a population study [217], abuse history was found to increase the odds of visiting a physician.

Possible Mechanisms
An abuse history is not etiologic for any of the functional gastrointestinal disorders but is associated with a tendency to communicate psychological distress through physical symptoms [204,218]. The co-occurrence of abuse and functional gastrointestinal disorder makes the symptoms more severe and refractory to usual treatment. This combination also increases the likelihood of comorbid psychiatric disorders and other psychological disturbances [219,220] (e.g., post-traumatic stress disorder, anxiety, depression, somatization).

Abuse or associated difficulties may: (1) lower the threshold of gastrointestinal symptom experience or increase intestinal motility; (2) modify the person's appraisal of bodily symptoms (i.e., increase medical help-seeking) through inability to control the symptoms; and (3) lead to unwarranted feelings of guilt and responsibility, making spontaneous disclosure unlikely [220].

Over time, the co-occurrence of these factors can produce a chronic state of symptom amplification originating either at the CNS level (hypervigilance to body sensations) or gut level (visceral hypersensitivity and conditioned hypermotility). Eventually, a "vicious cycle" of health care seeking, refractoriness, and repeated referral develops, if the health care system provides only symptomatic treatments and does not address the abuse issues.

Psychiatric Disorders

Our understanding of the relationship between functional gastrointestinal disorders and psychiatric disorders has advanced greatly since the early accounts [221,222], largely through the use of validated diagnostic criteria for psychiatric disorders such as the International Classification of Disease (ICD-10) [223], Classification of Mental and Behavioral Disorders (WHO 1992), and the American Psychiatric Diagnostic and Statistical Manual of Mental Disorders (DSM-IV) [36].

Methodological Issues
The arguments regarding assessment of psychiatric disorders by research interview or self-administered questionnaire are similar to those outlined above for assessment of life events. In general, rates of psychiatric disorders tend to be lower and more accurate when obtained by interview rather than self-administered questionnaires. Some structured interviews measure lifetime as well as current psychiatric disorders [36].

Among patients with IBS studied at medical centers [211,224], the most frequent diagnostic categories are: (1) anxiety disorders (Panic and Generalized Anxiety Disorder); (2) mood disorders (Major Depression and Dysthymic Disorder); and (3) somatoform disorders (Hypochondriasis and Somatization Disorder). Since anxiety and depressive disorders overlap so greatly, the term "psychiatric disorder" in this chapter will refer to anxiety, depressive, or mixed disorders.

Findings
The results of recent studies using standardized research interviews for current psychiatric diagnosis and an adequate sample size (730 patients) are reported in Table 1. It can be seen that between 42% and 61% of patients with functional bowel disorders seen in gastroenterology clinics have a current psychiatric diagnosis (usually anxiety or depression), and this is significantly greater than that seen in the control groups (<25%). The presence of psychiatric disorder is even higher (up to 94%) in studies from tertiary care centers when lifetime psychiatric diagnosis is considered [37,224].

Panic disorder has been frequently linked both to irritable bowel syndrome [224–226] and functional chest pain [226], and these gastrointestinal symptoms

Table 1. Prevalence of Psychiatric Disorder in Functional Bowel Disorder/ Irritable Bowel Syndrome Using Standardized Research Psychiatric Interviews

	Number of Subjects	Instrument for Psychiatric Disorder	Functional Bowel Disorders	Organic Gastrointestinal Disorder	Healthy Controls
McDonald, Boucher (1980) [387]	32 [FBD]	CIS	53%	20%	—
Colgan et al. (1988) [246]	37 [FBD]	CIS	57%	6%	—
Corney, Stanton (1990) [388]	48 [IBS]	CIS	48%	—	—
Craig, Brown (1984) [53]	79 [FBD]	PSE	42%	18%	—
Ford et al. (1987) [195]	44 [IBS]	PSE	42%	6%	8%
Toner et al. (1990) [38]	44 [IBS]	DIS	61%	—	14%
Blanchard et al. (1990) [389]	68 [IBS]	DIS	56%	25%	18%

Abbreviations: CIS = Clinical Interview Schedule; DIS = Diagnostic Interview Schedule; FBD = functional bowel disorder (i.e., consecutive non-organic gastrointestinal disorders in the clinic); IBS = irritable bowel syndrome; PSE = present state examination.

improve when the concomitant panic disorder is successfully treated [225,227]. However, less than 5% of patients with IBS seen by gastroenterologists meet criteria for panic disorder. It is possible that the bowel symptoms seen in panic disorder do not represent IBS, but rather a gastrointestinal response to extreme anxiety. It is also possible that patients with IBS with panic disorder are experiencing "incomplete panic attacks," where the physical (i.e., gastrointestinal symptoms) are more prominent than the behavioral symptoms of panic disorder.

Like abuse history, psychiatric disorder is greater among patients with IBS seen in referral centers than patients with IBS seen in community clinics. One population-based study [228] (part of the NIMH Epidemiological Catchment Area Study) demonstrated that the prevalence of psychiatric diagnosis among persons with symptoms typical of functional gastrointestinal disorder was higher than those without gastrointestinal symptoms. The former group were more likely to have experienced a lifetime episode of major depression (7.5% vs. 2.9%), panic disorder (2.5% vs. 0.7%), or agoraphobia (10.0% vs. 3.6%). Even higher rates of major depression (13.4%), panic (5.2%), and agoraphobia (17.8%) occurred in those subjects who complained of multiple gastrointestinal symptoms.

Other Psychological Factors

This section addresses other psychosocial domains, personality and psychological distress, in addition to those previously discussed (life stress, abuse, psychiatric diagnosis).

Methodological Issues

There are a number of measurement artifacts that can produce unreliable data from self-administered questionnaires of psychological distress.

Standardization of Measures for Functional Gastrointestinal Disorders
The majority of psychosocial questionnaires used in functional gastrointestinal disorders research were normalized to psychiatrically ill or healthy populations. They include items concerning diarrhea and pain, for example, which are regarded as measures of distress; in FGID patients, these symptoms may in fact be due to the bowel condition under study.

This problem may be partially resolved by comparing the results on FGID patients to norms that are available for patients with organic gastrointestinal disorders who also have abdominal pain, diarrhea and who seek medical treatment [229]. It is preferable to reanalyze results excluding the "somatic" items [230].

Patient Status
Some studies have addressed the issue that psychological factors may be more closely linked to patient status (i.e., seeking medical consultation) than to any specific gastrointestinal disorder [48,49,231].

Response or Presentation Style
Some patients with IBS have a greater need to portray themselves as having socially desirable characteristics than some psychiatric patient groups or normal controls. This may influence the way they answer questionnaires (by endorsing socially approved items), and it may affect the accuracy of certain psychological tests [38,232] or the extent of their placebo response [233]. These characteristics are also shown by patients with other physical disorders [234] and chronic pain [235].

Findings
Personality
Well controlled studies using healthy and/or medical patient groups as controls, with the Eysenck Personality Inventory (EPI), the Spielberger Trait Anxi-

ety Inventory (STAT-T), or the Minnesota Multiphasic Personality Inventory (MMPI) suggest that patients with IBS are more neurotic and anxious in their personality scores than people without health problems or a nonclinical population with similar gastrointestinal complaints [32,48,105,153,231,236–239]. However, these findings also hold for clinic patients with other medical disorders, so there is not support for a personality profile that is unique to IBS.

As stated before, the reported association between personality scores and IBS may reflect the selection factor, in which individuals with psychosocial difficulties who also have IBS come into health care facilities [48,49].The second explanation is that the experience of chronic symptoms of pain and bodily dysfunction leads to raised scores on personality measures [240].

Psychological State

Studies evaluating psychological distress (as symptoms of anxiety and depression) have used medical or psychiatric controls and the following questionnaires: Spielberger State Anxiety Inventory (STAT-S); the Middlesex Hospital Questionnaire (MHQ); Symptom Checklist-90 (SCL-90); and the Beck Depression Inventory (BDI) [37,105,153,192,231,236,241–244]. With psychiatric patients as the comparison group [33,38,234,239,245], the findings replicate those observed in the personality literature. Patients with IBS, like other medical patient groups, show elevated levels of depression, anxiety, and somatization relative to healthy controls. However, the psychological mechanisms operating to produce this association remain unclear [38].

Health Beliefs

The cognitive model attempts to explain why FGID patients develop and maintain concerns and beliefs that their gut symptoms indicate cancer or other serious illness even after a negative work-up or reassurance by the physician. An important methodological consideration is the tendency for people who are distressed or depressed to have increased anxiety about bowel symptoms and related health concerns [246].

Cognitive-Behavioral Theory. Cognitive-behavioral theory provides a framework for understanding a broad range of patient experiences, including physiological responses and observable behavior as well as health beliefs. Some beliefs relevant to gastrointestinal disorders include ideas about when it is appropriate to seek health care, what may be gained from a health care provider, whether friends or family support or criticize complaints, and beliefs about the seriousness of one's illness, such as "*I may lose control of my bowels*" or "*my bowel symptoms indicate serious gut disease/cancer.*" Typical of the inputs that may maintain these beliefs are (1) news of bowel disorder in a relative or reference to this in the media or (2) a normal twinge of abdominal discomfort, which is misinterpreted as representing disease. The consequent increase in health concerns may lead to a physiological response, e.g., diarrhea, which is further interpreted as indicating the veracity of the underlying fears of loss of control or serious pathology in the bowel. This increase in anxiety can also lead to behavioral changes, such as change in diet, refusal to go out or far away from a toilet, and seeking medical treatment [247,248]. This cognitive model is not confined to functional gastrointestinal disorders; it holds across a wide range of hypochondriacal and health concern presentations [248–252].

Selective Attention and Somatic Preoccupation. People may selectively attend to those cognitions and perceptions that confirm their explanatory model of illness. Thus abdominal sensations may be regarded as evidence of serious bowel pathology. In addition, the patient may selectively dismiss information or sensory input that is inconsistent with their beliefs [249]. The patient may ignore the fact that the pain ceases once the bowel is emptied, or the fact that serious pathology would have declared itself over the many years of the illness. Accordingly, the role of other contributing factors such as life stressors, psychological distress, overwork, interpersonal conflict, or loss may be minimized or selected out of their conceptualization of their condition. There is some empirical support for this model. Colgan et al. found that FGID patients with psychiatric disorders were more convinced that their symptoms represented physical disease than patients who actually had an organic gastrointestinal disorder. Patients with FGID also had more difficulty expressing their personal feelings [246]. Similarly, Drossman and colleagues [48] found that individuals with IBS seeing a gastroenterologist were significantly more likely to minimize psychological and stress related factors in their lives relative to a comparison group of individuals with IBS who did not consult specialists for their symptoms (i.e., IBS non-patients). More recently, Levy's group found that patients with IBS were less likely to report an association between IBS symptoms and stressors relative to IBS non-patients [253].

Illness Attitudes and Depression. Patients with IBS commonly have concerns, depression, and psychological symptoms [254], but do not see them as important as the physical symptoms. Toner et al. [234] found that patients with IBS presenting to a psychiatrist did not hold a pronounced negative view of themselves while patients with major depression did. This was in spite of the fact that both groups of patients were similarly depressed, based on a depression questionnaire. Patients with IBS have been found to have high moral standards and a heightened need for approval [232]. They are especially wary of the negative stigma and moral connotations associated with a psychological explanation for their symptoms.

Gomborone et al. found that patients with IBS, compared to depressed patients seeing a psychiatrist, showed higher scores on hypochondriacal beliefs, disease phobia, and bodily preoccupation scales of the Illness Attitude Scale [255].

Health Care Seeking. The primary factors differentiating patients with IBS seeking help from a gastroenterologist from those people in the community with IBS symptoms who do not consult (IBS non-consultors) are greater pain severity and greater duration of pain [48,49,256–258]. Once the severity of pain is accounted for, people who seek treatment for IBS have been shown to have increased psychological distress [48,238] or excessive anxiety that their symptoms indicate severe bowel disorder [258].

In addition, Thompson et al. [259] found that the subgroup of patients who choose to further consult specialists were less likely to see a link between stress and their IBS symptoms. Following investigations, even with specialists, some patients may still feel that something has been overlooked, and will seek out other gastrointestinal specialists or alternative treatments [260,261] in the persistent search for an answer.

A satisfactory consultation with the gastroenterologist leads to a reduction of overall anxiety, less fear that the symptoms represent cancer, and a reduction in the patient's preoccupation and helplessness in relation to the pain [262]. However, patients who have increased health concerns, together with anxiety and/or depression, may fail to be reassured by the doctor; they may interpret negative investigations according to their established beliefs that the illness cannot be detected by doctors, which in turn increases fear. Lack of a clear diagnosis and explanation from the doctor may therefore contribute to increased health concerns and the subsequent chance of further consultations.

Illness Behavior

The term "illness behavior" refers to the ways people perceive, interpret, and react to somatic sensations that may be interpreted as symptoms of disease. Although there is a wide range of "normal" behavior relating to illness, abnormal illness behavior of concern to the health care provider exists at two ends of a continuum. Denial of illness may lead some people with inflammatory bowel disease, cancer, or other serious illness to postpone medical consultation, when earlier detection could lead to more effective management. At the other extreme, persons interpret normal bodily sensations as evidence of disease, which leads them to seek medical treatment and report symptoms and disability inconsistent with the physician's assessment. This latter type of illness behavior may elicit negative feelings in the physician [263].

There may be a number of behaviors that are the result of interpreting normal bodily sensations as evidence of disease and seeking medical treatment repeatedly.

Symptom Reports. Patients with IBS report approximately twice as many non-gastrointestinal disorders as the general population [61,264]. The kinds of symptoms and disorders reported vary greatly, but disorders for which there is a well-documented association include fibromyalgia [265], dysmenorrhea [266, 267], and asthma [268]. Patients with IBS also score higher than healthy controls on the somatization scale of the SCL-90R [49], and on several subscales of the Illness Behavior Questionnaire [48,269].

Health Care Utilization. Patients with IBS make 2–3 times as many visits to physicians for non-gastrointestinal complaints [3,61,264]. Keeling and Fielding [270] reported that 50% of their patients with IBS had received two or more surgical procedures, and several investigators have documented an excess incidence of hospitalizations [61] and hysterectomy in patients with IBS [271,272].

Disability Days. In a recent survey of 5,400 United States households [3], people meeting criteria for IBS reported missing an average of 13.4 days from work or usual activities due to illness, compared to 4.9 days for the whole sample. Similar results were found for almost all of the functional gastrointestinal disorders.

Illness Behaviors Derived from Childhood Social Learning via Reinforcement and Modeling. Somatization or health care seeking behavior, including using illness to avoid unpleasant work or interpersonal situations [273], may be learned during childhood [60,61,274,275]. Adults with IBS are more likely to report that their parents gave them gifts or special privileges when they were ill as children and to report that their parents displayed illness behavior [60–62]. Moreover, the children of IBS parents are more likely to be brought to the pediatrician for abdominal pain and diarrhea [273].

Health-Related Quality Of Life (HRQOL)

What is Health-Related Quality of Life?

Health-related quality of life (HRQOL) is a broad concept that incorporates the patient's perception of the illness experience and of his/her functional status as related to the illness. It is influenced by social, cultural, physiological, and disease-related factors [276,277]. Some investigators have included symptom frequency and severity as a part of HRQOL [278], and some have focused on patients' concerns about the anticipated consequences of their illness (e.g., loss of bowel control or fear of cancer) [279] or on measures of psychological well-being [280]. However, what distinguishes HRQOL from other health outcome measures is the concept of the impact of the illness. This impact is assessed in relation to (1) the patient's role and function (i.e., ability to carry out activities of daily living such as work, social and family interaction, and self-care); (2) the patient's perceptions of what his/her needs are and whether they are being met (e.g., independence, attractiveness); (3) perceptions of the illness; and (4) concerns about the consequences of the illness.

Measurement Issues: Types of Health-Related Quality of Life Instruments

Two approaches have been taken to the measurement of health-related quality of life (HRQOL): (1) generic instruments that are designed to be applicable to all medical disorders; and (2) disease- specific instruments that assess the unique effects of specific diseases on quality of life [281,282]. Both approaches may be useful in assessing the impact of functional gastrointestinal disorders, but they have different strengths and weaknesses. Generic instruments such as the SF-36 [283] and the Sickness Impact Profile (SIP) [45] provide a way of comparing the relative impact of IBS (or any specific disorder) to the impact of other diseases such as congestive heart failure. For example, the SF-36 has been used to assess the impact of IBS [284] and functional dyspepsia [285] on quality of life and to compare those impacts to other medical conditions. Disease-specific instruments, on the other hand, are believed to be more responsive than generic instruments to the changes which may result from treatment of a specific disorder, but they do not permit one to compare the impact of the specific disease of interest to the impact of other common health concerns.

Methodological Considerations

Generic measures of HRQOL are highly correlated with measures of psychological distress. Some view this as appropriate, reasoning that a sense of psychological well being is a dimension of HRQOL [277,286]. However, other investigators view this as inappropriate, arguing that neuroticism is a stable personality trait leading people to take a negative or pessimistic view and that this negative outlook could lead people to rate their quality of life as poor independent of external events such as illness [284]. This could make the HRQOL measure less valid as a measure of the impact of illness, and it could make the measure less sensitive to the detection of change in response to treatment.

Whitehead and colleagues [284] examined this issue by giving the SF-36 [283], as well as the NEO Personality Inventory [287] and the SCL-90R [42], to three groups of college students: a group who had IBS symptoms for which they had consulted a physician, a group who had IBS but had not consulted a physician, and a third group that had no chronic bowel symptoms. All scales on the SF-36 were significantly correlated with the neuroticism scale of the NEO Personality Inventory and with the global symptom index of the SCL-90R [42]. The SF-36 still differentiated between patients with IBS, non-patients, and healthy controls after statistically adjusting for the mediating effects of neuroticism, but the strength of the association was substantially reduced. Investigators may want to consider adjusting for neuroticism or other personality traits in the interpretation of HRQOL measures.

Findings

Generic quality of life instruments have been used to show that patients with IBS [284] and functional dyspepsia [285] have impaired quality of life. In the Medical Outcomes Study comparing nine common chronic medical conditions, patients reporting gastrointestinal disorders had among the least desirable mental health, social functioning, and health perceptions as measured by the SF-36 [288]. Drossman and colleagues [192] used the SIP in a study of patients seen in an academic gastroenterology clinic and found greater impairment in patients with functional gastrointestinal disorders than in patients with structural abnormalities such as peptic ulcer and liver disease. There are no published data as yet on the relationship of disease-specific quality of life instruments to health outcomes in FGID.

Assessment

— Clinical Assessment

The previous sections of this chapter demonstrate that functional gastrointestinal disorders commonly have both physiological as well as psychosocial dimensions. To arbitrarily adopt a purely biomedical or psychological approach usually leads to less than optimal patient outcomes. A biopsychosocial approach to assessment is more productive, particularly for patients who are refractory to first-line medical therapy such as dietary fiber and antispasmodics. There is some evidence that taking a psychosocial history plays a part in reducing the frequency of visits [289].

Obtaining the History

The medical history is obtained by encouraging the patient to tell the story in his or her own way so that the psychosocial events contributing to the illness unfold naturally [290–293]. The questions should communicate the physician's willingness to address both biologic and psychological aspects of the illness. The clinician should also be sensitive to the patient's cultural background and understand that most cultures have unique beliefs about the significance of physical symptoms. Open-ended questions are used initially to encourage the patient to describe problems from their perspective and to generate hypotheses. Additional information is obtained with facilitating expressions: "Yes?", "Can you tell me more?", repeating the patient's previous statements, head nodding, or even silent pauses with an expectant look. As the data are obtained, they can be further elaborated and tested with more direct questions. In addition, a patient-centered style is recommended by maintaining eye contact, not interrupting the patient and adopting a "low control" style (Table 2 [291,294]).

Table 2. Physician Interaction Styles

High Control	Low Control
Frequently interrupts the patient	Allows patient to talk without interruptions
Asks closed-ended [yes/no] questions	Asks open-ended questions
Asks symptom-oriented questions	Asks patient-oriented questions
Ignores expressions of emotion	Acknowledges and supports the patient's feelings
Presents unemotionally	Projects own persona with jokes, compliments

Adapted from Ong et al., 1995 [294].

Evaluating the Role for Psychosocial Factors

A few questions can help the physician understand the role for psychosocial factors in a patient's illness [27,291,293,295].

(1) *Is the illness acute or chronic?* Chronic illness has greater psychosocial concomitants, either contributing to or resulting from the medical condition;

(2) *What is the patient's history of illness?* A lifelong history of physical complaints (somatization), multiple diagnostic procedures, and nonspecific treatments or poorly explainable symptoms (e.g., "thick-chart" or "fat-folder" patients) will usually predict future occurrences and should alert the clinician to the fact that psychological factors are contributing to the illness presentation;

(3) *Why is the patient coming now?* Particularly with chronic illness, psychosocial factors strongly influence health care seeking;

(4) *What is the impact of the illness?* The patient's health-related quality of life should be determined in terms of physical, psychological, and social functioning;

(5) *How does the family interact around the illness?* At times, family members may unwittingly impede successful treatment. This may be related to: (a) the adaptive value of the illness in "binding" family distress (making the patient's illness rather than the family's illness the focus of attention); (b) struggles for control between marital partners that are manifest through the illness; and/or (c) overprotectiveness (e.g., "enmeshment" by close family members who may be anxious about the medical condition);

(6) *What are the patient's psychosocial resources?* Clinical improvement also depends on a strong social support network and effective coping style.

In addition, there are certain issues that need to be addressed in some patients:

(1) *Is there a psychiatric diagnosis?* Disorders such as depression, somatization, and anxiety disorders, particularly panic disorder, are often highly responsive to psychological or psychopharmacologic treatments [21];

(2) *Is there a history of unresolved major loss or trauma?* Eliciting the initial details of an abuse/trauma history can be difficult for both patient and physician. A straightforward and empathic approach can elicit critical information in this area [204,220];

(3) *Does the patient exhibit unhelpful illness behavior?* This includes urgent or repeated requests for health care that are disproportionate to the physician's perception of disease severity and unrealistic expectations to validate an organic disease and find a cure.

Medical Tests

Diagnosis will depend on identifying symptoms consistent with a functional gastrointestinal disorder, performing limited diagnostic studies to exclude other disease, and re-evaluating the patient at another point in time (usually three to six weeks) [296]. Increasing evidence has shown the value of a "positive diagnosis" based on the Rome Criteria. Performing redundant endoscopies and/or imaging studies rarely yield new information [297]. The use of symptom-based diagnostic (e.g., "Rome") criteria, as discussed in this book, can help establish a positive diagnosis and minimize unneeded studies [298]. Studies should be based on the clinical need as determined by the objective data (e.g., blood in stool, abnormal blood studies, etc.) rather than the patient's insistence to "do something." Other equally important factors are safety, whether the results would make a difference in treatment, and whether the test is cost-effective. A key element to evaluating a patient with vague abdominal complaints is to proceed in a stepwise manner [296].

Additional work-up should be directed to evaluate symptoms that persist over time despite otherwise effective treatment for the functional gastrointestinal disorders. At times, when there is incomplete or nonspecific information and the condition is chronic, it is easier to tolerate the uncertainty of diagnosis and observe the patient for new developments. Two major concerns of physicians managing functional gastrointestinal patients is a fear of missing an organic diagnosis and the appearance of a new organic illness in the context of an ongoing functional gastrointestinal disorder. Initially using the Rome criteria for diagnosis and following the patient over time to take note of any change in the patient's symptoms (such as the development of new weight loss) or failure to respond to previously effective treatment can be an indication for additional work-up. However, clinicians should be reassured that overall, the long-term prognosis of these patients is quite good [289]. Experienced physicians make diagnostic and treatment decisions based on the "trajectory" of the illness: the change in the condition over time.

Evaluating for a Psychological Disorder

The association of an FGID with a co-morbid psychiatric disorder is associated with poorer health status. Therefore, the physician should screen for anxiety and depression using a few key questions: *Have you been worrying, had difficulty relaxing, had difficulty with sleep? Have you felt low in energy, losing interest and confidence in yourself and unable to concentrate?* If the answers to any of these questions are positive, the clinician must ask further questions to establish if a psychiatric disorder is present. There are a few psychiatric syndromes that are often associated with the functional gastrointestinal disorders, and the gastroenterologist should be able to make these diagnoses in everyday clinical practice—panic, depression, agoraphobia, and somatoform disorders. Recent diagnostic criteria have increased the reliability of making these diagnoses [36]. More complex diagnoses are usually made by a mental health professional.

— Psychosocial Evaluation Instruments

Psychological screening instruments can help in the evaluation of functional gastrointestinal disorders, although they are most often used for research purposes. There is a large spectrum of psychological and social instruments that have been used in the assessment of these patients [299]. A review of the most commonly used instruments is presented here (Table 3).

The various psychological measures used among patients with functional gastrointestinal disorders can be categorized into specific domains. These include:

(1) psychiatric diagnosis;
(2) psychological state (e.g., transient mood disturbance such as anxiety or depression or psychological distress);
(3) personality (e.g., psychological traits), a measure of relatively stable aspects of psychological status;
(4) illness behaviors and attitude scales;
(5) cognitive scales (e.g., attitudes and beliefs relating to illness);
(6) social support;
(7) coping; and
(8) quality of life.

Table 3 briefly describes the most frequently used measures for each of these domains.

Structured Interviews for Psychiatric Diagnosis

These are extensive, highly structured interviews with an interviewer who is specifically trained in the use of the instrument. A trained interviewer rates each symptom according to predetermined criteria, e.g., loss of weight greater than x, loss of sleep greater than y, depressed mood >50% of the time. The resulting data must meet specific criteria to provide a psychiatric diagnosis. These instruments come in many forms. The Diagnostic Interview Schedule (DIS) [300] is administered by clinicians with no formal training in psychiatry or psychology and requires 45–75 minutes. There is also a computerized, self-

Table 3. Commonly Used Measures of Psychological Domains

Psychosocial Domain	Measure	Descriptions	Comments
1. Structured Interviews For Psychiatric Diagnosis	DIS Diagnostic Interview Schedule [300]	Structured interview from which psychiatric diagnoses (DSM-IV Axis I) may be systematically obtained.	Lay people as well as health professional can be trained to conduct the interview. Computer-administered version is also available.
	SCID Structured Clinical Interview for DSM-III-R [390]	Semistructured interview for making Axis I and Axis II diagnoses.	The SCID requires specialized training and clinical experience.
	SCAN Schedule for Clinical Assessment in Neurophysiology [301]	Structured interview from which diagnoses (ICD-10 and DSM-IV) are made.	Requires prior mental health knowledge or specific training.
	CIDI Composite International Diagnostic Interview	Highly structured diagnostic interview for epidemiological studies of ICD-10 and DSM-IV diagnoses.	Can be used in a variety of cultures and does not require clinically experienced interviewers.
2a. Psychological State Self-Rating Scales [Generic]	SCL-90 Hopkins Symptom Checklist [42]	Consists of 90 items designed primarily to measure psychological symptom patterns of psychiatric and medical patients including somatization, obsessive-compulsive, interpersonal sensitivity, depression, anxiety, hostility, phobic anxiety, paranoid ideation and psychoticism. Each item is rated on a 5-point Likert scale ranging from not at all to extremely.	Widely used as both a screening device and an outcome measure in a broad spectrum of clinical research. Validity and reliability has been well established. Possible limitation is that it is relatively expensive to purchase.

Psychosocial Domain	Measure	Descriptions	Comments
2a. Psychological State Self-Rating Scales [Generic] *cont'd*	GHQ General Health Questionnaire [303]	The main version contains 60 items. It was designed for use in general population surveys in primary medical care settings. Covers 4 elements of distress: depression, anxiety, social adjustment and hypochondriasis.	Emphasis is on changes in condition, not on the absolute level of the symptom.
	MBHI Millon Behavioral Health Inventory [304]	Comprised of 20 scales grouped into four broad categories including basic coping styles, psychogenic attitudes, psychosomatic correlates and prognostic indices.	Good reliability and validity have been established. Developed and validated on medical patient samples.
	POMS Profile of Mood States [305]	This 65-item adjective rating scale includes six domains of mood including tension, depression, anger, vigor, fatigue and confusion.	Established reliability and validity in several studies.
2b. Psychological State Self-Rating Scales [Syndrome Specific]	STAI-S Spielberger State Anxiety Inventory [306]	Consists of 20 items which ask respondents to report how they feel at a particular moment in time. It is usually administered along with the STAI-T in the same scaling format.	It is the most widely used state anxiety scale. Acceptable reliability and validity estimates have been established in several studies.
	SPRAS Sheehan Patient Rated Anxiety Scale [307]	46 item scale for measuring presence of panic symptoms scored from not present to severe.	Limitations in using self-report for diagnosis.
	MOCI Maudsley Obsessive Compulsive Inventory [308,391]	30 item self-inventory designed to measure different types of obsessive-compulsive ritual.	Fair concurrent validity.

193

Table 3. Commonly Used Measures of Psychological Domains cont'd

Psychosocial Domain	Measure	Descriptions	Comments
2b. Psychological State Self-Rating Scales [Syndrome Specific] cont'd	BDI Beck Depression Inventory [309]	Consists of 21 items that assess cognitive or affective features of depressive symptoms. There are four graded statements for each item ranging from the most serious to the least serious level.	It provides a rapid assessment of the severity of depressive symptoms. It is one of the most frequently used measures of depressive symptoms and it has established validity and reliability in psychiatric, nonclinical and medical populations. Underates somatic symptoms.
	Zung Zung Depression Scale [310]	Respondents are asked to rate each of the 20 items as to how it applied to them at the time of testing along a four point scale from a little of the time to most of the time.	Quantitative scale of depression based on affect and its physiological and psychological concomitants.
	CES-D Center for Epidemiological Studies-Depression Scale [242]	The CES-D is a 20-item self-report scale which measures depression. Items are rated by the subject on a 4-point scale to reflect present affective state.	It has been validated for research use in the general population.
	HAD Scale Hospital Anxiety and Depression Scale [311]	Designed for medical populations. Consists of 14 items with subscales for anxiety and depression graded for severity.	Has "cut-off" scores for anxiety and depression each but not widely validated. Easy to use.
3. Personality Inventory (trait)	MMPI Minnesota Multiphasic Personality Inventory [313]	Comprises 550 statements to which one may answer true, false or cannot say. It contains ten clinical scales and four validity scales.	Most widely used empirically based personality inventory. Limitations include its length and poor reliability over longer time intervals.

Psychosocial Domain	Measure	Descriptions	Comments
3. Personality Inventory (trait) cont'd	EPI Eysenck Personality Inventory [314]	Consists of 57 items in a true-false format. It is designed to measure two dimensions of personality; neuroticism and extroversion-introversion.	Adequate test-retest reliabilities ranging from 0.84 to 0.94.
	NEO Neurotism Extroversion Openness Personality Inventory [287]	Measures five broad domains of personality including neuroticism, extroversion, openness, agreeableness and conscientiousness. The revised NEO (NEO-PI-R) has 240 items and uses a 5 point Likert scale ranging from strongly disagree to strongly agree.	The revised (NEO-PI-R) has acceptable validity and reliability. This inventory measures differences among personality domains among normal individuals, not intended to diagnose problems of mental health or adjustment.
	STAI-T Spielberger Trait Anxiety Inventory [306]	Consists of 20 statements which ask respondents to report how they generally feel. It is a 4 point Likert scale ranging from almost never to almost always.	Most widely used trait anxiety scale. Adequate internal consistency; test-retest reliability and validity have been established.
4. Illness Behaviors and Attitudes	Illness Behavior Questionnaire (Pilowsky [56])	Consists of 7 scales including two on hypochondriasis (disease phobia, disease conviction), three affect scales (affective inhibition, affective disturbance, and irritability), a denial scale, and a scale measuring psychological vs. somatic perception of illness.	Good reliability and validity. Oldest Scale. Not well accepted by patients presenting with a medical complaint because questions are mostly psychological.

Table 3. Commonly Used Measures of Psychological Domains *cont'd*

Psychosocial Domain	Measure	Descriptions	Comments
4. Illness Behaviors and Attitudes *cont'd*	Illness Attitude Scale (Kellner [315])	Consists of 9 scales similar to the IBQ but includes more behavioral scales (health habits, treatment experience, effects of symptoms). Test-retest reliabilities of 0.62 to 1.00 across subscales. Good correlation with other scales measuring similar constructs.	Relatively few questions for each scale (2–3), which limits reliability.
5. Cognitive Scales	IMIQ Implicit Models of Illness Questionnaire [316]	38 item self-report. Assesses respondents' attribution of their illness along four dimensions: seriousness of illness; personal responsibility for illness, controllability of illness; and its changeability.	IMIQ scales have discriminant validity and high reliability (r=0.68 to 0.92).
	DAS Dysfunctional Attitude Scale [317]	Consists of 40 items designed to measure dysfunctional attitudes that relate to cognitive vulnerability and depression. Respondents are required to endorse items that best describe how they think, using a 7-point Likert scale ranging from totally agree to totally disagree.	While this scale has been validated on psychiatric and non-clinical populations, this measure may be somewhat useful for functional GI since several dysfunctional attitudes on this scale have been reported in this group (e.g., high need for approval and perfectionism).

Psychosocial Domain	Measure	Descriptions	Comments
5. Cognitive Scales *cont'd*	CS-FBD [318]	25 item single factor Likert scale ranging from 1 (strongly disagree) to 7 (strongly agree). Designed to assess thoughts and concerns of relevance to patients with FBD. Total score for the scale ranges from 25 to 175.	Valid and reliable scale which can be used as an outcome measure in evaluating the efficacy of different forms of psychotherapeutic intervention for FBD, and can also serve as a helpful assessment tool for health professionals working with patients diagnosed with FBD.
6. Social Support	SSQ-6 Sarason Social Support Questionnaire (Brief Form) [319]	Brief questionnaire designed to measure respondent's number of social supports and the degree of satisfaction with them.	Most widely used social support scale.
7. Coping	Ways of Coping-R [44]	Includes items that assess styles of coping with an identified stressful encounter. Responses are grouped into eight coping styles including confronting behavior, emotional distancing, self-controlling behavior, seeking social support, accepting responsibility, escape-avoidance, planful problem solving and positive reappraisal.	One of the most highly used measure of coping style.
	CSQ Coping Strategies Questionnaire (CSQ) [320]	Consists of 6 subscales that relate to coping with painful condition. Also includes individual questions on perceived ability to control to decrease symptoms.	In a sample of female patients at a GI referral setting, the 6-item Catastrophizing scale of the CSQ, and the question "ability o decrease symptoms" was shown to predict adverse health outcome [193,322]

Table 3. Commonly Used Measures of Psychological Domains *cont'd*

Psychosocial Domain	Measure	Descriptions	Comments
8a. Health-Related Quality of Life (Generic)	SF-36 Short-Form 36-Item Health Survey [283]	36 Items that assess 8 domains including physical limitations, physical and mental role limitations, social activities, pain, general health perception, mental health, vitality. Physical and psychosocial subscales are available.	One of the most widely used means of HRQOL for health conditions.
	SIP Sickness Impact Profile [45]	136 Items that assess 12 different categories of behavioral dysfunction including work, eating behavior, recreations and pastimes, sleep and rest, alertness behavior, home management, emotional behavior, social interaction, body care and movement, mobility, ambulation, communication. Two psychological and physiological subscales are available.	Widely used in gastrointestinal disorders and other health conditions.
8b. Health-Related Quality of Life (Disease Specific)	IBS-QOL Quality of Life with IBS [286]	34 item self-report questions with 8 subscales: dysphoria, interference with activity, body image, health worry, food avoidance, social reaction, sexual relationship.	Developed from focus groups of IBS patients at 2 institutions. Has achieved good psychometric validation. Responsiveness has also been established.

Psychosocial Domain	Measure	Descriptions	Comments
8b. Health-Related Quality of Life (Disease Specific) *cont'd*	IBSQoL [324]	30 item self-report questionnaire with 9 sub-scales: emotional, mental health, sleep, energy, physical functioning, diet, social role, physical role, and sexual relations.	Development of items based on review of literature and interviews with physicians which was then modified by a sample of patients. Has achieved psychometric validation.
	SEIQoL [325]	Subjects define 5 areas of their lives and then rate on VAS.	Allows for individual preferences on QOL, but may be difficult for some subjects to understand.

administered version. The DIS has been well validated, and the results obtained by persons who are not mental health professionals correlate well with those of psychiatrists. The Structured Clinical Interview for DSM-IV (SCID) is a useful screening instrument in that it guides the interviewer through the major DSM-IV Axis I diagnoses (e.g., depression, anxiety, and somatoform disorders). The interview can be abbreviated to focus on only certain Axis I diagnoses [301]. The Schedules for Clinical Assessment in Neuropsychiatry (SCAN) provides DSM-IV and ICD-10 diagnoses. It is a very long interview that requires a trained mental health professional [223]. The Composite International Diagnostic Interview (CIDI) has been validated across different cultural settings and yields diagnosis by DSM-IV or ICD-10 criteria.

Psychological State Self-Rating Scales

Generic

These instruments measure generic distress. They have two uses. In a two-stage research protocol they are used as screening instruments, i.e., patients with a high score are interviewed at the second stage by a psychologist or psychiatrist to assess whether a specific psychiatric diagnoses is present. Alternatively, the mean scores on these instruments may be compared between different patient groups. The major advantage is that these instruments do not require staff involvement and are easy for the patient to complete. They can also be used to measure response to treatment. However, the disadvantages include the fact that patients with poor insight may under-report symptoms and that the severity of symptoms is hard to precisely measure.

The Symptom Checklist-90 (SCL-90) usually takes 15–30 minutes for patients to complete and is a well-validated and useful tool [42]. However, because of high intercorrelation between the subscales, it is best used as an overall measure of psychologic distress, rather than as a measure of discreet psychological symptoms as originally intended [302]. There are different versions of the General Health Questionnaire (GHQ) (composed of 60, 28 or 12 questions). This is a well validated self-reporting measure for the possible presence of psychiatric illness and requires 10–15 minutes to complete [303]. Other instruments include the Millon Behavioral Health Inventory (MBHI) [304] and Profile of Mood State (POMS) [305] (Table 3).

Syndrome Specific

These instruments include self-administered or interview-directed questionnaires, which assess symptoms of a specific psychiatric syndrome. Most of these instruments have been designed to evaluate patients for anxiety or mood disorders. The Spielberger State Trait Anxiety Inventory (STAI) [306] is a self-reporting instrument used to measure both anxiety resulting from acute stressors (state anxiety) as opposed to the patient's intrinsic level of anxiety irrespective of any particular acute stressor (trait anxiety). The Sheehan Patient Rated Anxiety Scale (SPRAS) [307] is a validated, easy-to-administer instrument for detection of panic disorder. Scores greater than 30 are correlated with the diagnosis of panic disorder. The Maudsley Obsessive Compulsive Inventory (MOCI) is an effective, validated patient self-reported questionnaire that effectively screens for obsessive-compulsive disorder [308]. The Beck Depression Inventory (BDI) is a self-administered questionnaire; a score greater than 14 is usually taken as an indication of at least mild depression [309]. The Zung Depression Self-Rating Scale [310] is accepted as a reasonable screening tool but has not been well validated. The Center for Epidemiologic Studies-Depression Scale (CES-D) is a short questionnaire frequently used in population studies [242].

The Hospital Anxiety and Depression Scale (HAD Scale) was developed for use in medical outpatients rather than psychiatric patients [311,312]. In the construction of this scale symptoms which might equally arise from somatic as from mental disorders were excluded, which means that the scale scores are not affected by bodily illness. The cutoff point with all these instruments for patients with functional gastrointestinal disorders has yet to be established.

Personality

Several instruments are available which assess more stable personality features that may affect illness behavior or response to treatment (Table 3). These include the MMPI [313], which is lengthy to complete, the EPI [314], and the NEO [287]. The Spielberger Trait Anxiety Inventory [306] also assesses more stable "Trait" anxiety—anxiety that persists independent of acute stressors—than the state scale.

Illness Behavior Questionnaires

The Illness Behavior Questionnaire [56] is a 62-item questionnaire that yields scores on the following scales: illness worry/general hypochondriasis, disease conviction, psychological versus somatic orientation to illness, affective inhibition, affective disturbance, denial, and irritability. The score on each scale is determined by the response to only four or five questions. Fourteen items have been used in the Whitely Index of hypochondriasis (WI) [56]. All scores tend to be highly correlated with psychiatric disorder. The Kellner Illness Attitude Scale [315] is a 29-item self report measure of attitudes towards illness. The instrument provides scores on nine scales, worry about illness, concern about pain, health habits, hypochondriacal beliefs, thanatophobia, disease phobia, bodily preoccupation, treatment experience and effect of symptoms. Patients with chronic disease tend to find it difficult to complete this questionnaire. However, the items' content is relatively independent of psychological distress.

Cognitive Scales

These instruments are designed to measure particular aspects of attitudes toward illness. They measure attitudes, beliefs, and attributions associated with illness and may be used as predictors of outcome, or as outcome measures of psychological treatment. The Implicit Model of Illness Scale (IMIQ) [316] assesses patient beliefs as related to the seriousness of the illness, its degree of personal controllability, and its changeability. Other scales include the Dysfunctional Attitudes Scale [317] and the newly developed FBD Cognitive Scale (CS-FBD) [318] (Table 3).

Social Support

Respondents indicate the quantity and quality of the social support they feel they receive. The original Sarason Social Support Questionnaire (SSQ) [43], which is easy to administer, but still provides essentially subjective data, has been reduced to six items (SSQ-6) [319].

Coping

There are numerous ways that individuals cope with illness. The Ways of Coping Questionnaire [44] is commonly used in medical research. More recently, the Coping Strategies Questionnaire (CSQ) [320], and particularly the Catastrophizing Scale [321] and questions about the patient's ability to decrease symptoms has been shown to be predictive of adverse health outcome among patients with gastrointestinal disorders [193,322].

Health-Related Quality of Life

Generic HRQOL Instruments
The following are examples of generic HRQOL instruments that have been used in patients with FGID.

Medical Outcomes Study Short Form (SF-36)
The SF-36 [283] is a brief measure of functional status and well-being which consists of eight scales: *physical functioning* (e.g., walking, climbing stairs, carrying groceries); *role physical* (limitations in ability to work or perform usual ac-

tivities); *bodily pain* (intensity of bodily pain or discomfort); *general health* (self-perception of current state of health, resistance to illness, and health outlook); *vitality* (energy level and fatigue); *social functioning* (impact of health or emotional problems on social activities); *role emotional* (impact of emotional problems on work or usual daily activities); and *mental health* (anxiety, depression, loss of control, sense of psychological well-being).

Sickness Impact Profile (SIP)
The SIP [45] is also a generic measure of the impact of illness on functional status and well being. It contains 136 questions as compared to 36 for the SF-36, and it is scored for 12 subscales instead of 8. The 12 subscales are grouped into three domains: *physical activities* , which include ambulation, mobility, and body care and movement; *psychosocial areas*, which include social interaction, alertness behavior, emotional behavior, and communication; and *independent categories*, including sleep and rest, eating, work, home management, and recreation and pastimes. Thus, the SIP provides a more detailed description than the SF-36 of the impact of illness.

Disease-Specific HRQOL Instruments
Irritable Bowel Syndrome Quality of Life Instrument (IBS-QOL).
Patrick, Drossman, and colleagues [286] developed a disease-specific quality of life scale which includes items highly specific to IBS, e.g., "*I am bothered by how much time I spend on the toilet,*" "*I feel unclean because of my bowel problems,*" and "*I worry about losing control of my bowels.*" This instrument shows very good convergent and discriminant validity with measures of symptom frequency and severity and measures of psychological well being. In addition, it had good test-retest reliability. A recent study showed that this instrument is responsive to changes in response to treatment [323].

Irritable Bowel Syndrome Quality of Life Questionnaire (IBSQOL)
Hahn and colleagues [324] developed a second disease specific instrument for IBS. Construct validity and split-half reliability are good to excellent for all the scales. Comparison of these scales to those of the IBS-QOL developed by Patrick and Drossman and QOL [286] suggests that the two questionnaires sample similar domains.

Schedule for the Evaluation of Individual Quality of Life (SEIQOL)
This scale has the advantage of being completely individualized, but a disadvantage is that the procedure is time consuming and may be difficult for some subjects to understand [325].

Treatment

— Approach to the Patient

This section reviews how the gastroenterologist and primary care physician can apply psychosocial principles in the management of patients with functional gastrointestinal disorders [291,296,394].

Establish a Therapeutic Relationship

The behavioral style of the physician can greatly influence the quality of the doctor-patient relationship. The ability to adopt a "care" vs. "cure" approach has been shown to be much more effective in eliciting a positive outcome for the patient [294]. Characteristics of the "care" model include the following:

(1) a focus on the patient's overall concerns about illness;
(2) physician and patient are egalitarian (e.g., physician calls patient by name); and
(3) a willingness to discuss diagnosis, prognosis, results of tests and treatment recommendations.

The physician can establish a therapeutic relationship when he or she:

(1) elicits and acknowledges the patient's beliefs, concerns and expectations;
(2) offers empathy when needed;
(3) clarifies misunderstandings;
(4) provides education; and
(5) negotiates the plan of treatment with the patient [326].

We believe that the physician should ask in a supportive manner what specific concerns the patient feels are still not resolved. Thorough information about the expectation of normal findings on clinical examination and diagnostic tests aimed at excluding organic disorders may also contribute to a confident and positive working alliance.

Addressing Psychosocial Factors

A good therapeutic relationship facilitates the patient's disclosure of psychosocial information. If the patient accepts or volunteers a link with stress, the reasons for this can be explored. Systematic evidence for the link should be sought; a bowel chart (see below) may be helpful. Sometimes this association is not immediately volunteered, since patients vary in their ability to report thoughts and emotions.

Some patients may be unwilling to accept a role for psychosocial factors in the illness even when it is evident to others. In this case, it is <u>not</u> helpful to discuss psychosocial and biological factors in terms of causation (e.g., *"it's due to stress"*) or as being separate (*"the work-up is negative; it must be psychiatric"*) [326]. The physician needs to help the patient to express their distress in a way that is consistent with their illness beliefs. Here it helps to focus on the psychosocial impact of the illness in terms of its emotional effects, impaired quality of life, and consequences on family and social dynamics.

On occasion, patients may make statements such as *"You don't think this pain is 'in my head,' do you?"* This highlights the need to understand the patient's perspective. It is important to explore with the patient the underlying meaning associated with the statement. Following this the physician and patient can work towards common understanding which can lead to the development of shared treatment goals [326].

At times fear of disapproval or lack of trust will prevent the patient from sharing thoughts and feelings. However, with the physician's non-judgmental behavior and concern, and continuing support this will improve. Furthermore, any recommended psychotherapeutic care should be presented in addition to the on-going care by the patient's primary care physician. This avoids recreating a mind-body dualism and gives the patient the clear message that they are not being dismissed [293].

Connecting Bowel Symptoms with Psychosocial Factors

In some cases, the use of a bowel symptom chart may help to connect symptoms with psychological precipitants. The patient is asked to record on each day the predominant symptoms (e.g., pain, bloating, nausea), and their severity along with the time of bowel movements. For premenopausal women it is important to include data on the menstrual cycle. Other columns can be used to record dietary, lifestyle changes, or stressors to assess whether these are associated with symptom exacerbation, and how the patient's mood state and thoughts or cognitions vary with the symptoms.

Notable variation of pain or bowel symptoms and its relationship with inciting factors as well as the patient's emotional and cognitive responses should be discussed with the patient on subsequent visits with a view to discerning a pattern if possible. It sometimes becomes clear that exacerbations are related to external events, and may be associated with catastrophic thought (e.g., *"It was so bad I didn't think I could live another day"*). This information can provide the basis for cognitive-behavioral strategies.

If the patient initially does not make a connection between bowel symptoms and psychosocial factors, the physician may use the patient's bowel chart as the first step to his/her increased understanding of this possible connection and to find ways to try to modify any stress-related responses. The times when the symptoms are less severe provide an opportunity for trying some helpful strategies or behaviors. If feelings of tension and anxiety occur when the symptoms are severe, these may be addressed. Unhelpful coping strategies may be identified—e.g. remaining in bed or focusing on the intensity of the symptom when they are severe. These should be discussed in detail and the increased rapport and trust between patient and doctor often permit the patient the opportunity to speak more freely of the psychosocial aspects of the disorder.

Reassurance and Reconceptualization

Many patients come to the physician with concerns about the severity and prognosis of their illness. Patients often have unique health beliefs, e.g., *"I know my colon is blocked. Why don't we just do surgery?"* or *"I worked in a chemical factory years ago. I know that is the cause of my illness."* The physician therefore needs to understand the patient's particular concerns first, and then to reassure him or her. Such fears and concerns can be addressed by emphasizing the overall favorable prognosis for the FGIDs. However, premature or inappropriate reassurance is perceived by the patient as insincere, or as a lack of thoroughness by the physician. When the symptoms are chronic and the evaluation is otherwise negative, the physician should reassure the patient of his or her willingness to help in the ongoing care rather than guaranteeing success. The patient should be helped to reconceptualize the nature of the illness as a set of troublesome symptoms rather than an indication of underlying pathology with patients.

Accept the Adaptations of Chronic Illness

In a small subgroup of patients, chronic illness may provide attention from others, release from usual responsibilities, and possibly social and financial compensation. In these situations, clinical improvement may take a long time, but may be advanced if the physician focuses more on improving the patient's function in the presence of illness rather than attempting to "cure." Adopting a collaborative approach to care involving behavioral interventions, collaborative definition of problems, use of self-care, and support services (particularly support groups) with sustained follow up by the principal care provider can maximize outcomes [327].

Reinforce Healthy Behaviors

If the physician focuses on symptoms at the exclusion of working toward psychosocial adaptation, illness behaviors may be reinforced. The patient will assume that the physician's interest is contingent on continued illness. The challenge for the physician is to reinforce positive coping behaviors and to move the patient gently away from focusing on physical symptoms, as a means to reduce diagnostic studies and symptomatic treatments. Successful strategies for management of these patients emphasize scheduling frequent, brief visits to the same physician, recognizing the value of the patient as a human being rather than having an illness based relationship ("the sick role") and screening for treatable mood and anxiety disorders [328]. Patients should be given more responsibility in their care, for example, by being given a choices in the treatment (e.g., selecting among several indicated medications or designing an exercise program). When the physician rewards these efforts (by praise and attention), patients learn that personal efforts toward health have positive impact on the physician. The patient, in turn, feels valued not because of symptoms but because of their health-promoting behavior [329].

— Role of the Mental Health Professional as a Consultant

Psychological Problems Requiring Referral

Problems which might require referral for consultation and treatment include:

(1) psychiatric disorders (e.g., major depression, panic disorder) which require specific treatments (e.g., antidepressants, cognitive-behavior or other psychotherapy);

(2) a history of abuse which comes to light during consultation and may be interfering with adjustment to the current illness;

(3) serious impairment in daily function which requires specific treatment to improve coping skills; and

(4) somatization, where multiple symptoms are leading to numerous consultations across specialties.

Clinical Evaluation

In order for the gastroenterologist to refer a patient to a mental health professional, the patient must acknowledge the relevance of the psychosocial aspects as they relate to his or her presenting problem (see previous section). The evaluation of symptoms of psychiatric diagnoses are previously discussed. When the patient also has multiple unexplained symptoms, somatization disorder should be suspected. High scores on psychological screening instruments (e.g., for SCL-90, GHQ, Beck) would suggest a depressive or anxiety disorder. These rating scales are important screening tools. Further, formal psychiatric evaluation may also be needed.

Preparing for a Referral to a Mental Health Professional

A patient seeing a gastroenterologist for a functional gastrointestinal disorder may be reluctant to be referred to a psychologist or a psychiatrist for several reasons. First, the patient may feel stigmatized by such a referral and lack knowledge of the benefits of psychological evaluation and treatment. Second, the patient may view his/her problem as "physical", and would prefer to visit a medical physician, since a mental health professional "logically" deals with psychological problems. Third, if the referral is made at the end of a medical evaluation, the patient may see it as a rejection ("the work up is negative, it must be nerves").

In our experience, usually it is not effective, to "turn over" the care to the mental health professional, since the patient will view such a referral as ignoring their somatic concerns and feel insulted and rejected. This can result in their seeking other doctors for second opinions. The extent of continued involvement of the gastroenterologist will vary from regular visits (assuming there are reasons for continued medical treatment) concurrent with the psychological treatment, to occasional visits for reassessment, to no scheduled visits but with continued availability as the need arises.

The major goal in preparing the patient for a referral to the mental health professional is to define the patient's complaints in terms of a biopsychosocial disorder rather than just a medical illness and to get the patient interested in and motivated to further explore the psychological factors involved.

Making the Referral

Assuming an effective patient-physician relationship, the physician should clearly explain the reason for the referral to a mental health professional. The mental health professional should be seen as a member of the team involved in the patient's over-all care: "*I have a colleague Dr. —, who sees many of my patients with these symptoms and we find that his/her treatment can help us with your care*".

The mental health professional will require a detailed referral letter from the medical physician, which states the nature of the presenting complaint, its duration, and any psychosocial factors that have been identified or suspected (e.g. a history of major loss, abuse, interpersonal difficulties), as contributing to the symptoms or their exacerbation. It is also important for the referring physician to report any fears or concerns (illness in the family, previous experience of a relative with symptoms developing cancer, etc.) that were identified, so the mental health professional can be alerted to their presence.

The Role of the Consultant Mental Health Professional

If the mental health professional believes that the patient has reservations about the referral, these should be explored before attempting any psychological or psychopharmacologic treatment. Sometimes the first consultation is taken up with this task. Patients will not attend the next appointment unless they feel that their view of the illness has been understood. Therefore, time spent reviewing the patient's gastrointestinal symptoms along with describing types of psychological treatment relevant to them will be rewarded by the patient's increased interest and compliance [330].

The mental health professional should review the problem in detail, while keeping an open mind regarding the relative importance of its physical and psychological aspects. He or she should explain that, in a multidisciplinary approach to treatment, there can be several goals:

(1) to alter the contents of the gut (e.g., diet or a bulking agent);
(2) to modify gut motility or pain threshold (e.g., antispasmodics or antinociceptives); or
(3) to reduce stress which can alter gut function;
(4) to help the patient cope with his/her symptoms; and/or
(5) to address the psychological problems that may be associated with the symptoms and thereby to improve quality of life.

Treatment of any anxiety or depressive symptoms alone may lead to some improvement of the bowel symptoms or at least improvement in general wellbeing. Combining antidepressants and psychological treatment may be more effective than either alone [331].

— Overview of Psychotherapies

While the mental health consultant can select from different types of psychological treatments (e.g., cognitive-behavioral therapy, dynamic psycho-

Table 4. Specific Psychological Treatment Techniques Used in Functional Bowel Disorders

	Psychodynamic	Cognitive behavioral	Relaxation	Biofeedback	Education	Hypnosis	Psychodramatic
Svedlund et al. [354]	X						
Guthrie et al.[352]	X						
Arn et al.[353]			X				X
Lynch and Zamble [344]		X	X				
Corney et al. [392]		X					
Bennett and Wilkinson [349]		X	X		X		
Shaw et al. [345]		X	X				
Rumsey [346]		X	X		X		
Blanchard, Schwarz [350]		X	X	X	X		
Neff, Blanchard [347]		X	X	X	X		
Blanchard et al.[351]		X	X	X	X		
Voirol, Hipolito[355]			X				
Blanchard et al. [356]			X				
Whorwell et al.[337]						X	
Whorwell et al.[357]						X	
Harvey et al.[338]						X	
Waxman [393]						X	
Greene, Blanchard [360]		X					
Payne, Blanchard [334]		X					
van Dulmen et al. [348]		X	X				
Toner et al. [332]		X	X				

Note: The Cognitive Behavioral category includes assertiveness training, exposure, stress management, and coping techniques.

therapy, hypnotherapy, and relaxation), experience and the empirical research suggests that no one treatment is superior for functional gastrointestinal disorders. The most important aspect of treatment is the patient's acceptance of the need for treatment and his/her motivation to engage in it. This can be enhanced if the gastroenterologist and psychologist/psychiatrist help the patient accept the treatment as a necessary part of an overall plan of care. Treatments include the following major types (Table 4).

Cognitive-Behavioral Therapy

Cognitive-behavioral techniques consist of a wide range of strategies and procedures designed to bring about alterations in patients' perceptions of their situation and their ability to control their gastrointestinal symptoms. The rationale for cognitive behavioral strategies assumes that individuals can learn new ways of thinking and behaving through personal experience and practice. In addition, it helps patients recognize the role played by illness beliefs and behavior in chronic pain [332].

Cognitive-behavioral treatment (CBT) may be particularly valuable for patients with IBS because studies have found: (a) a high prevalence of anxiety and depression [34,38,254,333]; (b) a high frequency of difficulties with appropriate assertiveness; (c) a high need for social approval; and (d) perfectionistic attitudes. All of the patterns are amenable to CBT. Relaxation/stress management is often incorporated into CBT packages because of its effect in reducing autonomic arousal and anxiety in IBS [334].

Dynamic Psychotherapy

This form of therapy (similar to brief interpersonal psychotherapy [335,336] requires a close relationship between the patient and therapist. A significant degree of psychological and physical distress is either caused, or exacerbated, by difficulties in interpersonal relationships, and within the therapy, these difficulties are mirrored or recur, leading the patient to perceive the therapist in a particular way based on previous personal experience. When this happens, increased anxiety or distress in the therapy may be recognized and dealt with. Psychological distress can usually be related to physical symptoms, and in extreme cases the patient may experience abdominal discomfort or the urge to defecate even within the therapy session. As the patient comes to understand the problems in his/her relationships, he or she may act upon these insights, which may lead to a reduction in psychological symptoms, and generally, a reduction in bowel symptoms.

Hypnotherapy

Hypnotherapy has become increasingly popular in England [154,337, 338]. The hypnotic "state" is a state of heightened suggestibility. Following induction, the hypnotherapist uses progressive muscular relaxation plus suggestions of relaxation to reduce striated muscle tension, and "gut directed" imagery and suggestions to relax gastrointestinal smooth muscle. Sessions end with the patient being told that he or she will feel positive and good about themselves. Patients are also asked to practice autohypnosis at home with an audio tape with the goal of being able to self-administer suggestions of relaxation.

Relaxation (Arousal Reduction) Training

Relaxation or arousal reduction techniques include a variety of different methods used to teach patients to counteract the physiological sequellae of stress or anxiety. The rationale for these techniques is the belief that if muscle tension or autonomic arousal decreases, subjective anxiety or tension will, as a consequence of this, also decrease. The most widely used arousal reduction techniques include: (1) progressive muscle relaxation training [58,339]; (2) biofeedback for striated muscle tension, skin temperature, or electrodermal activity [340]; (3) autogenic training [341]; and (4) transcendental or Yoga meditation [342]. Progressive muscle relaxation training and EMG biofeedback have as their primary aim the reduction of skeletal muscle tension, the assumption being that with reductions in skeletal muscle tension will come decreases in autonomic arousal and subjective tension or anxiety. Skin temperature and electrodermal biofeedback training attempt to reduce autonomic arousal directly, and autogenic training attempts to reduce smooth muscle activity through imagery in a technique closely resembling hypnosis. Transcendental meditation and Yoga aim to modify both skeletal muscle tension and autonomic arousal indirectly through cognitive focusing techniques. There is support for the effectiveness of all these techniques for anxiety or stress reduction.

— Empirical Support for Psychotherapies

It should be noted that most of the research to date has focused on IBS. One of the most difficult problems in reviewing the published literature is that, in general, studies have not adequately described their therapeutic procedures. In addition, most of the published research has involved multicomponent treatment packages including various combinations of cognitive-behavioral, relaxation, psychodynamic and biofeedback approaches. Accordingly, it is difficult to assess the effectiveness of the specific theoretical approach to treatment. It should be noted that patient selection differs across studies according to setting with a range from chronic attendees at a gastroenterology clinic to patients attending a mental health setting [335,340,343]. This section will briefly review the multicomponent treatments followed by studies that have used a single therapeutic approach.

Multicomponent Treatments

Nine studies [332,344–351] have combined progressive muscle relaxation training with cognitive-behavioral therapy, and all of them reported that the results from this treatment combination to be superior to those in the control group. In five instances, comparison was made to a waiting list control group. However, a waiting list group does not provide an equivalent expectation of improvement (placebo response). In four other studies, comparison was made to conventional medical therapy. Only two studies used an active placebo control. One found no difference between placebo and cognitive-behavioral therapy plus relaxation training. However, the second study found the combination of cognitive-behavioral therapy and relaxation to be superior to an educational control treatment.

In another study relaxation training combined with interpersonal psychotherapy was superior to medical management for both bowel symptoms and psychological symptoms [351]. However, relaxation training combined with psychodrama [353] was no better than standard therapy for bowel symptoms, but active treatment was more effective for anxiety reduction. A combination of behavioral techniques (exposure, education, and bowel retraining) was no better than standard medical treatment [353].

Individual Therapeutic Approaches

Psychodynamic Therapy

Svedlund et al. [354] compared psychodynamic therapy to continuation of routine medical care and found that bowel dysfunction and abdominal pain improved more in the psychotherapy than in controls. The difference became more pronounced one year later when the psychotherapy group showed further improvement on measures of anxiety and depression in addition to gastrointestinal symptoms, compared with the control group. Similar results were obtained by Guthrie [335].

Relaxation/Autogenic Training

There have been only two studies that looked at relaxation/autogenic training alone, i.e., not combined with psychotherapy or cognitive-behavioral therapy. Voirol and Hipolito [355] compared six months of treatment with conventional medical therapy to six months of treatment with relaxation exercises and reported that the relaxation group showed significantly fewer pain episodes and significantly fewer visits to medical clinics 40 months after treatment.

Blanchard's laboratory [356] recently reported a comparison of relaxation training alone to a symptom-monitoring control group. The relaxation group showed significantly more reduction in gastrointestinal symptoms than the control group. Fifty percent of the relaxation group improved by at least 50%, which is a figure comparable to previous reports with Blanchard's multicomponent treatment.

There is at present insufficient data to identify which characteristics of patients are predictive of the response to relaxation training, and there is very little information on the effectiveness of biofeedback, and none on the effectiveness of other forms of arousal reduction training in IBS.

Hypnosis

Whorwell, Prior, and Faragher [337] randomized patients to either hypnosis or a placebo control. The hypnotherapy group showed significantly greater reductions in bowel symptoms and improvements in the sense of well-being. Subsequently, Whorwell, Prior, and Colgan [357] reported follow-up data showing that patients given hypnosis maintained their treatment gains at 18 months. Age greater than 50 years and the presence of high levels of anxiety were predictors of poorer outcomes with hypnotherapy [358]. An independent research group [338] replicated the work of Whorwell and found hypnotherapy in groups to be as effective as individual hypnotherapy.

Whorwell and colleagues [359] recorded colonic motility from perfused catheters and showed that hypnosis significantly reduced the contractile activity. They speculate that this is the mechanism by which hypnosis improves bowel symptoms. Whorwell's laboratory [154] has also shown that hypnotherapy for IBS is associated with normalization of thresholds for pain from distension of a balloon in the rectum.

Cognitive Therapy

Blanchard's group [360] has completed a series of three studies using cognitive therapy alone. The first study found greater gastrointestinal symptom reduction for patients with IBS randomly assigned to cognitive therapy than for those in the symptom monitoring control group. The second study tested cognitive therapy against a self-help support group and found significant improvement in IBS symptoms, depression, and anxiety in the cognitive group [334]. The third study showed improvement on gastrointestinal symptoms in both individual and group cognitive therapy compared with a symptom monitoring group [361]. Results for all three studies held up at a three month follow-up assessment.

Summary of Findings from Psychological Treatment Studies

We reviewed 15 studies that used a controlled design to compare psychological treatment with conventional medical treatment. There are an inadequate number of well-designed studies to perform a meta-analysis. We excluded two studies with a participation rate of less than 40% [344,353]. In terms of reduction of bowel symptoms at the end of treatment, 10 of 13 studies showed significant superiority of psychological over conventional medical treatment. Of the nine studies with follow-up data (duration 9–40 months), eight showed superiority of psychological treatment [332,345–347,352,354,355, 357]. Only six studies also controlled for expectancy and time with therapist [332,337,340,348,352,361]. Five showed a significantly greater improvement in bowel symptoms in the psychological treatment groups [334,337,348,352,361]

There were no differences in outcome based on technique. Successful controlled studies have included exploratory psychotherapy, hypnosis, cognitive-behavior therapy, and relaxation training. Thus, given the current state of knowledge, the psychotherapist should use the technique with which they are most experienced.

— Psychopharmacology

The data concerning efficacy of psychopharmaceuticals in FGID is limited. The rationale for using psychotropic agents is: (a) approximately half of the patients with a FGID also have depression and/or anxiety disorders, which may respond to psychopharmacological intervention; (b) data support the efficacy of antidepressants in the relief of chronic pain [361]; (c) and an emerging body of data support the efficacy of psychotropic agents in FGIDs [362].

At least four studies have shown efficacy of psychopharmaceuticals in FGIDs. Non-cardiac chest pain is improved by imipramine, and the improvement is unrelated to change in mood [363]. Trazadone also leads to improvement in non-cardiac chest pain independent of changes in psychiatric symptoms and without change in esophageal motility [364]. Likewise, Greenbaum showed significant improvement of IBS symptoms with desipramine, which was independent of the anticholinergic and antidepressant effects of this drug [365]. Gorrard has shown significant slowing of transit time with imipramine and significant decrease in gastrointestinal transit time with paroxetine, but there was no measure of mood and gastrointestinal symptoms [366,367].

The following section: (a) provides guidelines for prescribing antidepressants in the gastroenterology or general medical setting; (b) describes basic properties of antidepressants and anxiolytic drugs to explain the pharmacology and side effect profiles; and (c) recommends that more serious or complex psychiatric problems or failure to respond to antidepressants should lead to treatment in conjunction with a psychiatrist.

Prescribing

The optimal use of psychopharmacology is best accomplished in the context of a strong doctor-patient relationship. Psychopharmacologic agents should be seen only as complementary to an overall multicomponent treatment plan. The physician needs to explain the rationale, possible side effects, and expected benefits from the prescribed medication carefully to the patient.

The response to antidepressant therapy is highly patient specific, i.e., there is no way to predict how an individual patient will respond either therapeutically or experience side effects to an individual drug [368]. The key to maximizing outcomes in these patients is to adopt an "alliance" or relationship-centered approach. This approach consists of explaining to the patient the rationale for antidepressant treatment, proposed target symptoms, and possible side effects. This includes:

(1) exploring the patient's beliefs and expectations relative to psycho pharmacologic treatment;
(2) addressing these factors relative to the rationale for antidepressant treatment and its proposed target symptoms and possible side effects; and
(3) negotiating a treatment plan; and
(4) continue a dialogue with the patient regarding symptom response and side effects.

The choice of antidepressants depends on the target symptoms, the overall clinical picture and the possible side effects (Table 5).

Patients are then started on a low dose of antidepressant medication and instructed to call the physician if they experience side effects. This procedure allows both the physician and patient to assess the benefits and side effects of the medication. Side effects usually occur early, i.e., within 1–2 days of initial dosage

Table 5. Antidepressants and Their Effects on CNS Receptor Sites

Antidepressant	Anticholinergic Effect	5-HT Receptor Uptake	Histaminic Effects	Daily Dosage Range	Side Effects
TCA's					
Amitriptyline	++++	+++	++++	50–300 mg	Sedation, Orthostasis, Dry Mouth, Constipation
Desipramine	+	+++	+	50–300 mg	Diaphoresis, Dry Mouth, Orthostasis
Doxepin	++	+++	++++	50–300 mg	Sedation, Dry Mouth
Maprotiline	+	Nil	++++	100–150 mg	Orthostasis, Dry Mouth, Seizure, Sedation
Nortriptyline	++	+	++	75–150 mg	Dry Mouth
SSRI's					
Fluoxetine	Nil	++++	Nil	10–60 mg	N + V, Bruxism, H.A. Diarrhea
Fluvoxamine	Nil	+++	Nil	50–300 mg	N + V, Bruxism, H.A. Diarrhea
Paroxetine	Nil	++++	Nil	20–60 mg	N + V, Bruxism, H.A. Diarrhea
Sertraline	Nil	++++	Nil	50–200 mg	N + V, Bruxism, H.A. Diarrhea
Clomipramine	++++	+++	+	25–250 mc	Sedation
ATYP					
Bupropion	—	Nil	Nil	200–450 mg	Seizures (>450mc/ day), Parkinsonian symptoms
Trazodone	Nil	+++	+++	50–600 mg 100–150 mg	Sedation, Priapism
Nefazodone	Nil	++	+++	200–600 mg 20–60 mg 50–200 mg	Sedation
Venlafaxine	Nil	+++	Nil	50–200 mg	Nausea + Vomiting, Diarrhea

Antidepressant Classes (Abbreviations): ATYP = Atypical antidepressants; NE/5-HT = Mixed adrenergic/serotonergic antidepressants; SSRI = Selective serotonin reuptake inhibitors; TCA = Tricyclic antidepressants.   N + V = nausea and vomiting administration of the drug. The development of side effects may warrant a change in medication. Often patients can be encouraged to continue their medication when reassured by the physician. Brown and others have found that patients who are intolerant of one drug within a class (SSRIs) can be switched effectively to a different agent within the same class [369,370]. Too often, drugs are changed because of side effects or presumed lack of effect before the optimal clinical response would normally occur. It is recommended that an appropriate dose level be established and maintained over a longer period of time (4–6 weeks) before changing medication. Generally, patients with FGIDs will benefit from lower dosages than that prescribed for major depression. Treatment must be individualized.

Pharmacology

The patient whose functional gastrointestinal complaint is characterized by prominent abdominal pain, diarrhea, or nausea would do better on a tricyclic antidepressant (TCA) than on a selective serotonin reuptake inhibitor (SSRI) because of the tendency of SSRIs to produce cramping, nausea and diarrhea due to their prokinetic effect. A patient with considerable anxiety might do better on an antidepressant that tends to be more sedating, i.e., one with a strong antihistaminic effect. The side effect profile of the various antidepressants is determined by their effect on various neurotransmitter symptoms (Table 5).

The utility of antidepressant medications in chronic pain suggests a "neuromodulation" effect that may be independent of their effect on depressed mood. The dosage needed to produce relief of pain is often considerably less than that routinely used for the treatment of depression. Furthermore, the onset of analgesia varies from immediately to up to ten weeks [362]. One study suggested that agents particularly effective in blocking norepinephrine reuptake are more likely to be effective in treating neuropathic pain than serotonin reuptake blockers such as fluoxetine [371]. The usefulness of the SSRIs for the treatment of visceral pain, as seen in the functional gastrointestinal disorders, is still uncertain.

Tricyclic Antidepressants

The oldest class of antidepressants is the tricyclic antidepressants (TCAs), which have been in use for over 30 years. They can lower the seizure threshold. These drugs have a "quinidine-like" effect and are arrhythmogenic. However, a recent review suggests that they are not as cardiotoxic as previously thought [372]. Tricyclic antidepressants have been used successfully in the treatment of a variety of non-visceral pain syndromes, including diabetic neuropathy

[371], arthritic back pain [362], and cancer pain [373]. Tricyclic antidepressants have also been the most widely studied of the antidepressants in the treatment of IBS [364,365,374,375] and functional chest pain [363]. Most have anticholinergic effects, but with some exceptions (see Table 5). One novel tricyclic antidepressant, clomipramine, has serotonin reuptake blocking properties and significant anticholinergic effects. Clomipramine and other agents have also been suggested as useful in treating a spectrum of obsessive-compulsive-like disorders [376,377].

Selective Serotonin Reuptake Inhibitors (SSRIs)

The SSRIs have revolutionized the psychopharmacologic treatment of depression. This new class of agents, which consists of fluoxetine, sertraline, fluvoxamine, and paroxetine, work by the inhibition of 5-HT receptors. The usefulness of the SSRIs in the treatment of chronic pain has not been conclusively demonstrated. One study found that fluoxetine was no better than a placebo for the treatment of neuropathic pain [371]. A recent meta-analysis reviewing 19 studies treating a variety of pain conditions did not show any definitive advantages to the SSRIs [378]

The SSRIs have not been extensively studied for their usefulness in the functional gastrointestinal disorders. They have been anecdotally reported to be useful in the treatment of chronic abdominal pain [379]. However, the SSRIs have a number of qualities that make them potentially useful in certain gastrointestinal settings. The prokinetic effects of SSRIs may make them particularly helpful in patients who have functional constipation and/or functional abdominal bloating. In addition, recent studies supporting a role for central 5-HT dysfunction in functional dyspepsia may suggest a use for these agents [366,380].

Other Antidepressants

Newer antidepressants have been developed which have both strong SSRI and adrenergic properties; an example of these is venlafaxine. "Mixed" agents are unique in that they lack the muscarinic, histaminic, and peripheral α-adrenergic blocking effects of the TCAs but at the same time, are potent 5-HT and adrenergic reuptake blockers in the brain [381]. Their usefulness has not yet been established in the functional gastrointestinal disorders, but they provide an alternative for patients who cannot tolerate SSRIs because of side effects.

Atypical antidepressants are so named because they do not act by the more common effect of blocking 5-HT or norepinephrine reuptake. Trazodone is a weak serotonin reuptake blocker. However, it also has some direct 5-HT agonist activity. It is completely devoid of anticholinergic, adrenergic or dopaminergic activity. One advantage of trazodone is its marked tendency to promote sedation. Trazodone's major side effects are to α-adrenergic blockade and include orthostatic hypotension and priapism in 1% of men who take the medication. This latter side effect makes it unacceptable for use in men [382]

Nefazodone is a novel antidepressant that blocks central $5-HT_{2\alpha}$ and norepinephrine reuptake. However, unlike trazodone, it does not block peripheral α_1-adrenergic receptors, making it unlikely to cause priapism [383]. It has no anticholinergic effect, has a very mild side effect profile and is well tolerated in elderly patients. Nefazodone has not been studied in the functional gastrointestinal disorders, but it is a reasonable agent for use in men.

Bupropion, a monocyclic antidepressant, acts via stimulation of norepinephrine pathways. The major precaution to be taken with bupropion is to be aware of the drug's tendency to induce seizures when used above the recommended therapeutic range (450 mg/day for adults). No formal studies have demonstrated a particular usefulness for bupropion in the functional gastrointestinal disorders. However, its lack of sexual and anticholinergic side effects makes it a potentially useful agent for patients struggling with these side effects.

Anxiolytics

Anxiolytic agents, most often represented by the benzodiazepines, can be used in certain situations, including treating patients with co-morbid generalized anxiety and panic disorders. Benzodiazepines are excellent anti-panic agents, but the CNS depressant effect of these agents is synergistic with other CNS depressants such as alcohol or barbiturates, and they need to be used with caution in these settings. Alprazolam has been successfully used in the treatment of IBS associated with panic disorder [225]. However, the risk of addiction with the benzodiazepines, their tendency to produce mild transient cognitive dysfunction, and their effect on gastrointestinal motility (e.g., decreased esophageal sphincter pressure and delayed gastric emptying) means that they have very limited use in the gastrointestinal setting. Benzodiazepine dependence is not common, but we recommend that a psychiatrist be consulted to evaluate patients in order to firmly establish the presence of a psychiatric diagnosis that may make prescribing benzodiazepines reasonable. Prescribing benzodiazepines on a chronic basis is unwise and alternative strategies for the treatment for anxiety should be utilized.

Azapirones

A newer class of anti-anxiety agents, the azapirones (e.g., buspirone) act by serotonin agonist activity at presynaptic 5-HT receptors [355,384]. Buspirone has no anti-panic activity but has been used as an adjunctive treatment to potentiate the action of antidepressants [385]. Buspirone is well tolerated, displaying only occasional serotonergic-related side effects. It has no addictive potential and is a reasonable alternative in treating anxious patients who cannot tolerate benzodiazepines [386].

Psychiatric Consultation for Psychopharmacological Treatment

Many times patients will display particularly troublesome side effects from antidepressants. It is usually best to encourage the patient to continue with the drug as side effects reduce with time and the beneficial effect becomes more prominent. If a patient cannot tolerate an antidepressant, it is reasonable change to another drug in the same class. If patients then do not improve, then referral to a psychiatrist is warranted. A psychiatrist can be particularly helpful in determining further drug changes or dosage regimen.

A very small number of patients report significant psychiatric symptoms such as depression or intense anxiety symptoms. Psychiatric consultation can be extremely helpful in these settings. Expert opinion is required to optimize drug regimens for these complex patients.

Recommendations for Future Research

— Methodology

(1) Address effects of certain subgroups:
   (a) Severity (mild, moderate, severe)
   (b) Refractory-to-treatment groups.
(2) Studies of psychological interventions should include session-by-session treatment manuals and measures of therapist adherence to treatment protocols.
(3) Psychological intervention studies should use trained and experienced therapists (not trainees).
(4) Appropriate placebo conditions should be used to address expectancy and attention, and measure credibility.
(5) The interaction between psychosocial traits (e.g., neuroticism) and HRQOL should be looked at.
(6) Current measures should be standardized and new instruments for FGID developed.
(7) Well-designed, randomized ,controlled psychopharmacologic trials should be developed.

— Mechanisms

(1) Determine the role of genetic factors on the presence of FGID and the selectivity to specific organ systems.
(2) Determine the influence of gender and sociocultural factors on the illness.
(3) Determine the influence of clinical setting (non-patients, primary care, gastrointestinal referral, psychiatric referral).
(4) Design prospective studies to assess populations at risk:
   (a) Children of parents with FGID;
   (b) Individuals who acquire enteric infections;
   (c) Victims of abuse.
(5) Perform studies that combine brain imaging (PET, fMRI), gastrointestinal physiology, and standardized psychosocial assessment.
(6) Study the influence of psychiatric diagnosis and other psychological factors as they affect symptom expression and outcome in FGID.
(7) Develop new conceptual models for the pathogenesis of FGID rather than continuing descriptive studies.

(8) Study psychoneuroimmunological and psychoneuroendocrinological effects on FGID.

(9) Study whether or not treatment effects (pharmacological and psychological) on symptoms are mediated by changes in gut/CNS physiology.

— Assessment

(1) Develop standardized instruments for FGIDs (e.g., HRQOL, cognitive scales, etc.).

— Treatment

(1) Study the effect of physician communication skills on:
    (a) Physician/patient satisfaction with care;
    (b) Adherence to treatment including in drug trial;
    (c) Outcome.

(2) Determine the patient characteristics that predict response to specific psychological treatments.

(3) Determine which components of psychological treatment packages (e.g., relaxation, cognitive restructuring, etc.) account for effectiveness.

(4) Study the efficacy of different classes of psychotropic drugs.

(5) Perform studies to show effects of multidisciplinary treatment programs for FGIDs.

(6) Consider effects of long-term treatment interventions.

(7) Assess long term effects (>1 year) of treatment interventions.

References

1. Drossman DA, Creed FH, Fava GA, et al. Psychosocial aspects of the functional gastrointestinal disorders. Gastroenterol Internat 1995;8:47–90.
2. Mitchell CM, Drossman DA. Survey of the AGA membership relating to patients with functional gastrointestinal disorders. Gastroenterology 1987;92:1282–84.
3. Drossman DA, Li Z, Andruzzi E, et al. U.S. householder survey of functional gastrointestinal disorders: prevalence, sociodemography and health impact. Dig Dis Sci 1993;38:1569–80.
4. Talley NJ, Gabriel SE, Harmsen WS, et al. Medical costs in community subjects with irritable bowel syndrome. Gastroenterology 1995;109:1736–41.
5. Drossman DA. Presidential address: gastrointestinal illness and biopsychosocial model. Psychosomat Med 1998;60(3):258–67.
6. Drossman DA. Psychosocial and psychophysiologic mechanisms in GI illness. In: Kirsner JB, Editors.The Growth of Gastroenterologic Knowledge in the 20th Century. Philadelphia:Lea & Febiger;1993;419–22.
7. Lipowski ZJ. Psychosomatic medicine: past and present: part 1: historical background. Can J Psychiatry 1986;31:2–7.
8. Rush B. Sixteen Introductory Lectures. Philadelphia:Bradford and Innskeep;1811.
9. Dubos R, Escande JP. Reflections on Medicine, Science and Humanity. New York:Harcourt Brace Jovanovich;1979.
10. Beaumont W. Experiments and Observations on the Gastric Juice and the Physiology of Digestion. Plattsburg, New York:F.P. Allen;1833.
11. Cannon WB. The movements of the intestine studied by means of roentgen rays. Am J Physiol 1902;6:251–77.
12. Pavlov I. In: Thompson WH, Editor. The Work of the Digestive Glands. London: C. Griffen and Company;1910.
13. Selye H. The general adaptation syndrome and the diseases of adaptation. J Clin Endocrinol Metab 1946;6:117–26.
14. Wolf S; Wolff HG. Human Gastric Function. New York:Oxford University Press;1943.
15. Engel GL, Reichsman F, Segal HL. A study of an infant with gastric fistula. I. behavior and the rate of total hydrochloric acid secretion. Psychosomat Med 1956;18:374–98.
16. Almy TP, Hinkle LEJ, Berle B, et al. Alterations in colonic function in man under stress: III: experimental production of sigmoid spasm in patients with spastic constipation. Gastroenterology 1949;12:437–49.
17. Almy TP. Experimental studies on the irritable colon. Am J Med 1951;10:60–67.
18. Alexander F. Psychosomatic Medicine: Its Principles and Applications. New York: W.W. Norton; 1950.
19. Drossman DA. Psychosocial factors in ulcerative colitis and Crohn's disease. In: Kirsner JB, Editor. Inflammatory Bowel Disease. Ed 5. Philadelphia: W.B. Saunders; 1999, in press.

20. Aronowitz R, Spiro HM. The rise and fall of the psychosomatic hypothesis in ulcerative colitis. J Clin Gastroenterol 1988;10:298–305.

21. Olden KW. Pyschosocial aspects of gastroenterology: doctor-patient interactions. Brandt LJ, Friedman LS, Editors. Clinical Practice of Gastroenterology. Philadelphia:1998:

22. Harvey RF, Read AE. Effect of cholecystokinin on colon motility and symptoms in patients with the irritable bowel syndrome. Lancet 1973;1:1–3.

23. Sullivan MA, Cohen S, Snape WJ. Colonic myoelectrical activity in irritable-bowel syndrome. New Engl J Med 1978;298:878–83.

24. Connell AM, Jones FA, Rowlands EN. Motility of the pelvic colon. IV. Abdominal pain associated with colonic hypermotility after meals. Gut 1965;6:105–12.

25. Snape WJ, Carlson GM, Cohen S. Colonic myoelectric activity in the irritable bowel syndrome. Gastroenterology 1976;70:326–30.

26. Latimer PR, Sarna SK, Campbell D, et al. Colonic motor and myoelectrical activity: a comparative study of normal patients, psychoneurotic patients and patients with irritable bowel syndrome (IBS). Gastroenterol 1981;80:893–901.

27. Drossman DA. Psychosocial factors in gastrointestinal disorders. In: Feldman M, Scharschmidt B, Editors. Sleisenger and Fordtran's Gastrointestinal Disease. Ed 6. Philadelphia:W.B. Saunders;1997:69–79.

28. Engel GL. The need for a new medical model: a challenge for biomedicine. Science 1977;196:129–36.

29. Engel GL. The clinical application of the biopsychosocial model. Am J Psychiatry 1980;137:535–44.

30. Engel GL. The biopsychosocial model and medical education. New Engl J Med 1981;306:802–805.

31. Mendeloff AI, Monk M, Siegel CI, et al. Illness experience and life stresses in patients with irritable colon and with ulcerative colitis: an epidemiologic study of ulcerative colitis and regional enteritis in Baltimore, 1960–1964. New Engl J Med 1970;282:14–17.

32. Esler MD, Goulston KJ. Levels of anxiety in colonic disorders. New Engl J Med 1973;288:16–20.

33. Palmer RL, Crisp AH, Sonehill E, et al. Psychological characteristics of patients with the irritable bowel syndrome. Postgrad Med J 1974;50:416-19.

34. Young SJ, Alpers DH, Norland CC, et al. Psychiatric illness and the irritable bowel syndrome: practical implications for the primary physician. Gastroenterology 1976;70:162-66.

35. Feighner JP, Robins E, Guze B, et al. Diagnostic criteria for use in psychiatric research. Arch Gen Psychiatry 1972;26:57–63.

36. American Psychiatric Association. Diagnostic and Statistical Manual of Mental Disorders—DSM-IV. Ed. 4. Washington, D.C.:American Psychiatric Association; 1994.

37. Walker EA, Roy-Byrne PP, Katon WJ, et al. Psychiatric illness and irritable bowel

syndrome: a comparison with inflammatory bowel disease. Am J Psychiatry 1990; 147:1656–61.

38. Toner BB, Garfinkel PE, Jeejeebhoy KN. Psychological factors in irritable bowel syndrome. Can J Psychiatry 1990;35:158–61.

39. Clouse RE, Lustman PJ. Psychiatric illness and contraction abnormalities of the esophagus. New Engl J Med 1983;309:1337–42.

40. Magni G, DiMario F, Bernasconi G, et al. DSM-III diagnoses associated with dyspepsia of unknown cause. Am J Psychiatry 1987;144:1222–23.

41. Fava GA and Wise TN, Editors. Research Paradigms in Psychosomatic Medicine. Basel:Karger;1987.

42. Derogatis LR. SCL-90-R: Administration, Scoring, and Procedures Manual II— For the R(evised) Version. Towson, Maryland:Clinical Psychometric Research; 1983.

43. Sarason IG, Levine HM, Basham RB, et al. Assessing social support: the Social Support Questionnaire. J Pers Soc Psychol 1983;44:127–39.

44. Lazarus RS, Folkman S. Stress, Appraisal and Coping. New York:Verlag;1984.

45. Bergner M, Bobbitt RA, Carter WB. The Sickness Impact Profile: development and final revision of a health status measure. Med Care 1981;19:787–805.

46. Drossman DA, Sandler RS, McKee DC, et al. Bowel patterns among subjects not seeking health care: use of a questionnaire to identify a population with bowel dysfunction. Gastroenterology 1982;83:529–34.

47. Thompson WG, Heaton KW. Functional bowel disorders in apparently healthy people. Gastroenterology 1980;79:283–88.

48. Drossman DA, McKee DC, Sandler RS, et al. Psychosocial factors in the irritable bowel syndrome: a multivariate study of patients and nonpatients with irritable bowel syndrome. Gastroenterology 1988;95:701–708.

49. Whitehead WE, Bosmajian L, Zonderman AB, et al. Symptoms of psychologic distress associated with irritable bowel syndrome: comparison of community and medical clinic samples. Gastroenterology 1988;95:709–14.

50. Holmes TH, Rahe RH. The social readjustment rating scale. J Psychosomat Res 1967;11:213–18.

51. Sarason IG, Johnson JH, Siegel JM. Assessing the impact of life changes: development of the life experiences survey. J Consult Clin Psychol 1978;46:932–46.

52. Paykel ES. Methodological aspects of life events research. J Psychosomat Res 1983;27:341–52.

53. Craig TKJ, Brown GW. Goal frustration and life events in the aetiology of painful gastrointestinal disorder. J Psychosomat Res 1984;28:411–21.

54. Brown GW; Harris TO. Social Origins of Depression: A Study of Psychiatric Disorder in Women. London:Tavistock;1978.

55. Creed FH, Craig T, Farmer RG. Functional abdominal pain, psychiatric illness and life events. Gut 1988;29:235–42.

56. Pilowski S. Manual for the Illness Behavior Questionnaire (IBQ). Ed. 2. Adelaide, Australia:University of Adelaide;1983.

57. Miller NE. Effect of learning on gastrointestinal functions. Clin Gastroenterol 1977;6:533–46.

58. Jacobsen E. Progressive Relaxation. Ed 2. Chicago:Univ Chicago Press;1938.

59. Fordyce WE, Fowler RS, Delateur B. An application of behavior modification technique to a problem of chronic pain. Behav Res Ther 1968;6:105–107.

60. Lowman BC, Drossman DA, Cramer EM, et al. Recollection of childhood events in adults with irritable bowel syndrome. J Clin Gastroenterol 1987;9:324–30.

61. Whitehead WE, Winget C, Fedoravicius AS, et al. Learned illness behavior in patients with irritable bowel syndrome and peptic ulcer. Dig Dis Sci 1982;27:202–208.

62. Whitehead WE, Crowell MD, et al. Modeling and reinforcement of the sick role during childhood predicts adult illness behavior. Psychosomat Med 1994;6:541–50.

63. Miller NE, Dworkin BR. Effects of learning on visceral functions—biofeedback. New Engl J Med 1977;296:1274–78.

64. Bueno-Miranda F, Cerulli M, Schuster MM. Operant conditioning of colonic motility in irritable bowel syndrome abstr.). Gastroenterol 1976;70:867.

65. Schuster MM, Nikoomanesh P, Welles D. Biofeedback control of lower esophageal sphincter contraction (abstr.). Clin Res 1973;21:521.

66. Marzuk PM. Biofeedback for gastrointestinal disorders: a review of the literature. Ann Intern Med 1985;103:240–44.

67. Whitehead WE, Devroede G, Habib FI, et al. Functional disorders of the anorectum. Gastroenterol Internat 1992;5:92–108.

68. Epstein AM. The outcomes movement: will it get us where we want to go? New Engl J Med 1990;323:266–70.

69. Camara EG, Danao TC. The brain and the immune system: a psychosomatic network. Psychosomatics 1989;30:140–46.

70. Ottoway CA. Role of the neuroendocrine system in cytokine pathways in inflammatory bowel disease. Aliment Pharmacol Ther 1996;10(suppl.2):10–55.

71. Chrousos GP. The hypothalamic-pituitary-adrenal axis and immune-mediated inflammation. New Engl J Med 1995;332(20):1351–62.

72. Frieling T, Enck P, Wienbeck M. Cerebral responses evoked by electrical stimulation of rectosigmoid in normal subjects. Dig Dis Sci 1994;34(2):202–205.

73. Castell DO, Wood JD, Frieling T, et al. Cerebral electrical potentials evoked by balloon distention of the human esophagus. Gastroenterology 1994;98:662–66.

74. Silverman DHS, Munakata JA, Ennes H, et al. Regional cerebral activity in normal and pathologic perception of visceral pain. Gastroenterology 1997;112(1):64–72.

75. Aziz Q, Thompson DG. Brain-gut axis in health and disease. Gastroenterology 1998;114:559–78.

76. Holtmann G, Enck P. Stress and gastrointestinal motility in humans: a review of the literature. J Gastrointest Motil 1991;3(4):245–54.

77. Esophagus. Castell JA, Gideon RM, Castell DO, et al., Editors. Atlas of Gastrointestinal Motility in Health and Disease. Baltimore:Williams & Wilkins;1993:134–57.

78. Stacher G, Steinringer H, Blau A, et al. Acoustically evoked esophageal contractions and defense reactions. Psychophysiology 1979;16:234–41.

79. Young LD, Richter JE, Anderson KO, et al. The effects of pscyhological and environmental stressors on peristaltic esophageal contractions in healthy volunteers. Psychophysiology 1987;24:132–41.

80. Moser G, Wenzel-Abatzi TA, Stelzeneder M, et al. Pharyngoesophageal function, psychometric and psychiatric findings, and follow-up in 88 patients. Arch Intern Med 1998;158:1365–73.

81. The Gallup Organization. A Gallup survey on hearburn across America. Princeton, NJ:The Gallup Organization;1988.

82. Bradley LA, Richter JE, Pulliam TJ, et al. The relationship between stress and symptoms of gastroesophageal reflux: the influence of psychological factors. Am J Gastroenterol 1993;88:11–19.

83. Richter JE, Bradley LA, Castell DO. Esophageal chest pain: current controversies in pathogenesis, diagnosis, and therapy. Ann Intern Med 1989;110:66–78.

84. Rao SSC, Gregersen H, Hayek B, et al. Unexplained chest pain: the hypersensitive, hyperactive, and poorly compliant esophagus. Ann Intern Med 1996;124:950–58.

85. Levenstein S, Prantera C, Varvo V, et al. Patterns of biologic and psychologic risk factors in duodenal ulcer patients. J Clin Gastroenterol 1995;21(2):110–17.

86. Klein KB, Spiegel D. Modulation of gastric acid secretion by hypnosis. Gastroenterology 1989;96:1383–87.

87. Black PH. Central nervous system-immune sytem interactions: psychoneuroendocrinology of stress and its immune consequences. Antimicrob Agents Chemother 1994;38:1–6.

88. Dotevall G. Peptic ulcer, noxious stress, and Campylobacter Pylori. Gastroenterology 1990;98:252–53.

89. Levenstein S. Stress and peptic ulcer: life beyond Helicobacter. Brit Med J 1998; 316:538–41.

90. Thompson DG, Richelson E, Malagelada JR. Perturbation of upper gastrointestinal function by cold stress. Gut 1983;24:277–83.

91. Stanghellini V, Malagelada JR, Zinsmeister AR, et al. Stress-induced gastroduodenal motor disturbances in man: possible humoral mechanisms. Gastroenterology 1983;85:83–91.

92. Kellow JE, Gill RC, Wingate DL. Prolonged ambulant recordings of small bowel motility demonstrate abnormalities in the irritable bowel syndrome. Gastroenterology 1990;98:1208–18.

93. Kellow JE, Eckersley GM, Jones M. Enteric and central contributions to intestinal dysmotility in irritable bowel syndrome. Dig Dis Sci 1992;37:168–74.

94. Frank JW, Sarr MG, Camilleri M. Use of gastroduodenal manometry to differentiate mechanical and functional intestinal obstruction: an analysis of clinical outcome. Am J Gastroenterol 1994;89:339–44.

95. Kellow JE, Phillips SF, Miller LJ, et al. Dysmotility of the small intestine in irritable bowel syndrome. Gut 1988;29:1236–43.

96. Kumar D, Wingate DL. The irritable bowel syndrome: a paraxysmal motor disorder. Lancet 1985;2:973–77.

97. Kellow JE, Langeluddecke PM, Eckersley GM, et al. Effects of acute psychologic stress on small-intestinal motility in health and the irritable bowel syndrome. Scand J Gastroenterol 1992;27:53–58.

98. Evans PR, Bennett EJ, Bak Y-T, et al. Jejunal sensorimotor dysfunction in irritable bowel syndrome: clinical and psychosocial features. Gastroenterology 1996;110: 393–404.

99. Cann PA, Read NW, Brown C, et al. Irritable bowel syndrome: relationship of disorders in the transit of a single solid meal to symptom patterns. Gut 1983;24: 405–11.

100. Almy TP, Tulin M. Alterations in colonic function in man under stress: experimental production of changes simulating the "irritable colon." Gastroenterology 1947;8:616–26.

101. Welgan P, Meshkinpour H, Hoehler F. The effect of stress on colon motor and electrical activity in irritable bowel syndrome. Psychosomat Med 1985;47:139–49.

102. Welgan P, Meshkinpour H, Beeler M. Effect of anger on colon motor and myoelectric activity in irritable bowel syndrome. Gastroenterology 1988;94:1150–56.

103. Whorwell PJ, Houghton LA, Taylor EE, et al. Physiological effects of emotion: assessment via hypnosis. Lancet 1992;340:69–72.

104. Whitehead WE, Engel BT, Schuster MM. Irritable bowel syndrome: physiological and psychological differences between diarrhea-predominant and constipation-predominant patients. Dig Dis Sci 1980;25:6:404–13.

105. Whitehead WE, Holtkotter B, Enck P, et al. Tolerance for rectosigmoid distention in irritable bowel syndrome. Gastroenterology 1990;98:1187–92.

106. Sullivan MA, Cohen S, Snape WJ. Colonic myoelectrical activity in irritable bowel syndrome: effect of eating and anticholinergics. New Engl J Med 1978; 298:878–83.

107. Chasen R, Tucker H, Palmer D, et al. Colonic motility in irritable bowel syndrome and diverticular disease. Gastroenterology 1982;82:A1031.

108. Whitehead WE, Crowell MD, Davidoff AL, et al. Pain from rectal distension in women with irritable bowel syndrome: relationship to sexual abuse. Dig Dis Sci 1997;42(4):796–804.

109. Bell AM, Pemberton JH, Camilleri M, et al. The effect of acute stress on rectal tone and anal sphincter pressure. Gastroenterology 1989;96:A38.

110. Erckenbrecht JF, Lefhalm C, Wallstein U, et al. The gastrocolonic response to eating is not only a motor but also a sensory event. Gastroenterology 1989;96:A141.

111. Steadman CJ, Phillips SF, Camilleri M, et al. Variation of muscle tone in the human colon. Gastroenterology 1991;101:373–81.

112. Whitehead WE, Chami TN, Crowell MD, et al. Aerophagia: association with gastrointestinal and psychological symptoms. Gastroenterology 1991;100:A508.

113. Soykan I, Chen J, Bradley LA. The rumination syndrome: clinical and manometric profile, therapy, and long-term outcome. Dig Dis Sci 1997;42:1866–72.

114. Fonagy P, Calloway SP. The effect of emotional arousal on spontaneous swallowing rates. J Psychosomat Res 1986;30:183–88.

115. Calloway SP, Fonagy P, Pounder RE, et al. Behavioural techniques in the management of aerophagia in patients with hiatus hernia. J Psychosomat Res 1983;27: 499–502.

116. Solyom L, Sookman D. Fear of choking and its treatment. Can J Psychiatry 1980; 25:30–34.

117. DiScipio WJ, Kaslon K, Ruben RJ. Traumatically acquired conditioned dysphagia in children. Ann Otol Rhinol Laryngol 1978;87:509–14.

118. DiScipio WJ, Kaslon K. Conditioned dysphagia in cleft palate children after pharyngeal flap surgery. Psychosomat Med 1982;44:247–57.

119. Richter JE, Baldi F, Clouse RE, et al. Functional oesophageal disorders. Gastroenterol Internat 1992;5:3–17.

120. DeMeester TR, Johnson LF, Guy JJ, et al. Patterns of gastroesophageal reflux in health and disease. Ann Surg 1976;184:459–70.

121. Chatoor I, Dickson L, Einhorn A. Rumination: etiology and treatment. Pediatr Ann 1984;13:924–29.

122. Parry-Jones B. Merycism or rumination disorder: a historical investigation and current assessment. Brit J Psychiatry 1994;165:303–14.

123. Einhorn AH. Rumination syndrome (mercycism or cerycasm). In:. Barnett HL, Editor.Pediatrics. New York:Appleton-Century-Crofts;1972:1576–8.

124. Richmond JB, Eddy E, Green M. Rumination: a psychosomatic syndrome of infancy. Pediatrics 1958;59:371–77.

125. Toister RP, Condron CJ, Worley L, et al. Faradic therapy of chronic vomiting in infancy: a case study. J Behav Ther Exp Psych 1975;6:55–59.

126. Whitehead WE; Schuster MM. Gastrointestinal Disorders: Behavioral and Physiological Basis for Treatment. San Diego:Academic Press;1985.

127. O'Brien MD, Bruce BK, Camilleri M. The rumination syndrome: clinical features rather than manometric diagnosis. Gastroenterology 1995;1088:1024–29.

128. Whitehead WE, Drinkwater D, Cheskin LJ, et al. Constipation in the elderly living at home: definition, prevalence and relationship to lifestyle and health status. J Am Geriatr Soc 1989;37:423–29.

129. Sandler RS, Drossman DA. Bowel habits in young adults not seeking health care. Dig Dis Sci 1987;32:841–45.

130. Johanson JF. Geographical distribution of constipation in the United States. Am J Gastroenterol 1998;93(2):188–91.

131. Romero Y, Evans JM, FLeming KC, et al. Constipation and fecal incontinence in the elderly population. Mayo Clin Proc 1996;71:81–92.

132. Preston DM, Lennard-Jones JE. Anismus in chronic constipation. Dig Dis Sci 1985;30(5):413–18.

133. Devroede G, Girard G, Bouchoucha M, et al. Idiopathic constipation by colonic dysfunction. Dig Dis Sci 1989;34:1428–33.

134. Tucker DM, Sandstead HH, Logan GMJ, et al. Dietary fiber and personality factors as determinants of stool output. Gastroenterology 1981;81:879–83.

135. Wald A, Hinds JP, Caruana BJ. Psychological and physiological characteristics of patients with severe idiopathic constipation. Gastroenterology 1989;97:932–37.

136. Whitehead WE. Illness behavior. In: Kamm MA, Lennard-Jones JE, Editors. Constipation. Petersfield,UK:Wrightson Biomedical Publishing;1994:95–100.

137. Leroi AM, Bernier C, Watier A, et al. Prevalence of sexual abuse among patients with functional disorders of the lower gastrointestinal tract. Internat J Colorect Dis 1995;10(4):200–206.

138. Grimaud JC, Bouvier M, Naudy B, et al. Manometric and radiologic investigations and biofeedback treatment of chronic idiopathic anal pain. Dis Colon Rectum 1991;34:690–95.

139. West L, Abell TL, Cutts T. Long-term results of pelvic floor muscle rehabilitation of constipation. Gastroenterology 1992;102:A533.

140. Mayer EA, Raybould HE. Role of visceral afferent mechanisms in functional bowel disorders. Gastroenterology 1990;99:1688–1704.

141. Mayer EA, Gebhart GF. Basic and clinical aspects of visceral hyperalgesia. Gastroenterology 1994;107(1):271–93.

142. Richter JE, Barish CF, Castell DO. Abnormal sensory perception in patients with esophageal chest pain. Gastroenterology 1986;91:845–52.

143. Marbet UA, Stalder GA, Faust H, et al. Endoscopic sphincterotomy and surgical approaches in the treatment of the 'sump syndrome'. Gut 1987;28:142–45.

144. Bradley LA, Richter JE, Scarinci IC, et al. Mechanisms of altered pain perception in non-cardiac chest pain patients. Gastroenterology 1993;104:A482.

145. Whitehead WE, Delvaux M, Working Team. Standardization of procedures for testing smooth muscle tone and sensory thresholds in the gastrointestinal tract. Dig Dis Sci 1994;42(2):223–41.

146. Bradette M, Pare P, Douville P, et al. Visceral perception in health and functional dyspepsia: crossover study of gastric distension with placebo and domperidone. Dig Dis Sci 1991;36:52–58.

147. Mearin F, Cucala M, Azpiroz F, et al. The origin of symptoms on the brain-gut axis in functional dyspepsia. Gastroenterology 1991;101:999–1006.

148. Lemann M, Dederding JP, Flourie B, et al. Abnormal perception of visceral pain in response to gastric distension in chronic idiopathic dyspepsia: the irritable stomach syndrome. Dig Dis Sci 1991;36:1249–54.

149. Notivol R, Coffin B, Azpiroz F, et al. Gastric tone determines the sensitivity of the stomach to distention. Gastroenterology 1995;108:330–36.

150. Coffin B, Azpiroz F, Guarner F, et al. Selective gastric hypersensitivity and reflex hyporeactivity in functional dyspepsia. Gastroenterology 1994;107(5):1345–51.

151. Accarino AM, Azpiroz F, Malagelada JR. Attention and distraction: effects on gut perception. Gastroenterol 1997;113:415–22.

152. Ritchie J. Pain from distension of the pelvic colon by inflating a balloon in the irritable bowel syndrome. Gut 1973;6:105–12.

153. Cook IJ, van Eeden A, Collins SM. Patients with irritable bowel syndrome have greater pain tolerance than normal subjects. Gastroenterology 1987;93:727–33.

154. Prior A, Colgan SM, Whorwell PJ. Changes in rectal sensitivity after hypnotherapy in patients with irritable bowel syndrome. Gut 1990;31:896–98.

155. Accarino AM, Azpiroz F, Malagelada JR. Selective dysfunction of mechanosensi-

tive intestinal afferents in irritable bowel syndrome. Gastroenterology 1995;108: 636–43.

156. Greenwood B, Rodriguez S, Decktor D, et al. Irritable bowel syndrome: a study to investigate the mechanism(s) of visceral hypersensitivity. Med J Austral 1996; 89(2):47–50.

157. Stein MB, Koverola C, Hanna C, et al. Hippocampal volume in women victimized by childhood sexual abuse. Psychol Med 1997;27(4):951–59.

158. Costantini M, Sturniolo GC, Zaninotto G, et al. Altered esophageal pain threshold in irritable bowel syndrome. Dig Dis Sci 1993;38:206–12.

159. Trimble KC, Farouk R, Pryde A, et al. Heightened visceral sensation in functional gastrointestinal disease is not site-specific: evidence for a generalized disorder of gut sensitivity. Digestive Diseases & Sciences 1995;40(8):1607–13.

160. Kellow JE, Eckersley GM, Jones MP. Enhanced perception of physiological intestinal motility in the irritable bowel syndrome. Gastroenterology 1991;101:1621–27.

161. Prior A, Maxton DG, Whorwell PJ. Anorectal manometry in irritable bowel syndrome: differences between diarrhoea and constipation predominant subjects. Gut 1990;31:458–62.

162. Lembo T, Munakata J, Mertz H, et al. Evidence for the hypersensitivity of the lumbar splanchnic afferents in irritable bowel syndrome. Gastroenterology 1994;107: 1686–96.

163. Mertz H, Naliboff B, Munakata J, et al. Altered rectal perception is a biological marker of patients with irritable bowel syndrome. Gastroenterology 1995;109(1): 40–52.

164. Ford MJ, Camilleri M, Zinsmeister AR, et al. Psychosensory modulation of colonic sensation in the human transverse and sigmoid colon. Gastroenterology 1995;109:1772–80.

165. Whitehead WE, Palsson OS. Is rectal pain sensitivity a biological marker for irritable bowel syndrome: psychological influences on pain perception. Gastroenterology 1998 (in press).

166. Whitehead WE, Diamant NE, Meyer K, et al. Pain thresholds measured by the barostat predict the severity of clinical pain in patients with irritable bowel syndrome. Gastroenterology 1998;114:A859.

167. Sternberg EM, Chrousos GP, Wilder RL, et al. The stress response and the regulation of inflammatory disease. Ann Intern Med 1992;117:854–66.

168. Shavit Y, Martin FC. Opiates, stress and immunity: animal studies. Ann Behav Med 1987;9:11–15.

169. Burks TF, Galligan JJ, Hirning LD, et al. Brain, spinal cord and peripheral sites of action of enkephalins and other endogenous opioids on gastrointestinal motility. Gastroenterol Clin Biol 1987;11:44B–51B.

170. Baile CA, McLaughlin CL, Della Fera MA. Role of cholecystokinin and opioid peptides in control of food intake. Physiol Rev 1986;66:172–234.

171. Shavit Y, Terman GW, Martin FC, et al. Stress, opioid peptides, the immune system, and cancer. J Immunol 1985;135 (2):834s–37s.

172. Smith GP. Satiety effect of gastrointestinal hormones. In: Beers RFJ, Bassett EG, Editors. Polypeptide Hormones. New York:Raven Press;1980:413–20.

173. Geracioti TDJ, Liddle RA. Impaired cholecystokinin secretion in bulimia nervosa. New Engl J Med 1988;319:683–88.

174. Sanger GJ. 5-Hydroxytryptamine and functional bowel disorders. Neurogastroenterol Motil 1996;8(4):319–31.

175. Goldberg PA, Kamm MA, Setti-Carraro P, et al. Modification of visceral sensitivity and pain in irritable bowel syndrome by 5-HT$_3$ antagonism (ondansetron). Digestion 1996;57:478–83.

176. Banner SE, Sanger GJ. Differences between 5-HT$_3$ receptor antagonists in modulation of visceral hypersensitivity. Brit J Pharmacol 1995;114(2):558–62.

177. The Subcutaneous Sumatriptan International Study Group. Treatment of migraine attacks with sumatriptan. New Engl J Med 1991;325:316–21.

178. Eison MS. The new generation of serotonergic anxiolytics: possible clinical roles. Psychopathology 1989;22(Suppl 1):13–20.

179. Collins SM. The immunomodulation of enteric neuromuscular function: implications for motility and inflammatory disorders. Gastroenterology 1996;111(6): 1683–99.

180. Shanahan F. The intestinal immune system., Johnson LR, Editor. Physiology of the Gastrointestinal Tract. Ed. 3. New York:Raven Press;1994:643–84.

181. Sternberg EM, Parker CW. Pharmacologic aspects of lymphocyte regulation. In: Marchalonis JJ, Editor.The Lymphocyte: Structure and Function. New York: Marcel Dekker, Inc.;1988.:1–54.

182. Coderre TJ, Katz J, Vaccarino AL, et al. Contribution of central neuroplasticity to pathological pain: review of clinical and experimental evidence. Pain 1993;52: 259–85.

183. Drossman DA. The functional gastrointestinal disorders and their diagnosis: a coming of age. In: Drossman DA, Richter JE, Talley NJ, Editors. The Functional Gastrointestinal Disorders: Diagnosis, Pathophysiology and Treatment. McLean, VA:Degnon Associates;1994:1–23.

184. Drossman DA; Richter JE; Talley NJ, et al. The Functional Gastrointestinal Disorders: Diagnosis, Pathophysiology and Treatment. McLean,VA:Degnon Associates;1994.

185. Drossman DA, Whitehead WE, Camilleri M. Irritable bowel syndrome: a technical review for practice guideline development. Gastroenterology 1997;112(6): 2120–37.

186. Richter JE, Barish CF, Castell DO. Abnormal sensory perception in patients with esophageal chest pain. Gastroenterology 1986;91:845–52.

187. Clouse RE, Lustman PJ, McCord GS, et al. Clinical correlates of abnormal sensitivity to intraesophageal balloon distention. Dig Dis Sci 1991;36:1040–45.

188. Mearin F, Cucala M, Azpiroz F, et al. The origin of symptoms on the brain-gut axis in functional dyspepsia. Gastroenterology 1991;101:999–1006.

189. Valori RM, Kumar D, Wingate DL. Effects of different types of stress and or

"prokinetic" drugs on the control of the fasting motor complex in humans. Gastroenterology 1986;90:1890–1900.

190. Kumar D, Thompson PD, Wingate DL, et al. Abnormal REM sleep in the irritable bowel syndrome. Gastroenterol 1992;103:12–17.

191. Fukudo S, Nomura T, Muranaka M, et al. Brain-gut response to stress and cholinergic stimulation in irritable bowel syndrome. J Clin Gastroenterol 1993; 17:133–41.

192. Drossman DA, Li Z, Leserman J, et al. Health status by gastrointestinal diagnosis and abuse history. Gastroenterology 1996;110(4):999–1007.

193. Drossman DA, Li Z, Leserman J, et al. Association of coping pattern and health status among female GI patients after controlling for GI disease type and abuse history: a prospective study (abstr.). Gastroenterology 1997;112(4):724.

194. Whitehead WE. Assessing the effects of stress on physical symptoms. Health Psychol 1994;13:99–102.

195. Ford MJ, Miller PM, Eastwood J, et al. Life events, psychiatric illness and the irritable bowel syndrome. Gut 1987;28:160–65.

196. Ellard K, Beaurepaire J, Jones M, et al. Acute and chronic stress in duodenal ulcer disease. Gastroenterology 1990;99:1628–32.

197. Gilligan I, Fung L, Piper DW, et al. Life event stress and chronic difficulties in duodenal ulcer: a case control study. J Psychosomat Res 1987;31(1):117–23.

198. Jenkins CD, Hurst MW, Rose RM. Life changes: Do people really remember? Arch Gen Psychiatry 1979;36:379–84.

199. Klein DN, Rubovits DR. Relativity of subjects' reports on stressful life events inventories—longitudinal studies. J Behav Med 1987;10:501–12.

200. Brown GW, Harris TO. Fall-off in the reporting life events. Soc Psychiatry 1982; 17:23–28.

201. Neilson E, Brown GW, Marmot M. Myocardial infarction. In: Brown GW, Harris TO, Editors. Life Events and Illness. New York:The Guilford Press;1989:313–43.

202. Thomas J, Greig M, Paper DW. Chronic gastric ulcer and life events. Gastroenterology 1980;78:905–11.

203. Whitehead WE, Crowell MD, Robinson JC, et al. Effects of stressful life events on bowel symptoms: subjects with irritable bowel syndrome compared to subjects without bowel dysfunction. Gut 1992;33:825–30.

204. Drossman DA, Talley NJ, Olden KW, et al. Sexual and physical abuse and gastrointestinal illness: review and recommendations. Ann Intern Med 1995;123(10): 782–94.

205. Talley NJ, Owen B, Bai J, et al. Does psychological distress account for the apparent association between abuse and irritable bowel syndrome? A population-based study. Gastroenterology 1995;110:A767.

206. Peters SD, Wyatt GE, Finkelhor D. Prevalence. Finkelhor D, Editor. A Sourcebook on Child Sexual Abuse. Beverly Hills:Sage Publications;1986:15–59.

207. Leserman J, Drossman DA, Li Z, et al. Sexual and physical abuse in gastroenterology practice: how types of abuse impact health status. Psychosomat Med 1996;58:4–15.

208. Leserman J, Li Z, Drossman DA, et al. Impact of sexual and physical abuse dimensions on health status: development of an abuse severity measure. Psychosomat Med 1997;59:152–60.
209. Drossman DA, Leserman J, Nachman G, et al. Sexual and physical abuse in women with functional or organic gastrointestinal disorders. Ann Intern Med 1990;113:828–33.
210. Talley NJ, Fett SL, Zinsmeister AR. Self-reported abuse and gastrointestinal disease in outpatients: association with irritable bowel-type symptoms. Am J Gastroenterol 1995;90(3):366–71.
211. Walker EA, Katon WJ, Roy-Byrne PP, et al. Histories of sexual victimization in patients with irritable bowel syndrome or inflammatory bowel disease. Am J Psychiatry 1993;150:1502–1506..
212. Delvaux M, Denis P, Allemand H, French Club of Digestive Motility. Sexual and physical abuses are more frequently reported by IBS patients than by patients with organic digestive diseases or controls: results of a multicenter inquiry. Eur J Gastroenterol Hepat 1997;9:345–52.
213. Scarinci IC, McDonald-Haile JM, Bradley LA, et al. Altered pain perception and psychosocial features among women with gastrointestinal disorders and history of abuse: a preliminary model. Am J Med 1994;97:108–18.
214. Leserman J, Toomey TC, Drossman DA. Medical consequences of sexual and physical abuse in women. Humane Med 1995;11(1):23–28.
215. Laws A. Does a history of sexual abuse in childhood play a role in women's medical problems? A review. J Women's Health 1993;2:165–72.
216. Longstreth GF, Wolde-Tsadik G. Irritable bowel-type symptoms in HMO examinees: prevalence, demographics, and clinical correlates. Dig Dis Sci 1993;38:1581–89.
217. Talley NJ, Fett SL, Zinsmeister AR, et al. Gastrointestinal tract symptoms and self-reported abuse: a population-based study. Gastroenterology 1994;107:1040–49.
218. Drossman DA. Physical and sexual abuse and gastrointestinal illness: what is the link? Am J Med 1994;97:105–107.
219. Walker EA, Katon W, Roy-Byrne PP, et al. Psychiatric illness and irritable bowel syndrome: a comparison with inflammatory bowel disease. Am J Psychiatry 1990;147:1656–61.
220. Drossman DA. Irritable bowel syndrome and sexual/physical abuse History. Eur J Gastroenterol Hepat 1997;9:327–30.
221. White BV, Jones CM. Mucous colitis: a deliniation of the syndrome with certain observations on its mechanism and on the role of emotional tension as a precipitating factor. Ann Intern Med 1940;14:845–72.
222. Chaudhary NA, Truelove SC. The irritable colon syndrome: a study of the clinical features, predisposing causes, and prognosis in 130 cases. Quart J Med 1962;31:307–22.
223. World Health Organization Schedules for Clinical Assessment in Neuropsychiatry. Washington DC:American Psychiatric Association Press, Inc.;1994.

224. Lydiard RB, Fossey MD, Marsh W, et al. Prevalence of psychiatric disorders in patients with irritable bowel syndrome. Psychosomatics 1993;34:229–34.
225. Noyes RJ, Cook B, Garvey M, et al. Reduction of gastrointestinal symptoms following treatment for panic disorder. Psychosomatics 1990;31:75–79.
226. Zaubler TS, Katon W. Panic disorder and medical comorbidity: a review of the medical and psychiatric literature. Bull Menninger Clin 1996;60(suppl A):A12–38.
227. Lydiard RB, Greenwald S, Weissman MM, et al. Panic disorder and gastrointestinal symptoms: findings from the NIMH Epidemiologic Catchment Area project. Am J Psychiatry 1994;151:64–70.
228. Walker EA, Katon WJ, Jemelka RP, et al. Comorbidity of gastrointestinal complaints, depression, and anxiety in the Epidemiologic Catchment Area (ECA) Study. Am J Med 1992;92:26s–30s.
229. Guthrie E, Creed FH. Severe sexual dysfunctioning in women with IBS: comparison with IBD and duodenal ulceration. Brit Med J 1987;295:577–78.
230. Hurwicz ML, Berkanovic E. The stress process in rheumatoid arthritis. J Rheumatol 1993;20:1836–44.
231. Smith RC, Greenbaum DS, Vancouver JB, et al. Psychosocial factors are associated with health care seeking rather than diagnosis in irritable bowel syndrome. Gastroenterology 1990;98:293–301.
232. Toner BB, Segal ZV, Emott SD, et al. Cognitive-Behavioral Treatment of Irritable Bowel Syndrome: The Brain-Gut Connection. London, New York: Guilford Press; 1999:1–188.
233. Crookes TG, Pearson PR. The lie scale as a predictor of placebo response. Personality Indiv Diff 1981;2:341–42.
234. Toner BB, Garfinkel PE, Jeejeebhoy KN et al. Self-schema in irritable bowel syndrome and depression. Psychosomat Med 1990;52:149–55.
235. Turk DC; Meichenbaum D; Genest M. Pain and Behavioural Medicine: A Cognitive-Behavioral Perspective. New York:Guilford Press;1978.
236. Blanchard EB, Radnitz CL, Evans ED, et al. Psychological comparisons of irritable bowel syndrome to chronic tension and migraine headache and non-patient controls. Biofeedback Self Reg 1986;11:221–30.
237. Talley NJ, Phillips SF, Bruce B, et al. Relation among personality and symptoms in nonulcer dyspepsia and the irritable bowel syndrome. Gastroenterology 1990;99 (2):327–33.
238. Heaton KW. What makes people with abdominal pain consult their doctor? In: Creed FH, Mayou R, Hopkins A, Editors. Medical Symptoms Not Explained by Organic Disease. London:Royal Colleges of Physicians and Psychiatrists;1992: 1–8.
239. Lolas R, Heerlein A. Content category analysis of affective expression in irritable bowel, duodenal ulcer, and anxiety disorder patients. Psychopathology 1986;19: 309–16.
240. Creed F, Guthrie E. Relation among personality and symptoms in nonulcer dyspepsia and the irritable bowel syndrome (letter). Gastroenterology 1991;100: 1154–55.

241. Ryan WA, Kelly MG, Fielding JF. Personality and the irritable bowel syndrome. Irish Med J 1983;76:140–41.

242. Radloff LS. The CES-D scale: a self-report depression scale for research in the general population. App Psychol Measur 1977;1:385–401.

243. Attanasio V, Ankrasik F, Blanchard EG, et al. Psychosomatic properties of the SUNYA revision of the Psychosomatic Symptom Checklist. J Behav Med 1984;7: 245–59.

244. Main J. The modified somatic perception questionnaire (MSPQ). J Psychosomat Res 1983;27:503–14.

245. Latimer PR, Campbell D, Latimer M, et al. Irritable bowel syndrome: a test of the colonic hyperalgesia hypothesis. J Behav Med 1979;2:285–95.

246. Colgan S, Creed FH, Klass SH. Psychiatric disorder and abnormal illness behaviour in patients with upper abdominal pain. Psychol Med 1988;18:887–92.

247. Sharpe M, Peveler R, Mayou R. The psychological treatment of patients with functional somatic symptoms: a practical guide. J Psychosomat Res 1992;36(6): 515–29.

248. Salkovskis P. The cognitive-behavioural approach. In: Creed FH, Mayou R, Hopkins A, Editors. Medical Symptoms *Not Explained* by Organic Disease. London: Royal College of Psychiatrists and Royal College of Physicians;1992:70–84.

249. Barsky AJ, Geringer E, Wool CA. A cognitive-educational treatment for hypochondriasis. Gen Hosp Psychiatry 1988;10:322–7.

250. Beck AT, Emery G, Greenberg R. Anxiety Disorders and Phobias: A Cognitive Perspective. New York:Basic Books;1985.

251. Mayou R. Invited review: atypical chest pain. Psychsomat Res 1989;33:393–406.

252. Warwick HMC, Salkovskis P. Hypochondriasis. Behav Res Ther 1990;28:105–18.

253. Levy RL, Cain KC, Jarrett M, et al. The relationship between daily life stress and gastrointestinal symptoms in women with irritable bowel syndrome. J Behav Med 1997;20(2):177–93.

254. Walker EA, Roy-Byrne PP, Katon WJ. Irritable bowel syndrome and psychiatric illness. Am J Psychiatry 1990;147 (5):565–72.

255. Gombrone J, Dewsnap P, Libby G, et al. Abnormal illness attitudes in patients with irritable bowel syndrome. J Psychosomat Res 1995;39(2):227–30.

256. Heaton KW, O'Donnell LJD, Braddon FEM, et al. Symptoms of irritable bowel syndrome in a british urban community: consulters and nonconsulters. Gastroenterology 1992;102:1962–67.

257. Talley NJ, Boyce PM, Jones M. Predictors of health care seeking for irritable bowel syndrome: a population based study. Gut 1997;41(3):394-8.

258. Kettell J, Jones R, Lydeard S. Reasons for consultation in irritable bowel syndrome: symptoms and patient characteristics. Brit J Gen Pract 1992;42:459–61.

259. Thompson WG, Heaton KW, Smyth T, et al. Irritable bowel syndrome: The view from general practice. Gastroenterology 1996;A769.

260. Verhoef MJ, Sutherland LR, Brkich L. Use of alternative medicine by patients attending a gastroenterology clinic. Can Med Assoc J 1990;142:121–25.

261. Smart HL, Mayberry JF, Atkinson M. Alternative medicine consultations and remedies in patients with the irritable bowel syndrome. Gut 1986;27:826–28.

262. Van Dulmen AM, Fennis JFM, Mokkink HGA, et al. Doctor-dependent changes in complaint-related cognitions and anxiety during medical consultations in functional abdominal complaints. Psychol Med 1995;25:1011–18.

263. Groves JE. Taking care of the hateful patient. New Engl J Med 1978;298:883–87.

264. Sandler RS, Drossman DA, Nathan HP, et al. Symptom complaints and health care seeking behavior in subjects with bowel dysfunction. Gastroenterology 1984;87: 314–18.

265. Triadafilopoulos G, Simms RW, Goldenberg DL. Bowel dysfunction in fibromyalgia syndrome. Dig Dis Sci 1991;36:59–64.

266. Prior A, Wilson K, Whorwell PJ, et al. Irritable bowel syndrome in the gynecological clinic. Dig Dis Sci 1989;34:1820–24.

267. Crowell MD, Dubin NH, Robinson JC, et al. Functional bowel disorders in women with dysmenorrhea. Am J Gastroenterol 1994;89(11):1973–77.

268. White A, Upton A, Collins SM. Is irritable bowel the asthma of the gut? Gastroenterology 1988;94:A494.

269. Whitehead WE, Enck P, Anthony JC, et al. Psychopathology in patients with irritable bowel syndrome. In: Singer MV, Goebell H, Editors. Nerves and the Gastrointestinal Tract. Lancaster:Kluwer Academic Publishers;1989:465–76.

270. Keeling PWN, Fielding JR. The irritable bowel syndrome: a review of 50 consecutive cases. J Irish Coll Phys Surg 1975;4:91–94.

271. Whitehead WE, Cheskin LJ, Heller BR, et al. Evidence for exacerbation of irritable bowel syndrome during menses. Gastroenterology 1990;98:1485–89.

272. Prior A, Whorwell PJ. Gynaecological consultation in patients with the irritable bowel syndrome. Gut 1989;30:996–98.

273. Levy RL, Whitehead WE, Von Korff MR, et al. Intergenerational transmission of GI illness behavior. Am J Gastroenterol (in press).

274. Whitehead WE, Crowell MD, Heller BR, et al. Modeling and reinforcement of the sick role during childhood predicts adult illness behavior. Psychosomat Med 1994;6:541–50.

275. Wooley SC, Blackwell B, Winget C. A learning theory model of chronic illness behavior: theory, treatment and research. Psychosomat Med 1978;40:379–401.

276. Garrett JW, Drossman DA. Health status in inflammatory bowel disease: biological and behavioral considerations. Gastroenterology 1990;99:90–96.

277. Guyatt GH, Feeny DH, Patrick DL. Measuring health-related quality of life. Ann Intern Med 1993;118:622–29.

278. Guyatt G, Mitchell A, Irvine EJ, et al. A new measure of health status for clinical trials in inflammatory bowel disease. Gastroenterology 1989;96:804–10.

279. Drossman DA, Patrick DL, Mitchell CM, et al. Health related quality of life in inflammatory bowel disease: functional status and patient worries and concerns. Dig Dis Sci 1989;34:1379–86.

280. Drossman DA. Quality of life in IBD: methods and findings. In: Rachmilewitz D,

Editor. Falk Symposium #72: Inflammatory Bowel Diseases—1994. Dordrecht: Kluwer Academic Publishers;1994:105–16.

281. Patrick DL, Deyo RA. Generic and disease-specific measures in assessing health status and quality of life. Med Care 1989;27:s217–32.

282. Guyatt GH, Cook DJ. Health status, quality of life and the individual. JAMA 1994;272(8):630–31.

283. Ware JE, Sherbourne CD. The MOS 36-item short form Health Survey (SF-36): I. conceptual framework and item selection. Med Care 1992;30(6):473–83.

284. Whitehead WE, Burnett CK, Cook E, III, et al. Health related quality of life in IBS: patients compared to IBS non-consulters and asymptomatic individuals (abstr.). Am J Gastroenterol 1994;89:1700.

285. Talley NJ, Weaver AL, Zinsmeister AR. Impact of functional dyspepsia on quality of life. Dig Dis Sci 1995;40(3):584–89.

286. Patrick DL, Drossman DA, Frederick IO, et al. Quality of life in persons with irritable bowel syndrome: development of a new measure. Dig Dis Sci 1998;43(2): 400–11.

287. Costa PTJ; McCrae RR. The NEO Personality Inventory Manual. Odessa, Florida:Psychological Assessment Resources;1985.

288. Stewart AL, Greenfield S, Hays RD, et al. Functional status and well-being of patients with chronic conditions. JAMA 1989;262:907–13.

289. Owens DM, Nelson DK, Talley NJ. The irritable bowel syndrome: long term prognosis and the physician-patient interaction. Ann Intern Med 1995;122: 107–12.

290. Lipkin, MJ. The Medical Interview and Related Skills. In: Branch WT, Editor. Office Practice of Medicine. 3rd ed. Philadelphia:W.B. Saunders;1994:970–86.

291. Drossman DA. Psychosocial factors in the care of patients with gastrointestinal disorders. In: Yamada T, Editor.Textbook of Gastroenterology. Ed 3. Philadelphia:Lippincott-Raven;1999:638–59.

292. Drossman DA. Struggling with the "controlling" patient. Am J Gastroenterol 1994;89(9):1441–46.

293. Olden KW. Approach to the patient with irritable bowel syndrome. In: Stern TA, Herman JB, Slavin PL, Editors. The MGH Guide to Psychiatry in Primary Care. New York:McGraw-Hill; 1998:113–20.

294. Ong LM, de Haes JC, Hoos AM, et al. Doctor-patient communication: a review of the literature. Soc Sci Med 1995;40(7):903–18.

295. Rockemann MG, Seeling W, Bischof C, et al. Prophylactic use of epidural mepivacaine/morphine, systemic diclofenac, and metamizole reduces postoperative morphine consumption after major abdominal surgery. Anesthesiol 1996;84(5): 1027–34.

296. Drossman DA. Diagnosing and treating patients with refractory functional gastrointestinal disorders. Ann Intern Med 1995;123(9):688–97.

297. Longstreth GF. Irritable bowel syndrome: diagnosis in the managed care era. Dig Dis Sci 1997;42(6):1105–11.

298. Vanner SJ, Depew WT, Paterson WG, et al. Predictive value of the Rome criteria for diagnosing Irritable Bowel Syndrome. Gut 1999;94:2912–17.

299. Naifeh K. Psychometric testing in functional GI disorders. In: Olden KW, Editor. Handbook of Functional Gastrointesinal Disorders. New York:Marcel Dekker; 1996:79–126.

300. Robins LN, Helzer JE, Croughan J, et al. National Institute of Mental Health diagnostic interview schedule. Arch Gen Psychiatry 1981;38:381–89.

301. Marder SR. Psychiatric rating scales. In: Kaplan HJ, Sadock BJ, Editors. Comprehensive Textbook of Psychiatry/VI. Ed. 6. Baltimore:Williams and Wilkins;1995: 619–35.

302. Bonynge ER. Unidimensionality of SCL-90-R scales in adult and adolescent crisis samples. J Clin Psychol 1993;49(2):212–15.

303. Morris PL, Goldberg RJ. Validity of the 28-item General Health Questionnaire in hospitalized gastroenterology patients. Psychosomat 1989;30:290–95.

304. Millon T; Green CJ; Meagher RB. Millon Behavioral Health Inventory Manual. Ed. 3. Minneapolis, Minnesota:National Computer Systems;1982.

305. McNair DM; Lorr M; Dropplemon LF. Profile of Mood States. San Diego:Educational and Industrial Testing Service;1971.

306. Spielberger CD. Manual for the State-Trait Anxiety Inventory (Form Y). Palo Alto, California:Consulting Psychologists Press;1983.

307. Sheehan DV. Sheehan patient-related anxiety scale. In: McGlynn TJ, Metcalf HL, Editors. Diagnosis and Treatment of Anxiety Disorders: A Physician's Handbook. Washington DC:American Psychiatric Press;1989:98–99.

308. Rating scales for OCD and related disorders. In: Jenike MA, Baer L, Minichiello WE. Obsessive-Compulsive Disorders: Theory and Management. Chicago:Year Book Publishers; 1990: 394–425.

309. Beck AT, Ward CH, Mendelson M, et al. An inventory for measuring depression. Arch Gen Psychiatry 1961;4:561–71.

310. Zung WWK. A self-rating depression scale. Arch Gen Psychiatry 1965;12:63–70.

311. Zigmond AS, Snaith RP. The hospital anxiety and depression scale. Acta Psychiatr Scand 1983;67:361–70.

312. Talley NJ et al. Optimal design of Treatment Trials. In: Drossman DA, Richter JE, Talley NJ, et al., Editors. The Functional Gastrointestinal Disorders: Diagnosis, Pathophysiology, and Treatment—A Multinational Consensus. McLean, VA: Degnon Associates; 1994:265–309.

313. Dahlstrom WG, Welsh GS, Dahlstrom LE. An MMPI Handbook. Rev. Ed. Minneapolis:University of Minnesota;1972.

314. Eysenck JH and Eysenck SBG, Editors. Eysenck Personality Inventory. San Diego: Educational and Industrial Testing Service;1968.

315. Kellner R. Somatization and Hypochondriasis. New York:Prager-Greenwood; 1986.

316. Turk DC, Rudy TE, Salovey P. Implicit models of illness. J Behav Med 1986;9: 453–74.

317. Weissman AN. The Dysfunctional Attitudes Scale: A validation scale. Unpub-

lished doctoral dissertation, University of Pennsylvania, Philadelphia, Pennsylvania; 1979.

318. Toner BB, Stuckless N, Ali A, et al. The development of a cognitive scale for functional bowel disorders. Psychosomat Med 1998;60:492–97.

319. Sarason IG, Sarason BR, Shearin EN, et al. A brief measure of social support: practical and theoretical implications. J Soc Personal Relat 1987;4:497–510.

320. Rosenstiel AK, Keefe FJ. The use of coping strategies in chronic low back pain patients: relationship to patient characteristics and current adjustment. Pain 1983; 17:33–40.

321. Keefe FJ, Brown GK, Wallston KA, et al. Coping with rheumatoid arthritis pain: catastrophizing as a maladaptive strategy. Pain 1989;37:51–56.

322. Drossman DA, Li Z, Leserman J, et al. Association of coping patterns and health status among female GI patients after controlling for GI disease type and abuse history. Gastroenterology 1997;112:A724.

323. Drossman DA, Patrick DL, Whitehead WE, et al. Responsiveness of the IBS-QOL: further validation of a disease specific quality of life measure for IBS. Gastroenterology 1999;116:A988.

324. Hahn BA, Kirchdoerfer LJ, Fullerton S, et al. Evaluation of a new quality of life questionnaire for patients with irritable bowel syndrome. Aliment Pharmacol Therapeut 1997;11(3):547–52.

325. McGee HM, O'Boyle CA, Hickey A, et al. Assessing the quality of life of the individual: the SEIQoL with a healthy and a gastroenterology unit population. Psychol Med 1991;3:749–59.

326. Drossman DA. Psychosocial Sound Bites: exercises in the patient-doctor relationship. Am J Gastroenterol 1997;92(9):1418–23.

327. Von Korff M, Gruman J, Schaefer J. Collaborative management of chronic illness. Ann Intern Med 1997;127:1097–1102.

328. Barsky A, Borus JF. Somatization and medicalization in the era of managed care. JAMA 1995;274:1931–34.

329. Barsky AJ. Hypochondriasis: medical management and psychiatric treatment. Psychosomatics 1996;37(1):48–56.

330. Nemiah J, Sifneos P. Psychosomatic illness: a problem in communication. Psychother Psychosomat 1970;18:154–60.

331. Pilowsky I, Barrow CG. A controlled study of psychotherapy and amitriptyline used individually and in combination in the treatment of chronic intractable, 'psychogenic' pain. Pain 1990;40:3–19.

332. Toner BB, Segal ZV, Emmott S, et al. Cognitive behavioral group therapy for patients with irritable bowel syndrome. Internat J Group Psychother 1998;48(2): 215–43.

333. Latimer P. Functional Gastrointestinal Disorders: A Behavioural Approach. New York:Springer Publishing Company;1983.

334. Payne A, Blanchard EB. A controlled comparison of cognitive therapy and self-help support groups in the treatment of irritable bowel syndrome. J Consult Clin Psychol 1995;63(5):779–86.

335. Guthrie E, Creed F, Dawson D, et al. A randomised controlled trial of psycho-therapy in patients with refractory irritable bowel syndrome. Brit J Psychiatry 1993;163:315–21.
336. Elkin I, Parloff MB, Hadley SW, et al. NIMH Treatment of Depression Collaborative Research Program. Arch Gen Psychiatry 1985;42:305–16.
337. Whorwell PJ, Prior A, Faragher EB. Controlled trial of hypnotherapy in the treatment of severe refractory irritable bowel syndrome. Lancet 1984;2:1232–33.
338. Harvey RF, Hinton RA, Gunary RM, et al. Individual and group hypnotherapy in treatment of refractory irritable bowel syndrome. Lancet 1989;1:424–25.
339. Bernstein DA, Borkovec TD. Progressive Relaxation Training. Champaign: Champaign Illinois Research Press;1973.
340. Blanchard EB, Schwarz SP, Suls JM, et al. Two controlled evaluations of multicomponent psychological treatment of irritable bowel syndrome. Behav Res Ther 1992;30:175–89.
341. Mayer EA; Raybould HE. Mayer EA, et al., Editors. Basic and Clinical Aspects of Chronic Abdominal Pain. Ed. 9. Amsterdam:Elsevier;1993.
342. Benson H. The Relaxation Response. New York:William Morrow;1975.
343. Toner BB. Cognitive-behavioral treatment of functional somatic syndromes: integrating gender issues. Cognit Behav Pract 1994;1:157–78.
344. Lynch PM, Zamble E. A controlled behavioral treatment study of irritable bowel syndrome. Behavior Ther 1989;20:509–23.
345. Shaw G, Srivastava ED, Sadlier M, et al. Stress management for irritable bowel syndrome: a controlled trial. Digestion 1991;50:36–42.
346. Rumsey N. Group stress management programmes vs pharmacological treatment in the treatment of the irritable bowel syndrome. In: Heaton KW, Creed F, Goeting NLM, Editors. Current Approaches Towards Confident Management of Irritable Bowel Syndrome. Lyme Regis:Lyme Regis Printing Company;1991: 33–39.
347. Neff DF, Blanchard EB. A multi-component treatment of irritable bowel syndrome. Behavior Ther 1987;18:70–83.
348. Van Dulmen AM, Fennis JF, Bleijenberg G. Cognitive-behavioral group therapy for irritable bowel syndrome: effects and long-term follow-up. Psychosomat Med 1996;58(5):508–14.
349. Bennett P, Wilkinson S. A comparison of psychological and medical treatment of the irritable bowel syndrome. Brit J Clin Psychol 1985;24:215–16.
350. Blanchard EB, Schwarz SP. Adaptation of a multicomponent treatment for irritable bowel syndrome to a small-group format. Biofeedback Self Regul 1987;12: 63–69.
351. Blanchard EB, Schwarz SP, Neff DF. Two-year follow-up of behavioral treatment of irritable bowel syndrome. Behav Ther 1988;19:67–73.
352. Guthrie E, Creed F, Dawson D, et al. A controlled trial of psychological treatment for the irritable bowel syndrome. Gastroenterology 1991;100:450–57.
353. Arn I, Theorell T, Uvnas-Moberg K, et al. Psychodrama group therapy for patients with functional gastrointestinal disorders. Psychother Psychosomat 1989;51: 113–19.

354. Svedlund J. Psychotherapy in irritable bowel syndrome: a controlled outcome study. Acta Psychiatr Scand 1983;67(Suppl 306):1–86.

355. Voirol MW, Hipolito J. [Anthropo-analytical relaxation in irritable bowel syndrome: results 40 months later]. Schweiz Med Wochenschr 1987;117:1117–19.

356. Blanchard EB, Greene B, Scharff L, et al. Relaxation training as a treatment for irritable bowel syndrome. Biofeedback Self Regul 1993;18(3):125–32.

357. Whorwell PJ, Prior A, Colgan SM. Hypnotherapy in severe irritable bowel syndrome: further experience. Gut 1987;28:423–25.

358. Whorwell PJ. Hypnotherapy in severe irritable bowel syndrome (Letter). Lancet 1989;1:622.

359. Whorwell PJ, Houghton LA, Taylor EE,35 al. Physiological effects of emotion: assessment via hypnosis. Lancet 1992;340:69–72.

360. Greene B, Blanchard EB. Cognitive therapy for irritable bowel syndrome. J Consult Clin Psychol 1994;62(3):576–82.

361. Vollmer A, Blanchard EB. Controlled comparison of individual versus group cognitive therapy for irritable bowel syndrome. Behavior Ther 1998;29:19–33.

362. Egbunike IG, Chaffee BJ. Antidepressants in the management of chronic pain syndromes. Pharmacotherapy 1990;10(4):262–70.

363. Cannon RO, Quyyumi AA, Mincemoyer R, et al. Imipramine in patients with chest pain despite normal coronary angiograms. New Engl J Med 1994;20:1411–17.

364. Clouse RE, Lustman P, Geisman RA. Antidepressant therapy in 138 patients with irritable bowel syndrome: a five-year clinical experience. Aliment Pharmacol Ther 1994;8:409–16.

365. Greenbaum DS, Mayle JE, Vanegeren LE, et al. The effects of desipramine on IBS compared with atropine and placebo. Dig Dis Sci 1987;32:257–66.

366. Gorard DA, Libby GW, Farthing MJG. Effect of a tricyclic antidepressant on small intestinal motility in health and diarrhea-predominant irritable bowel syndrome. Dig Dis Sci 1995;40:86–95.

367. Gorard DA, Libby GW, Farthing JG. Influence of antidepressants on whole gut orocaecal transit times in health and irritable bowel syndrome. Aliment Pharmacol Ther 1994;8:159–66.

368. Gruber AJ, Hudson JI, Pope HG, Jr. The management of treatment-resistant depression in disorders on the interface of psychiatry and medicine: fibromyalgia, chronic fatigue syndrome, migraine, irritable bowel syndrome, atypical facial pain, and premenstrual dysphoric disorder. Psychiatr Clin North Am 1996;19(2):351–69.

369. Brown WA, Harrison W. Are patients who are intolerant to one serotonin selective reuptake inhibitor intolerant to another? J Clin Psychiatry 1995;56:30–34.

370. Zarate CA, Kando JC, Tohen M. Does intolerance or lack of response with fluoxetine predict the same will happen with sertraline? J Clin Psychiatry 1996;57:67–71.

371. Max MB, Lynch SA, Muir J, et al. Effects of desipramine, amitriptyline, and fluoxetine on pain in diabetic neuropathy. New Engl J Med 1992;326:1250–56.

372. Glassman AH, Roose SP, Bigger JT. The safety of tricyclic antidepressants in cardiac patients. JAMA 1993;269:2673–75.

373. McDaniel JS, Musselman DL, Porter MR. Depression in patients with cancer. Arch Gen Psychiatry 1995;52:89–99.

374. Clouse RE. Antidepressants for functional gastrointestinal syndromes. Dig Dis Sci 1994;39(11):2352–63.

375. Myren J, Lovland B, Larssen S-E, et al. A double-blind study of the effect of trimipramine in patients with the irritable bowel syndrome. Scand J Gastroenterol 1984;19:835–43.

376. Zola SM. The neurobiology of recovery memory. J Neuropsych Clin Neurosci 1997;9(3):449–59.

377. Hollander E, Kwon JH, Stein DJ. Obsessive-compulsive and spectrum disorders: overview and quality of life issues. J Clin Psychiatry 1996;57:3–6.

378. Jung AC, Staiger T, Sullivan M. The efficacy of selective serotonin reuptake inhibitors for the management of chronic pain. J Gen Intern Med 1997;12:384–89.

379. Eisendrath SJ, Kodama KT. Fluoxetine management of chronic abdominal pain. Psychosomatics 1992;33(227):229.

380. Gorard DA, Dewsnap DA, Medbak SH. Central 5-hydroxytryptaminergic function in irritable bowel syndrome. Scand J Gastroenterol 1995;30:994–99.

381. Feighner JP. The role of venlafaxine in rational antidepressant therapy. J Clin Psychiatry 1994;44:62–68.

382. Golden RN, Bebchuk JM, Leatherman ME. Trazodone and other antidepressants. In:. Schatzberg AF, Nemeroff CB, Editors. The American Psychiatric Press Textbook of Psychopharmacology. Washington,DC:APA Press;1995:195–213.

383. Pecknold JC, Langer SF. Priapism: trazodone versus nefazodone (letter). J Clin Psychiatry 1996;57(11):547–48.

384. Farley M, Keaney JC. Physical symptoms, somatization, and dissociation in women survivors of childhood sexual assault. Women and Health 1997;25(3):33–45.

385. Blier P, Bergeron R, DeMontigny C. Selective activation of postsynaptic 5-HT_{1alpha} receptors produces a rapid antidepressant response. Neuropsychopharm 1997;16:333–38.

386. Rakel RE. The use of buspirone in primary care. J Clin Psychiatry 1994;12:22–26.

387. MacDonald AJ, Bouchier IAD. Non-organic gastrointestinal illness: a medical and psychiatric study. Brit J Psychiatry 1980;136:276–83.

388. Corney RH, Stanton R. Physical symptom severity, psychological and social dysfunction in a series of outpatients with irritable bowel syndrome. J Psychosomat Res 1990;34:483–91.

389. Blanchard EB, Scharff L, Schwartz SP, et al. The role of anxiety and depression in the irritable bowel syndrome. Behav Res Ther 1990;28:401–405.

390. Spitzer RL, Williams JB, Gibbon M, et al. Structured Clinical Interview for DSM-III Disorders (SCID) and SCID-NP. New York:Biometrics Research Department, New York State Psychiatric Institute;1988.

391. Hodgson R, Rachman S. Obsessive compulsive complaints. Behav Res Ther 1977; 15:389–95.
392. Corney RH, Stanton R, Newell R, et al. Behavioural psychotherapy in the treatment of irritable bowel syndrome. J Psychosomat Res 1991;35:461–69.
393. Waxman D. The irritable bowel: a pathological or a psychological syndrome. J Roy Soc Med 1988;81:718–20.
394. Drossman DA. A Biopsychosocial Approach to Irritable Bowel Syndrome: Improving the Physician-Patient Relationship (videotape). Ed. 1. Toronto:Zancom International;1997.

Chapter 5

A. Functional Esophageal Disorders

Ray E. Clouse, Chair,
Joel E. Richter, Co-Chair, *with*
Robert C. Heading,
Jozef Janssens,
and Janet A. Wilson

Introduction

As a group, functional esophageal disorders represent chronic unexplained symptoms typifying esophageal disease that have no readily identified structural or metabolic basis (Table 1). With the exception of rumination syndrome, the disorders are most commonly encountered in adults and collectively represent a major strain on health care resources. Physiologic mechanisms underlying symptom production are poorly understood. A combination of physiologic and psychosocial factors probably is responsible for escalating the symptoms to a level requiring medical attention, and most available information arises from studies of patients who have sought medical care. Consequently, basic mechanisms that initiate symptoms remain unknown and understudied in all the functional esophageal disorders.

Rumination syndrome has important distinctions from the other functional esophageal disorders, whereas the latter have remarkable similarities. Symptom overlap in patients presenting with functional globus, chest pain, heartburn, or dysphagia, and the fact that each can be produced by singular distal esophageal diseases (e.g., gastroesophageal reflux disease) suggest that these syndromes may not be independent functional disorders. Since the introduction of a nosology for functional esophageal disorders and formation of diagnostic criteria, little additional data have appeared to help establish their individual importance, particularly from the standpoint of management [1]. Distinctions appear most relevant in exclusion of structural diseases—cardiac disease, for example, in the case of chest pain, and neck or pharyngeal diseases in the case of globus. In this second edition, the disorders and their criteria remain separate, but further studies will be required to substantiate the importance of the distinctions.

Several diagnostic requirements are uniform across the functional esophageal disorders. *First* is exclusion of structural or metabolic disorders that might be producing the symptoms, a principal criterion for all functional gastrointestinal disorders [2]. Careful consideration and investigation of otolaryngological, pulmonary and cardiac causes may be required. *Second* is the presence of symptoms for at least three months (12 weeks in a 12-month period), an arbitrary criterion in the case of the functional esophageal disorders. Considering the lack of specific symptoms, except for rumination syndrome, this limit decreases the risk of overlooking a structural lesion. Evidence-based research supporting an adjustment in this time constraint is lacking. *Third* is a confident stance that gastroesophageal reflux disease or an esophageal motor disorder is not the primary problem. This final criterion requires a degree of definition, as both reflux and motor events are potential contributors to symptoms in several functional esophageal disorders.

The threshold required in the first edition has been retained: both pathologic

Table 1. Functional Gastrointestinal Disorders

A. Esophageal Disorders

A1. Globus	A4. Functional Heartburn
A2. Rumination syndrome	A5. Functional Dysphagia
A3. Functional Chest Pain of Presumed Esophageal Origin	A6. Unspecified Functional Esophageal Disorder

B. Gastroduodenal Disorders

B1. Functional Dyspepsia	B2. Aerophagia
B1a. Ulcer-like Dyspepsia	B3. Functional Vomiting
B1b. Dysmotility-like Dyspepsia	
B1c. Unspecified (nonspecific) Dyspepsia	

C. Bowel Disorders

C1. Irritable Bowel Syndrome	C4. Functional Diarrhea
C2. Functional Abdominal Bloating	C5. Unspecified Functional Bowel Disorder
C3. Functional Constipation	

D. Functional Abdominal Pain

D1. Functional Abdominal Pain Syndrome
D2. Unspecified Functional Abdominal Pain

E. Functional Disorders of the Biliary Tract and the Pancreas

E1. Gallbladder Dysfunction
E2. Sphincter of Oddi Dysfunction

F. Anorectal Disorders

F1. Functional Fecal Incontinence
F2. Functional Anorectal Pain
F2a. Levator Ani Syndrome
F2b. Proctalgia Fugax
F3. Pelvic Floor Dyssynergia

G. Functional Pediatric Disorders

G1. Vomiting	G2b. Irritable bowel syndrome
G1a. Infant regurgitation	G2c. Functional abdominal pain
G1b. Infant rumination syndrome	G2d. Abdominal migraine
G1c. Cyclic vomiting syndrome	G2e. Aerophagia
G2. Abdominal pain	G3. Functional diarrhea
G2a. Functional dyspepsia	G4. Disorders of defecation
G2a1. Ulcer-like dyspepsia	G4a. Infant dyschezia
G2a2. Dysmotility-like dyspepsia	G4b. Functional constipation
	G4c. Functional fecal retention
G2a3. Unspecified (nonspecific) dyspepsia	G4d. Functional non-retentive fecal soiling

gastroesophageal reflux and pathology-based esophageal motor disorders must be eliminated from consideration before establishing the presence of a functional esophageal disorder, whereas reflux-provoked symptoms and lesser degrees of motor dysfunction are not exclusionary criteria [1]. Pathologic gastroesophageal reflux is defined as evidence of esophagitis or abnormal acid exposure time on an ambulatory, 24-hour pH study. Some may argue that symptoms closely associated with reflux events in the face of normal esophageal acid exposure also represent reflux disease rather than a functional disorder. Further studies are needed, however, to firmly extricate this subject group from the remainder, the symptoms of which are less reliably associated with reflux events; symptoms induced by physiologic degrees of gastroesophageal reflux are considered functional in this chapter. Symptoms that persist despite treatment of pathologic gastroesophageal reflux disease and normalization of objective measures may qualify toward a functional diagnosis. Like pathologic reflux, esophageal motor dysfunction of the type and severity found in pathology-based disorders (e.g., achalasia, scleroderma involvement of the esophagus) is an exclusionary criterion. High-amplitude peristaltic contractions (nutcracker esophagus) and other spastic disorders, in contrast, do not preclude a functional diagnosis. The distinction is based on failure to establish a disease basis for this type of motor dysfunction, the indirect relationship of motor events with symptoms in the average case, and the unsatisfactory response to treatments directed solely at abnormal motility.

The original criteria evolved from consensus opinion of several international working teams charged with initiating a structured diagnostic approach to functional syndromes [3]. The present criteria for functional esophageal disorders have few substantive differences from the original (see Appendix A in this book). They remain as guidelines for the categorization and investigation of patients and maintain previous limitations in clinical application. Summary information for each disorder is subdivided by epidemiology, physiologic features, psychologic features, clinical evaluation, and treatment. This information should be of benefit to the investigator and clinician interested in the functional esophageal disorders, and it is hoped, will stimulate further investigation in this field. Important focuses for future research work were identified by the subcommittee and are outlined in the final section of the chapter.

A1. Globus

— Definition

Globus (globus pharyngis, globus pharyngeus) is a sensation of something stuck or of a lump or tightness in the throat. The symptom is considered functional when no organic explanation is detected. The ancients attributed the symptom to the uterus (indicating early associations of this symptom with women), despite acknowledging that the uterus resided in the pelvis except during pregnancy [4]. Today patients are typically referred for initial investigation to otolaryngologists and gastroenterologists, even though globus has been identified as the fourth most discriminating symptom of somatization disorder [5]. The practice, while based on a proper concern to exclude sinister pathology, has resulted in a plethora of potential physical disease explanations, including sinusitis, tonsillitis, cervical spondylitis, dental malocclusion, and cricopharyngeal hypertonicity [6–9].

Many such proposals were based on very small numbers of subjects and probably represent casual rather than causal associations. Patients presenting with the conditions mentioned above and other common otolarygologic or cervical disorders rarely complain of globus, and such associations would not explain the female preponderance of patients seeking medical attention for this symptom. Nevertheless, at least major structural lesions must be excluded by appropriate clinical examination of the larynx, pharynx, and neck. A more recent study using high resolution thyroid ultrasound claims a significantly greater prevalence of impalpable thyroid nodules in globus patients (72% of 43 patients) than in controls [10], but the difference may be due to an abnormally low prevalence in the controls (33%). The two most popular definable organic explanations for the symptom are that globus can be an atypical manifestation of gastroesophageal reflux [11,12] or caused by esophageal dysmotility [13,14]; for this reason, pathologic gastroesophageal reflux and pathology-based motor disorders must be excluded. Potential organic causes may need appropriate treatment before establishing globus as a functional diagnosis.

— Epidemiology

Up to 45% of the general population have intermittent symptoms resembling globus [15]. More severe and distressing symptoms account for up to 4% of laryngological referrals [16]. Symptoms persist for at least two years [17] in the majority of patients with more severe complaints and last as long as seven years in 45% of subjects [18]. Persistence of globus may be related to the degree of associated psychological distress [17]. Peak incidence of the symptom is in middle age. Older subjects can report a globus sensation, but it is difficult to extricate the contribution of mucous membrane inflammation that can occur in this age group. The symptom is very uncommon in subjects under the age of 20 years. Detailed examination of so-called globus in adolescents reveals that the symptoms are more typical of dysphagia or food aversion. [19,20].

Since ancient times, globus has been regarded a disorder of women, but the everyday experience of globus is reported similarly by both sexes [15]. In contrast, three of four subjects seeking health care and reporting the symptom to physicians are women. Males with globus, consequently, are subject to an exclusion bias, making much less known about male patients with this symptom. A UK community survey of over 1150 middle aged women shoppers [21] found that 6% of the sample described a persistent feeling over the prior 3 months of something caught in the throat. The likelihood of seeking medical advice was related statistically only to the perceived severity of the symptom.

— Diagnostic Criteria

At least 12 weeks, which need not be consecutive, in the preceding 12 months of:

(1) The chronic or intermittent sensation of a lump or foreign body in the throat;

(2) Occurrence of the sensation between meals;

(3) Absence of dysphagia and odynophagia; *and*

(4) Absence of pathologic gastroesophageal reflux, achalasia, or other motility disorder with a recognized pathologic basis (e.g., scleroderma of the esophagus).

The actual sensation varies greatly among subjects. Classically a lump, it may be a hair- or crumb-like (foreign body) sensation, a constriction, or a choking. Many patients "feed" globus, as the sensation is less prominent when buffered by bolus than during interprandial dry swallows. One in five, however, note something abnormal during food swallows [22]. This awareness of the same foreign body sensation should not be regarded as true dysphagia, as there is no sense of or actual interference with the passage of food. The symptom is often maximal in the evening when the subject has fewest distractions.

— Justification for Change in Criteria

Globus sensation most often occurs centrally in the neck, but may migrate in location and is reported in a lateral position in more than 20% of patients [12]. The remainder reports a midline symptom, most often at the laryngeal level but not infrequently at the hyoid level or the suprasternal notch. The prior restrictions in location were removed. Although implicit in the definition of the functional esophageal disorders, the criterion that pathologic gastroesophageal reflux and pathology-based motor disorders be excluded is now stated distinctly.

— Clinical Evaluation

The clinical evaluation centers around a full history that includes psychosocial factors such as recent major life events, history of anxiety or affective disorders, and social support. Specific inquiry should be made about panic attacks, particularly in those who are awakened from sleep with "choking" or a sense of difficult breathing as part of the presentation. Such symptoms can also suggest gastroesophageal reflux disease (GERD), and other symptoms supporting this diagnosis or presence of a significant distal esophageal motility disorder should also be sought. It is often worthwhile to grade symptom severity, a maneuver that can be useful in long-term follow-up or for clinical reports. Deary et al. [23] published a self-report globus symptom scale, the Glasgow Edinburgh Throat Scale derived from 105 consecutive patients completing a 10-item questionnaire (see appendix to this chapter). Factor analysis of the responses on this questionnaire showed that the true globus symptoms (wanting to swallow all the time, feeling of something in the throat) could be segregated from dysphagia or pain.

The history is followed by a thorough examination of the neck, larynx and pharynx. Those sensations localized above the cricoid arise in areas clearly visible to the otolaryngologist at flexible laryngoscopy in the office. (If facilities allow, patient reassurance may be enhanced by sharing these images with the patient on a video monitor screen.) Very rarely, globus may be a presentation of hypopharyngeal malignancy. These tumors almost always are accompanied by other symptoms, e.g., pain, dysphagia, altered voice quality. The post-cricoid region cannot be examined adequately with a flexible endoscope. Although the technique is useful in incriminating esophageal disorders in globus patients, the post-cricoid area remains a blind zone [24]. Rigid laryngoscopy may have a role in the investigation of some patients. A series of 120 globus patients undergoing rigid examinations under general anesthesia showed hypopharyngeal cancer in two, both of whom had associated symptoms including dysphagia and hoarseness [25]. Malignancy is rare, however. A seven-year follow up of 74 globus patients failed to reveal any instance of upper aerodigestive tract malignancy [18].

Radiological evaluation is of limited utility. A barium swallow may miss an early hypopharyngeal lesion, especially if double-contrast technique is not employed. By the time hypopharyngeal carcinomas are radiographically visible, other symptoms accompany the presentation. Radiologic studies of the pharynx are typically normal, as are contrast studies of the remainder of the esophagus. Abnormalities when detected are often nonspecific, including reflux during the study, nonspecific motility abnormalities, and cricopharyngeus indentations [22,26]. On occasion, significant reflux disease and distal motor disorders, including achalasia, can be detected, emphasizing the utility of a clinical evaluation directed toward pathologic reflux and pathology-based motor disorders when the clinical presentation favors the presence of such diagnoses. Pathologic reflux can be demonstrated in as many as a third of unselected globus patients who undergo comprehensive evaluations for this disorder [22,27,28].

— Physiologic Features

The relationships of gastroesophageal reflux, upper esophageal sphincter dysfunction, and esophageal dysmotility to globus have been studied in some detail. Population studies support an association between reflux symptoms and globus. [29,15]. As many as 30–50% of globus patients report heartburn, even in populations where gastroesophageal reflux is uncommon [15,29,30]. These data must be interpreted, however, in light of the fact that nearly 10% of non-patients in population surveys report heartburn as often as once per month [15]. Potential mechanisms whereby reflux events could produce globus include referred sensation to the neck (vagal afferents), direct inflammation of the upper esophagus, esophagopharyngeal reflux or reflex cough and throat clearing in response to distal or proximal esophageal acid, or supraglottic penetration. Results from ambulatory pH monitoring have been instrumental in demonstrating the relationship of pathologic reflux or reflux events to globus in a substantial minority of patients. Wilson et al. [22], using ambulatory pH monitoring and distal esophageal biopsy in a large number of globus patients determined that pathologic reflux was present in less than 30%. Other studies suggest that pathologic reflux may be present in 30–40% of patients [27,28]. Additionally, reflux episodes precede globus symptoms more than half the time in many globus patients without pathologic reflux [27]. Consequently, globus can accompany reflux disease and may be at least partially provoked by reflux events in a substantial number of patients with no evidence of pathologic reflux.

Although early studies suggested abnormally elevated upper esophageal sphincter pressures in some globus patients [9], subsequent work with high fidelity manometric equipment did not confirm this result [22]. The upper sphincter in globus is normotensive and normally coordinated with pharyngeal contraction. Likewise the increment in upper sphincter pressure in response to acute experimental stress is similar in globus patients and healthy volunteers [31]. Despite the location of the symptom, a consistent abnormality in upper sphincter function has not been detected. Pharyngoesophageal deglutition contraction amplitudes are somewhat elevated in globus patients, but this may represent a reaction to rather than a cause of globus sensation. The interprandial dry swallow frequency increases as the subject ties to "dislodge" the sensation of a foreign body. Paradoxically, this dry swallow habit has been postulated as an indirect cause of globus—or at least a contributory factor, perhaps building up a column of air periodically trapped beneath the upper sphincter [32].

A number of recent studies have revisited the association of globus-like symptoms with dysmotility in the esophageal body. The possibility that globus is a proximal symptom of more distal motor disorders is particularly provoked by the finding of achalasia in 7 of 30 patients with persistent globus who had been referred to a psychosomatic clinic; an additional 10 demonstrated poor lower esophageal sphincter (LES) relaxation in conjunction with nonspecific spastic motor abnormalities [33]. Other nonspecific findings with normal LES relaxation were found in 7 other subjects. This report is atypical. Others rarely report achalasia but have detected nonspecific spastic disorders and abnormalities associated with reflux disease in large proportions of patients [30,14], although even these findings are inconsistently present [22]. Distal esophageal motor dysfunction may participate in symptom production in some patients, but a reliable physiologic marker for globus has not been detected.

— Psychologic Features

Disorders of mood are common in globus. This might be expected given the analogous sensation in everyday life—a "lump in the throat"—as an emotional response, often taken colloquially to mean suppression of tears. Patients of both sexes have been shown in a small series to have Beck Depression Inventory scores suggestive of significant depressive symptomatology [34]. Likewise, anxiety disorders are common in globus patients; 9 of 30 patients in one study met DSM-III-R lifetime criteria for panic disorder and/or agoraphobia

[35]. In another series, female patients were found to have high levels of free-floating anxiety and somatic concern [36]. These findings do not necessarily invoke causality and might affect healthcare resource use.

Life events studies have attempted to discover associations of life events with symptom onset or persistence. Deary et al. [34] found that 13 of 25 patients, but only 2 of 25 controls, had significant life events within 2 months of symptom onset, namely death of or serious illness in a close relative, birth in the close family, or loss of job. Globus patients also had higher hassles ratings on Kanner's hassles scale that scores 117 stressful events over the preceding month. In a subsequent more detailed controlled study of life events, Harris et al. [37] found that globus patients reported significantly more severe life events than controls over the preceding year. They also described fewer close confiding relationships than controls.

Others have measured personality features, persistent psychologic characteristics that might influence response to life events or transient psychiatric disorders. A substantial psychometric study of personality traits in 121 globus patients found low extraversion levels in females but largely normal personality traits in males [36]. Hysteroid traits have been consistently absent from globus patients. Recent work characterizing alexithymia, difficulty in expressing emotions, has identified specific factors that are common among patients with globus and other medically unexplained symptoms. An alexithymia scale, along with a range of other psychological measures, was completed by 244 otolaryngology referrals, primary care patients, and healthy volunteers [38]. The experience of medically unexplained symptoms, such as globus, was correlated with neuroticism, poor coping, depression, and two subscales of the alexithymia measure: difficulty in identifying and describing feelings to others and the capacity to distinguish between feelings and bodily symptoms of emotion. The authors propose that a negative affect influences symptom detection whereas alexithymia influences symptom discrimination, a theory proposed for globus and somatization in general.

— Treatment

Reassurance is an important measure. When possible, the negative findings on flexible laryngoscopy should be demonstrated on monitor to the patient. The vicious cycle of dry swallow, possible role of GERD and throat clearing should be explained, and persistence of symptoms for years, perhaps at a low level, should be predicted. At least a third of globus patients have pathologic reflux, and potential benefit from antireflux therapy cannot be easily predicted by symptoms [16]. Consequently, a trial of antireflux therapy is logical. Unfortunately, the only controlled trial of antireflux therapy in globus [39] showed no significant difference between placebo and an H2 receptor antagonist. Small subject numbers and the short treatment course may have interfered with a positive finding.

Successful treatment with antidepressants has been reported at the anecdotal level [40]. A controlled study of amitriptyline was prematurely terminated when 10 of 12 patients in the active drug limb dropped out because of unacceptable side effects [35]. Compliance may preclude the use of psychopharmacologic agents in many patients, but the approach has not been thoroughly studied. Cognitive behavioral techniques coupled with anxiety management and relaxation strategies may be helpful. It is not clear if psychologic treatments reduce globus symptoms or solely reduce accompanying anxiety.

A2. Rumination Syndrome

— Definition

Rumination syndrome is defined, in the absence of structural disease, as a regurgitation of recently ingested food into the mouth with subsequent remastication and reswallowing or spitting out. Regurgitation is effortless, is not associated with abdominal discomfort, heartburn, or nausea, and sometimes has the features of a voluntary pleasurable experience. It usually occurs within 15 minutes of eating and may last for several hours. The symptoms characteristically cease when the food becomes acid to the taste, and they do not occur during sleep. Despite the characteristic presentation, patients and many physicians describe these symptoms as "chronic vomiting" or "regurgitation." Lack of physician familiarity with this diagnosis prevents identifying the typical history and delays diagnosis [41].

— Epidemiology

Rumination syndrome occurs more often in males than in females by a ratio of 2:1 [42]. The diagnosis is made most frequently in infants and the mentally retarded [43,44] (see Chapter 10 for further discussion of infant rumination syndrome). A familial predisposition has been demonstrated, but a role for genetic factors in the pathogenesis is not established [42,43]. The true prevalence of rumination is unknown because few people seek medical attention and physician awareness is poor [45,41]. However, rumination accounts for about 0.05 to 0.07% of admissions to children's hospitals [43,46] and occurs in 6 to 10% of institutionalized retarded children [47]. Rumination in adults is not a rarity, especially in the presence of eating disorders (e.g., bulimia nervosa) wherein up to 20% of patients may ruminate [48]. Rumination syndrome may result in life-threatening complications including malnutrition and aspiration pneumonia. In mentally retarded patients, mortality rates of 15% to 20% are reported [46]. Even in less serious cases, ruminated acidic material can lead to dental erosions, esophagitis, and Barrett's metaplasia [49,50].

— Diagnostic Criteria

At least 12 weeks, which need not be consecutive, in the preceding 12 months of:

(1) Persistent or recurrent regurgitation of recently ingested food into the mouth with subsequent remastication and swallowing or spitting it out;
(2) Absence of nausea and vomiting;
(3) Cessation of the process when the regurgitated material
becomes acidic; *and*
(4) Absence of pathologic gastroesophageal reflux, achalasia,
or other motility disorder with a recognized pathologic
basis as the primary disorder.

— Clinical Evaluation

Identifying the characteristic clinical features in the absence of other organic esophageal or gastric diseases is the key to diagnosis. Medical conditions including gastroesophageal reflux disease, gastric outlet obstruction, and gastric
or esophageal motility disorders should be excluded. Disorders most typically
confused with rumination syndrome are gastroesophageal reflux disease and
bulimia [51]. Reflux disease is further distinguished by the fact that (1) solid
food is rarely brought back; (2) reflux may occur at any time, not primarily after
meals; and (3) reflux symptoms are more common when lying down or bending
over, whereas rumination is not. Bulimia is distinguished by the absence of
rechewing and reswallowing digesta.

Diagnostic studies may include upper gastrointestinal contrast studies with
fluoroscopy, endoscopy, and esophageal motility testing, depending on the
clinical suspicion and accompanying symptoms. Radiologic studies in rumination are typically normal; persistent contraction bands in the body of the stomach have been described in a few patients [52]. Gastrointestinal motility studies
are more suitable for documenting the pathophysiology of rumination than for
diagnosis [53].

— Physiologic Features

The mechanism of rumination in animals is well known: a negative intrathoracic pressure with simultaneous contractions of the abdomen induces
gastroesophageal reflux while esophageal antiperistalsis allows transport of the
fluid into the mouth [54]. In humans, reversed esophageal or gastric peristalsis
has not been reported. Rumination is occasionally initiated by inserting the

fingers into the throat or by stimulation of the palate with the tongue. The process is more often initiated by a belch or swallow, whereby the lowered LES pressure creates a common cavity between the stomach and the esophagus [45,55]. The voluntary contraction of abdominal wall muscles and the diaphragm is the primary force producing regurgitation of ingested food [55,56]. The performance of a Mueller maneuver (deep inspiration against a closed glottis) facilitates reflux of gastric contents into the esophagus because intraabdominal pressure rises while intrathoracic pressure becomes more negative.

Several groups have assessed esophageal and gastric motility in ruminators. Levine et al. [45] detected no motility abnormalities during rumination while monitoring esophageal and fundic pressures. Likewise, Amarnath et al. [56] reported no abnormalities of esophageal motility or the gastric phasic migrating motor complexes in 12 patients with rumination. However, all these latter patients, but no healthy control subjects, showed a characteristic "pressure spike wave" motor pattern associated with regurgitation that was recorded simultaneously along the gastric antrum and proximal duodenum with sudden decreases in intraesophageal pH (fig. 1). The spikes were more common postprandially than during fasting, in agreement with the timing of the symptoms. Also, the spike waves almost invariably coincided with visible regurgitation of food into the patient's mouth.

Some of the failure of Levine et al. to detect these abnormalities may be related to technical factors dampening pressure effects in the proximal part of the stomach. However, more recent manometric evaluations of adults with rumination syndrome suggest that gastroduodenal studies will detect the reported spike wave abnormalities in only a third of subjects [53]. Other physiological characteristics may better define this disorder. Some subjects with rumination demonstrate markedly reduced compliance of the proximal stomach, another finding that may help explain the occurrence of symptoms [57]. A convincing singular explanation is not available.

— Psychologic Features

The process of rumination provides a good example of the combined contributions of psychological and psychosocial factors to gastrointestinal dysfunction. In mentally retarded individuals, the degree of neuropsychiatric impairment largely determines the importance of rumination. In nonretarded children, two distinct hypotheses underlying psychological mechanisms are proposed. Some authors [46,58] state that rumination is a somatic symptom resulting from a poor mother-infant relationship. Mothers of ruminating infants

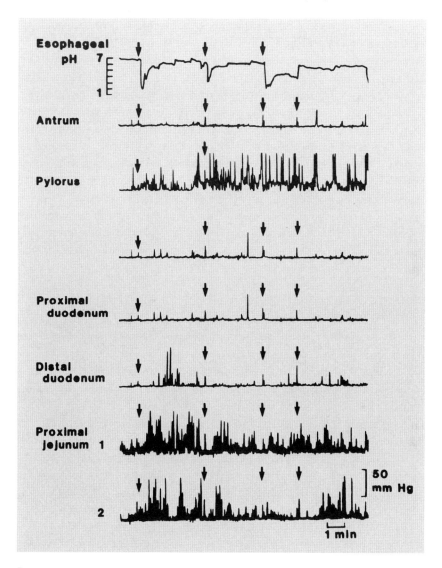

Figure 1. Gastroduodenal motility pattern in a rumination patient. Postprandial manometry with simultaneous esophageal pH monitoring shows several synchronous pressure spikes (arrows) associated with simultaneous decreases in esophageal pH. The manometric probe had three antroduodenal sites 1 cm apart and five intestinal sites 10 cm apart. The most distal jejunal recording site has been excluded. (Reproduced with permission from Amarnath RP, Abell TL, Malagelada JR. The rumination syndrome in adults: a characteristic manometric pattern. Ann Intern Med 1986;105:513–18.)

are often characterized as having difficulty in enjoying their babies (possibly related to personality problems or marital conflicts) and in sensing what gives the baby satisfaction, resulting in the infants turning to self-stimulating behavior. Numerous authors [46,58,59] have described the appearance of infants during rumination as "withdrawn and self-absorbed," as though they were deriving gratification from the process. An alternative theory in nonretarded children is that the behavior is a learned, conditioned response maintained by the reward of increased parental attention or by the pleasure associated with the taste of regurgitated food [60]. In intellectually intact adults, the most plausible explanation for rumination is that it is a learned habit. In patients who have ruminated since childhood, the habit may have persisted with parental approval. Although not distinctly linked to psychiatric disorder, rumination in adults with normal intelligence has been associated with obsessional personality and anxiety reaction to stressful events [45,56].

— Treatment

Treatment of rumination syndrome varies depending on the age of the patient and the presence of mental deficits. In children, several treatment methods are used, assuming that rumination is either a learned habit or a somatic symptom from lack of reciprocity between parent and child. Those who think rumination is a learned habit use punishment techniques to stop the habit. Electric shock applied to the calf muscle [61], adverse taste stimuli (e.g., lemon juice or hot sauce) placed on the infant's tongue [62], and excluding the child from play or social interactions for 3 to 10 minutes [63] all have been suggested punishments. Time out from social interaction and electric shock have resulted in the best outcomes [64]. Proponents of the theory that rumination results from the disruption of the emotional bond between mother and infant suggest a psychodynamic approach based on increased holding or increased "mothering" by a surrogate [43,58,59]. An integration of psychodynamic and behavioral theories into a single approach also has been suggested [65].

The different procedures used for managing mentally retarded patients with rumination can be classified as medical, behavioral, or nutritional. Medical or surgical procedures (antiemetic drugs, fundoplication) unfortunately are rarely effective [66,67]. Behavioral therapies have included extinction procedures, correction, and overcorrection [68,69]. Nutritional procedures include satiation techniques, decreasing the amount of food during each meal, giving clear liquids, and withholding fluids during mealtime [70]. Unfortunately, some of these nu-

Table 2. Outcome in 12 Patients with Rumination Syndrome

Type of treatment	No. of patients	Follow-up duration	Outcome, number
Eating habits regulation program	7	6–41 mo	Asymptomatic, 2 Improved, 4 No improvement, 1
Biofeedback and jacobsonian relaxation	3	3–31	Asymptomatic, 2 No improvement, 1 (patient declined therapy)
Psychotherapy	1	27 mo	Asymptomatic, 1
Lost to follow-up	1		

Modified from Amarnath RP, Abell RL, Malagelada JR. The rumination syndrome in adults: a characteristic manometric pattern. Ann Intern Med 1986;105:513–18, with permission.

tritional treatments cause weight loss and dehydration, whereas satiation techniques may result in obesity.

Adults with normal intelligence can "unlearn" this condition by nonadversive behavioral treatment (Table 2). Regulation of eating habits associated with strong encouragement not to vomit is reportedly successful [71], and chewing gum in the postprandial period is of anecdotal benefit [72]. Biofeedback techniques may be helpful by teaching the patient to relax the abdominal muscle during and after eating [73,74]. Jacobsonian progressive relaxation also has been shown to be effective [75,76]. In patients with severe psychiatric disturbances, psychotherapy and psychotropic drugs may be required.

A3. Functional Chest Pain of Presumed Esophageal Origin

— Definition

Functional chest pain of presumed esophageal origin is characterized by episodes of unexplained chest pain that are usually midline, of visceral quality, and therefore, potentially of esophageal origin. The pain is easily confused with cardiac angina or pain from other esophageal disorders including achalasia and gastroesophageal reflux disease. A careful exclusion of these esophageal and nonesophageal disorders is required to establish the diagnosis.

— Epidemiology

The prevalence of functional chest pain of presumed esophageal origin is unknown, because many subjects with this symptom do not complete the evaluation required to establish the diagnosis. Inferential data suggest this is a common disorder. Between 15% and 30% of coronary angiograms performed in chest pain patients are normal, and coronary artery spasm rarely explains the symptom [77]. Considering that at least 500,000 coronary angiograms are performed in the United States annually for chest pain of recent onset, a functional disorder may be present in 75,000 to 150,000 patients per year. These figures underestimate the total because many patients less than 40 years of age do not undergo cardiac catheterization. An exclusionary criterion is subsequently detected in no more than a third of patients with negative cardiac evaluations [78]. Although once considered a diagnosis of elderly women, chest pain without specific diagnosis was reported in a householder survey twice as commonly by subjects 15–34 years of age than by subjects more than 45 years old with equal gender representation [79]. Using survey responses to estimate rates of functional chest pain and other functional esophageal disorders, however, is confounded by the fact that the diagnoses depend heavily on medical exclusionary criteria. Patients with functional chest pain of presumed esophageal origin have a favorable prognosis; very low rates of myocardial infarction and death from cardiac causes (less than 1% for each) occurs over 10 years of observation once the diagnosis is established [80–84].

─ Diagnostic Criteria

At least 12 weeks, which need not be consecutive, in the preceding 12 months of:

(1) Midline chest pain or discomfort that is not of burning quality; *and*

(2) Absence of pathologic gastroesophageal reflux, achalasia, or other motility disorder with a recognized pathologic basis.

─ Justification for Criteria Change

To avoid diagnostic overlap with functional heartburn, pain or discomfort with burning quality is now excluded. By definition, establishing a functional esophageal disorder requires the exclusion of structural or metabolic explanations for the symptoms. In the case of functional chest pain, exclusion of cardiac disease is particularly important.

─ Clinical Evaluation

Initial studies are directed at excluding cardiac disease. The history and clinical presentation are inaccurate in predicting the presence of coronary artery disease [85], and the extent of investigation is typically determined by the patient's age, family history, and risk factors. Some patients with cardiac disease have pain that is poorly explained by the cardiac findings [86], but making a concurrent diagnosis of functional chest pain requires careful consideration. The diagnosis of "microvascular angina," characterized by small vessel coronary artery disease and increased coronary artery resistance, is no longer considered a tenable explanation for chest pain in patients without other cardiac findings [87,88]. Identifying gastroesophageal reflux disease is also of primary importance, because this is an easily treated, common cause of pain. Endoscopy is abnormal in less than 30% of patients with negative cardiac evaluation, usually showing only a hiatal hernia or mild esophagitis [89]. Esophagitis provides only inferential evidence that reflux disease is the cause of pain yet is a sufficient indication for instituting and continuing antireflux treatment.

Other studies can better define the relationship of reflux events to pain. The acid perfusion (Bernstein) test has been popular but is insensitive compared to ambulatory pH monitoring. For example, one study compared results from 75 consecutive patients with noncardiac chest pain who underwent an acid perfusion test and experienced chest pain during ambulatory monitoring. The acid perfusion test was specific (90%) but poorly sensitive (36%) for acid-related pain, using the ambulatory study as the standard. Thus, a positive test reliably indicated that the patient's chest pain was related to acid reflux events. However, a negative test did not exclude acid-provoked pain [90]. Ambulatory pH monitoring also helps identify acid-related pain in the subset without pathological reflux, a finding noted in 10%–15% of patients with functional chest pain and one that is helpful in management [91–93]. When combining subjects with or without pathological reflux, up to half of patients with normal coronary angiograms may have acid-related pain [85, 90, 94–102]. Treadmill testing during ambulatory pH monitoring may be further revealing if the pain has an exertional component [103]. Although objective tests can help identify the subset with acid-provoked pain during investigation, symptom relief during antireflux therapy may be the best method of proving an important clinical association of reflux and chest pain. For this reason, a brief therapeutic trial with a high dose of a proton pump inhibitor (omeprazole 40 mg PO QAM and 20 mg PO QPM) can be very cost effective [104].

Other diagnostic tests rarely provide results that exclude the diagnosis of functional chest pain. Manometric testing has a low yield for significant motor disorders that mandate specific intervention [105]. During the course of investigation, however, physiologic abnormalities may be discovered that identify mechanisms potentially involved in pain production. These observations may have a role in patient reassurance. For example, serial intraesophageal balloon inflation during ECG monitoring may reinforce for the patient that the esophagus, rather than the heart, is the likely source of symptoms. Such tests have had little other effect on diagnosis or treatment and are described in the following section as physiologic features of the disorder.

— Physiologic Features

Physiologic abnormalities of several types have been identified, especially motility abnormalities and hypersensitivity to acid, cholinergic agents, and an intraluminal distention stimulus. No singular feature characterizes all subjects. Up to half of subjects have esophageal motility abnormalities, particularly high amplitude peristaltic contractions (nutcracker esophagus) and other nonspecific spastic abnormalities [78,105,106]. A direct relationship of the motility abnormalities to pain is not demonstrable in the majority of cases. The patients are usually asymptomatic when the motility abnormalities are defined, and chest pain improvement correlates poorly with improvement in manometry either by medical or surgical approaches [107,108]. Ambulatory motility studies suggest that, on the average, pain could conceivably be attributed to motor events in <15% of episodes, but the definition of a pain-producing motor event is less established than the definition of reflux (Table 3) [109]. Recent data show that esophageal wall thickness can be demonstrated by ultrasonography during spontaneous and provoked chest pain [110]. These "sustained esophageal contractions" were not accompanied by definable intraluminal pressure abnormalities and may reflect longitudinal muscle contraction. Consequently, motor abnormalities other than those usually defined and identified by conventional manometric techniques may still have an important role in pain production, but further studies are required to clarify this point.

Investigations combining ambulatory pH monitoring with ambulatory motility measurement, as first described by Janssens and Vantrappen [94], have shed the most light on the relative contributions of usual motor abnormalities and intraluminal provocation by acid reflux events. Acid-related pain is far more common, although at least half of pain episodes are not preceded by either motility or reflux events (Table 3). Timing of the investigative study may in-

Table 3. Ambulatory Esophageal Studies of Patients with Non-cardiac Chest Pain

Investigators [Reference]	Number of Patients	Pain with Abnormal Motility	Abnormal Acid Exposure Time	Pain with Acid Reflux Event
Janssens [94]	60	8 (13%)	13 (22%)	13 (22%)
DeCaestecker [95]	50	ND	14 (28%)	6 (12%)
Hewson [96]	45	10 (22%)	20 (44%)	14 (31%)
Soffer [97]	20	1 (5%)	ND	9 (45%)
Richter [90]	100	ND	48 (48%)	50 (50%)
Ghillebert [98]	50	4 (8%)	ND	15 (30%)
Neuvens [85]	37	1 (3%)	15 (41%)	5 (14%)
Paterson [99]	25	7 (28%)	ND	10 (40%)
Voskuil [101]	28	0 (0%)	12 (43%)	10 (36%)
Total	415	31 (12%)	122 (38%)	132 (32%)

fluence the results. Lam and colleagues studied 45 patients admitted to the coronary care unit for chest pain [100], immediately after a cardiac cause was excluded as causing their chest pain. Of the 30 patients having one or more chest pain episodes during intraesophageal monitoring, 27 (90%) had an esophageal abnormality. Acid reflux was associated with chest pain in 14 patients (47%), abnormal motility in 12 patients (40%), and both in 1 patient (3%). On the other hand, the same group using similar techniques failed to find any evidence of esophageal motility disorders causing chest pain in patients with chronic relapsing chest pain seen in the gastroenterology clinic [111] or in patients with chest pain newly referred to a cardiology clinic [101]. This study may represent a special exception, and alternative mechanisms for pain production must be implicated in the average situation.

A variety of stimuli other than acid can provoke pain in some patients, including hot and cold liquids [112], pentagastrin [113], vasopressin [98], solid food bolus [114], ergonovine [115], bethanechol [116], and edrophonium. Edrophonium hydrochloride, a cholinesterase inhibitor, has been most studied. The agent, when injected intravenously (80–200 mcg/kg), can induce chest pain in 20% to 30% of patients, yet rarely in asymptomatic volunteers [117, 118]. Pain provocation correlates poorly with manometric changes and occurs in the same patients who respond to intraluminal balloon distension [119]. A positive response, however, does not distinguish which subjects appear to have acid-related pain by other testing methods, and coaching may unduly influence the report of pain following the injection [120]. Thus, although once promoted as a useful diagnostic test, the value of edrophonium injection rests more as a maneuver demonstrating physiologic abnormalities in some patients with functional chest pain.

Intraesophageal balloon distension is a nonpharmacologic method of provoking pain, and observations from using this maneuver have been most instrumental in suggesting a sensory abnormality in patients with functional chest pain. In an initial report by Richter et al. [121], 50% of patients meeting criteria for functional chest pain developed pain at balloon volumes of 8 ml or less, while control subjects began developing pain only at volumes of 9 ml or more (fig. 2). Later studies demonstrated that hypersensitivity to balloon distension also identified sensitivity to other stimuli, including acid and edrophonium [119]. More recently, Rao and associates used impedance planimetry to measure the sensory, motor, and biomechanical properties of the esophagus in healthy controls and patients with functional chest pain [122]. Pain thresholds were significantly lower in the chest pain patients confirming presence of a hypersensitive esophagus. Unlike earlier investigators, they also found the esophagus to be

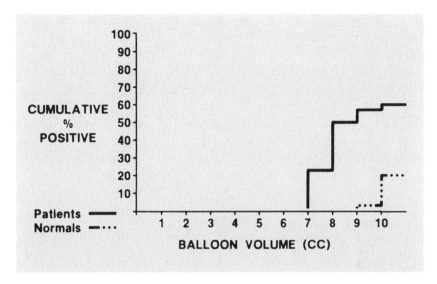

Figure 2. Intraesophageal balloon distension outcome in 30 patients with functional chest pain and 30 age-matched controls. Sixty percent of chest pain patients (solid line) experienced pain compared to only 20% of controls (broken line, p<0.005). Pain in the patients also occurred at smaller balloon volumes, suggesting a lower visceral pain threshold to intraluminal distension. (Reproduced with permission from Richter JE, Barish CF, Castell DO. Abnormal sensory perception in patients with esophageal chest pain. Gastroenterology 1986;91:845–52.)

less compliant and more reactive to luminal stretching in chest pain patients. Like edrophonium injection, balloon distension has demonstrated physiologic abnormalities in some patients but has not directed therapy.

Sensitivity to intraluminal stimuli, including acid and distension, has overshadowed motility abnormalities in mechanistic importance. Reflux events may be precipitants not only through acid sensitivity, but also through sensitivity to other refluxate ingredients (e.g., bile salts) and distension from the reflux episode. Other factors of potential importance include hydrogen ion concentration [123] and acid burden (summated acid exposure) one hour before the chest pain episode [124], the latter suggesting that recurrent acid exposure can sensitize mucosal chemoreceptors. Evidence does not favor usual motor abnormalities as the pain-producing response to acid. Besides reflux-related distension, spontaneous painful distension could result from belching against a closed upper esophageal sphincter [125] or could accompany food bolus trapping or impaction [126]. The underlying mechanisms responsible for lowered visceral pain sensitivity may be similar to those responsible in other functional gastrointestinal disorders [121,122]. Most studies suggest the defect is central rather than peripheral, possibly in the caudate, thalamus, anterior insular cortex, and anterior cingulate gyrus [127,128]. The esophagus is very accessible to instrumentation, and future studies using cerebral evoked potentials, positron emission tomography, and functional magnetic resonance should be helpful in better understanding the relevant pathophysiologic processes. Some data suggest that a stretch receptor, linked to the longitudinal muscle, mediates the sensory response [129]. Such observations may help integrate motor and sensory abnormalities noted in these patients.

— Psychologic Features

Cross-sectional studies in subjects with unexplained chest pain who seek health care demonstrate that at least 60% of these patients carry psychiatric diagnoses, the most common being anxiety disorders, depression, and somatization disorder [130–133]. Panic attacks are reported by 30% to 60% of patients [134,135]; chest pain associated with panic attacks may account for 25% of chest pain patients seen in the emergency room setting [136]. Rates of psychiatric diagnoses are unrelated to presence or absence of physiologic features including nonspecific motor disorders and balloon distention sensitivity [137]. For example, more than 75% of patients with spastic motility disorders had psychiatric diagnoses in two studies [130,138], a rate two to three times higher than that expected in the general population or found in patients with achalasia.

Higher ratings on anxiety and depression scales influence pain reporting and may contribute to the psychosocial morbidity suffered by these patients. The psychological characteristics are accompanied by a perceived vulnerability to serious heart disease. Lantinga and associates found that non-cardiac chest pain patients had higher levels of neuroticism and psychiatric morbidity before and after cardiac catherization than patients with coronary artery disease [139]. This appears to have prognostic significance, because these patients display less improvement in pain, more frequent pain episodes, greater social maladjustment, and more anxiety disorders at one year follow-up than individuals with relatively low initial levels of psychological disturbances.

Central nervous system influences can modulate esophageal motor activity and potentially exacerbate a vicious cycle of psychophysiologic interaction. At a minimum, central factors influence the rates of physiologic abnormalities noted in cross-sectional studies. Eliciting the stress response with acute stressors (e.g., startling noises, stressful interviews, hyperventilation) is accompanied by simultaneous contractions, modest increases in distal contraction amplitude, and impaired lower esophageal sphincter relaxation, but the relationship to chest pain is inconsistent [140–142]. A longitudinal study of alcoholics undergoing withdrawal demonstrated marked manometric changes occurring in parallel with changes in measures of stress [143]. During early alcohol withdrawal, contraction wave amplitudes consistent with the diagnosis of nutcracker esophagus (greater than 180 mm Hg), often with hypertensive lower esophageal sphincter pressures, were found in 9 of 14 patients. Thirty days after alcohol abstinence, the initial manometric high pressures reverted to normal in all subjects. The mechanism by which stress may affect esophageal motility is unknown but likely relates to neuropeptides release (e.g., corticotropin releasing factor). Although not established, it could be postulated that, in some patients, spastic motility disorders are manometric markers of a clinical stress syndrome rather than having direct responsibility for symptoms.

A prospective case control study by Bradley and colleagues explored pain thresholds and psychosocial factors among chest pain patients and four groups of control subjects [144,145]. The control groups consisted of healthy individuals and patients with gastroesophageal reflux disease, coronary artery disease, and irritable bowel syndrome. Pain thresholds for both somatic (finger) and visceral (esophagus) sites were assessed. Sensory decision theory was used to determine whether differences in pain thresholds resulted from discrimination problems (a neurosensory process) or response bias—the tendency to set either high or low standards for reporting pain (a cultural and emotional process) [146]. Patients with functional chest pain had significantly lower esophageal pain thresholds but not somatic pain thresholds than healthy subjects or patients with other painful gastrointestinal disorders. Discrimination was similar among groups, but chest pain patients tended just to set lower standards for judging esophageal distension stimuli as painful (Table 4). Psychological factors possibly contributing to this lower response bias included greater use of negative pain coping strategies, less ability to perform specific behaviors to decrease their pain, and reinforcement of pain behavior by spouses or significant others.

These controlled studies suggest that psychosocial factors may well have a contribution to the presentation of functional chest pain that exceeds similar relationships in pathologically based esophageal disorders including achalasia and gastroesophageal reflux disease. Generalization to a causative role remains unsubstantiated.

Table 4. Pain Thresholds and Sensory Decision Theory Parameters by Subject Groups

	Subject groups			
Variable	Chest pain n = 50	Irritable bowel n = 23	Reflux n = 42	Healthy controls n = 37
Esophageal distension pain threshold (ml) [a]	10.89± 1.09*	12.26 ± 1.29	13.15 ± 0.82	12.96 ± 0.96
Discrimination ability [b]	29.7 ± 0.9	27.7 ± 1.3	28.5 ± 1.0	28.1 ± 1.0
Response bias [c]	9.0 ± 0.2	9.5 ± 0.3	9.8 ± 0.2	9.9 ± 0.2

* Mean + SEM

[a] $p = 0.005$ Patients with chest pain of unknown etiology exhibited significantly lower balloon distension threshold for pain than other groups.
[b] $p = 0.20$ No significant difference in discrimination ability across groups.
[c] $p = 0.002$ Patients with chest pain exhibited significantly lower response bias than other groups.

Modified from Bradley LA, Scarinci IC, Richter JE. Pain threshold levels and coping strategies among patients who have chest pain and normal coronary arteries. Med Clin North Am 1991;75:1189–1202, with permission.

— Treatment

Treatment is not well established, mainly because pain-producing mechanisms are poorly understood and may differ from episode to episode and across patients. Simply providing a diagnosis may have some therapeutic importance, because reassurance solely about the noncardiac nature of the pain rarely results in definitive relief of concern [139,147,148]. Patients who are told that an esophageal source can explain the pain have significantly reduced health resource use and improved work functioning [147–150]. Pharmacologic therapy can be initially directed by testing results, but empirical therapeutic trials also are reasonable. Because a modest proportion of chest pain episodes are reflux-related in many patients, an aggressive trial of acid suppression for one to two months is recommended; more than three-fourths of patients unselected by presence or absence of documented reflux disease will respond to high-dose acid suppression in the first week [104]. Proton pump inhibitors relieve acid related chest pain nearly as well as typical reflux symptoms [151,152]. This response is independent of nonspecific motility abnormalities. Other therapeutic trials that might be contemplated in this patient group (e.g., psychotropic medications and smooth-muscle relaxants) may exacerbate unrecognized reflux disease.

Drugs directed at improving spastic motility disorders are popular in these patients, but evidence supporting this approach is largely anecdotal. Short- and long-acting nitrates [153,154], anticholinergic agents [155–157], and hydralazine [158] produce inconsistent results. The most carefully studied medications are the calcium-channel antagonists, particularly nifedipine and diltiazem. These drugs decrease esophageal pressures in healthy subjects [159], patients with chest pain and diffuse esophageal spasm [160], and patients with nutcracker esophagus [107]. Four controlled studies have been performed, but the results are inconclusive and not encouraging. In the initial study, Richter et al. found that nifedipine was no better than placebo in the relief of chest pain in 20 patients with nutcracker esophagus, although the drug significantly decreased distal esophageal contraction amplitude and duration [107]. A subsequent study in patients with diffuse esophageal spasm had similar findings [160]. Results with diltiazem are conflicting, one study finding symptomatic efficacy in a group of patients with nutcracker esophagus [161] while another showing no effect on pain in a group with mixed motility abnormalities [162]. These studies have a number of methodologic limitations. Subject groups were small; short-acting smooth-muscle relaxants were used; and all studies used standard manometry to identify the nonspecific motility disorders. The results might have been different if ambulatory pressure monitoring had been used to select patients in whom motility disturbances appeared related to chest pain episodes, but this is not the conventional method of evaluating patients. Both chest pain and dysphagia have also responded anecdotally to botulinum toxin injection in patients with spastic esophageal motility disorders [163]. The high response rate at one month (73%) declined to 33% by 11 months in this uncontrolled report. Controlled data will be required to determine if this approach has any diagnostic or therapeutic potential.

The most encouraging outcomes have come from psychotropic drugs and behavioral interventions. For antidepressants, the best studied agents, treatment effect is independent of depression or anxiety modulation by the medications. Potential benefits include direct effect on pain and sleep, but mechanism of action remains unknown. Clouse and associates found that low doses of the heterocyclic antidepressant trazodone (100–150 mg daily) produced global improvement and reduced distress ratings from esophageal symptoms over six weeks in patients with chest pain and nonspecific spastic esophageal motility disorders [138]. Symptom improvement was not related to changes in manometric parameters. Similarly, Cannon and colleagues found imipramine (50 mg at bedtime for two months) superior to clonidine or placebo in the treatment of unexplained chest pain [164]. The response to imipramine was not predicted by baseline psychologic or physiologic abnormalities, including esophageal manometry or balloon distension studies, and not dependent on their change. Because these antidepressant doses are lower than those used in treating psychiatric disorders, an unconventional mechanism or analgesic effect may be responsible for improvement. Other psychotropic agents (including other tricyclics, contemporary antidepressants, and anxiolytics) have enjoyed anecdotal use and the newer agents may be most helpful if active psychiatric symptoms are present. This remains conjectural, but the medications are capable of treating other uncomfortable symptoms that may be interfering with global improvement or coping abilities.

Behavioral therapy also is effective in patients with chest pain of functional origin. Hegel and colleagues [165] reported outcome of three chest pain patients with anxiety disorders who were treated with relaxation training and controlled diaphragmatic breathing exercises, practicing the techniques during increasingly complex activities. Two had substantial reductions in frequency and intensity of chest pain, a response that was maintained for 12 months after treatment ceased. Klimes and colleagues performed a controlled study of behavioral treatment in 31 patients with chest pain [166]. The intervention consisted of education, controlled breathing, training in relaxation and diversion of attention from pain, and practice of newly learned skills in the home environment. Active intervention, compared with a waiting-list control, produced significant improvement in chest pain episodes, functional capacity, and psychological distress that was maintained for 46 months after treatment. Some reported benefit potentially could be attributed to methodologic factors in the design of this investigation. The value of psychological management was recently confirmed in an 8-week treatment trial of 60 patients with continuing chest pain despite negative cardiologic evaluations [167]. Besides reducing chest pain episodes, the combination package of cognitive and behavioral treatments improved anxiety and depression scores, disability ratings, and exercise tolerance—effects maintained at 6-month follow-up.

A4. Functional Heartburn

— Definition

Functional heartburn is defined as episodic retrosternal burning in the absence of pathologic gastroesophageal reflux, pathology-based motility disorders, or structural explanations. Symptoms related to acid reflux events in the absence of pathologic gastroesophageal reflux are not excluded from consideration toward the diagnosis. This straightforward definition has practical applicability. The diagnosis of functional heartburn is constrained, however, by uncertainties in recognition of the symptom, artifact and error associated with 24-hour pH monitoring, and by the fact that a majority of individuals who experience heartburn never seek medical attention, let alone undergo gastrointestinal evaluation.

— Epidemiology

Twenty to thirty percent of subjects in Western populations claim to suffer from heartburn, depending on the thresholds for a positive response [168,169]. Heartburn occurring at least once per month is reported by 20% of responders, the rates being similar in males and females irrespective of age (in the range of 20–70 years). A minority of individuals with heartburn seek medical attention. Allowing for variation in definition of heartburn, consultation rates approximate 20–40%. Consequently, most information about the relationship between heartburn and objective tests of pathologic reflux is obtained from this minority. Additionally, an increasing proportion of patients with reflux symptoms have received prior treatment that may have healed esophagitis before index evaluation. Considering these caveats, functional heartburn probably accounts for less than 20% of patients complaining of heartburn to gastroenterologists.

— Diagnostic Criteria

At least 12 weeks, which need not be consecutive, in the preceding 12 months of:

(1) Burning retrosternal discomfort or pain; *and*

(2) Absence of pathologic gastroesophageal reflux, achalasia, or other motility disorder with a recognized pathologic basis.

— Justification for Criteria Change

Evidence-based data are absent to determine the specific symptom features of functional heartburn, including diurnal characteristics, exacerbating factors, and ameliorating maneuvers. The criteria were revised to acknowledge this lack of information and include all subjects with unexplained heartburn until further scientific data become available.

— Clinical Evaluation

Clarification of the nature of the symptom is an essential first step. Heartburn is typically assumed to resemble the cardinal manifestation of gastroesophageal reflux disease, characterized by pain or discomfort of burning quality that originates high in the epigastrium with intermittent cephalad retrosternal radiation. The feeling may be associated with salivation, voluntary swallowing, and regurgitation of sour-tasting fluid, and exacerbated by meals, certain foods, and postural changes. Not all these characteristics are required for diagnosing heartburn, and stringent criteria are associated with high specificity (yet relatively low sensitivity) for pathologic reflux [170]. In contrast, less rigorous criteria used by most practicing clinicians will include more patients with functional heartburn. Functional heartburn usually occurs during the day and, like the heartburn of reflux disease, may be elicited or exacerbated by certain foods and by lying down or bending over. Functional heartburn responds less predictably than classic reflux-related heartburn to antireflux treatment, but this feature is seldom helpful in diagnosis or management.

Little is required in the way of formal diagnostic work up for subjects with episodic, short-lasting, typical symptoms that are responsive to antacids or alginates. Patients with longer lasting, troublesome symptoms that have a limited response to medication require assessment, and the investigative sequence is straightforward. Clinical history, upper gastrointestinal endoscopy, and 24-hour ambulatory esophageal pH monitoring study provide the required information. False negative results from 24-hour ambulatory pH monitoring can occur, partially related to probe recording error; the possibility of overlooking pathologic reflux remains after thorough investigation. Alternative esophageal and non-esophageal explanations (e.g., achalasia or coronary artery disease) should be carefully considered when atypical esophageal symptoms, unusual symptom characteristics (e.g., exercise exacerbation), or a paucity of typical characteristics are found in the presentation [171].

— Physiologic Features

Within the group who meet criteria for functional heartburn are those having a high (>50%) association of heartburn episodes with acid reflux events as well as those having less consistent associations [92,93]. Reflux may play a more important physiologic role in symptom production for the former, but careful comparisons of characteristics across groups have not been performed in prospective fashion. In some subjects with symptom association indices (% of esophageal symptoms preceded by acid reflux events) approaching the high values seen in patients with esophagitis, pathologic reflux may have been underdiagnosed because of falsely negative results, for example, from ambulatory pH monitoring.

A degree of hypersensitivity to intraluminal stimuli has been proposed for this disorder and has been demonstrated in several ways. Heartburn sufferers with normal esophageal acid exposure times can be shown to have lower thresholds to pain from intraesophageal balloon distension [93]. Likewise, at least a third of heartburn episodes are preceded by acid reflux events indicating that sensitivity to acid may be one factor in symptom production [172]. Heartburn and reflux events are also partially related in patients with functional dyspepsia, another disorder wherein visceral hypersensitivity has a presumed pathogenetic role. Small et al. reported a symptom association index >50% in one-quarter of patients with functional dyspepsia in whom total esophageal acid exposure times on ambulatory 24-hour pH monitoring were normal, implying that these patients experience heartburn from a degree of acid reflux not perceived by normal subjects [173]. Dyspeptic patients without heartburn have lower symptom association indices, adding some specificity to the findings.

— Psychologic Features

Psychologic features in patients with functional heartburn have been poorly characterized. Nevertheless, the contribution of psychologic factors may be significant in the reporting of this discomfort as they can be in other pain syndromes. They may help explain some of the variability in symptom association indices in patients with reflux disease as well as functional heartburn [127,174, 175]. Heartburn not correlated with acid reflux events on pH monitoring predicts heightened anxiety, emotional lability, and poor social support compared with correlated symptoms [176]. In contrast, illness behavior has not differentiated functional heartburn patients from others with bona fide reflux disease [177].

Experimental stress can enhance the perception of reflux events in susceptible (anxious) individuals without influencing objective measures of reflux [178]. This may be relevant to the clinical arena in that nearly two-thirds of heartburn sufferers responding to a population poll declare that stress induces or exacerbates the symptoms [179]. Relaxation training appears to have an attenuating capacity by reducing symptoms in response to stressful tasks, but the effect may be partially related to a reduction in objective reflux induced by the behavioral intervention [180]. Despite laboratory evidence that stress can modify the reporting of symptoms, the relevance of stress experiments toward understanding potential effects of more persistent psychologic factors remains unknown.

— Treatment

The therapeutic approach initially follows principles for treating gastroesophageal reflux disease under the assumption that pathologic reflux may have been overlooked in the evaluation and/or that symptoms may respond to antireflux treatment. Lifestyle modifications should be encouraged before relying solely on medications. Pharmacotherapy data are limited, and outcome from antisecretory or prokinetic agents is expectedly less predictable. For example, proton pump inhibitor treatment provides better symptom control than placebo, but the response is attenuated compared to that in conventional reflux disease [181,182]. Limited information suggests that heartburn also decreases with low-dose antidepressant therapy. Based on limited data in patients with pathologic reflux, relaxation training may have a role in reducing symptom perception in some patients [180]. Other psychologic approaches have not been well studied in this disorder. Symptom persistence is documented in the subset of functional heartburn patients having high association of symptoms with reflux events [183]. The majority remains symptomatic over years of follow-up, substantiating the importance of treatment approaches having safe long-term profiles.

A5. Functional Dysphagia

— Definition

The diagnosis is restricted to patients with esophageal rather than oropharyngeal dysphagia, the hallmark symptom being a sensation of abnormal bolus transit through the esophageal body. Dysphagia is considered functional when there is no structural abnormality, pathological reflux, or pathology-based motility disturbance to explain the symptom. Comprehensive evaluation is required to exclude structural lesions.

— Epidemiology

Little information is available to determine the epidemiology of this disorder. In the householders survey for functional disorders, between 7% and 8% of respondents reported dysphagia that was unexplained by the exclusionary criteria [79]. Forty-one percent of these had seen a physician for the complaint. Diagnosis of the functional esophageal disorders depends heavily on objective testing, and consequently, some of these patients may have had another explanation for the symptoms (*e.g.,* gastroesophageal reflux disease). By survey methods, functional dysphagia is the least prevalent of the functional esophageal disorders [79].

— Diagnostic Criteria

At least 12 weeks, which need not be consecutive, in the preceding 12 months of:

(1) **Sense of solid and/or liquid foods sticking, lodging, or passing abnormally through the esophagus;** *and*
(2) **Absence of pathologic gastroesophageal reflux, achalasia, or other motility disorder with a recognized pathologic basis.**

— Clinical Evaluation

The diagnosis of functional dysphagia is established only after fastidious exclusion of a host of structural disorders that might be responsible for the symptom (Table 5). Evaluation begins with a targeted barium esophagram (usually with videofluoroscopy) and endoscopy. These studies also help identify pathologic reflux, and in the case of fluoroscopy, screen for motility disorders. Barium-impregnated bolus challenge during fluoroscopy (e.g., tablets, food) can help identify mucosal rings or strictures that may be overlooked with standard radiographic studies [184]. Evaluations negative for structural lesions including esophagitis should be followed by manometry. Ambulatory 24-hour pH monitoring generally is reserved for patients in whom dysphagia is associated with heartburn or regurgitation. A more thorough work-up including the diagnostic tests listed in the third step in Table 5 may be required for evaluating the isolated symptom.

A variety of nonspecific spastic motility abnormalities including peristaltic disturbances (intermittent simultaneous contractions, segmental aperistalsis), contraction wave abnormalities (increased wave durations and/or amplitude, multipeak waves), and hypertension or poor relaxation of the LES is found in 34% to 70% of patients with dysphagia who have no other explanation for this symptom [105]. The great variation in published reports is likely related to differences in manometric techniques and interpretations. These motor abnormalities do not have a recognized pathologic cause, and their presence does not preclude the diagnosis of functional dysphagia. The manometric abnormalities

Table 5. Stepwise Method for Establishing the Diagnosis of Functional Dysphagia

Step 1	Exclude intrinsic or extrinsic structural esophageal lesions (including esophagitis)	Double-contrast barium esophagram Upper endoscopy Barium impregnated solid bolus challenge during fluoroscopy
Step 2	Exclude achalasia or other pathology-based motility disorder	Barium videofluoroscopy Esophageal manometry
Step 3*	Further evaluation for pathologic gastroesophageal reflux and intermittent motor disorder	24-hour ambulatory pH monitoring ? Intensive antireflux trial Food provocation testing (during manometry or barium study) Manometry with balloon distension

*Steps 1 and 2 should be taken in all patients, as the identified disorders are easily treated. The extent of further testing (Step 3) is driven by the severity of symptoms, presence of associated symptoms (e.g., heartburn), or desire to demonstrate physiologic disturbances in some patients with functional dysphagia.

Source: Modified from Richter JE, et al. Functional oesophageal disorders. Gastroenterol Internat 1992;5:3–17.

of diffuse esophageal spasm also do not prevent a diagnosis of functional dysphagia, as their distinction from nonspecific motility disorders is not well substantiated in many cases [106,185].

— Physiologic Features

Several mechanisms may be responsible for functional dysphagia, and the intermittent complaints in some patients limit their clarification. Concurrent manometry and fluoroscopy has shown that simultaneous contraction sequences characterizing diffuse esophageal spasm (propagation velocity > 8 cm/sec) are invariably accompanied by poor barium clearance that may be perceived as dysphagia [96]. Simultaneous contraction sequences are found in a minority of patients during stationary manometric evaluation for dysphagia, but are more frequently detected during ambulatory pressure monitoring. Simultaneous contractions can be induced in 70% of subjects with presumed functional dysphagia but not in asymptomatic controls using intraesophageal balloon distension [186]. Induced simultaneous sequences frequently are accompanied by a reproduction of dysphagia.

In contrast, peristaltic dysfunction caused by failed contraction sequences or low-amplitude contractions (i.e., < 30–35 mm Hg) may also cause symptoms, but these events are less typically quantitated during manometric studies [187]. This type of peristaltic dysfunction is possibly responsible for nonobstructive dysphagia accompanying gastroesophageal reflux disease [188]. Failed contraction sequences or markedly reduced peristaltic activity also can be produced by feeding patients during manometry, and the induced motor abnormality correlates well with sensation of dysphagia [189]. Considering the frequency with which this type of abnormality could be induced in patients with otherwise unexplained dysphagia, persitaltic failure may be an important physiologic explanation in many patients with intermittent functional dysphagia [189].

Abnormal intraesophageal sensory perception may be a third physiologic factor in the report of dysphagia. A feeling of "food sticking" as well as pain is induced in some normal subjects with intraesophageal balloon distension in the distal esophagus [186]. Likewise, dysphagia is reported during acidification of the distal esophagus in some patients with reflux esophagitis [188]. Because dysphagia can be produced by various intraluminal stimuli, an error in visceral perception could be operational in patients with functional dysphagia as it is in patients with functional chest pain [121]. The studies by Deschner et al. demonstrating peristaltic dysfunction related to intraesophageal balloon distension could be interpreted as showing increased sensitivity to balloon distension [186]. The concordance of provoked dysphagia and peristaltic dysfunction was high but imperfect (87%), and peristaltic dysfunction might have represented an epiphenomenon. Other data indicate that abnormal sensitivity to balloon distension (using pain as the endpoint) is significantly associated with dysphagia as a presenting symptom in patients with functional esophageal symptoms [190]. Taken together, the observations in functional dysphagia favor both abnormal motility and abnormal visceral sensitivity as contributory mechanisms toward symptom production.

— Psychologic Features

Little information is available for review. Acute stress experiments suggest that central factors can precipitate motor abnormalities potentially responsible for dysphagia. Barium transit is adversely altered in asymptomatic and symptomatic subjects during recollection of unpleasant topics or stressful, unpleasant interviews [191,192]. Noxious auditory stimuli or difficult cognitive tasks alter manometry by increasing contraction wave amplitude and occasionally inducing simultaneous contraction sequences [141]. Extrapolating acute stress experiments to chronic symptoms in a functional esophageal disorder, however, is conjectural. Studies that have examined associations of psychiatric and psychologic factors with motility abnormalities in patients with functional chest pain may also have relevance to functional dysphagia [137]. Anxiety, depression, and somatization disorders are significantly more common in the subset with dysphagia and nonspecific motility disorders compared with patients having other explanations for the symptom [1].

— Treatment

The management of patients with functional dysphagia generally involves reassurance, avoidance of precipitating factors, careful chewing of food, and modification of physiologic and psychologic abnormalities that might be amenable to intervention. Functional dysphagia may regress over time, and an overzealous treatment approach is unwarranted in patients with mild symptoms. Patients with more severe symptoms warrant a comprehensive medical evaluation and pharmacologic trials. A trial of antireflux therapy should be considered in all patients but terminated if ineffective and pathologic reflux has not been demonstrated. Other medications commonly used are similar to those given to patients with functional chest pain of presumed esophageal origin, including smooth-muscle relaxants, anticholinergic drugs, and anxiolytics/antidepressants. None has proved efficacy for treatment of functional dysphagia, but nevertheless can be tried. The mechanisms by which these medications might influence the pathophysiology is unclear. Smooth muscle relaxants conceivably could improve symptoms if nonspecific spastic motor abnormalities (including poor LES relaxation) were interfering with transit. Some conflicting evidence is available regarding the effects of tricyclic antidepressants on visceral hypersensitivity [193,194].

Mechanical interventions should be considered in some patients. Dilation with a mercury-filled bougie (e.g., 54F Maloney) can be tried for patients presenting with intermittent food dysphagia, as a stricture or ring can be overlooked [195]. This technique has anecdotal use in some patients with dysphagia associated with nonspecific spastic motor disorders [196]. Similar to the treatment of achalasia, patients with incomplete LES relaxation and associated nonspecific motility disorders may respond to a pneumatic dilation. This procedure should be reserved for patients with a documented delay of distal esophageal emptying as defined by barium esophagram or scintigraphic studies [197]. Surgical interventions such as myotomy for functional dysphagia are almost never indicated because the symptoms usually improve over time, in contrast to achalasia [198].

A6. Unspecified Functional Esophageal Disorder

— Definition

This diagnosis is reserved for poorly described esophageal complaints or complaints that differ from the other functional disorders, such as belching or gurgling. The diagnosis should not be used if the principal symptoms meet criteria for another functional esophageal disorder. No data are available for epidemiology, diagnosis, physiologic features, or management.

— Diagnostic Criteria

At least 12 weeks, which need not be consecutive, in the preceding 12 months of:

(1) Unexplained symptoms attributed to the esophagus that do not fit into the previously described categories; *and*

(2) Absence of pathologic gastroesophageal reflux, achalasia, or other motility disorder with a recognized pathologic basis.

Recommendations for Future Research

The need for further investigation of the functional esophageal disorders cannot be overemphasized. Validation studies are lacking. Studies enhancing the sensitivity and specificity of the diagnostic criteria for each functional esophageal disorder would be welcomed. With the exception of rumination syndrome, the functional esophageal disorders rely entirely on the exclusion of organic diseases, including pathologic reflux and pathology-based motility disorders. Methods of improving the accuracy of symptom-based criteria alone should be sought. The importance of the individual diagnoses (excepting rumination) over a combined "functional esophageal syndrome" should be critically evaluated. Accuracy of diagnosis using symptom-based criteria might be enhanced if the criteria were inclusive rather than restrictive, encompassing a broader definition within the esophagus and considering other gastrointestinal and nongastrointestinal symptoms in the presentations.

Other important and underexplored areas in the functional esophageal disorders are identified in three categories.

1. Fundamental mechanisms of symptom production. Despite clear delineation of the individual symptoms and relative ease of esophageal instrumentation and investigation, the mechanisms responsible for symptom production remain poorly understood. Further examination of the contributions of motor and sensory dysfunction to symptoms should be undertaken; initiating and perpetuating processes should be investigated. The independent contribution of psychological factors, including personality, should be studied in well-designed fashion. Despite the similarity among the functional esophageal disorders in psychologic and physiologic associations (excluding rumination), explanations for site specificity should be sought.

2. Treatment approaches. Randomized trials of short- and long-acting treatments affecting the esophageal environment (e.g., antisecretory medications) are needed over anecdotal reports. The relative utility of such intraluminal modification over approaches affecting perception and reporting of symptoms remains understudied. Although short-term benefits of psychopharmacologic treatments in some functional esophageal disorders have been determined, long-term outcome is unreported and treatment mechanisms have been poorly delineated. Outcomes from psychologic and behavioral interventions remain unknown in most functional esophageal disorders, yet these approaches may be very effective considering the nature of the disorders and associated psychologic features. The best behavioral approaches for managing rumination syndrome in the developmentally impaired have yet to be determined.

3. *Health economics and quality of life.* Important indictors of morbidity from functional esophageal disorders are measures of health-care resource use and social dysfunction (e.g., both time off work and quality of life impairment). Treatment interventions should include measures of functional outcome when determining both short-term and long-term effects. The value of testing over empirical treatment for most functional esophageal disorders remains understudied.

Difficulties in studying the functional esophageal disorders are fully recognized. Investigations that consider these recommendations individually for future research are encouraged. Because of the interaction of factors involved in the pathogenesis of symptoms, however, studies of multidimensional design and capable of multivariate analysis are likely to provide important results.

CHAPTER 5: APPENDIX
The Glasgow-Edinburgh Throat Scale (GETS)

Name _____   Date _____

Throat Questionnaire

Do you have any of the following sensations?
  Please indicate by circling the figure which best describes how much you are affected.
  Answer all items please

	None						Unbearable	
Feeling of something in the throat	0	1	2	3	4	5	6	7
Pain in the throat	0	1	2	3	4	5	6	7
Discomfort / irritation in the throat	0	1	2	3	4	5	6	7
Difficulty in swallowing food	0	1	2	3	4	5	6	7
Throat closing off	0	1	2	3	4	5	6	7
Swelling in throat	0	1	2	3	4	5	6	7
Catarrh down throat	0	1	2	3	4	5	6	7
Can't empty throat when swallowing	0	1	2	3	4	5	6	7
Want to swallow all the time	0	1	2	3	4	5	6	7
Food sticking when swallowing	0	1	2	3	4	5	6	7

	None						All the time	
How much time do you spend thinking about your throat?	0	1	2	3	4	5	6	7

	Not at all						Extremely	
At present how annoying do you find your throat sensation?	0	1	2	3	4	5	6	7

References

1. Richter JE, Baldi F, Clouse R, et al. Functional esophageal disorders. In: Drossman DA et al., Editors. The Functional Gastrointestinal Disorders: Diagnosis, Pathophysiology, and Treatment. Boston: Little, Brown and Company;1994:25–70.
2. Drossman DA, Richter JE, Talley NJ,et al., Editors. The Functional Gastrointestinal Disorders: Diagnosis, Pathophysiology, and Treatment. Boston: Little, Brown and Company;1994.
3. Richter JE , Baldi F, Clouse RE, et al. Functional oesophageal disorders. Gastroenterol Internat 1992;5:3–17.
4. Merskey H, Merskey SJ. Hysteria, or "suffocation of the mother." Can Med Assoc J 1993;148:399–405.
5. Othmer E, Desouza CA. A screening test for somatisation disorder (hysteria). Am J Psychiatry 1985;142:1146–49.
6. Mills CP. A "lump" in the throat. J Laryngol Otol 1956;70:530–34.
7. Tremble GE. Hypertrophied lingual tonsils. Laryngoscope 1956;67:785–95.
8. Counter RT. Globus hystericus and cervical osteophytes. J Roy Nav Med Serv 1977;63:81–84.
9. Watson WC, Sullivan SN. Hypertonicity of the upper oesophageal sphincter: a cause of globus sensation. Lancet 1974;2:1417–19.
10. Marshall JN, McGann G, Cook JA, et al. A prospective controlled study of high resolution thyroid ultrasound in patients with globus pharyngeus. Clin Otolaryngol 1996;21:228–31.
11. Mair IWS, Schroder KE, Modalsli B, et al. Aetiological aspects of the globus symptom. J Laryngol Otol 1974;88:1033–40.
12. Batch AJG. Globus pharyngeus (pts I & II). J Laryngol Otol 1988;102:152–58; 227–30.
13. Flores TC, Cross FS, Jones RD. Abnormal oesophageal manometry in globus hystericus. Ann Otol Rhinol Laryngol 1981;90:83–86.
14. Farkkila MA, Ertama L, Katila H, et al. Globus pharyngis, commonly associated with esophageal motility disorders. Am J Gastroenterol. 1994;89:503–8.
15. Thompson WG, Heaton KW. Heartburn and globus in healthy people. Can Med Assoc J 1982;126:46–48.
16. Moloy PJ, Charter R. The globus symptom. Arch Otolaryngol 1982;108:740–44.
17. Wilson JA, Deary IJ, Maran AGD. The persistence of symptoms in patients with globus pharyngis. Clin Otolaryngol 1991;16:202–205.
18. Rowley H, O'Dwyer TP, Jones AS, et al. The natural history of globus pharyngeus. Laryngoscope 1995;05:1118–21.
19. Culbert TP, Kajander RL, Kohen DP, et al. Hypnobehavioral approaches for school–age children with dysphagia and food aversion: a case series. J Dev Behav Ped 1996;17:335–41.
20. Donohue B, Thevenin DM, Runyon MK. Behavioral treatment of conversion disorder in adolescence. A case example of globus hystericus. Behav Modification 1997;21:231–51.

21. Deary IJ, Wilson JA, Kelly SW. Globus and psychological distress in the general population. Psychosomat 1995;36:570–77.

22. Wilson JA, Pryde A, Macintyre CCA, et al. Pharyngoesophageal dysmotility in globus sensation. Arch Otolaryngol Head Neck Surg 1989;115:1086–90.

23. Deary IJ, Wilson JA, Harris MB, et al. Globus pharyngis: development of a symptom assessment scale. J Psychomat Res 1995;39:203–13.

24. Lorenz R, Jorysz G, Clasen M. The globus syndrome: value of flexible endoscopy of the upper gastrointestinal tract. J Laryngol Otol 1993;107:535–37.

25. Wilson JA, Murray JM, Haacke NPV. Rigid endoscopy in ENT practice: appraisal of the diagnostic yield in a district general hospital. J Laryngol Otol 1987;101: 286–92.

26. Ott DJ, Ledbetter MS, Koufman KA, et al. Globus pharyngeus: radiographic evaluation and 24-hour pH monitoring of the pharynx and esophagus in 22 patients. Radiology 1994;191(1):95–7.

27. Curran AJ, Barry MK, Callanan V, et al. A prospective study of acid reflux and globus pharyngeus using a modified symptom index. Clin Otolaryngol 1995;20: 552–54.

28. Walther EK, Schmidt C. Globus pharyngis and gastroesophageal equivalents. Laryngo- Rhino-Otologie 1997;76:225–28.

29. Lindgren S, Janzon L. Prevalence of swallowing complaints and clinical findings among 50–79-year-old men and women in an urban population. Dysphagia 1991; 6:187–92.

30. Leelamanit V, Geater A, Sinkitjaroenchai W. A study of 111 cases of globus hystericus. J Med Assoc Thailand 1996;79:460–67.

31. Cook IJ, Dent J, Collins SM. Upper esophageal sphincter tone and reactivity in patients with a history of globus sensation. Dig Dis Sci 1989;34:672–76.

32. Gray L. The relationship of the 'inferior constrictor swallow' and 'globus hystericus' or the hypopharyngeal syndrome. J Laryngol Otolaryngol 1093;97:607–18.

33. Moser G , Vacariu-Granser GV, Schneider C, et al. High incidence of esophageal motor disorders in consecutive patients with globus sensation. Gastroenterology 1991;101:1512–21.

34. Deary IJ, Smart A, Wilson JA. Depression and 'hassles' in globus pharyngis. Br J Psychiatry 1992;161:115–117.

35. Deary IJ, Wilson JA. Problems in treating globus pharyngis. Clin Otolaryngol 1994;19:55–60.

36. Deary IJ, Wilson JA, Mitchell L, et al. Covert psychiatric disturbance in patients with globus pharyngis. Br J Med Psychol 1989;62:381–89.

37. Harris MB, Deary IJ, Wilson JA. Life events and difficulties in relation to globus pharyngis onset. J Psychosomat Res 1996;40:603–15.

38. Deary IJ, S Scott, Wilson JA. Alexithymia and medically unexplained symptoms. J Personality Indiv Diff 1997; 22:551–64.

39. Kibblewhite DJ, Morrison MD. A double-blind controlled study of the efficacy of cimetidine in the treatment of the cervical symptoms of gastro-oesophageal reflux. J Otolaryngol 1990;19:103–9.

40. Brown SR, Schwartz JM, Summergrad P, et al. Globus hystericus syndrome responsive to antidepressants. Am J Psychiatry 1986;143:917–18.

41. Malcolm A, Thumshirn MB, Camilleri M, et al. Rumination syndrome. Mayo Clin Proc 1997;72:646–52.

42. Kanner L. Historical notes on rumination in man. Med Life 1936;27:27–32.

43. Whitehead WE, Schuster MM. Rumination syndrome, vomiting, aerophagia, and belching. In: Whitehead WE, Schuster MM, Editors. Gastrointestinal disorders: behavioral and physiological basis for treatment. Orlando, FL:Academic; 1985: 67–90.

44. Sullivan PB. Gastrointestinal problems in the neurologically impaired child. Baillieres Clin Gastroenterology 1997;11:529–46.

45. Levine DF, Wingate DL, Pferrer JM, et al. Habitual rumination: a benign disorder. Br Med J 1983;287:255–56.

46. Einhorn AH. Rumination syndrome (merycism or merycasm). In: Barnett HL, Editor. Pediatrics. New York: Appleton-Century-Crofts; 1972:1576–78.

47. Singh NN. Rumination. Internat Rev Res Ment Retard 1981;10:139–82.

48. Larocca FE, Della Fera MA. Rumination: its significance in adults with bulimia nervosa. Psychosomat 1986;27:209–12.

49. Roberts IM, Curtis RL, Madara JL. Gastroesophageal reflux and Barrett's esophagus in developmentally disabled patients. Am J Gastroenterol 1986;86:519–23.

50. Scheutzel P. Etiology of dental erosion–intrinsic factors. Eur J Oral Sci 1996;104: 178–90.

51. Herbst J, Friedland GW, Zboralski FF. Hiatal hernia and "rumination" in infants and children. J Pediatr 1971;78:261–65.

52. Brown WR. Rumination in the adult: a study of two cases. Gastroenterology 1968;54:933–39.

53. O'Brien BD, Bruce BK, Camilleri M. The rumination syndrome: clinical features rather than manometric diagnosis. Gastroenterology 1995;108:1024–29.

54. Winship DH, Zboralske FF, Weber WN, et al. Esophagus in rumination. Am J Physiol 1964;207:1189–94.

55. Reynolds RPE, Lloyd DA. Manometric study of a ruminator. J Clin Gastroenterol 1986;8:127–30.

56. Amarnath RP, Abell RL, Malagelada JR. The rumination syndrome in adults: a characteristic manometric pattern. Ann Intern Med 1986;105:513–18.

57. Thumshirn M, Camilleri M, Hanson RB, et al. Gastric mechanosensory and lower esophageal sphincter function in rumination syndrome. Am J Physiol 1998;275: G314–21.

58. Stein ML, Rusen AR, Blau A. Psychotherapy of an infant with rumination. JAMA 1959;171:2309–12.

59. Richmond JB, Eddy E, Green M. Rumination: a psychosomatatic syndrome of infancy. Pediatrics 1958;22:49–55.

60. Ferholt J, Provence S. Diagnosis and treatment of an infant with psychophysiological vomiting. Psychoanal Study Child 1976;31:439–59.

61. Lang PJ, Melamed BJ. Avoidance conditioning therapy of an infant with chronic ruminative vomiting. J Abnorm Psychol 1969;74:1–8.

62. Becker JV, Turner SM, Sajwaj TE. Multiple behavioral effects on the use of lemon juice with a ruminating toddler-age child. Behav Modif 1978;2:267–72.

63. Lavigne JV, Burns WJ. Rumination in infancy: recent behavioral approaches. Internat J Easting Disord 1981;1:70–82.

64. Davis PK, Cuvo AJ. Chronic vomiting and rumination in intellectually normal and retarded individuals: review and evaluation of behavioral research. Behav Res Severe Disabil 1980;1:31–59.

65. Whitehead WE, Dreschev VM, Morrill-Corbin E, et al. Rumination syndrome in children treated by increased holding. Pediatr Gastroenterol Nutr 1985;4:550–56.

66. Munford PR, Pally R. Outpatient contingency management of operant vomiting. J Behav Ther Exp Psychiatry 1979;10:135–37.

67. Welsley JR, Coran AG, Sarahan TM, et al. The need for evaluation of gastroesophageal reflux in brain damaged children referred for feeding gastrostomy. J Pediatr Surg 1981;16:866–70.

68. Pazulinec R, Sajwau T. Psychological treatment approaches to psychogenic vomiting and rumination. In: Holzl R, Whitehead WE, Editors. Psychophysiology of the Gastrointestinal Tract: Experimental and Clinical Applications. New York: Plenum; 1983:43–63.

69. Holvoet JF. The etiology and managment of rumination and psychogenic vomiting: a review. Monogr Am Assoc Defic 1982;5:29–77.

70. Rast J, Johnston JM, Drum C, et al. The relation of food quantity to rumination behavior. J Appl Behav Anal 1981;14:121–30.

71. Latimer PR, Malmud LS, Fisher RS. Gastric stasis and vomiting: behavioral treatment. Gastroenterology 1982;83:684–88.

72. Weakley MM, Petti TA, Karwisch G. Case study: chewing gum treatment of rumination in an adolescent with an eating disorder. J Am Acad Child Adol Psychiatry 1997;36:1124–27.

73. Schuster MM. Biofeedback control of gastrointestinal motility. In: Basmaijian JV, Editor. Biofeedback: Principles and Practice for Clinicians. Baltimore: Williams & Wilkins; 1983:2275–81.

74. Johnson LF. 24 hour pH monitoring in the study of gastroesophageal reflux. J Clin Gastroenterol 1980;2:387–399.

75. Morrow GR, Morrell C. Behavioral treatment for the anticipatory nausea and vomiting induced by cancer chemotherapy. N Engl J Med 1982;307:1476–1480.

76. Soykan I, Chen J, Kendall BJ, et al. The rumination syndrome: clinical and manometric profile, therapy, and long-term outcome. Dig Dis Sci 1997;42:1866–72.

77. Kemp HG, Vokonas PS, Cohn PF, et al. The anginal syndrome associated with normal coronary arteriogram. Report of a six-year experience. Am J Med 1973; 54:735–42.

78. Richter JE. Bradley LA, Castell DO. Esophageal chest pain: current controversies in pathogenesis, diagnosis and treatment. Ann Intern Med 1989;110:66–78.

79. Drossman DA, Li Z. Andruzzi E, et al. US householder survey of functional GI disorders: prevalence, sociodemography and health impact. Dig Dis Sci 1993;38: 1569–80.

80. Kemp HG, Kronmal RA, Vlietstra RE, et al. Seven year survival of patients with normal or near normal coronary arteriograms. A CASS registry study. J Am Coll Cardiol 1986;7:479–83.

81. Pasternak RC, Thibault GE, Savoia M, et al. Chest pain with angiographically insignificant coronary arterial obstruction:clinical presentation and long-term follow-up. Am J Med 1980;68:813–17.

82. Wielgosz AT, Gletcher RH, McCants CB, et al. Unimproved chest pain in patients with minimal or no coronary disease: a behavioral problem. Am Heart J 1984;108: 67–72.

83. Brushke AVG, Proudfit WL, Sones FM. Clinical course of patients with normal, and slightly or moderately abnormal coronary angiogram. A follow-up study on 500 patients. Circulation 1973;47:936–45.

84. Proudfit WL, Bruschke AVG, Sones FM. Clinical course of patients with normal or slightly or moderately abnormal coronary arteriograms: 10 year follow-up of 521 patients. Circulation 1980;62:712–17.

85. Nevens F, Janssen J, Piessens J, et al. Prospective study on prevalence of esophageal chest pain in patients referred on an elective basis to a cardiac unit for suspected myocardial ischemia. Dig Dis Sci 1991;36:229.

86. Lux G, Van Els J, The GS, et al. Ambulatory esophageal pressure, pH and ECG recording in patients with normal and pathological coronary angiography and intermittent chest pain. Neurogastroenterol Motil 1995;7:23–30.

87. Cannon RO, Epstein JE. "Microvascular angina" as a cause of chest pain with angiographically normal coronary arteries. Am J Cardiol 1988;61:1338–43.

88. Cannon RO, Quyyumi AA, Schenke WH, et al. Abnormal sensitivity in patients with chest pain and normal coronary arteries. J Am Coll Cardiol 1990;16:1359–66.

89. Frobert O, Funch-Jensen P, Jacobsen NO, et al. Upper endoscopy in patients with angina and normal coronary angiograms. Endoscopy 1995;27:365–70.

90. Richter JE, Hewson EG, Sinclair JW, et al. Acid perfusion test and 24-hour esophageal pH monitoring with symptom index: comparison of tests for esophageal sensitivity. Dig Dis Sci 1991;36:565–71.

91. DeMeester TR, Johnson LF, Joseph GJ, et al. Patterns of gastroesophageal reflux in health and disease. Ann Surg 1976;184:459–70.

92. Shi G, Varannes SB, Scarpignato C, et al. Reflux related symptoms in patients with normal oesophageal exposure to acid. Gut 1995;37:457–64.

93. Trimble KC, Pryde A, Heading RC. Lowered oesophageal sensory thresholds in patients with symptomatic but not excess gastro-oesophageal reflux: evidence for a spectrum of visceral sensitivity. Gut 1995;37:7–12.

94. Janssen J, Vantrappen G, Ghillibert G. 24-hour recording of esophageal pressure and pH in patients with non-cardiac chest pain. Gastroenterology 1986;90:1978–84.

95. de Caestecker JS, Brown J, Blackwell JN, et al. The oesophagus as a cause of recur-

rent chest pain: which patients should be investigated and which tests should be used? Lancet 1985;2:1143–46.

96. Hewson EG, Dalton CB, Richter JE. Comparison of esophageal manometry, provocative testing and ambulatory monitoring in patients with unexplained chest pain. Dig Dis Sci 1990;35:302–309.

97. Soffer EE, Scalabrini P, Wingate DL. Spontaneous non-cardiac chest pain: value of ambulatory esophageal pH and motility monitoring. Dig Dis Sci 1989;34:1651–55.

98. Ghillebert G, Janssen J, Vantrappen G, et al. Ambulatory 24-hour intraesophageal pH and pressure recordings vs provocative tests in the diagnosis of chest pain of oesophageal origin. Gut 1990;31:738–44.

99. Paterson WG, Abdollah, Beck IT, et al. Ambulatory esophageal manometry, pH-metry and Holter monitoring in patients with atypical chest pain. Dig Dis Sci 1993;38:795–802.

100. Lam HG, Dekker W, Kan G, et al. Acute noncardiac chest pain in a coronary care unit: evaluation by 24-hour pressure and pH recording of the esophagus. Gastroenterology 1992;102:453-60.

101. Voskuil JH, Cramer MJ, Breumelhof R, et al. Prevalence of esophageal disorders in patients with chest pain newly referred to the cardiologist. Chest 1996;189:1210–14.

102. DeMeester TR, O'Sullivan GC, Bermudez G, et al. Esophageal function in patients with angina-type chest pain and normal coronary angiogram. Ann Surg 1982;196: 488–98.

103. Schofield PM, Bennett DH, Whorwell PJ, et al. Exertional gastroesophageal reflux: a mechanism for symptoms in patients with angina pectoris and normal coronary angiograms. Brit Med J 1987;294:1459–61.

104. Fass R, Fennerty MB, Ofman JJ, et al. The clinical and economic value of a short course of omeprazole in patients with noncardiac chest pain. Gastroenterology 1998;115:42–49

105. Kahrilas PJ, Clouse RE, Hogan WJ. American Gastroenterological Association technical review on the clinical use of esophageal manometry. Gastroenterology, 1994;107:1865–84.

106. Clouse RE. Spastic disorders of the esophagus. Gastroenterologist. 1997; 5:112–27.

107. Richter JE, Dalton CB, Bradley LA, et al. Oral nifedipine in the treatment of non-cardiac chest pain patients with the nutcracker esophagus. Gastroenterology 1987; 93:21–28.

108. Ellis FH, Crozier RE, Shea JA. Long esophagomyotomy for diffuse esophageal spasm and related disorders. In: Siewert JR, Holschen AH, Editors. Diseases of the Esophagus: Pathophysiology, Diagnosis, Conservative and Surgical Treatment. New York: Springer-Verlag; 1988:913–17.

109. Richter JE, Castell DO. 24-hour ambulatory esophageal motility monitoring: how should motility data be analyzed? Gut 1989;30:1040–47.

110. Balaban DH, Yamamoto Y, Liu J, et al. Sustained esophageal contraction: a marker of esophageal chest pain idenitfied by intraluminal ultrasonography. Gastroenterology 1999;116:29–37.

111. Breumelhof R, Nasdorp JHSM, Smout AJPM, et al. Analysis of 24-hour esophageal pressure and pH data in unselected patients with non-cardiac chest pain. Gastroenterology 1990;99:1257–64.

112. Catalano CJ, Bozymski EM, Orlando RC. Temperature dependent symptoms in a patient with esophageal motor disease. Gastroenterology 1982;85:1407–10.

113. Orlando RC, Bozymski EM. The effect of pentagastrin in achalasia and diffuse esophageal spasm. Gastroenterology 1979;472–77.

114. Allen ML, Orr WC, Mellow MH, et al. Water swallows versus food ingestion as manometric tests for esophageal dysfunction. Gastroenterology 1988;95:831–37.

115. Eastwood GL, Weiner BH, Dickerson WJ 2nd, et al. Use of ergonovine to identify esophageal spasm in patients with esophageal chest pain. Ann Intern Med 1981; 94:768–71.

116. Nostrant TT, Saver J, Haber T. Bethanechol increases the diagnostic yield in patients with esophageal spasm. Gastroenterology 1986;91:1141–46.

117. Richter JE, Hackshaw BT, Wu WC, et al. Edrophonium: a useful provocative test for esophageal chest pain. Ann Intern Med 1985;103:14–21.

118. Lee CA, Reynolds JC, Ouyang A, et al. Esophageal chest pain: value of high-dose provocative testing with edrophonium chloride in patients with normal manometrics. Dig Dis Sci 1987;32:682–88.

119. Barish CF, Castell DO, Richter JE. Graded esophageal balloon distension: a new provocative test for non-cardiac chest pain. Dig Dis Sci 1986;31:1292–98.

120. Rose S, Achkar EA, Falk GW, et al. Interaction between patient and test administrator may influence the results of edrophonium provocation testing in patients with non-cardiac chest pain. Am J Gastroenterol 1993;88:20–24.

121. Richter JE, Barish CF, Castell DO. Abnormal sensory perception in patients with esophageal chest pain. Gastroenterology 1986;91:845–54.

122. Rao SSC, Gregersen H, Hayek B, et al. Unexplained chest pain: the hypersensitive, hyperactive, and poorly compliant esophagus. Ann Intern Med 1996;124:950–58.

123. Smith JL, Lankai E, Opekum AR, et al. Sensitivity of the esophageal mucosa to pH in gastroesophageal reflux disease. Gastroenterology 1989;96:683–89.

124. Weusten BL, Akkerman LMA, vanBerge-Hennegouwen GP, et al. Symptom perception in gastroesophageal reflux disease is dependent on spatiotemporal reflux characteristics. Gastroenterology 1995;108:1739–44.

125. Kahrilas PJ, Dodds WJ, Hogan WJ. Dysfunction of the belch reflux: a cause of incapitating chest pain. Gastroenterology 1987;93:818–22.

126. Howard PJ, Pryde A, Heading RC. Oesophageal manometry during eating in the investigation of patients with chest pain or dysphagia. Gut 1989;30:1179–86.

127. McDonald-Haile J, Bradley LA, Bailey MA, et al. Low regional cerebral blood flow to caudate nuclei is associated with chest pain of undetermined etiology. Gastroenterology 1994;106:1038A.

128. Aziz Q, Anderson JLR, Valind S, et al. Indentification of human brain loci processing esophageal sensation using positron emission tomography. Gastroenterology 1997;113:5059.

129. de Caestecker JS, Pryde A, Heading RC. Site and mechanism of pain perception with esophageal balloon distension and intravenous edrophonium in patients with esophageal chest pain. Gut 1992;33:580.

130. Clouse RE, Lustman PJ. Psychiatric illness and contraction abnormalities of the esophagus. N Engl J Med 1983;309:1387–92.

131. Richter JE, Obrecht WF, Bradley LA, et al. Psychological comparison of patients with nutcracker esophagus and irritable bowel syndrome. Dig Dis Sci 1986;31:131–38.

132. Bass C, Wade C. Chest pain with normal coronary arteries: a comparative study of psychiatric and social morbidity. Psychol Med 1984;14:51–61.

133. Alexander PJ, Prabhu SAS, Krishnamoorthy ES, et al. Mental disorders in patients with noncardiac chest apin. Acta Psychiatr Scand 1994;89:291–93.

134. Beitman BD, Basha I, Flaker G, et al. Atypical or non-anginal chest pain: panic disorder or coronary artery disease? Arch Intern Med 1987;147:1548–52.

135. Katon W, Hall ML, Russo J, et al. Chest pain: relationship of psychiatric illness to coronary arteriographic results. Am J Med 1988;84:1–9.

136. Fleet RP, Dupuis G, Marchand A, et al. Panic disorder in emergency department chest pain patients: prevalence, comorbidy, suicidal ideation and physician recognition. Am J Med 1996;101:371–80.

137. Clouse RE, Carney RM. The psychologic profile of non-cardiac chest pain patients. Eur J Gastroenterol Hepatol 1995;7:1160–65.

138. Clouse RE, Lustman PJ, Eckert TC, et al. Low-dose trazodone for symptomatic patients with esophageal contraction abnormalities: double-blind, placebo-controlled trial. Gastroenterology 1986;92:1027–36.

139. Lantinga LJ, Sprafkin RP, McCroskery JH, et al. One-year psychosocial follow-up of patients with chest pain and angiographically normal coronary arteries. Am J Cardiol 1988;62:209–13.

140. Rubin J, Nagler R, Sprio HM, et al. Measuring the effect of emotions on esophageal motility. Psychosomat Med 1962;24:170–74.

141. Stacher G, Schmieeser C, Landgraf M. Tertiary esophageal contractions evoked by acoustic stimuli. Gastroenterology 1979;44:49–54.

142. Anderson KO, Dalton CB, Bradley LA, et al. Stress: a modulator of eosphageal pressures in healthy volunteers and non-cardiac chest pain patients. Dig Dis Sci 1989;34:83–91.

143. Keshavarzian A, Iber FL, Ferguson Y. Esophageal manometry and radionuclide emptying in chronic alcoholics. Gastroenterology 1987;92:751–57.

144. Bradley LA, Scarinci IC, Richter JE. Pain threshold levels and coping strategies among patients who have chest pain and normal coronary arteries. Med Clinic North Am 1991;75:1189–1202.

145. Bradley LA, Scarinci IC, Richter JE, et al. Psychosocial and psychophysical assessments of patients with unexplained chest pain. Am J Med 1992;92(suppl 5A): 65–78.

146. Clark WC. Pain sensitivity and the report of pain: an introduction to sensory decision theory. Anesthesiology 1974;40:272–87.

147. Ward BW, Wu WC, Richter JE, et al. Long-term follow-up of symptomatic status of patients with non–cardiac chest pain: is diagnosis of esophageal etiology helpful? Am J Gastroenterol 1987;82:215–18.

148. Ockene IS, Shay MJ, Alpart JA, et al. Unexplained chest pain in patients with normal coronary arteriograms: a follow-up study of functional status. New Engl J Med 1980;303:1249–52.

149. Schofield PM. Follow-up study of morbidity in patients with angina pectoris and normal coronary angiograms and the value of investigation for esophageal dysfunction. Angiology 1990;41:286-96.

150. Swift GL, Alban-Davies N, McKirdy H, et al J. A long term clinical review of patients with esophageal pain. Quart J Med 1994;29:937–44.

151. Richter JE, Schan C, Burgard S, et al. Placebo controlled trial of omeprazole in the treatment of acid-related non-cardiac chest pain. Am J Gastroenterol 1992;87:1255A.

152. Achem SR, Koltz BE, MacMath T, et al. Treatment of acid related non-cardiac chest pain: a double blind placebo controlled trial of omeprazole vs placebo. Dig Dis Sci 1997;42:2138–45.

153. Orlando RC, Bozymski EM. Clinical and manometric effects of nitroglycerin in diffuse esophageal spasm. N Engl J Med 1973;289:23–25.

154. Kikendall JW, Mellow MH. Effect of sublingual nitroglycerine and long-acting nitrate preparations on esophageal motility. Gastroenterology 1980;79:703–706.

155. Hongo M, Traube M, McCallum RW. Comparison of effects of nifedipine, probantheline bromide, and the combination on esophageal motility. Dig Dis Sci 1984;29:300–304.

156. Blackwell JN, Dalton CB, Castell DO. Oral pirenzipine does not affect esophageal pressures in man. Dig Dis Sci 1986;31:230–35.

157. Bassotti G. Manometric evaluation of cimetropium bromide activity in patients with nutcracker esophagus. Scand J Gastroenterol 1988;23:1079–84.

158. Mellow MH. Effect of isosorbide and dydralazine in painful esophageal motility disorders. Gastroenterology 1982;83:364–70.

159. Richter JE, Dalton CB, Castell DO. Nifedipine a potent inhibitor of contractions in the esophageal body of the human esophagus. Gastroenterology 1985;9:549–54.

160. Alban-Davie H, Blackwell JB. Trial of nifedipine for prevention of esophageal spasm. Digestion 1987;36:81–83.

161. Cattau EL, Castell DO, Johnson DA, et al. Diltiazem therapy of symptoms associated with the nutcracker esophagus. Am J Gastroenterol 1991;86:272–76.

162. Frachtman RL, Botoman VA, Pope CE. A double-blind crossover trial of diltiazem shows no benefit in patients with dysphagia and/or chest pain of esophageal origin. Gastroenterology 1986;90:140A.

163. Miller LS, Parkman HP, Schiano TD, et al. Treatment of nonachalasia esophageal motor disorders with botulinum toxin injection. Dig Dis Sci 1996;41:2025–31.

164. Cannon RO III, Quyyumi A, Mincemoyer R, et al. Imipramine in patients with chest pain despite normal coronary angiograms. N Engl J Med 1996;330:1411–17.

165. Hegel MT, Abel GG, Etscheidt M, et al. Behavioral treatment of angina-like chest pain in patients with hyperventilation syndrome. J Behav Ther Exp Psychiatry 1989;20–31.

166. Klimes I, Mayou RA, Pearce MJ, et al. Psychological treatment of atypical non-cardiac chest pain: a controlled evaluation. Psychol Med 1990;20:605–11.

167. Potts SG, Lewin R, Fox KAA, et al. Group psychological treatment for chest pain with normal coronary arteries. Quart J Med 1999;92:81–86.

168. Kennedy T, Jones R. Gastro-oesophageal reflux symptoms in the community. Gut 1998;42(suppl 1):A64.

169. Talley NJ, Boyce P, Jones M. Identification of distinct upper and lower gastrointestinal symptom groupings in an urban population. Gut 1998;42:690–95.

170. Carlsson R, Dent J, Bolling-Sternevalde E, et al. The usefulness of a structured questionnaire in the assessment of symptomatic gastroesophageal reflux disease. Scand J Gastroenterol 1998;33:1023–29.

171. Spechler SJ, Souza RF, Rosenberg SJ, et al. Heartburn in patients with achalasia. Gut 1995;37:305–308.

172. Baldi F, Ferrarini F, Longanesi A, et al. Acid gastroesophageal reflux and symptom occurrence: analysis of some factors influencing their association. Dig Dis Sci 1989;34:1890–93.

173. Small PK, Loudon MA, Waldron B, et al. The importance of reflux symptoms in functional dyspepsia. Gut 1995;36:189–92.

174. Hennessy TPJ. Clinical features of reflux. In: Hennessy TPJ, Cuschieri A, Bennett JR, Editors. Reflux Oesophagitis. London:Butterworths;1989;123–41.

175. Singh S, Richter JE, Bradley LA, et al. The symptom index: differential usefulness in suspected acid–related complaints of heartburn and chest pain. Dig Dis Sci 1993;38:1402–1408.

176. Johnston BT, Lewis SA, Collins JSA, et al. Acid perception in gastro-oesophageal reflux disease is dependent on psychosocial factors. Scand J Gastroenterol 1995;30:1–5.

177. Tew S, Jamieson GG, Pilowsky I, et al. The illness behavior of patients with gastroesophageal reflux disease with and without endoscopic esophagitis. Diseases of the Oesophagus 1997;10:9–15.

178. Bradley LA, Richter JE, Pulliam TJ, et al. The relationship between stress and symptoms of gastroesophageal reflux: the influence of psychological factors. Am J Gastroenterol 1993;88:11–19.

179. A gallup survey on hearburn across America. Princeton, NJ: The Gallup Organization, 1988.

180. McDonald-Haile J, Bradley LA, Bailey MA, et al. Relaxation training reduces symptom reports and acid exposure in patients with gastroesophageal reflux disease. Gastroenterology 1994;107:61–69.

181. Lind T, Havelund T, Carlsson R et al. Heartburn without oesophagitis: efficacy of omeprazole therapy and features determining a therapeutic response. Scand J Gastroenterol 1997;32:974–79.

182. Watson RGP, Tham TCK, Johnston BT, et al. Double blind cross-over placebo controlled study of omeprazole in the treatment of patients with reflux symptoms and physiological levels of acid reflux–the "sensitive oesophagus." Gut 1997;40:587–90.

183. Trimble KC, Douglas S, Pryde A, et al. Clinical characteristics and natural history of symptomatic but not excess gastroesophageal reflux. Dig Dis Sci 1995;40: 1098–1104.

184. Davies HA, Evans KT, Butler F, et al. Diagnostic value of "bread–barium" swallow in patients with esophageal symptoms. Dig Dis Sci 1983;28:1094–1100.

185. Richter JE, Castell DO. Diffuse esophageal spasm: a reappraisal. Ann Intern Med 1984;100:242–45.

186. Deschner WK, Maher KA, Cattau El Jr, et al. Manometric responses to balloon distention in patients with nonobstructive dysphagia. Gastroenterology 1989;97: 1181–85.

187. Jacob P, Kahrilas PJ, Vanagunas A. Peristaltic dysfunction associated with nonobstructive dysphagia in reflux disease. Dig Dis Sci 1990;35:939–42.

188. Triadafilopoulos G. Nonobstructive dysphagia in reflux esophagitis. Am J Gastroenterol 1989;84:614–18.

189. Howard PJ, Maher L, Pryde A, et al. Esophageal motor patterns during episodes of dysphagia for solids. J Gastrointest Motil 1991;3:123–30.

190. Clouse RE, McCord GS, Lustman PJ, et al. Clinical correlates of abnormal sensitivity to intraesophageal balloon distention. Dig Dis Sci 1991;36:1040–45.

191. Faulkner WB, Rudenbaugh FH, O'Neill Jr. Influence of the emotions on esophageal function: comparison of esophagoscopic and roentgenologic findings. Radiology 1942;37:443–47.

192. Wolf S. Almy RP. Experimental observation on cardiospasm in man. Gastroenterology 1949;13:401–402.

193. Gorelick AB, Koshy SS, Hooper FG, et al. Differential effects of amitriptyline on perception of somatic and visceral stimulation in healthy humans. Am J Physiol 1998;275:G460–66.

194. Peghini PI, Katz PO, Castell DO. Imipramine decreases oesophageal pain perception in human male volunteers. Gut 1998;42:807–13.

195. Marshall JB. Dysphagia: diagnostic pitfalls and how to avoid them. Postgrad Med 1989;85:243–60.

196. Winters C, Artnak EJ, Banjamin SB, et al. Esophageal bougienage in symptomatic patients with the nutcracker esophagus. JAMA 1984;252:363–66.

197. Ebert EC, Ouyang A, Wright SH, et al. Pneumatic dilatation in patients with symptomatic diffuse esophageal spasm and lower esophageal sphincter dysfunction. Dig Dis Sci 1983;28:481–85.

198. Aliperti GA, Clouse RE. Incomplete lower esophageal sphincter (LES) relaxation in subjects without aperistalsis: prevalence and clinical outcome. Am J Gastroenterol 1991;86;609–14.

Chapter 6

B. Functional Gastroduodenal Disorders

Nicholas J. Talley, Chair,
Vincenzo Stanghellini, Co-Chair, *with*
Robert C. Heading,
Kenneth L. Koch,
Juan-R. Malagelada,
and Guido N. J. Tytgat

Introduction

An important group of patients with functional gastrointestinal disorders have chronic symptoms that, somewhat arbitrarily, are attributed to the gastroduodenal region (Tables 1 and 2). This includes patients who complain of epigastric or upper abdominal pain or discomfort in the absence of peptic ulceration or other organic upper gastrointestinal diseases, patients who complain of excess belching and are air swallowers, and patients who have recurrent unexplained vomiting. Based on the consensus opinion of an international panel of clinical investigators who reviewed the available evidence, a classification of the functional gastroduodenal disorders into functional dyspepsia (category B1), aerophagia (category B2) and functional vomiting (category B3) is recommended. In addition, symptom subgroups for functional dyspepsia are proposed, namely ulcer-like dyspepsia (B1a) and dysmotility-like dyspepsia (B1b), based on patient ranking of the most bothersome complaint. The evidence in support of this classification is summarized here, and an approach to management reviewed.

Table 1. Functional Gastrointestinal Disorders

A. Esophageal Disorders

A1. Globus
A2. Rumination syndrome
A3. Functional Chest Pain of Presumed Esophageal Origin

A4. Functional Heartburn
A5. Functional Dysphagia
A6. Unspecified Functional Esophageal Disorder

B. Gastroduodenal Disorders

B1. Functional Dyspepsia
B1a. Ulcer-like Dyspepsia
B1b. Dysmotility-like Dyspepsia
B1c. Unspecified (nonspecific) Dyspepsia

B2. Aerophagia
B3. Functional Vomiting

C. Bowel Disorders

C1. Irritable Bowel Syndrome
C2. Functional Abdominal Bloating
C3. Functional Constipation

C4. Functional Diarrhea
C5. Unspecified Functional Bowel Disorder

D. Functional Abdominal Pain

D1. Functional Abdominal Pain Syndrome
D2. Unspecified Functional Abdominal Pain

E. Functional Disorders of the Biliary Tract and the Pancreas

E1. Gallbladder Dysfunction
E2. Sphincter of Oddi Dysfunction

F. Anorectal Disorders

F1. Functional Fecal Incontinence
F2. Functional Anorectal Pain
F2a. Levator Ani Syndrome
F2b. Proctalgia Fugax
F3. Pelvic Floor Dyssynergia

G. Functional Pediatric Disorders

G1. Vomiting
G1a. Infant regurgitation
G1b. Infant rumination syndrome
G1c. Cyclic vomiting syndrome
G2. Abdominal pain
G2a. Functional dyspepsia
G2a1. Ulcer-like dyspepsia
G2a2. Dysmotility-like dyspepsia
G2a3. Unspecified (nonspecific) dyspepsia

G2b. Irritable bowel syndrome
G2c. Functional abdominal pain
G2d. Abdominal migraine
G2e. Aerophagia
G3. Functional diarrhea
G4. Disorders of defecation
G4a. Infant dyschezia
G4b. Functional constipation
G4c. Functional fecal retention
G4d. Functional non-retentive fecal soiling

B1. Functional Dyspepsia

— Definition

It is self evident that no definition of functional dyspepsia can be given without first considering what the term dyspepsia means.

Definition of Dyspepsia

Many different sets of symptoms have been used synonymously with the term dyspepsia, which has caused enormous confusion. The term dyspepsia is not recognized by most patients and historically physicians have interpreted the meaning of dyspepsia very variably [1–5]. Some authorities have restricted dyspepsia to refer to meal related symptoms [6–8], but this is inadequate as conditions such as peptic ulcer disease, which is considered to be a classical cause of dyspepsia, do not cause symptoms that are confined to the pre- or post-prandial period [9–12]. Others have suggested that the symptoms of dyspepsia should be believed to emanate from the proximal gut [3,7], but such beliefs are open to substantial observer bias and are impossible to measure.

Here, the following definition is recommended. *Dyspepsia refers to pain or discomfort centered in the upper abdomen.*

"Centered" refers to pain or discomfort mainly in or around the midline. Pain in the right or left hypochondrium is not considered to be representative of dyspepsia. "Discomfort" refers to a subjective, negative feeling that the patient does not interpret as pain and which if fully assessed can include a number of specific symptoms. "Discomfort" may be characterized by or associated with upper abdominal fullness, early satiety, bloating, belching, nausea, retching, or vomiting; these symptoms typically are accompanied by a component of upper abdominal distress (Table 2). Unless specifically asked about, some of these symptoms may or may not be labeled as pain by the patient, which may depend on cultural factors and possibly education level.

There remains disagreement in the literature over whether discomfort represents part of the spectrum of pain or not. For example, itching and skin pain are distinct symptoms; while the sensations are transmitted via the same pain pathways, the processing depends on the stimulus thresholds. Hence, these are distinct yet interrelated symptoms. In the English language, pain and discomfort are not clearly distinguished; discomfort is considered to be a part of mild pain, although pain does not have to be present [13]. Thus, in the United Kingdom, Australia, and the United States, many subjects who have mild pain may call this discomfort rather than pain unless specifically asked, but in parts of Europe the terms pain and discomfort are commonly clearly distinguished by patients

Table 2. The Spectrum of Dyspepsia Symptoms and Recommended
Definitions

Symptom	Definition
Pain centered in the upper abdomen	Pain refers to a subjective, unpleasant sensation; some patients may feel that tissue damage is occurring. Other symptoms may be extremely bothersome without being interpreted by the patient as pain. By questioning the patient, pain should be distinguished from discomfort.
Discomfort centered in the upper abdomen	A subjective, unpleasant sensation or feeling that is not interpreted as pain according to the patient and which, if fully assessed, can include any of the symptoms below.
Early satiety	A feeling that the stomach is overfilled soon after starting to eat, out of proportion to the size of the meal being eaten, so that the meal cannot be finished.
Fullness	An unpleasant sensation like the persistence of food in the stomach; this may or may not occur post-prandially (slow digestion).
Bloating in the upper abdomen	A tightness located in the upper abdomen; it should be distinguished from visible abdominal distension.
Nausea	Queasiness or sick sensation; a feeling of the need to vomit.
Retching	Heaving as if to vomit but no gastric contents are forced up.

[14,15]. This Working Team concluded that pain and discomfort should be considered separate concepts at this time; hence, patients may have both painful and nonpainful sensations (discomfort).

Duration is not specified as part of the definition because patients may present immediately following the onset of symptoms, or may wait months or years before being evaluated. In research studies, investigators may opt for a specified duration of symptoms to define dyspepsia (e.g., two weeks, four weeks or 12 weeks), and this should depend on the study setting and objectives so as to improve homogeneity of the patients being studied. The painful or uncomfortable symptoms may be intermittent or continuous, and may or may not be related to meals.

"Heartburn" has been defined by a consensus committee on gastroesophageal reflux disease [16]. Burning pain confined to the epigastrium is not considered to be heartburn. Heartburn (and acid regurgitation) have often been included as sufficient on their own to define dyspepsia [4]. However, there is growing consensus based on 24-hour esophageal pH testing that patients with a history of typical heartburn, when this is a dominant complaint, almost invariably have gastroesophageal reflux disease (GERD) [16,17] and should be distinguished from patients with dyspepsia. There is reasonably good evidence that predominant heartburn is highly specific for GERD and hence the positive predictive value for heartburn is high in countries where GERD is a common disease [10,17]. How many patients with burning epigastric pain alone have GERD is unknown. Retrosternal pain suggestive of esophageal disease, or of a type embraced by the term "non-cardiac chest pain," should also be excluded from dyspepsia.

Uninvestigated vs. Investigated Dyspepsia

It is important to distinguish the patient who presents with dyspepsia that has not been investigated (uninvestigated dyspepsia) from patients with a diagnostic label after investigation, with an identified causal abnormality (such as peptic ulcer or GERD), or with functional dyspepsia (fig. 1).

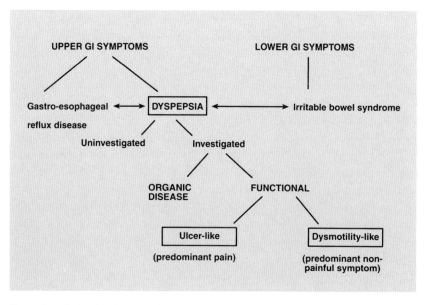

Figure 1. Relationship between dyspepsia and functional dyspepsia. GI = gastrointestinal

Causes of Dyspepsia

From an etiological viewpoint, patients with dyspepsia can be subdivided into three main categories:

(1) Those with an identified cause for the symptoms where if the disease improves or is eliminated, symptoms also improve or resolve (e.g., chronic peptic ulcer disease, gastroesophageal reflux disease with or without esophagitis, malignancy, pancreatico-biliary disease, and medications);
(2) Those with an identifiable pathophysiological or microbiologic abnormality of uncertain clinical relevance (e.g., *Helicobacter pylori* gastritis, histologic duodenitis, gallstones, visceral hypersensitivity, gastroduodenal dysmotility); and
(3) Those with no identifiable explanation for the symptoms.

It is those patients who have no definite structural or biochemical explanation for their symptoms (i.e., categories 2 and 3) who are considered to have functional dyspepsia. While many consider this term to imply that a disturbance of function, or an awareness of disturbed function, is present in the upper abdomen, other mechanisms may be operating, or no disturbances may be documented with current technology. For this reason, some authors prefer to use the term *essential* or *idiopathic* dyspepsia. The term *"non-ulcer dyspepsia"* remains in popular usage but is not recommended here because some patients with functional dyspepsia will have symptoms typical of ulcer disease while others will have symptoms not at all like an ulcer, and peptic ulcer is not the only disease of exclusion in patients with dyspepsia.

— Epidemiology

The prevalence of uninvestigated dyspepsia in the general population is now well documented. If predominant heartburn is not included in dyspepsia, then approximately 25% of people in the community each year report chronic or recurrent pain or discomfort in the epigastrium or upper abdomen [18–22]. This is reasonably consistent around the world [23]. Only a minority of the subjects have a history of chronic peptic ulcer disease, and hence it is reasonable to assume that the majority of these individuals have a diagnosis of functional dyspepsia [23–26]. The prevalence of dyspepsia is lower in the elderly and is slightly higher in men than in women overall.

The incidence of dyspepsia is substantially lower than the prevalence estimates. Based on prospective studies of subjects who report dyspepsia for the first time, the incidence is approximately 1% per year [21,27]. Those who appear to develop symptoms are balanced by a similar number of people who lose their symptoms over time, a fact which accounts for the prevalence being stable from year to year.

The majority with a diagnosis of functional dyspepsia continue to be symptomatic over the long term despite periods of remission [28]. Approximately one third of patients lose their symptoms spontaneously [21,27]. In patients with a diagnosis of functional dyspepsia, the risk of developing peptic ulcer disease appears to be no different from the rate in the background asymptomatic population [28,29].

Only some dyspepsia sufferers present for medical care; in the United States and United Kingdom, only one in four consult [18,19] but the rate is higher in Australia [30]. Pain severity and anxiety (including fear of serious disease) appear to be factors associated with consulting behavior [30].

— Diagnostic Criteria

At least 12 weeks, which need not be consecutive, in the preceding 12 months of:

(1) Persistent or recurrent dyspepsia (pain or discomfort centered in the upper abdomen);

(2) No evidence of organic disease (including at upper endoscopy) that is likely to explain the symptoms; _and_

(3) No evidence that dyspepsia is exclusively relieved by defecation or associated with the onset of a change in stool frequency or stool form (i.e., not irritable bowel).

Rationale for Dyspepsia Criteria

Symptom patterns alone are unable to adequately discriminate organic from functional dyspepsia [9,30]. Patients need to be investigated to rule out relevant organic disease, and there should be no evidence of structural or metabolic abnormalities that definitely explain the symptoms. Functional dyspepsia therefore remains a diagnosis of exclusion. There is agreement that symptoms should run a chronic course before a patient is labeled as having functional dyspepsia. It is therefore recommended that functional dyspepsia be defined as presented above in the Diagnostic Criteria.

The committee agreed that functional dyspepsia is a chronic condition.

Table 3. Investigation of Functional Dyspepsia in the Research Setting

Priority	Test
Essential	Upper endoscopy during a symptomatic period off ulcer healing medications
Recommended*	H. pylori testing Psychometric testing
Not routine	Ultrasonography Gastric emptying study Electrogastrogram Gastroduodenal manometry Gastroduodenal sensory testing 24-hour esophageal pH testing Autonomic function testing Gastrointestinal hormone assays Gastric acid secretion

*May affect study outcome depending on the research question.

However, the 12 week criterion is purely arbitrary and is set as a standard for re-search to reduce the probability of a misclassification error. Clinicians may choose a shorter period depending on the clinical setting. "Organic" includes metabolic and systemic disease. The minimum diagnostic work-up required to sustain a diagnosis of functional dyspepsia in the research context is a careful history and physical examination, and an upper endoscopy during a symptomatic period. In the research setting, additional investigations depend on the research question (Table 3).

Patients with a past history of documented chronic peptic ulcer disease should generally not be classified as having functional dyspepsia because even in the absence of an ulcer crater, symptoms conceivably are related to the underlying cause of the ulcer itself. However, patients who have had ulcer disease cured by H. pylori eradication may remain symptomatic; a subset of these patients probably have functional dyspepsia, although this remains poorly documented.

— **Diagnostic Criteria:** Functional Dyspepsia Subgroups

B1a. Ulcer-like Dyspepsia
Pain centered in the upper abdomen is the predominant (most bothersome) symptom.

B1b. Dysmotility-like dyspepsia
An unpleasant or troublesome nonpainful sensation (dis-

comfort) centered in the upper abdomen is the predominant symptom; this sensation may be characterized by or associated with upper abdominal fullness, early satiety, bloating, or nausea.

B1c. Unspecified (Nonspecific) Dyspepsia
Symptomatic patients whose symptoms do not fulfill the criteria for ulcer-like or dysmotility-like dyspepsia.

Development and Rationale for Functional Dyspepsia Subgroups

The concept of subdividing dyspepsia into subsets based on distinctive symptom patterns continues to be controversial but has become entrenched in clinical practice [32]. Four working teams have independently proposed that functional dyspepsia be subdivided into symptom subgroups [4,5,33,34], but the definitions of the subgroups have not been uniform [35]. In contrast to other groups, the previous Rome Criteria proposed *not* to include the reflux-like subgroup in functional dyspepsia as these patients have GERD until proven otherwise [35].

Two main hypothetical subgroups were identified in all the reports: "ulcer-like" and "dysmotility-like" dyspepsia. The former has usually been characterized by several aspects of pain, the latter by distinct symptoms different from pain and suggestive of impaired gastroduodenal motility. Two working team reports introduced numeric limitations by requiring the concomitant presence of at least two [34] or three [35] specific symptoms to be included in a subgroup, thus introducing the concept of "symptom clusters." All these definitions of dyspepsia subgroups were totally arbitrary but were proposed in order to direct future research so that more homogeneous populations could be identified and rational treatment prescribed.

Epidemiologic, pathophysiologic, and clinical studies over the last decade however have demonstrated that the symptom cluster classification is probably of no clinical utility [10,18,36,37]. Nevertheless, the concept of functional dyspepsia subgroups has gained popularity among doctors [33].

The dyspepsia subgroup classification proposed here is therefore based not on symptom clusters but on the predominant (or most bothersome) single symptom identified by the patient as defined above.

The classification in the Diagnostic Criteria has the advantage of substantially reducing overlap and the number of patients who cannot be classified. Patients usually are able to describe their most bothersome complaint even when they have multiple complaints [15]. It may be that patients with predominant nausea, retching, and vomiting comprise a distinct subset within dysmotility-like dyspepsia [15], as do patients with early satiety [38], but this needs to be prospectively evaluated. The subgroup classification does not mean that those with ulcer-like functional dyspepsia have or have had an ulcer, or indeed that dysmotility-like functional dyspepsia identifies a motor disorder [10].

Recent studies support the existence of such subgroups, as defined by the presence of a predominant (or most bothersome) single symptom identified by the patient. Stanghellini et al. showed that female gender, postprandial fullness severe enough to influence usual activities and vomiting severe enough to change usual activities were independently associated with delayed gastric emptying. On the other hand, neither the presence nor absence of symptoms or clusters of symptoms, nor the global symptom score were associated with delayed gastric emptying in functional dyspepsia [14]. This suggests that an approach based on identifying the predominant complaint may be of value [14]. Tack et al. have shown that impaired gastric accommodation is specifically linked to the symptom "early satiety" in functional dyspepsia [38].

The response to proton pump inhibitor therapy was predicted by subgrouping based on the most bothersome symptom; those with epigastric pain but not discomfort had a statistically significant response to omeprazole over placebo [15]. On the other hand, symptom subgroups have not been of predictive value for treatment outcome in large trials with the prokinetic cisapride, but these were uncontrolled studies, and the approach of using the predominant complaint to identify subgroups was not tested [39]. A trial with cisapride or nizatidine versus placebo for two weeks surprisingly failed to document any benefit of either treatment, and the predominant complaint did not identify treatment responders [40]. The subgroups, therefore, represent a working hypothesis but must be subjected to further careful testing before being widely accepted.

— Overlap Syndromes

Heartburn

Patients in whom heartburn (i.e., burning retrosternal pain) is the predominant symptom are excluded from dyspepsia (and therefore functional dyspepsia) by definition; such patients almost invariably have GERD. However, patients with functional dyspepsia very often have heartburn as an additional symptom subordinate to their abdominal pain or discomfort [18,22]. In many of these the heartburn is so minor or infrequent that it cannot be considered abnormal (indeed, physiological acid reflux is a normal event). A small minority of others with frequent heartburn and dyspepsia, if fully investigated, are found to have pathological acid reflux on ambulatory esophageal pH monitoring; they have GERD and their inclusion in functional dyspepsia is then recognized to be mistaken [41]. Another group of patients with functional dyspepsia and frequent heartburn have a normal 24-hour esophageal pH study and may or may not have GERD [41]; some of these will have a positive symptom index or evidence of microscopic esophageal damage (e.g., on electron microscopy) if investigated [42].

Irritable Bowel Syndrome

Dyspepsia occurs commonly in patients with symptoms otherwise compatible with irritable bowel syndrome (IBS). Despite this overlap, approximately 70% of patients with functional dyspepsia do not have major bowel symptoms [10], and dyspepsia is likely to be a distinct syndrome based on factor analysis studies [43]. However, it is possible for individuals to have both functional dyspepsia and IBS, or have upper abdominal pain or discomfort exclusively related to IBS. Therefore, if upper abdominal pain or discomfort is exclusively relieved by defecation and/or associated with a change in bowel pattern, irritable bowel syndrome is the diagnosis by definition. On the other hand, if there is pain or discomfort in the upper abdomen that is unrelated to bowel pattern and there is other pain or discomfort that is related to bowel pattern, then functional dyspepsia and IBS can be considered to coexist.

— Rationale for Changes in Diagnostic Criteria

The definition of functional dyspepsia is essentially unchanged. It was, however, not felt to be useful to restrict the definition arbitrarily to a set number of days over a three-month period in research or practice, and thus this part was deleted. While patients with predominant heartburn are excluded from the functional dyspepsia category, patients with coexistent IBS are not in the new classification based on the evidence described above.

The definitions of the dyspepsia subgroups have been altered based on new clinical, epidemiological and therapeutic evidence that the original concept of symptom "clusters" was of little or no value [10,18,36,37]. Recent data suggest that identification of the predominant symptom may identify true subgroups with different underlying pathophysiological mechanisms and response to treatment [14,15,38,44,45] although this remains to be firmly established.

— Clinical Evaluation

The management of the patient with uninvestigated dyspepsia should not be confused with the approach to the patient with functional dyspepsia.

Uninvestigated Dyspepsia

The current best first test for excluding structural causes of dyspepsia is upper endoscopy. However, there is growing consensus that *H. pylori* testing is a useful approach for triaging new patients without alarm features [36, 46,47]. Among those with uninvestigated upper gastrointestinal tract symptoms who are *H. pylori* positive, a substantial number will have peptic ulcer disease [23,36,48]. Those who are *H. pylori* negative (and those who are not taking NSAIDs) are unlikely to have peptic ulcer disease and usually can be safely labeled provisionally as having functional dyspepsia if there are no alarm features [23]. Hence, while symptoms are not sensitive or specific enough to help discriminate functional from structural disease, noninvasive *H. pylori* testing represents an advance. Endoscopy can now generally be reserved for patients who present with symptoms for the first time in older age or who have alarm features such as weight loss, vomiting, progressive dysphagia, or bleeding, any of which strongly suggests structural disease may be present. The test and treat strategy for *H. pylori* for younger patients without alarm features is also supported by decision analyses [49,50] and has been endorsed by the American Gastroenterological Association [23], a European ad hoc consensus meeting [47], an Asian Pacific consensus meeting [46], and a working team for the World Congresses of Gastroenterology [51]. In case of symptomatic failure after *H. pylori* eradication or failure of empiric therapy to relieve symptoms in *H. pylori* negative patients, endoscopy is generally recommended.

Functional Dyspepsia

Performance of an upper endoscopy during a symptomatic period off acid suppressant therapy is essential to appropriately identify functional dyspepsia by excluding other important structural diseases. A barium meal study is less sensitive and specific than upper endoscopy and hence is not generally recommended [23]. Ultrasonography is not recommended as a routine clinical test, as in outpatient studies most patients have no detectable abnormality in the absence of symptoms or biochemical tests suggestive of biliary tract or pancreatic disease [26,52,53]. Barium x-ray study of the small bowel is useful if there is any suspicion of mechanical obstruction.

A gastric emptying study (e.g., scintigraphy) is not currently recommended as a routine clinical test because the results uncommonly alter management. Indeed, there is no convincing evidence that prokinetics are more efficacious in those patients with functional dyspepsia who have delayed versus those with normal gastric emptying [54], although conflicting results have been published [55]. In patients with resistant symptoms, a gastric emptying test may be considered. If gastroparesis is found on a gastric emptying study, then specific causes of gastroparesis need to be excluded, and in particular, intestinal obstruction, diabetes mellitus, connective tissue disease, and drugs. Gastroduodenal manometry and electrogastrography (EGG) provide objective evidence of neuromuscular dysfunction in selected patients, but their role in clinical medicine is evolving at this time.

Patients with chronic or severe symptoms may benefit from an appropriate psychiatric history being taken to exclude depression, somatoform disorder and an eating disorder.

— Physiologic Features

Pathophysiologic abnormalities potentially associated with functional dyspepsia symptoms are gastric acid hypersecretion, *H. pylori* infection, gastrointestinal dysmotility, and visceral hypersensitivity (fig. 2). Linking symptoms to pathophysiology remains problematical in part because most of the studies investigating gastric acid secretion and *H. pylori* status have been carried out on patients complaining mainly of ulcer-like dyspepsia, and conversely, patients with dysmotility-like dyspepsia have been more frequently included in studies investigating gastroduodenal motility.

Gastric Acid

Patients with functional dyspepsia have, on average, normal basal and pentagastrin stimulated gastric acid secretion regardless of their *H. pylori* status [56–58]. However, *H. pylori* positive patients with functional dyspepsia may have gastrin-releasing peptide (GRP)-stimulated acid secretion responses that are lower than *H. pylori* duodenal ulcer patients, but higher than *H. pylori* negative healthy controls [59]. These results remain to be replicated but suggest that some subjects with functional dyspepsia and *H. pylori* have acid dysregulation. On the other hand, *H. pylori* status has not been linked to symptom response to proton pump inhibitor therapy [15]

Few studies have investigated whether or not instilling gastric acid contents

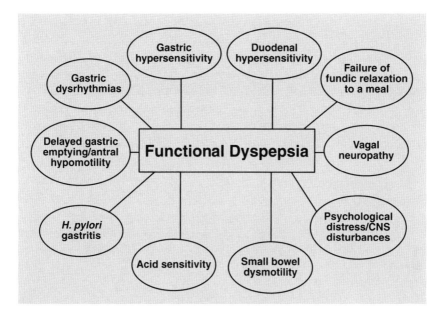

Figure 2. Putative mechanisms linked to functional dyspepsia.

onto the mucosa will induce symptoms in functional dyspepsia. Intragastric infusion of acid failed to elicit dyspeptic symptoms in patients with functional dyspepsia reliably [60,61], but interestingly, induced a perception of symptoms in a selected group of patients with ulcer-like dyspepsia [62]. Acid perfusion results may result in mechanical hyperalgesia in the stomach [63].

Helicobacter Pylori *and Chronic Gastritis*

Theoretically, *H. pylori* gastritis could sensitize visceral afferents both in the periphery and at the spinal level; interleukin 8 for example is overexpressed in gastritis and has a stimulatory effect on enteric neurone expression of sensory neuropeptides [37]. However, down-regulation of central arousal systems and descending pain inhibitory pathways may account for the lack of symptoms in most people infected.

Seroconversion from negative to positive has been reported to be associated with the development of dyspepsia [64,65]. No specific symptom profile has been identified that can help to distinguish *H. pylori* positive from *H. pylori* negative patients [37].

Monitoring the effects of *H. pylori* eradication and of the subsequent changes in mucosal inflammation should provide the most convincing evidence for or against a link with functional dyspepsia. Past studies were flawed by important limitations and, therefore, are difficult to interpret [66]. The most recent large randomized double-blind controlled trials with a follow-up period of one year have been weakly positive [67–69] or negative [70–73]. Symptom improvement may be observed in 20% of patients, at the most, over placebo after eradication therapy. A majority of the patients cured of the infection remain symptomatic, and medical therapy is frequently reintroduced.

Duodenitis

Erosive duodenitis very likely represents part of the spectrum of duodenal ulcer disease and is strongly associated with *H. pylori* infection [74]. It is uncertain whether nonerosive duodenitis alone causes symptoms. Intraduodenal infusion of acid invariably reproduced typical epigastric pain in patients with duodenal ulcer or duodenitis, but not in dyspeptic patients with a normal duodenal mucosa, but this was based on uncontrolled observations [75]. Moreover, duodenitis may occur occasionally in asymptomatic, otherwise healthy persons [24,25].

Gastrointestinal Dysmotility

Gastrointestinal dysmotility is complex, characterized by myoelectrical and smooth muscle activity, gut wall movements, intraluminal phasic and tonic pressure changes, and movement of intraluminal contents. No single technique is available to measure all these events simultaneously, and we have only fragmentary information in both health and disease.

Inability of the meal to stimulate antral contractions can be found in both functional and structural dyspepsia [76]. Studies of upper gastrointestinal tract motility in patients with functional dyspepsia have demonstrated delayed gastric emptying and antral hypomotility following meals in up to 50% of patients [14]. In healthy controls, postprandial fullness was found to be directly related to gastric emptying times of the aqueous phase (more full when gastric emptying was slower), and postprandial hunger was inversely related to gastric emptying rates of oil (less hungry when more oil was emptied into the small bowel); in this experimental setting, cisapride accelerated gastric emptying of both oily and aqueous meal components and concomitantly decreased fullness and increased hunger [77].

Measurement of gastric emptying provides only a broad and indirect indication of the complex series of motor events necessary to empty the stomach of its contents. Recent studies have demonstrated an abnormal distribution of intragastric contents in functional dyspepsia characterized by a rapid emptying from the proximal stomach because of impaired accommodation with a sudden and prolonged distension of the antrum [78,79]. These studies were carried out exclusively on patients with dysmotility-like dyspepsia, and whether this regional motor dysfunction can also be evidenced in patients complaining of epigastric pain is unknown.

The results of the studies investigating scintigraphic gastric emptying in *H. pylori* positive and negative dyspeptic patients have generally failed to detect any difference between the two groups. Moreover, *H. pylori* eradication does not influence gastric emptying [80]. A link between *H. pylori* and manometric abnormalities is also unconvincing [81]. Testoni et al. manometrically recorded fasting and postprandial motility of the gastric antrum and proximal small bowel in 38 patients with functional dyspepsia [82]. *H. pylori* infected patients had decreased gastric phase IIIs of the migrating motor complex compared to *H. pylori* negative patients. Pieramico et al. failed to detect significant differences between *H. pylori* positive and negative patients, but reported normalization of interdigestive motility after eradication [83]. Most studies, however, have failed to confirm a link between *H. pylori* and manometric abnormalities [81].

There is also evidence that the duodenal bulb is hypersensitive to acid in functional dyspepsia, impairing acid clearance and inducing symptoms. Sampson et al. infused acid and saline intraduodenally; acid infusion significantly reduced duodenal pressure waves and reproducibly induced nausea in patients with functional dyspepsia, but not controls [84].

Intestinal dysmotility is uncommon in functional dyspepsia in the absence of the irritable bowel syndrome, intestinal pseudo-obstruction, or extraintestinal diseases such as diabetes mellitus and autonomic neuropathies, even when ambulatory 24-hour intestinal manometry is used [85]. The major exception may be very severe cases with vomiting and weight loss [6].

Reflex inhibition of upper-gut motility triggered by nutrients reaching the ileum (the "ileal brake") may be disturbed in some patients [86]. Duodenogastric reflux is probably not an important mechanism in the induction of symptoms in unoperated patients [87,88].

Perception Threshold

The gut wall contains three kinds of neural receptors: chemoreceptors, in the mucosa, which respond to chemical stimuli; mechanoreceptors, in the smooth muscle layer, which respond to stretch or compression; and nociceptors, in all layers, and the most numerous receptors, which are commonly silent, but can be "recruited" by any stimulus strong enough to induce pain

[89]. The stomach and duodenum are dually innervated by vagal and spinal afferents.

A subset of dyspeptic patients have gastric [90–92] or duodenal [93–96] hypersensitivity to balloon distension. Visceral hypersensitivity is not influenced by age or gender. There is some evidence that patients with functional dyspepsia have hypersensitivity to esophageal and rectal distension [97]. In contrast, patients with functional dyspepsia do not have a lower somatic pain threshold than do healthy volunteers [91].

The mechanisms that explain visceral hypersensitivity in functional dyspepsia remain poorly understood. *H. pylori* infection has not been linked to hypersensitivity in the stomach [92] or duodenum [93]. Proximal stomach compliance is not altered [92]. The sensations induced by changes in intragastric pressure and volumes have been shown to be independent of gastric emptying times, although coexisting motor abnormalities theoretically may favor perception of symptoms. Duodenal lipid infusion can induce fullness and nausea and can decrease pressures at which gastric sensations were reported [98].

Autonomic Dysfunction

Vagal afferents on activation may enhance or inhibit visceral sensations mediated by spinal afferents. Feinle et al. have shown that loxiglumide (a CCK-A receptor antagonist) reduced meal-like sensations induced by gastric distension with intraduodenal lipid infusion, presumably because CCK released from enterochromaffine cells was blocked from acting on CCK-A receptors on mucosal vagal afferents [98].

Vagal efferent dysfunction occurs in a subset of patients with functional dyspepsia [96,99]. Moreover, vagal efferent function (as measured by the pancreatic polypeptide response to insulin hypoglycemia) has been correlated with small intestinal hypersensitivity in functional dyspepsia [96].

A vagal neuropathy could induce disturbed motor function due to loss of efferent neural control. Moreover, vagal denervation hypersensitivity could induce an exaggerated response to afferent signals.

Gastric Accommodation

Most studies suggest that in dyspepsia gastric accommodation is normal during fasting but is impaired in response to a meal because there is failure of proximal relaxation [100,101]. This could be due to vagal neuropathy; similar findings occur in vagotomized patients [78]. The increased wall tension could conceivably increase visceral afferent traffic. It is also possible that increased "squeezing" in the proximal stomach tends to lead to normal or near normal liquid gastric emptying in many patients with functional dyspepsia, who might otherwise have an abnormality of both solids and liquids. Other studies [38] suggest that reduced proximal relaxation is associated with symptoms of early satiety and weight loss, and these symptoms are relieved by agents (e.g., the $5HT_1$ agonists, sumatriptan, buspirone) that specifically increase fundal compliance. Future studies may target the treatment of functional dyspepsia symptoms based on the need to increase gastric emptying (with prokinetics) and/or increased fundal compliance.

Gastric Myoelectric Activity

Gastric dysrhythmias are myoelectrical abnormalities originating in the corpus or antrum. The normal gastric pacesetter potential frequency ranges from 2.4–3.6 cpm, i.e., approximately 3 cpm. During gastric dysrhythmias the normal rhythm is suppressed and tachygastrias (3.6–9.9 cpm) or bradygastrias (flatline pattern or 1.0–2.4 cpm) may appear to be present [102].

Gastric dysrhythmias have been recorded in some patients with functional dyspepsia symptoms [102,103]. However, the results are inconstant and often minor [104]. While some studies suggest that myoelectrical abnormalities can precede the onset of nausea and epigastric discomfort, the exact prevalence of these abnormalities remains obscure, and measurement error with commercially available electrography programs continues to be a problem.

Hormonal Changes

Abnormalities of circulating hormones have not been established to be important in functional dyspepsia. A significant reduction of circulating motilin levels and of the number of motilin peaks has been observed in a group of dyspeptic patients who exhibited abnormal antroduodenal motility [105]. Cholecystokinin (CCK) may induce satiety by acting both in the central nervous system and peripherally in the gut, via afferent vagal fibers [106], but CCK at physiological concentrations has a similar action on gastric emptying in functional dyspepsia and health [107]. Other experimental data suggest that progesterone, estradiol, and prolactin affect smooth muscle contractility and delay transit times [108]. Basal but not postprandial levels of circulating gastrin have been found to be slightly higher in patients with functional dyspepsia compared to healthy controls, but *H. pylori* status was not assessed [109]. Endogenous opiates might also contribute to motility derangements in functional dyspepsia

[110]. The prolactin response to buspirone, which is an indirect measure of central 5-hydroxytryptamine sensitivity, has been reported to be increased in patients with functional dyspepsia [111]. These data remain fragmentary, however, and well-defined subgroups have not been evaluated.

Diet and Environmental Factors

Food intolerance has been reported to occur more commonly in patients with functional dyspepsia than in control subjects, but a relationship between diet and functional dyspepsia remains to be established by carefully conducted, double-blind, food challenge studies [112,113]. Eating patterns appear not to be affected [114]. Smoking and alcohol are probably not causally linked with functional dyspepsia [115].

Psychologic Features

Acute stress can alter gastrointestinal function and induce symptoms in healthy subjects. Wolf was the first to observe that a marked decrease of gastric contractility preceded the onset of nausea in response to centrally acting stressful stimuli [116], and others subsequently confirmed these observations [117]. However, it is uncertain whether chronic dyspeptic symptoms can be explained by such a mechanism. Indeed, in one small study, patients with functional dyspepsia with or without antral hypomotility were shown to have normal autonomic and humoral responses to experimental stress [118], although other data suggest that the autonomic reaction to experimental stress was suppressed in functional dyspepsia [119].

The role of life event stress in the pathogenesis of functional dyspepsia remains controversial. Studies that compared the frequency of stressful major life events (e.g., bereavement or divorce) preceding diagnosis found that patients with functional dyspepsia did not differ from control subjects [120,121]. The interpretation of these findings has been limited, however, because of possible recall bias and the failure of these studies to take into account individual differences in the interpretation of events as stressful. Thus, a study of Chinese subjects in Hong Kong using the Life Experiences Survey showed that dyspeptic patients were distinguished from normal control subjects by the perceived magnitude of negative life events [122]. In other case-control studies, the more sophisticated Life Events and Difficulties Schedule has been used, where independent assessment is made of the severity of acute and chronic stressors, and their impact; these researchers found that events that were highly threatening or led to frustration of goals were associated with functional dyspepsia [123,124]. However, these types of patient-based studies are potentially subject to selection bias, as psychosocially disturbed patients may be more likely to present to tertiary referral centers where such research is being conducted.

Sociodemographic factors may be linked to functional dyspepsia. In a study of socioeconomic and marital status, childhood environment, family structure, and family migration, there were no major differences between patients and control subjects except for an increased risk of functional dyspepsia with social status incongruity; those who lived in a community where the other residents were of a higher occupational status were twice as likely to have functional dyspepsia [125]. Social support and coping style can modify a patient's adjustment to illness, and "buffer" the adverse effects of stress. One study found that "less mature" coping strategies, and less availability of emotional support through social relationships were associated with functional dyspepsia, although this relationship was not as strong as the relationship was for life stress [123]. While it is conceivable that the gut in a sensitized subject may react more vigorously to stress, this has not been established.

No characteristic personality profile is demonstrable in patients with functional dyspepsia [124,126–128]. Higher scores for neuroticism, state and trait anxiety, depression, hostility and tension have been variously documented in patients compared with controls. In general, however, the scores are not very different from those for patients with structural disease such as peptic ulcer, and scores are similar to those for patients with other functional gastrointestinal disorders. Patients with functional dyspepsia may have high frequencies of psychiatric diagnoses, but adequate studies are lacking [129].

Patients with functional dyspepsia exhibited more abdominal illness behaviors in one study than did a control group with ulcer disease; they had an average of three times as many sick days requiring compensation, and were more likely to report nonabdominal complaints suggesting a somatization tendency [56]. Illness behaviors in adults may also be shaped by childhood experiences. For example, a relationship between sexual abuse and functional dyspepsia has been reported [130]. Another study found that dyspeptic patients tended to recall a more unhappy childhood [125]. Patients with abnormal psychological features may have a lower incidence of gastrointestinal motility disorders [6] and visceral hypersensitivity [90] than those with psychological scores within the normal range, but this remains to be confirmed by appropriate population-based studies.

While psychosocial factors are not of diagnostic value, it is important that they be identified since they often contribute to the patient's poor adjustment to illness. Eliciting and treating comorbid psychological disturbances should help improve clinical outcomes.

— Treatment

General Measures

The range of therapies prescribed for functional dyspepsia reflects its uncertain pathogenesis and the lack of satisfactory treatment options. Management is further confounded by high placebo response rates; between 20% and 60% of patients with functional dyspepsia have symptom improvement on placebo [131].

Reassurance and explanation represent the first step in treatment (Table 4). Coffee can aggravate symptoms in some cases and, if implicated, should be avoided [132]. Stopping smoking and ceasing consumption of alcohol are suggested to be helpful, but there is no convincing evidence that these factors are important in the pathogenesis of functional dyspepsia [115]. The avoidance of aspirin and other nonsteroidal anti-inflammatory drugs is commonly recommended; although not of established value, this seems sensible advice as these drugs may cause symptoms that are confused with functional dyspepsia [133,134]. If the patient has a coexistent anxiety disorder or depression, appropriate treatment should be considered.

Diet

Anecdotally, postprandial symptoms may be lessened by avoiding offending foods; spicy and fatty foods are common offenders. If early satiety, postprandial fullness or bloating, or nausea is dominant, taking six small low-fat meals per day may help decrease the intensity of the symptoms. When the neuromuscular function of the stomach is abnormal, the normal work of mixing and emptying ingested food can be seriously impaired. Dietary recommendations in this situation aim at maintaining adequate hydration and varying the gastric workload [135].

Medications

Antacids

While antacids are commonly taken by patients with dyspepsia, double-blind controlled trials have shown that antacids are not superior to placebo in functional dyspepsia [136,137]. However, this may reflect selection bias since subjects who would have responded to over-the-counter medications are unlikely to present for clinical trials.

Table 4. An Approach to the Management of Patients
with Functional Dyspepsia

General Guidelines

1. Make a positive clinical diagnosis as early as possible.

2. Determine why the patient having chronic symptoms has presented on this occasion, and allay any unwarranted fears that the patient may have.

3. Do not over investigate—an empiric therapeutic trial may be appropriate initially especially in the younger patient in the absence of risk factors for serious organic disease.

4. After the evaluation, reassure the patient regarding the absence of serious disease and reinforce that the diagnosis represents a recognized entity.

5. Explain the pathogenesis of the dyspepsia symptoms as far as possible.

6. Psychological factors may contribute to the morbidity of the disorder; these issues should be explored and counselling offered.

7. Advise the patient to avoid possible precipitating factors where appropriate (e.g., alcohol, non-steroidal anti-inflammatory drugs, dietary factors).

8. Inquire if the patient would like medication for their problem—not all patients want or require further treatment following reassurance, explanation, advice about precipitating factors, and exploration of psychological issues.

9. Follow up with the patient at least once to determine the natural history or response to treatment.

10. Do not repeat investigations based on symptoms alone. Diagnostic studies should depend on new or objective findings (e.g. new onset of vomiting or weight loss, blood in the stool).

11. Some patients with severe symptoms or multisystem complaints may benefit from counselling, particularly by a specialist interested in chronic pain syndromes.

12. Referral to a specialist in motility disorders and/or referral for formal psychological, psychiatric, and/or eating disorder evaluation may be indicated for some patients.

Adapted from Gastroenterol Internat, 1991 [35].

H$_2$ Blockers

H$_2$-receptor antagonists are widely prescribed for dyspeptic patients, but the results of double-blind controlled trials have been conflicting. Nyren et al. failed to detect any effect of cimetidine or antacids on ulcer-like dyspepsia [136] while other studies showed minor benefit of doubtful clinical significance [138] which was restricted to a positive effect on pain [137]. A meta-analysis has suggested a therapeutic gain of 20% over placebo, but a substantial number of studies could not be included [139] and the quality of many of the trials has been questioned [131]. Different inclusion criteria may account for the different results; responders to H_2 blockers may be restricted to the subset with unrecognized GERD [140].

Proton Pump Inhibitors

Proton pump inhibitors (PPI) appear to be modestly superior to placebo in functional dyspepsia, possibly because most trials of functional dyspepsia have included some patients with unrecognized GERD [15,141,142]. While patients with dysmotility-like dyspepsia or predominant nausea do not respond, there appears to be a benefit in ulcer-like dyspepsia [15].

Bismuth

Bismuth subcitrate and bismuth subsalicylate suppress but usually do not eradicate *H. pylori* infection. Statistically significant improvement over placebo was demonstrated for some symptoms in some trials in *H. pylori*-positive patients [143,144] but was not shown in other studies [145,146]. All of these investigations had several shortcomings [66]. In particular, study blinding was difficult as bismuth causes black discoloration of the tongue and stools.

Cytoprotection

Sucralfate has been inadequately tested in functional dyspepsia, with one positive [147] and one negative study [148]. Misoprostol is of uncertain efficacy; in the only controlled trial reported, patients with erosive prepyloric changes and dyspepsia had a worsening of symptoms [149].

Prokinetics

Metoclopramide
Metoclopramide has multiple mechanisms of action, including dopamine D_2 receptor antagonism and serotonin (5-HT$_3$) antagonism. Metoclopramide appears to be efficacious in functional dyspepsia but has been poorly studied [150,151], and the side effect profile limits it use.

Cisapride
Cisapride is a substituted benzamide approved for the treatment of nocturnal heartburn in the United States. It is a 5-HT$_4$ receptor agonist that releases acetylcholine from cholinergic motor neurons; it is also a 5HT$_3$ antagonist.

Cisapride improves symptoms in functional dyspepsia. A recent meta-analysis suggests it produces a therapeutic gain two-fold increased over placebo [152], confirming previous results [139]. However its mode of action in this condition is unclear. Treatment response failed to correlate with gastric emptying improvement in one large trial [54]. On the other hand, cisapride can eradicate gastric dysrhythmias [153] and improve the impaired gastric accommodation response to a meal [154].

The combination of cisapride with erythromycin, other macrolide antibiotics, and antifungal agents, is contraindicated. These drugs compete for the liver cytochrome enzyme P450 3A4, and when given together, result in an increase in blood levels of cisapride. High plasma levels of cisapride have been associated with cardiac dysrhythmias, in particular Q–T prolongation, which can evolve to arrhythmias such as torsades des pointe, ventricular tachycardia, and ventricular fibrillation, and syncope [155]. Fatal arrhythmias can occur very rarely without other concurrent medications [155].

Domperidone

Domperidone is a substituted benzamide and peripheral dopamine D_2 antagonist [156]. Unlike metoclopramide, domperidone does not cross the blood-brain barrier. Domperidone binds D_2 receptors in the circumventricular organs in the fourth ventricle, however, especially in the area postrema and at gastric D_2 receptors [156]. Because domperidone does not readily cross the blood-brain barrier, central nervous system symptoms are rare.

Davis et al. showed that domperidone improved symptoms in patients with functional dyspepsia and idiopathic gastroparesis, but did not increase the rate of gastric emptying [157], suggesting that the domperidone may improve symptoms by reducing gastric dysrhythmias [158] and/or alter the area postrema to induce symptom improvement. A number of other trials suggest that domperidone is superior to placebo in reducing symptoms [152].

Domperidone increases plasma prolactin levels, which is associated with breast tenderness and galactorrhea in less than 5% of patients.

Motilin Agonists

Erythromycin is a macrolide antibiotic; administered by mouth or intravenously, erythromycin increases the rate of gastric emptying in patients with diabetic and idiopathic gastroparesis [159,160]. The erythromycin molecule acts at motilin receptor sites on nerve and smooth muscle to produce strong antral contractions. Macrolide compounds also increase small bowel contractions and may produce abdominal cramps and diarrhea. In one report, 30% of the patients who were given erythromycin for gastroparesis were not able to tolerate the drug because of these side effects [160]. Synthetic motilin-like molecules that increase gastric emptying and possess no antibacterial activity are being developed but do not appear to be of value in functional dyspepsia.

Combination Therapy

Combinations of the drugs mentioned above have been little studied but may have theoretical advantages [161]. The combination of metoclopramide and cisapride provides D_2 antagonism and 5-HT$_4$ agonist actions. Similarly, the combination of cisapride and domperidone would yield D_2 receptor antagonism and 5-HT$_4$ agonist activity. Because specific pathophysiological mechanisms remains poorly understood, empiric trials of combinations of drugs can be helpful in difficult cases.

Visceral Analgesics

The kappa agonist fedotozine has been shown to reduce gastric hypersensitivity in volunteer studies. Two randomized controlled trials demonstrated that fedotozine improved symptoms over placebo in functional dyspepsia [162,163] but the absolute improvement was very small and of questionable clinical significance [164]. A number of newer visceral analgesics are currently under testing, including 5HT$_3$ antagonists.

5HT$_1$ Agonists

These drugs appear to reduce fundic disaccommodation and may improve meal-related symptoms [38]. Sumatriptan and buspirone have been tested and are promising; new drugs are in development.

Antispasmodics

The antispasmodic drug dicyclomine was no better than placebo in reducing global symptoms in dyspeptic patients in two crossover studies [165,166]. Likewise, a double-blind trial with a 4-week crossover protocol showed that trimebutine was no better than placebo in 24 dyspeptic patients [167]. Newer, more selective M3 antispasmodics have been developed but have not been tested in functional dyspepsia yet.

Antinauseants

Ondansetron

The 5-HT$_3$ antagonist drugs have been remarkably successful in controlling nausea and vomiting specifically related to cancer chemotherapy agents and post-operatively. The exact mechanism of beneficial action of the 5-HT$_3$ antagonists is not known, although blockade of 5-HT$_3$ receptors in the area postrema and vagal afferent fibers in the stomach and duodenum has been reported [168]. The serotonin-type 3 receptor antagonists may block afferent signals. Modest symptom improvement in functional dyspepsia has been shown with ondansetron in one trial over placebo [169]; more potent agents are yet to be tested.

Perchlorperazine
Perchlorperazine is an anti-nauseant drug with nonspecific actions in the central nervous system. The side effects can be formidable and range from hypotension to spastic torticollis and dystonia.

Antihistamines
Dimenhydrinate and Cyclizine
Dimenhydrinate and cyclizine are anti-motion sickness drugs. These H_1 antagonists have not been studied for efficacy in controlling nausea due to gastrointestinal disorders. Dimenhydrinate and cyclizine, however, decrease gastric dysrhythmias and motion sickness symptoms, suggesting that a portion of the drug action is at a peripheral site, namely the stomach [170].

Promethazine
Promethazine is used to treat mild, nonspecific nausea. These drugs frequently induce unacceptable drowsiness.

Antidepressants
There is only one small controlled trial of a tricyclic antidepressant in functional dyspepsia [171]. Amitryptiline in low dose improved symptoms but not visceral hypersensitivity or sleep. Mianserin has been tested in a broad group of functional bowel disease patients with promising results over placebo [172]. Selective serotonin re-uptake inhibitors have not been evaluated in functional dyspepsia.

Choice of Drug Therapy
Drug therapy is not always required; a proportion of patients will respond to reassurance and explanation. It seems logical to individualize drug therapy in functional dyspepsia when it is required. This Rome II committee believes that it is acceptable in general to consider either antisecretory or a prokinetic agent as first-line treatment. However, in the literature there is only limited evidence to support the view that different symptom subgroups respond to a specific type of pharmacologic intervention [15,173,174]. For the patient with documented ulcer-like functional dyspepsia initially, an acid suppressant may be preferred over a prokinetic agent. For the patient with dysmotility-like dyspepsia, a prokinetic agent may initially be preferred over an acid suppressant. In case of failure, the alternative therapy can be tried.

Long-term drug treatment may be needed in some patients. For those patients with frequent relapses, short intermittent treatment courses (e.g., 1–2 weeks) may be considered when no other management is successful and symptoms significantly impact on the patient's quality of life. In the rare patient whose symptoms are unremitting and incapacitating in the absence of medication, continuous therapy may be required; in such patients, drug holidays can help to determine if the medication is still needed.

There is evidence that symptoms in most patients with *H. pylori* positive functional dyspepsia do not improve with eradication of the organism. The physician faced with the problem of a patient with functional dyspepsia symptoms who is tempted to give eradication therapy should proceed to treatment only after explaining to the patient that there can be no confident expectation of symptomatic benefit and that there is a small risk of adverse reactions. The physician should also be aware of other potential problems with therapy such as the emergence of microbial resistance to the antibiotics [175]. Although all therapeutic decisions must be taken on a case-by-case basis with a fully informed patient, many physicians currently give eradication therapy in these circumstances.

Novel Approaches

In patients with difficult symptoms other options may be worth exploring.

Acupuncture, Acupressure and Acustimulation
Acupuncture stimulates a specific site during insertion and rotation of the acupuncture needle. In acupressure treatment, pressure with fingers or other devices is applied to the specific acupuncture point. Acupuncture and acupressure decrease nausea and vomiting related to cancer chemotherapy [176]. Dundee et al. showed that acupuncture and acustimulation were significantly better in reducing these symptoms postoperatively compared with placebo stimulation [177]. Acustimulation and acupressure also decrease the nausea that is part of motion sickness induced by illusory self motion [178,179]. Acupressure and acupuncture have not been systematically evaluated in patients with functional dyspepsia.

Gastric Electrical Stimulation
Pacing the stomach with electrodes sutured onto the serosa was a technique directed initially toward entraining the gastric pacemaker rhythm and/or improving gastric contractions. Kelly et al. showed that the gastric slow wave rhythm could be entrained with pacing electrodes sutured to the gastric serosa,

but that gastric emptying was not accelerated [180]. However, McCallum was successful in patients with gastroparesis [181]. Further studies are needed to define the efficacy of gastric electrical stimulation in these patients.

Psychologic Treatment

Very few trials of behavioral therapy in functional dyspepsia are available. One study demonstrated a clear benefit of cognitive behavioral therapy over standard care [182]. Another study compared psychotherapy with no treatment; both groups improved at one year of follow-up although the psychotherapy group did better on some of the symptomatic outcomes [183].

B2. Aerophagia

— Definition

Aerophagia is an unusual presenting complaint. It refers to a repetitive pattern of swallowing or ingestion of air and belching.

— Epidemiology

Belching, presumably due to air swallowing, is common but if this symptoms is not troublesome, it cannot be considered a disorder [20]. The epidemiology of aerophagia in the general population remains to be carefully defined, but clinical impression suggests it is rare.

— Diagnostic Criteria

At least 12 weeks, which need not be consecutive, in the preceding 12 months of:

(1) Air swallowing that is objectively observed; *and*
(2) Troublesome repetitive belching.

— Rationale for Diagnostic Criteria

Patients with aerophagia may belch to try and relieve abdominal discomfort. It is usually an unconscious act unrelated to meals. The belching must be troublesome as belching is a normal phenomenon. Repetitive belching alone is common and may be due to causes other than aerophagia; observation of air swallowing and belching is unequivocal evidence of aerophagia. There should be no evidence of structured or metabolic abnormalities to explain the symptoms.

The committee concluded, based on a strong clinical impression, that aerophagia cannot be definitively diagnosed without observing that excessive air swallowing or ingestion is occurring (which may or may not be obvious at the office assessment). As belching is a normal phenomenon, the committee concluded that the symptom must be troublesome to be clinically relevant. As visible abdominal distension is often part of the irritable bowel syndrome rather than a gastroduodenal disorder and as belching may not reduce distension, the requirement that belching relieve visible distension was considered unlikely to be of value.

— Clinical Evaluation

A positive diagnosis is based on a careful history and observation of air swallowing. In addition to belching, excess rectal flatus may occur with excessive air ingestion [184]. In typical cases no investigation is required. Rumination can usually be distinguished by the history and observation. Patients with GERD have increased air swallowing, but GERD is usually clearcut clinically. It is important to screen for psychiatric disease, including depression and anxiety.

— Physiologic Features

Belching is not aerophagia. Air swallowing is normal; approximately 10–15 ml is swallowed with a liquid meal [185]. Postprandial belching is also normal, with 3–4 belches per hour occurring with a normal diet. To belch, certain key reflex events need to occur: The lower esophageal sphincter has to relax in response to distension of the stomach from gas, and this has to be followed by relaxation of the upper esophageal sphincter, which can occur when a large volume of gas abruptly distends the esophagus. The motility patterns of belching are similar to those found in gastroesophageal reflux [185].

The patient with aerophagia ingests air into the esophagus by expanding the chest and lowering the diaphragm against a closed glottis. The air is then released, often with a loud noise. The maneuvre may relieve abdominal discomfort or even be pleasurable. While usually unconscious, presumably the habit is learned. Aerophagia may be equally common in patients with functional and organic dyspepsia [186].

Data on habitual air swallowers are lacking but excess gas is probably not present in patients with aerophagia, based on inert gas washout studies [187]. It has been suggested that disturbed upper gastrointestinal tract motility may account for the symptoms, but this has not been carefully studied [187]. Whether or not an incompetent or abnormal upper esophageal sphincter is present in some of these patients has not been evaluated.

— Psychological Features

Changes in emotional state can lead to increases in spontaneous swallowing in health [188]. Psychological factors have been presumed to be of importance in aerophagia, but there is no objective evidence of excess major psychopathology in aerophagia [186]. However, this does not rule out a role for psychiatric disease in some patients.

— Treatment

General Measures

Explanation of the symptoms and reassurance are important. It is probably useful to demonstrate chest expansion and air ingestion as the patient belches. The habit if not established can sometimes be unlearned. Treatment of associated psychiatric disease or employment of stress reduction techniques theoretically may be of benefit.

Diet

Dietary modification (avoiding sucking hard candies or chewing gum, eating slowly and encouraging small swallows at mealtime, and avoiding carbonated beverages) is often recommended but has not been rigorously tested and is usually disappointing in practice.

Medications

While tranquilizers [189] may occasionally be useful in severe cases, drug therapy is not generally recommended. Simethicone and activated charcoal preparations are usually ineffective [190].

Psychologic Treatment

Sustained improvement has been reported with hypnotherapy in a case report [191]. The value of other psychologic interventions is unknown.

B3. Functional Vomiting

— Definition

Nausea is a subjective symptom that most people describe as a queasy, sick to the stomach sensation that may progress to a feeling of the need to vomit. Three dimensions of nausea have been identified; epigastric discomfort and queasiness, systemic symptoms including sweating and light-headedness, and emotional symptoms including fatigue and depression [192]. Vomiting is the forceful expulsion of gastric contents from the stomach. In functional vomiting, recurrent vomiting is the presenting complaint, and all known medical and psychiatric causes for the problem have been excluded.

— Epidemiology

Functional vomiting is a rare condition in clinical practice. It should be distinguished from occasional vomiting that occurs in patients with documented functional dyspepsia. Recurrent vomiting in the general population is uncommon. A population-based study from Olmsted County, Minnesota reported that vomiting once a month or more occurred in 2% of women and 3% of men [18]. The epidemiology of functional vomiting is essentially undefined.

— Diagnostic Criteria

At least 12 weeks, which need not be consecutive, in the preceding 12 months of:

(1) Frequent episodes of vomiting, occurring on at least three separate days in a week over three months;

(2) Absence of criteria for an eating disorder, rumination, or major psychiatric disease according to DSM-IV;

(3) Absence of self-induced and medication-induced vomiting; *and*

(4) Absence of abnormalities in the gut or central nervous system, and metabolic diseases to explain the recurrent vomiting.

A working definition of frequent episodes of vomiting adapted by this Committee is at least one vomiting episode on a minimum of three separate days in a week every three months. The term psychogenic vomiting has no standard definition in the literature [193–196]. The Committee recommends its use be abandoned in favor of functional vomiting as defined above. Cyclical vomiting where there are clear symptom-free periods between discrete episodes may occur as part of functional vomiting but is more often observed in children (see Chapter 10).

— Clinical Evaluation

The differential diagnosis of recurrent vomiting is extensive. Drugs that may cause nausea and vomiting should be stopped. Rumination and eating disorders must be excluded on clinical grounds.

Rumination

This occurs in normal adults as well as in mentally impaired children. Classically there is daily effortless regurgitation of undigested food after every meal [197–199]. This can occur during or soon after finishing the meal. The food is not sour or bitter (suggesting no acid regurgitation as occurs in reflux disease). The patient may spit out or reswallow the food. There may be weight loss associated, but normal weight is often maintained. A suggestive history combined with a normal gastric emptying study and normal 24-hour esophageal pH monitoring is sufficient for diagnosis [198]. A full discussion of rumination is provided in Chapter 5.

Eating Disorders

It is beyond the scope of this chapter to describe the current DSM-IV diagnostic criteria for the eating disorders [200,201]. Patients with bulimia may have self-induced vomiting associated with binge episodes and generally a distorted body image. A careful clinical evaluation is essential to avoid overlooking an eating disorder [202,203].

Diagnostic Tests

It is particularly important to exclude either mechanical obstruction of the gastrointestinal tract or central nervous system disease. Initial relevant tests include an upper endoscopy and small bowel enema to exclude gastroduodenal diseases and small bowel obstruction. A metabolic screen is essential to exclude electrolyte and other abnormalities. A CT scan or ultrasound of the abdomen may also be indicated to exclude other intra-abdominal disease depending on the clinical setting. If these tests are normal, then an assessment of gastric neuromuscular function (gastric emptying of solids and liquids, preferably by scintigraphy) is required.

If gastric emptying is delayed, then exclusion of intestinal pseudo-obstruction needs consideration. Gastroduodenal manometry is useful to exclude a myopathic or neuropathic process and can help identify a missed obstructive disorder of the intestine. Autonomic function testing, if abnormal, may point to a central nervous system process which may be confirmed by an MRI of the brain.

The EGG may be helpful when combined with gastric emptying assessment to evaluate otherwise unexplained nausea and vomiting although this remains to be convincingly confirmed [102]; subsets include those patients with gastroparesis and normal gastric myoelectrical activity, those with normal gastric emptying but a gastric arrhythmia, and those where both gastric emptying and gastric myoelectrical rhythm are normal. If patients have gastroparesis with normal myoelectrical activity, pyloric channel or small bowel obstruction may have been missed and needs to be carefully reconsidered. In patients with normal gastric emptying and a gastric arrhythmia, the gastric rhythm disturbance may be the prime feature responsible for the nausea and vomiting due to autonomic nervous system abnormalities, smooth muscle dysfunction, interstitial cell of Cajal dysfunction or abnormalities in gastrointestinal hormone secretion. If gastric emptying and EGG activity are both normal, then extragastric causes of nausea and vomiting need to be considered, although abnormalities of antral dilatation, antroduodenal dyscoordination, or duodenal contractual abnormalities may cause the symptoms in a few.

It is unknown how commonly gastric emptying disturbances and EGG abnormalities occur in patients with a clinical diagnosis of functional vomiting. Vomiting conceivably could be an atypical presentation of GERD which may require 24-hour esophageal pH testing to detect [204]. Psychiatric disease as the primary cause also needs to be excluded.

— Physiological Features

Vomiting usually occurs after nausea reaches a severe and intolerable level. It is unknown how many patients with functional vomiting have nausea, but some certainly do, while others deny nausea. After a threshold for vomiting is exceeded, stereotypic events occur in multiple organ systems to induce a vomiting episode. Features of a vomiting episode include the mouth opening, salivation, inhibition of gastric motility, retroperitoneal contractions in the small bowel and stomach, breath holding, posturing, contraction of the abdominal muscles, and the ejection of the gastric contents from the mouth. Vomiting is coordinated in the reticular areas of the medulla and the dorsal vagal complex. The vomiting center actually includes a variety of brainstem nuclei that are required to integrate responses. The mechanisms explaining functional vomiting are completely unknown and could be central or peripheral, or both.

— Psychological Features

Major depression has been linked to habitual postprandial and irregular vomiting, while conversion disorder may explain some cases of continuous vomiting [205]. No information is available on the psychological profile of patients with functional vomiting where major psychiatric disease has been excluded and there is no evidence of a structural or metabolic explanation for the symptoms.

— Treatment

Dietary and pharmacological therapy may have a role but have not been specifically tested in this condition.

General Measures

Psychosocial support is important. Assessment of nutritional status is vital and appropriate intervention provided if there is a need.

Diet

There is no evidence that dietary therapy is of value in reducing or preventing vomiting.

Medications

There is no evidence that medications are of use in this group. Anecdotally, antidepressants can be helpful in full doses. Antinauseants are usually of little value but are worth a trial.

Psychologic Treatment

One case report has documented the value of cognitive and social skills training [206]. Self-monitoring has also been reported to be of value [207]. Data are otherwise lacking on the value of behavioral or psychotherapy, but these approaches may be worthwhile trying.

Recommendations for Future Research

— Mechanisms of Symptom Production in Functional Dyspepsia

(1) The development of animal models applying inflammation of the gastric or duodenal mucosa may help to better understand the neural pathways involved in perception of symptoms in a subset of patients.

(2) PET studies will increase our understanding our understanding of the CNS areas involved in perception of dyspeptic symptoms, if applied in appropriate human studies.

(3) The relationship between ultrastructural abnormalities in the esophagus and duodenum and symptoms needs to be determined.

— Diagnostic Issues in Functional Dyspepsia

(1) The validity of the predominant symptom subgrouping needs to be rigorously tested. Furthermore, the differentiation of functional dyspepsia from other poorly differentiated illnesses in primary care needs study.

(2) Future studies will require a thorough evaluation of symptoms. Quantitative analysis of severity and frequency of individual dyspeptic symptoms by validated questionnaires is needed. Instruments must be developed to reliably explore localization, nature and temporal features of individual symptoms. Esophageal and lower gastrointestinal symptoms should also be analyzed in all studies, in order to clarify overlap syndromes.

(3) Optimization of screening tests for clinical practice and study entry is needed.

(4) The relationship between diet (including food intolerance) and functional dyspepsia needs to be explored.

(5) Gastrointestinal dysmotility and visceral hypersensitivity are complex and often very subtle abnormalities that can be only partially investigated by the available technology. The clinical utility of the available noninvasive technology such as region-specific nuclear medicine studies, ultrasound and electrogastrography needs to be explored.

— Therapeutic Issues in Functional Dyspepsia

(1) Evaluation of empiric therapies in dyspepsia in primary care is recommended.

(2) Head-to-head comparisons of prokinetics vs. acid suppressants should be evaluated in different subgroups.

(3) *H. pylori* eradication requires further investigation in different subgroups and in overlapping syndromes.

(4) Drugs modifying visceral sensitivity need to be appropriately investigated.

— Health Economics in Functional Dyspepsia

(1) The economic impact of functional dyspepsia in different health care systems needs to be documented.

— Aerophagia

(1) Studies of air swallowing in health and disease and evaluation of upper gastrointestinal tract motility (including upper esophageal sphincter function) in aerophagia are needed.

(2) The link between psychological distress and aerophagia requires careful study.

(3) Because this syndrome appears to be so resistant to standard treatments, investigation of psychological treatments such as hypnotherapy in controlled trials is suggested.

— Functional Vomiting

(1) The validity of functional vomiting as a separate syndrome requires confirmation.

(2) The prevalence needs to be established in different medical settings (psychiatric versus gastrointestinal clinics).

(3) More data are needed regarding the clinical, physiologic, and psychologic characteristics of these patients.

(4) Investigation of the value of psychological treatments and antidepressants is suggested.

References

1. Kingham JGC, Fairclough PD, Dawson AM. What is indigestion? J Royal Soc Med 1983;76:183–86.
2. Talley NJ, Phillips SF. Non-ulcer dyspepsia: potential causes and pathophysiology. Ann Intern Med 1988;108:865–79.
3. Testoni PA, Bagnolo F, Bologna P, et al. *Helicobacter pylori* infection in dyspeptic patients who do not have gastric III phase of the migrating motor complex. Scand J Gastroenterol 1996;31:1063–68.
4. Colin-Jones DG, Bloom B, Bodemar G. Management of dyspepsia: report of a working party. Lancet 1988;1:576–79.
5. Heading RC. Definitions of dyspepsia. Scand J Gastroenterol 1991;26[suppl 182]: 1–6.
6. Malagelada J-R, Stanghellini V. Manometric evaluation of functional upper gut symptoms. Gastroenterology 1985;88:1223–1231.
7. Thompson WG. Nonulcer dyspepsia. Can Med Assoc J 1984;130:565–69.
8. Barbara L, Camilleri M, Corinaldesi R. Definition and investigation of dyspepsia: consensus of an international ad hoc working party. Dig Dis Sci 1989;34:1272–76.
9. Talley NJ, McNeil D, Piper DW. Discriminant value of dyspeptic symptoms: a study of the clinical presentation of 221 patients with dyspepsia of unknown cause, peptic ulceration and cholelithiasis. Gut 1987;28:40–46.
10. Talley NJ, Weaver AL, Tesmer DL. Lack of discriminant value of dyspepsia subgroups in patients referred for upper endoscopy. Gastroenterology 1993;105: 1378–86.
11. Earlam R. A computerized questionnaire analysis of duodenal ulcer symptoms. Gastroenterology 1976;71:314–17.
12. Crean GP, Holden RJ, Knill-Jones RP. A database on dyspepsia. Gut 1994; 35:191–202.
13. Oxford English Dictionary.
14. Stanghellini V, Tosetti C, Paternico A, et al. Risk indicators of delayed gastric emptying of solids in patients with functional dyspepsia. Gastroenterology 1996;110: 1036–42.
15. Talley NJ, Meineche-Schmidt V, Pare P, et al. Efficacy of omeprazole in functional dyspepsia: double-blind, randomised placebo-controlled trials with omeprazole (the Bond and Opeca studies). Aliment Pharmacol Ther 1998;12:1055–65.
16. Beck IT, Champion MC, Lemire S, et al. The Second Canadian Consensus Conference on the management of patients with gastroesophageal reflux disease. Can J Gastroenterol 1997;11(suppl)B:7–20B.
17. Klauser AG, Schindlbeck NE, Muller-Lissner SA. Symptoms in gastro-esophageal reflux disease. Lancet 1990;335:205–208.
18. Talley NJ, Zinsmeister AR, Schleck CD, et al. Dyspepsia and dyspepsia subgroups: a population based study. Gastroenterology 1992;102:1259–68.
19. Jones RH, Lydeard SE, Hobbs FDR, et al. Dyspepsia in England and Scotland. Gut 1990;31:401–405.

20. Drossman DA, Li Z, Andruzzi E, et al. U.S. householder survey of functional gastrointestinal disorders: prevalence, sociodemography and health impact. Dig Dis Sci 1993;38:1569–80.

21. Agreus L, Svardsudd K, Nyren O, Tibblin G. Irritable bowel syndrome and dyspepsia in the general population: overlap and lack of stability over time. Gastroenterology 1995;109:671–80.

22. Locke GR III, Talley NJ, Fett S, Zinsmeister AR, Melton LJ III. Prevalence and clinical spectrum of gastroesophageal reflux in the community. Gastroenterology 1997;112:1448-1456.

23. Talley NJ, Silverstein M, Agreus L, et al. AGA Technical Review: evaluation of dyspepsia. Gastroenterology 1998;114:582–95.

24. Jonsson K-A, Gotthard R, Bodemar G, et al. The clinical relevance of endoscopic and histologic inflammation of gastroduodenal mucosa in dyspepsia of unknown origin. Scand J Gastroenterol 1989;24:385–95.

25. Johnsen R, Bernersen B, Straume B, et al. Prevalences of endoscopic and histological findings in subjects with and without dyspepsia. Brit Med J 1991;302: 749–52.

26. Klauser AG, Voderholzer WA, Knesewitsch PA, et al. What is behind dyspepsia? Dig Dis Sci 1993;38:147–54.

27. Talley NJ, Weaver AL, Zinsmeister AR, et al. Onset and disappearance of gastrointestinal symptoms and functional gastrointestinal disorders. Am J Epidemiol 1992;136:165–77.

28. Lindell GH, Celebioglu F, Graffner HO. Non-ulcer dyspepsia in the long-term perspective. Eur J Gastroenterol Hepatol 1995;7:829–33.

29. Talley NJ, McNeil D, Hayden A,et al. Prognosis of chronic unexplained dyspepsia: a prospective study of potential predictor variables in patients with endoscopically diagnosed nonulcer dyspepsia. Gastroenterology 1987;92:1060–66.

30. Talley NJ, Boyce P, Jones M. Dyspepsia and health care seeking in a community: how important are psychological factors? Dig Dis Sci 1998;43:1016–22.

31. Jones R, Lydeard S. Factors affecting the decision to consult with dyspepsia: comparison of consulters and non-consulters. J Royal Coll Gen Pract 1989;39:495–98.

32. Bytzer P, Hansen JM, Schaffalitzky de Muckadell OB,et al. Predicting endoscopic diagnosis in dyspeptic patients: the value of predictive score models. Scand J Gastroenterol 1997;32:118–25.

33. Chiba N, Bernard L, O'Brien BJ. A Canadian physician survey of dyspepsia management. Can J Gastroenterol 1998;12:83–90.

34. Drossman DA, Thompson GW, Talley NJ, et al. Identification of subgroups of functional gastrointestinal disorders. Gastroenterol Internat 1990;3:159–72.

35. Talley NJ, Colin-Jones D, Koch KL. Functional dyspepsia: a classification with guidelines for diagnosis and management. Gastroenterol Internat 1991;4:145–60.

36. Agreus L, Talley N. Dyspepsia management in general practice. Brit Med J 1997; 315:1284–88.

37. Talley NJ, Hunt RH. What role does *Helicobacter pylori* play in non-ulcer dyspep-

sia? arguments for and against *H. pylori* being associated with dyspeptic symptoms. Gastroenterology 1997;113 [6 suppl S]:s67–77.

38. Tack J, Piessevaux H, Coulie B, et al. Role of impaired gastric accommodation to a meal in functional dyspepsia. Gastroenterology 1998;115:1346–52.

39. Heading RC, Barrison IC, Brown RC, et al. Upper gastrointestinal symptoms in general practice: a multicentre UK study. Internat J Drug Devel 1995;7:109–17.

40. Hansen JM, Bytzer P, Demuckadell OBS. Placebo-controlled trial of cisapride and nizatidine in unselected patients with functional dyspepsia. Am J Gastroenterol 1998;93:368–74.

41. Small PK, Loudon MA, Waldron B, et al. Importance of reflux symptoms in functional dyspepsia. Gut 1995;36:189–92.

42. Tobey NA, Carson JL, Alkiek RA, et al. Dilated intercellular spaces: a morphological feature of acid reflux-damaged human esophageal epithelium. Gastroenterology 1996;111:1200–1205.

43. Talley NJ, Boyce P, Jones M. Identification of distinct upper and lower gastrointestinal symptom groupings in an urban population. Gut 1998;42:690–95.

44. Muth ER, Koch KL, Bingaman SA, et al. Clinical utility of symptom assessment in patients with functional dyspepsia. Gastroenterology 1998;114:A1079.

45. Tack J, Piessevaux H, Coulie B, et al. *Helicobacter pylori*, symptom severity and pathophysiological mechanisms in functional dyspepsia. Gastroenterology 1998; 114:A997.

46. Lam SK, Talley NJ. Report of the 1997 Asia Pacific consensus guidelines on the management of *H. pylori*. J Gastroenterol Hepatol 1998;13:1–12.

47. Malfertheiner P, Megraud F, O'Morain C, et al. Current European concepts in the management of *Helicobacter pylori* infection—the Maastricht Consensus Report: The European *Helicobacter pylori* Study Group [EHPSG]. Eur J Gastroenterol Hepatol 1997;9:1–2.

48. McColl KE, el-Nujumi A, Murray L, et al. The *Helicobacter pylori* breath test: a surrogate marker for peptic ulcer disease in dyspeptic patients. Gut 1997;40: 302–306.

49. Ofman JJ, Etchason J, Fullerton S, et al. Management strategies for *Helicobacter pylori*: seropositive patients with dyspepsia: clinical and economic consequences. Ann Intern Med 1997;126:280–91.

50. Fendrick MA, Chernew ME, Hirth RA, et al. Alternative management strategies for patients with suspected peptic ulcer disease. Ann Intern Med 1995;123:260–68.

51. Talley NJ, Axon A, Bytzer P, et al. Management of univestigated and functional dyspepsia: a working party report for the World Congresses of Gastroenterology. Aliment Pharmacol Ther (in press).

52. Heikkinen M, Pikkarainen P, Takala J, et al. Etiology of dyspepsia: four hundred unselected consecutive patients in general practice. Scand J Gastroenterol 1995;30: 519–23.

53. Talley NJ. Gallstones and upper abdominal discomfort: innocent bystander or cause of dyspepsia? J Clin Gastroenterol 1995;20:182–83.

54. Kellow JE, Cowan H, Shuter B, et al. Efficacy of cisapride therapy in functional dyspepsia. Aliment Pharmacol Ther 1995;9:153–60.

55. Jian R, Ducrot F, Ruskone A, et al. Symptomatic, radionuclide and therapeutic assessment of chronic idiopathic dyspepsia: a double-blind placebo-controlled evaluation of cisapride. Dig Dis Sci 1989;34:657–64.

56. Nyren O, Adami H-O, Gustavsson S, et al. The "epigastric distress syndrome": a possible disease entity identified by history and endoscopy in patients with nonulcer dyspepsia. J Clin Gastroenterol 1987;9:303–309.

57. Collen MJ, Loebenberg MJ. Basal gastric acid secretion in nonulcer dyspepsia with or without duodenitis. Dig Dis Sci 1989;34:246–50.

58. Tucci A, Corinaldesi R, Stanghellini V, et al. *Helicobacter pylori* infection and gastric function in patients with chronic idiopathic dyspepsia. Gastroenterology 1992;103:768–74.

59. El-Omar E, Penman I, Ardill JE, et al. A substantial proportion of non-ulcer dyspepsia patients have the same abnormality of acid secretion as duodenal ulcer patients. Gut 1995;36:534–38.

60. George AA, Tsuchiyose M, Dooley CP. Sensitivity of the gastric mucosa to acid and duodenal contents in patients with nonulcer dyspepsia. Gastroenterology 1991; 101:3–6.

61. Bates S, Sjoden PO, Fellenius J, et al. Blocked and unblocked acid secretion and reported pain in ulcer, nonulcer dyspepsia, and normal subjects. Gastroenterology 1989;97:376–83.

62. Son HJ, Rhee PL, Kim JJ, et al. Hypersensitivity to acid in ulcer-like functional dyspepsia. Korean J Intern Med 1997;12:188–92.

63. Coffin B, Azpiroz F, Guarner F, et al. Selective gastric hypersensitivity and reflex hyporeactivitiy in functional dyspepsia. Gastroenterology 1994;107:1345–51.

64. Parsonnet J, Blaser MJ, Perez-Perez GI, et al. Symptoms and risk factors of *Helicobacter pylori* infection in a cohort of epidemiologists. Gastroenterology 1992; 102:41–6.

65. Rosenstock S, Kay L, Andersen LP, et al. Relation between *Helicobacter pylori* infection and gastrointestinal symptoms and syndromes. Gut 1997;41:169–76.

66. Talley NJ. A critique of therapeutic trials in *Helicobacter pylori*-positive functional dyspepsia. Gastroenterology 1994;106:1174–83.

67. McColl K, Murray L, El-Omar E, et al. Symptomatic benefit from eradicating *Helicobacter pylori* infection in patients with nonulcer dyspepsia. New Engl J Med 1998;339:1869–74.

68. Gilvarry J, Buckley MJ, Beattie S, et al. Eradication of *Helicobacter pylori* affects symptoms in non-ulcer dyspepsia. Scand J Gastroenterol 1997;32:535–40.

69. Sheu BS, Lin CY, Lin XZ, et al. Long term outcome of triple therapy in *Helicobacter pylori* related nonulcer dyspepsia: a prospective controlled assessment. Am J Gastroenterol 1996;91:441–47.

70. Greenberg PD, Cello JP. Prospective, double-blind treatment of *Helicobacter pylori* in patients with non-ulcer dyspepsia. Gastroenterology 1996;109:A123.

71. Talley NJ, Janssens J, Lauritsen K, et al. Eradication of *Helicobacter pylori* in functional dyspepsia: randomised double blind placebo controlled trial with 12 months' follow up: the Optimal Regimen Cures Helicobacter Induced Dyspepsia (ORCHID) Study Group. Brit Med J 1999;318:833–37.

72. Koelz HR, Arnold R, Stolte M, et al. Treatment of *Helicobacter pylori* does not improve symptoms of functional dyspepsia. Gastroenterology 1998;114:182A.

73. Blum AL, Talley NJ, O'Morain C, et al. Lack of effect of treating *Helicobacter pylori* infection in patients with nonulcer dyspepsia: omeprazole plus clarithromycin and amoxicillin effect one year after treatment: (OCAY) Study Group. New Engl J Med 1998;339:1875–81.

74. Gisbert JP, Boixeda D, Martin de Argila C, et al. Erosive duodenitis: prevalence of *Helicobacter pylori* infection and response to eradication therapy with omeprazole plus two antibiotics. Eur J Gastroenterol Hepatol 1997;9:957–62.

75. Joffe SN, Primrose JN. Pain provocation test in peptic duodenitis. Gastrointest Endoscop 1983;29:282–84.

76. Stanghellini V, Ghidini C, Maccarini MR, et al. Fasting and postprandial gastrointestinal motility in ulcer and non-ulcer dyspepsia. Gut 1992;33:184–90.

77. Jones KL, Horowitz M, Carney BI,et al. Effects of cisapride on gastric emptying of oil and aqueous meal components, hunger, and fullness. Gut 1996;38:310–15.

78. Troncon LE, Thompson DG, Ahluwalia NK, et al. Relations between upper abdominal symptoms and gastric distension abnormalities in dysmotility like functional dyspepsia and after vagotomy. Gut 1995;37:17–22.

79. Ahluwalia NK, Thompson DG, Mamtora H, et al. Evaluation of gastric antral motor performace in patients with dysmotility-like dyspepsia using real-time high-resolution ultrasound. Neurogastroenterol Motil 1996;8:333–38.

80. Scott AM, Kellow JE, Shuter B, et al. Intragastric distribution and gastric emptying of solids and liquids in functional dyspepsia: lack of influence of symptom subgroups and *H. pylori* associated gastritis. Dig Dis Sci 1993;38:2247–54.

81. Pantoflickova D, Blum AL, Koelz HR, et al. *Helicobacter pylori* and functional dyspepsia: a real causal link? Bailliere's Clin Gastroenterol 1998;12:503–32.

82. Testoni PA, Bagnalo F, Colombo E, et al. The correlation in dyspeptic patients of *Helicobacter pylori* infection with changes in interdigestive gastroduodenal motility patterns but not in gastric emptying. Helicobacter 1996;1:229–39.

83. Pieramico O, Ditschuneit H, Malfertheiner P. Gastrointestinal motility in patients with non-ulcer dyspepsia: a role for Helicobacter pylori infection? Am J Gastroenterol 1993;88:364–68.

84. Samson M, Verhager MA, van Berge-Henegouwen GP, et al. Abnormal clearance of exogenous acid and increased acid sensitivity of the proximal duodenum in dyspeptic patients. Gastroenterology 1999;116:515–20.

85. Jebbink HJA, Vanberge-Henegouwen GP, Akkermans LMA, et al. Small intestinal motor abnormalities in patients with functional dyspepsia demonstrated by ambulatory manometry. Gut 1996;38:694–700.

86. Jain NK, Boivin M, Zinsmeister AR, et al. Effect of ileal perfusion of carbohy-

drates and amylase inhibitor on gastrointestinal hormones and emptying. Gastroenterology 1989;96:377–87.

87. Bost R, Hostein J, Valenti M, et al. Is there an abnormal fasting duodenogastric reflux in nonulcer dyspepsia? Dig Dis Sci 1990;35:193–99.

88. Mearin F, De Ribot X, Balboa A, et al. Duodenogastric bile reflux and gastrointestinal motility in pathogenesis of functional dyspepsia: role of cholecystectomy. Dig Dis Sci 1995;40:1703–1709.

89. Mayer EA, Gebhart GF. Basic and clinical aspects of visceral hyperalgesia. Gastroenterology 1994;107:271–93.

90. Lemann M, Dederding JP, Flourie B, et al. Abnormal perception of visceral pain in response to gastric distension in chronic idiopathic dyspepsia: the irritable stomach syndrome. Dig Dis Sci 1991;36:1249–54.

91. Mearin F, Cucala M, Azpiroz F, et al. The origin of symptoms on the brain-gut axis in functional dyspepsia. Gastroenterology 1991;101:999–1006.

92. Mearin F, de Ribot X, Balboa A, et al. Does *Helicobacter pylori* infection increase gastric sensitivity in functional dyspepsia? Gut 1995;37:47–51.

93. Holtmann G, Goebell H, Talley NJ. Impaired small intestinal peristaltic reflexes and sensory thresholds are independent functional disturbances in patients with chronic unexplained dyspepsia. Am J Gastroenterol 1996;91:485–91.

94. Holtmann G, Talley NJ, Goebell H. Association between *Helicobacter pylori*, duodenal mechanosensory thresholds and small intestinal motility in chronic unexplained dyspepsia. Dig Dis Sci 1996;41:1285–91.

95. Holtmann G, Goebell H, Talley NJ. Functional dyspepsia and irritable bowel syndrome: Is there a common pathophysiological basis? Am J Gastroenterol 1997;92: 954–59.

96. Holtmann G, Goebell H, Jockenhoevel, et al. Altered vagal and intestinal mechanosensory function in chronic unexplained dyspepsia. Gut 1998;42:501–506

97. Trimble KC, Farouk R, Pryde A, et al. Heightened visceral sensation in functional gastrointestinal disease is not site-specific: evidence of a generalized disorder of gut sensitivity. Dig Dis Sci 1995;40:1607–13.

98. Feinle C, D'Amato M, Read NW. Cholecystokinin-A receptors modulate gastric sensory and motor responses to gastric distension and duodenal lipid. Gastroenterology 1996;110:1379–85.

99. Greydanus MP, Vassallo M, Camilleri M, et al. Neurohormonal factors in functional dyspepsia: insights on pathophysiological mechanisms. Gastroenterology 1991; 100:1311–18.

100. Gilja OH, Hausken T, Wilhelmsen I, et al. Impaired accommodation of proximal stomach to a meal in functional dyspepsia. Dig Dis Sci 1996;41:689–96.

101. Berstad A, Hauksen T, Gilja OH, et al. Gastric accommodation in functional dyspepsia. Scand J Gastroenterol 1997;32:193–97.

102. Koch KL. Dyspepsia of unknown origin: pathophysiology, diagnosis and treatment. Dig Dis 1997;15:316–29.

103. Parkman HP, Miller MA, Trate D, et al. Electrogastrography and gastric emptying

scintigraphy are complementary for assessment of dyspepsia. J Clin Gastroenterol 1997;24:214–19.

104. Jebbink HJ, Van Berge-Henegouwen GP, Bruijs PP, et al. Gastric myoelectrical activity and gastrointestinal motility in patients with functional dyspepsia. Eur J Clin Invest 1995;25:429–37.

105. Labo G, Bortolotti M, Vezzadini P,et al. Interdigestive gastroduodenal motility and serum motilin levels in patients with idiopathic delay in gastric emptying. Gastroenterology 1986;90:20–26.

106. Raybould HE, Zittel TT, Holzer HH, et al. Gastroduodenal sensory mechanisms and CCK in inhibition of gastric emptying in response to a meal. Dig Dis Sci 1994;39(suppl):41s–43s.

107. Cote F, Pare P, Friede J. Physiological effect of cholecystokinin on gastric emptying of liquid in functional dyspepsia. Am J Gastroenterol 1995;90:2006–2009.

108. Kamm MA, Farthing MJ, Lennard-Jones JE. Bowel function and transit rate during the menstrual cycle. Gut 1989;30:605–608.

109. Nyren O, Adami H-O, Bergstrom R, et al. Basal and food-simulated levels of gastrin and pancreatic polypeptide in non-ulcer dyspepsia and duodenal ulcer. Scand J Gastroenterol 1986;21:471–77.

110. Narducci F, Bassotti G, Granata MT, et al. Functional dyspepsia and chronic idiopathic gastric stasis. Role of endogenous opiates. Arch Intern Med 1986;146: 716–20.

111. Chua A, Keating J, Hamilton D, et al. Central serotonin receptors and delayed gastric emptying in non-ulcer dyspepsia. Brit Med J 1992;305:280–82.

112. Kaess H, Kellermann M, Castro A. Food intolerance in duodenal ulcer patients, non-ulcer dyspeptic patients and healthy subjects: a prospective study. Klin Wochenschr 1988;66:208–11.

113. Ferguson A. Food sensitivity or self-deception? New Engl J Med 1990;323:476–78.

114. Cuperus P, Keeling PW, Gibney MJ. Eating patterns in functional dyspepsia: a case control study. Eur J Clin Nutr 1996;50:520–23.

115. Talley NJ, Zinsmeister AR, Schleck CD, et al. Smoking, alcohol and analgesics in dyspepsia and among dyspepsia subgroups: lack of association in a community. Gut 1994;35:619–24.

116. Wolf S. The relation of gastric function to nausea in man. J Clin Invest 1943; 22:877–82.

117. Thompson DG, Richelson E, Malagelada J-R. Perturbation of gastric emptying and duodenal motility through the central nervous system. Gastroenterology 1982; 83:1200–1206.

118. Camilleri M, Malagelada J-R, Kao PC, et al. Gastric and autonomic responses to stress in functional dyspepsia. Dig Dis Sci 1986;31:1169–77.

119. Jorgensen LS, Bonlokke L, Christensen NJ. Life strain, life events and autonomic response to a psychological stressor in patients with chronic upper abdominal pain. Scand J Gastroenterol 1986;21:605–13.

120. Talley NJ, Piper DW. Major life event stress and dyspepsia of unknown cause: a case-control study. Gut 1986;27:127–34.

121. Hafeiz HB, al-Quorain A, al Mangoor S, et al. Life events stress in functional dyspepsia: a case control study. Eur J Gastroenterol Hepatol 1997;9:21–26.

122. Hui WM, Shiu LP, Lam SK. The perception of life events and daily stress in nonulcer dyspepsia. Am J Gastroenterol 1991;86:292–96.

123. Bennett E, Beaurepaire J, Langeluddecke P, et al. Life stress and non-ulcer dyspepsia: a case-control study. J Psychosom Res 1991;35:579–90.

124. Bennett EJ, Piesse C, Palmer K, et al. Functional gastrointestinal disorders: psychological, social, and somatic features. Gut 1998;42:414–20.

125. Talley NJ, Jones M, Piper DW. Psychosocial and childhood factors in essential dyspepsia: a case-control study. Scand J Gastroenterol 1988;23:341–46.

126. Langeluddecke P, Goulston K, Tennant C. Psychological factors in dyspepsia of unknown cause: a comparison with peptic ulcer disease. J Psychosomat Res 1990; 34:215–22.

127. Talley NJ, Phillips SF, Bruce B, et al. Relation among personality and symptoms in nonulcer dyspepsia and the irritable bowel syndrome. Gastroenterology 1990; 99:327–33.

128. Wilhelmsen I, Haug TT, Ursin H, et al. Discriminant analysis of factors distinguishing patients with functional dyspepsia from patients with duodenal ulcer: significance of somatization. Dig Dis Sci 1995;40:1105–11.

129. Olden K. Are psychosocial factors of aetiological importance in functional dyspepsia? In: Talley NJ, Editor. Bailliere's Clin Gastroenterol 1998;12:557–71.

130. Talley NJ, Helgeson SL, Zinsmeister AR, et al. Gastrointestinal tract symptoms and self-reported abuse: a population-based study. Gastroenterology 1994;107: 1040–49.

131. Veldhuyzen van Zanten SJO, Cleary C, Talley NJ, et al. Drug treatment of functional dyspepsia: a systematic analysis of trial methodology with recommendations for the design of future trials: report of an international working party. Am J Gastroenterol 1996;91:660–73.

132. Elta GH, Behler EM, Colturi TJ. Comparison of coffee intake and coffee-induced symptoms in patients with duodenal ulcer, nonulcer dyspepsia and normal controls. Am J Gastroenterol 1990;85:1339–42.

133. Holtmann G, Goebell H, Talley NJ. Dyspepsia in consulters and non-consulters: prevalence, health care seeking behaviour and risk factors. Eur J Gastroenterol Hepatol 1994;6:917–24.

134. Nandurkar S, Talley NJ, Xia H H-X, et al. Dyspepsia in the community is linked to smoking and aspirin use and not *Helicobacter pylori*. Arch Intern Med 1998;158: 1427–33.

135. Koch KL. Approach to the patient with nausea and vomiting. In: Textbook of Gastroenterology, Ed. 2. T. Yamada, Editor. Philadelphia: J.B. Lippincott Co; 1995:731–49.

136. Nyren O, Adami H-O, Bates S, et al. Absence of therapeutic benefit from antacids or cimetidine in non-ulcer dyspepsia. New Engl J Med 1986;314:339–43.

137. Gotthard R, Bodemar G, Brodin U, et al. Treatment with cimetidine, antacid or placebo in patients with dyspepsia of unknown origin. Scand J Gastroenterol 1988; 23:7–18.

138. Talley NJ, McNeil D, Hayden A, et al. Randomized, double-blind, placebo-controlled crossover trial of cimetidine and pirenzepine in nonulcer dyspepsia. Gastroenterology 1986;91:149–56.

139. Dobrilla G, Comberlato M, Steele A, et al. Drug treatment of functional dyspepsia: meta analysis of randomized controlled clinical trials. J Clin Gastroenterol 1989; 11:169–77.

140. Farup PG, Hovde O, Breder O. Are frequent short gastro-esophageal reflux episodes the cause of symptoms in patients with non-ulcer dyspepsia responding to treatment with ranitidine? Scand J Gastroenterol 1995;30:829–32.

141. Blum AL, Arnold R, Koelz HR, et al. Treatment of functional dyspepsia (FD) with omeprazole and ranitidine. Gastroenterology 1997;110:A73.

142. Jones RH, Baxter G. Lansoprazole 30mg daily versus ranitidine 150mg bd in the treatment of acid-related dyspepsia in general practice. Aliment Pharmacol Ther 1997;11:541–46.

143. Rokkas T, Pursey C, Uzoechina E, et al. Non-ulcer dyspepsia and short term De-Nol therapy: a placebo controlled trial with particular reference to the role of *Campylobacter pylori*. Gut 1988;29:1386–91.

144. Kang JY, Tay HH, Wee A, et al. Effect of colloidal bismuth subcitrate on symptoms and gastric histology in non-ulcer dyspepsia: a double-blind placebo controlled study. Gut 1990;31:476–80.

145. McNulty CAM, Gearty JC, Crump B, et al. *Campylobacter pyloridis* and associated Gastritis: investigator blind, placebo controlled trial of bismuth salicylate and erythromycin ethylsuccinate. Brit Med J 1986;293:645–49.

146. Loffeld RJLF, Potters HVJP, Stobberingh E, et al. *Campylobacter* associated gastritis in patients with non-ulcer: a double-blind placebo controlled trial with colloidal bismuth subcitrate. Gut 1989;30:1206–1212.

147. Kairaluoma MI, Hentilae R, Alavaikko M, et al. Sucralfate versus placebo in treatment of non-ulcer dyspepsia. Am J Med 1987;83(Suppl 3B):51–55.

148. Gudjonsson H, Oddsson E, Bjornsson S, et al. Efficacy of sucralfate in treatment of non-ulcer dyspepsia: a double-blind placebo-controlled study. Scand J Gastroenterol 1993;28:969–72.

149. Hausken T, Stene-Larsen G, Lange O, et al. Misoprostol treatment exacerbates abdominal discomfort in patients with non-ulcer dyspepsia and erosive prepyloric changes: a double-blind placebo-controlled multicentre study. Scand J Gastroenterol 1990;25:1028–1033.

150. Johnson AG. Controlled trial of metoclopramide in the treatment of flatulent dyspepsia. Brit Med J 1971;2:25–26.

151. Perkel MS, Moore C, Hersh T, et al. Metoclopramide therapy in patients with de-

layed gastric emptying: a randomized, double-blind study. Dig Dis Sci 1979;24: 662–66.

152. Veldhuyzen van Zanten S, Talley NJ. Cisapride for treatment of non-ulcer dyspepsia (NUD): a meta-analysis of randomized controlled trials. Gastroenterology 1998;114:A323.

153. Rothstein RD, Alavi A, Reynolds J. Electrogastrography in patients with gastroparesis: effects of long-term cisapride. Dig Dis Sci 1993;38:1518–24.

154. Tack J, Piessevaux H, Coulie B, et al. In functional dyspepsia, impaired gastric accommodation is associated with early satiety and weight loss. Neurogastroenterol Motil 1998;10:A102.

155. Bran S, Murray WA, Hirsch IB, et al. Long QT syndrome during high dose cisapride. Arch Intern Med 1995;155:765–68.

156. Brogden RN, Carmine AA, Heel RC, et al. Domperidone: a review of its pharmacological activity, pharmacokinetics and therapeutic efficacy in the symptomatic treatment of chronic dyspepsia and as an antiemetic. Drugs 1982;24:360–400.

157. Davis RH, Clench MH, Mathias JR. Effects of domperidone in patients with chronic unexplained upper gastrointestinal symptoms: a double-blind, placebo-controlled study. Dig Dis Sci 1988;33:1505–11.

158. Koch KL, Stern RM, Stewart WR, et al. Gastric emptying and gastric myoelectrical activity in patients with symptomatic diabetic gastroparesis: Effects of long-term domperidone treatment. Am J Gastroenterol 1989;84:1069–75.

159. Janssens J, Peeters Tl, Vantrappen G, et al. Improvement of gastric emptying in diabetic gastroparesis by erythromycin: preliminary studies. New Engl J Med 1990; 322:1028–31.

160. Richards RD, Davenport K, McCallum RW. The treatment of idiopathic and diabetic gastroparesis with acute intravenous and chronic oral erythromycin. Am J Gastroenterol 1993; 88:203–206.

161. Tatsuta M, Iishi H, Nakaizumi A, Okuda S. Effect of treatment with cisapride alone or in combination with domperidone on gastric emptying and gastrointestinal symptoms in dyspeptic patients. Aliment Pharmacol Ther 1992;6: 221–28.

162. Read NW, Abitbol JL, Bardhan KD, et al. Efficacy and safety of the peripheral kappa agonist fedotozine versus placebo in the treatment of functional dyspepsia. Gut 1997;41:664–68.

163. Fraitag B, Homerin M, Hecketsweiler P. Double-blind dose-response multicenter comparison of fedotozine and placebo in treatment of nonulcer dyspepsia. Dig Dis Sci 1994;39:1072–77.

164. Talley NJ. Visceral analgesics and functional dyspepsia: Have we found the Holy Grail? Gut 1997;41:717–18.

165. Kagan G, Huddlestone L, Wolstencroft P. Comparison of dicyclomine with antacid and without antacid in dyspepsia. J Internat Med Res 1984;12:174–78.

166. Stephens CJM, Level L, Hoare AM. Dicyclomine for idiopathic dyspepsia (letter). Lancet 1988;1:1004.

167. Walters JM, Crean P, McCarthy CF. Trimebutine, a new antispasmodic in the treatment of dyspepsia. Irish Med J 1980;73:380–81.
168. Talley NJ. Functional dyspepsia: Should treatment be targeted on disturbed physiology? Aliment Pharmacol Ther 1995;9:107–15.
169. Maxton DG, Morris J, Whorwell PJ. Selective 5-hydroxytryptamine antagonism: A role in irritable bowel syndrome and functional dyspepsia? Aliment Pharmacol Ther 1996;10:595–99.
170. Muth ER, Jokerst M, Stern RM, et al. Effects of dimenhydrinate on gastric tachyarrhythmia and symptoms of vection-induced motion sickness. Aviat Space Environ Med 1995;66:1041–45.
171. Mertz H, Fass R, Kodner A, et al. Effect of amitriptyline on symptoms, sleep, and visceral perception in patients with functional dyspepsia. Am J Gastroenterol 1998;93:160–65.
173. Tanum L, Malt UF. A new pharmacologic treatment of functional gastrointestinal disorder: a double-blind placebo-controlled study with mianserin. Scand J Gastroenterol 1996;31:318–25.
173. Halter F, Miazza B, Brignoli R. Cisapride or cimetidine in the treatment of functional dyspepsia: results of a double-blind, randomized, Swiss multicentre study. Scand J Gastroenterol 1994;29:618–23.
174. Carvalhinhos A, Fidalgo P, Freire A, et al. Cisapride compared with ranitidine in the treatment of functional dyspepsia. Eur J Gastroenterol Hepatol 1995;7:411–17.
175. Xia H H-X, Kalantar J, Talley NJ. Metronidazole-and-clarithromycin-resistant *Helicobacter pylori* in dyspeptic patients in western Sydney as determined by testing multiple isolates from different gastric sites. J Gastroenterol Hepatol 1998; 13:1027–32.
176. Dundee JW, Yang J, McMillan C: Non-invasive stimulation of the P6 (Neiguan) antiemetic acupuncture point in cancer chemotherapy. Royal Soc Med 1993; 8: 603–606.
177. Dundee JW, Ghaly RG, Bill KM, et al. Effect of stimulation of the P6 antiemetic point on postoperative nausea and vomiting. Brit J Anaesthesiol 1989;63:612–18.
178. Hu S, Stern RM, Koch KL. Electrical acustimulation relieves vection-induced motion sickness. Gastroenterology 1992;102:1854–58.
179. Hu S, Stritzel R, Chandler A, et al. P6 acupressure reduces symptoms of vection-induced motion sickness. Aviat Space Environ Med 1995;66:631–34.
180. Kelly KA. Pacing the gut. Gastroenterology 1992;103:1967–69.
181. McCallum RW, Chen JDZ, et al. Gastric pacing improves emptying and symptoms in patients with gastroparesis. Gastroenterology 1998;114:456–61.
182. Bates S, Sjoden P, Nyren O. Behavioural treatment of non-ulcer dyspepsia. Scand J Behav Ther 1988;17:155–65.
183. Haug TT, Wilhelmsen I, Svebak S, et al. Psychotherapy in functional dyspepsia. J Psychosomat Res 1994;38:735–44.
184. Levitt MD, Furne J, Aeolus MR, et al. Evaluation of an extremely flatulent patients: case report and proposed diagnostic and therapeutic approach. Am J Gastroenterol 1998;93:2276–81.

185. Anonymous. Physiology of belch. Lancet 1991;1:23–24.
186. Talley NJ, Piper DW. Comparison of the clinical features and illness behaviour of patients presenting with dyspepsia of unknown cause (essential dyspepsia) and organic disease. Austral N Z J Med 1986;16:352–59.
187. Lasser RB, Bond LH, Levitt MD. The role of intestinal gas in functional abdominal pain. New Engl J Med 1975;293:524–26.
188. Cuevas JL, Cook EW III, Richter JE, et al. Spontaneous swallowing rate and emotional state: possible mechanism for stress-related gastrointestinal disorders. Dig Dis Sci 1995;40:282–86.
189. Baume P, Tracey M, Dawson L. Efficacy of two minor tranquillizers in relieving symptoms of functional gastrointestinal distress. Austral N Z J Med 1975;5: 503–506.
190. Friis H, Bode S, Rumessen JJ, et al. Effect of simethicone on lactulose-induced H_2 production and gastrointestinal symptoms. Digestion 1991;49:227–30.
191. Spiegel SB. Uses of hypnosis in the treatment of uncontrollable belching: a case report. Am J Clin Hypnosis 1996;38:263–70.
192. Muth ER, Stern RM, Thayer JF, et al. Assessment of multiple dimensions of nausea: the nausea profile [NP]. J Psychosom Res 1996;40:511–20.
193. Anonymous. Psychogenic vomiting: A disorder of gastrointestinal motility? Lancet 1992;339:279.
194. Morgan HG. Functional vomiting. J Psychosom Res 1985;29:341–52.
195. Wruble LD, Rosenthal RH, Webb WL Jr. Psychogenic vomiting: a review. Am J Gastroenterol 1982;77:318–21.
196. Rosenthal RH, Webb WL, Wruble LD. Diagnosis and management of persistent psychogenic vomiting. Psychosomatics 1980;21:722–30.
197. O'Brien MD, Bruce BK, Camilleri M. Rumination syndrome: clinical features rather than manometric diagnosis. Gastroenterology 1995;108:1024–29.
198. Soykan I, Chen JD, Kendall BJ, et al. The rumination syndrome: clinical and manometric profile, therapy and long-term outcome. Dig Dis Sci 1997;42: 1866–72.
199. Malcolm A, Thumshirn MB, Camilleri M, et al. Rumination syndrome. Mayo Clin Proc 1997;72:646–52.
200. Waldholtz BD, Andersen AE. Gastrointestinal aspects of eating disorders. In: Olden KW, Editor. Handbook of Functional Gastrointestinal Disorders. New York: Marcel Dekker;1996:229–53.
201. Fichter MM, Herpetz S, Quadflieg N, et al. Structured interview for anorexic and bulimic disorders for DSM-IV and ICD-10: Updated (Third) revision. Internat J Eat Dis 1998;24:227–49.
202. Wiseman CV, Harris WA, Halmi KA. Eating disorders. Med Clin N Am 1998; 82:145.
203. McGilley BM, Pryor TL. Assessment and treatment of bulimia nervosa. Am Fam Physic 1998;57:2743–50.
204. Brzana RJ, Koch KL. Gastroesophageal reflux disease presenting with intractable nausea. Ann Intern Med 1997;126:704–707.

205. Muraoka M, Mine K, Matsumoto K, et al. Psychogenic vomiting: the relation between patterns of vomiting and psychiatric diagnoses. Gut 1990;31:526–28.
206. Stravynski A. Behavioral treatment of psychogenic vomiting in the context of social phobia. J Nerv Ment Dis 1983;171:448–51.
207. Dura JR. Successful treatment of chronic psychogenic vomiting by self-monitoring. Psychol Rep 1988;62:239–42.

Chapter 7

C. Functional
Bowel Disorders
and D. Functional
Abdominal Pain

W. Grant Thompson, Chair,
George Longstreth, Co-Chair, *with*
Douglas A. Drossman,
Kenneth Heaton,
E. Jan Irvine,
and Stefan Muller-Lissner

C. Functional Bowel Disorders

A functional bowel disorder is a functional gastrointestinal disorder with symptoms attributable to the mid or lower gastrointestinal tract.

The functional bowel disorders include the *irritable bowel syndrome* (IBS), *functional abdominal bloating, functional constipation, functional diarrhea,* and *unspecified functional bowel disorders.*

Following an IBS symposium at the 12th International Congress of Gastroenterology in 1984, a working team was established to define and establish internationally agreed upon criteria for the diagnosis of IBS. After two years of deliberation and a preliminary meeting in Rome, this first working team presented its work at the 13th International Congress in Rome [1]. Subsequently, several working teams met to define and develop criteria for all the functional gastrointestinal disorders [2]. As part of that process, one working team dealt with the functional bowel disorders and functional abdominal pain (Table 1) [2,3]. The existing "Rome" criteria date from that process and were published in 1992.

The Rome Criteria for IBS are widely used in research, but are less employed in research involving other functional gastrointestinal disorders. In the "Rome II" process, new data need serious consideration. Since many functional bowel studies are ongoing using the existing criteria, any changes should not result from consensus, but rather from scientific evidence. The present working team on functional bowel disorders corresponded as a group and gathered evidence over a year before meeting in Rome. In Rome new data were considered judiciously, and then a draft document was circulated to six gastroenterologists interested in the functional bowel disorders worldwide. The results of these deliberations are the subject of this chapter.

Subjects with functional bowel disease (FBD) may be divided into the following groups:

(1) *Non-patients.* Those who have never sought health care for the FBD.
(2) *Patients.* Those who have sought health care for the FBD.
   (a) *Incident Cases.* Those who have sought health care for the FBD for the first time in the past year;
   (b) *Prevalent Cases.* Those who have ever sought health care for the FBD.

To separate these chronic conditions from transient gut symptoms, they must have been present for 12 weeks or more within the preceding 12 months, and the 12 weeks need not be consecutive. In the case of functional abdominal pain, the symptom must have been present at least six months. The diagnosis of a functional bowel disorder or functional abdominal pain always presumes the absence of a structural or biochemical disorder.

Table I. Functional Gastrointestinal Disorders

A. Esophageal Disorders

A1. Globus
A2. Rumination syndrome
A3. Functional Chest Pain of Presumed Esophageal Origin

A4. Functional Heartburn
A5. Functional Dysphagia
A6. Unspecified Functional Esophageal Disorder

B. Gastroduodenal Disorders

B1. Functional Dyspepsia
B1a. Ulcer-like Dyspepsia
B1b. Dysmotility-like Dyspepsia
B1c. Unspecified (nonspecific) Dyspepsia

B2. Aerophagia
B3. Functional Vomiting

C. Bowel Disorders

C1. Irritable Bowel Syndrome
C2. Functional Abdominal Bloating
C3. Functional Constipation

C4. Functional Diarrhea
C5. Unspecified Functional Bowel Disorder

D. Functional Abdominal Pain

D1. Functional Abdominal Pain Syndrome
D2. Unspecified Functional Abdominal Pain

E. Functional Disorders of the Biliary Tract and the Pancreas

E1. Gallbladder Dysfunction
E2. Sphincter of Oddi Dysfunction

F. Anorectal Disorders

F1. Functional Fecal Incontinence
F2. Functional Anorectal Pain
F2a. Levator Ani Syndrome
F2b. Proctalgia Fugax
F3. Pelvic Floor Dyssynergia

G. Functional Pediatric Disorders

G1. Vomiting
G1a. Infant regurgitation
G1b. Infant rumination syndrome
G1c. Cyclic vomiting syndrome
G2. Abdominal pain
G2a. Functional dyspepsia
G2a1. Ulcer-like dyspepsia
G2a2. Dysmotility-like dyspepsia
G2a3. Unspecified (nonspecific) dyspepsia

G2b. Irritable bowel syndrome
G2c. Functional abdominal pain
G2d. Abdominal migraine
G2e. Aerophagia
G3. Functional diarrhea
G4. Disorders of defecation
G4a. Infant dyschezia
G4b. Functional constipation
G4c. Functional fecal retention
G4d. Functional non-retentive fecal soiling

C1. Irritable Bowel Syndrome

— Definition

Irritable Bowel Syndrome comprises a group of functional bowel disorders in which abdominal discomfort or pain is associated with defecation or a change in bowel habit, and with features of disordered defecation.

— Epidemiology

Functional gastrointestinal symptoms occur in a large proportion of adolescent and adult Westerners, and about 10 to 20% have symptoms consistent with a diagnosis of IBS [4–20]. The prevalence of IBS in these epidemiological studies is higher in women than men, and it occurs throughout adulthood. The prevalence appears similar in whites and blacks, but single surveys suggest it is lower in Texas Hispanics [16] and California Asians [15]. The disorder accounts for 20 to 50% of referrals to gastroenterology clinics [21–25]. Some studies suggest that females may be more likely to consult a physician [4,11,21–23,25,26], while others do not [18,19]. Symptoms of IBS come and go over time and often overlap with dyspepsia [27,28] (see Chapter 6 covering gastroduodenal disorders).

Social and cultural factors may influence the prevalence of IBS in clinical practice. Irritable bowel syndrome is common in the Indian subcontinent [29–33] and Japan [34,35]. It seems as prevalent in China [36] as in Western countries, and is also common in Nigerian medical students [37]. It is less common in Thailand [38]. In South African blacks, it is unusual in rural areas but appears to be common in cities [39]. Female patients predominate in Western countries but represent only 20 to 30% of IBS patients in India and Sri Lanka [29–33].

The cost to society in terms of direct medical expenses and indirect costs, such as work absenteeism, is considerable [4,40,41]. There are between 2.4 and 3.5 million physician visits annually for IBS in the United States, during which 2.2 million prescriptions are written [42]. In a national survey of US households, those with IBS by the Rome Criteria and lacking history of structural disease were compared to those without the syndrome [4]. People with any functional gastro-intestinal disorder were more likely to be too sick to work, had missed more days of work in the past year, and had more physician visits for gut complaints as well as for nongastrointestinal complaints. Undergraduate students with IBS showed at least as much impairment on multiple indices of quality of life as patients with congestive heart failure [43], and elderly people also reported that functional status and quality of life were impaired by functional colonic symptoms [44]. A survey of Minnesota residents, including calculation of their inpatient and outpatient health services charges exclusive of outpatient drug costs, revealed overall median charges incurred by subjects with IBS were $472 compared with $429 for controls. Extrapolation of the results yielded estimated excess charges for IBS in the US white population of eight billion dollars yearly [41]. Unnecessary tests, inappropriate management, and even unnecessary surgery account for some of these costs [45–48].

Thus IBS affects a substantial percentage of adults in all regions of the world. While point prevalences are estimated at 10 to 20%, lifetime prevalences are much higher. The sheer numbers bespeak a very important disorder from well-being and economic points of view. In addition, IBS patients' discomfort and worry about the meaning of symptoms generate many consultations, tests, and treatment that draw resources from more serious gut disorders.

— Development of the Rome I IBS Diagnostic Criteria

In 1978, Manning et al., using questionnaire data from 32 patients with IBS and 33 patients with organic diseases, found four symptoms were more common in those with IBS [49] (Table 2). Although the proportions with mucus per rectum and feeling of incomplete emptying were not statistically different, discrimination between the two groups was increased when these factors were combined with the other four symptoms. In 1984, Kruis et al. found that the combination of abdominal pain, flatulence, bowel irregularity, the presence of symptoms for more than two years, and diarrhea alternating with constipation were more common in IBS [50]. In a later survey, the four independently significant Manning symptoms discriminated IBS from peptic ulcer; however, only abdominal distension (and the non-Manning symptoms, straining at stool and presence of scybala) distinguished IBS from inflammatory bowel disease [26]. The four core Manning symptoms have also been found to be useful in India [51] and Korea [52], and the more Manning symptoms that are present, the greater their diagnostic value [53], particularly in younger patients [54]. Interpretation of validation studies has been complicated by the large proportion of patients with upper gastrointestinal disease in the organic disease comparison groups [50,53,55].

Gender comparisons have found the value of the Manning symptoms in men to vary from similarly reliable [53] to less reliable [54] to unreliable [56]. A study of individual Manning symptoms in 130 female and 26 male IBS patients

Table 2. Symptoms More Likely To Be Found In Irritable Bowel Syndrome (IBS) Than In Organic Abdominal Disease

	Organic	IBS	Significance
Manning et al. [49]			
Pain eased after bowel movement	9/30	25/31	p < 0.01
Looser stools at onset of pain	8/30	25/31	p < 0.001
More frequent bowel movements at onset of pain	9/30	23/31	p < 0.01
Abdominal distension	7/33	17/32	p < 0.01
Mucus per rectum	7/33	15/32	0.05 < p < 0.1
Feeling of incomplete emptying	11/33	19/32	0.05 < p < 0.1
Kruis et al. [50]			
n (sample size)	299	108	
A. Abdominal pain	55%	96%	p < 0.61
B. Flatulence	50%	85%	p < 0.4
C. Irregularity	42%	85%	p < 0.025
A + B + C	0%	70%	p < 0.0005
Symptoms more than 2 yrs	39%	70%	p < 0.0005
Diarrhea and constipation	30%	65%	p < 0.0005
Pellety stools or mucus	38%	76%	p < 0.0001

revealed that the three pain-related symptoms were similarly present in women and men: pain relief by defecation, 77% versus 85%; looser stools at onset of pain, 65% versus 65%; and more frequent stools at onset of pain, 64% versus 65%. However, the other three symptoms, in addition to scybala, were less prevalent in males [57]. Both the Manning criteria (abdominal pain plus at least two Manning symptoms) and the 1992 Rome criteria [3] were more sensitive for diagnosing IBS in women than men, but the differences were not statistically significant. Therefore, less reporting of the non-pain-related symptoms could contribute to the reduced sensitivity of the Manning and Rome Criteria as well as the lower reported prevalence of IBS in men.

Factor analysis identified symptom clusters in three groups (Table 3). Twenty-three bowel symptoms including the Manning symptoms were evaluated. The first four Manning symptoms covaried (bloating loaded weakly) in 351 women visiting Planned Parenthood clinics and in 149 women recruited through church women's societies [58], and three of them (excluding bloating) covaried. A gastrointestinal reaction to food loaded weakly in both groups. In a similar study conducted in university psychology students, clustering of three of

Table 3. IBS Defined by Factor Analysis in Three Groups

	Group 1				Group 2	Group 3
	Males	Females	Whites	Blacks	Females	Females
Manning Symptoms						
Loose BM,						
pain onset	X	X	X	X	X	X
Frequent BM,						
pain onset	X	X	X	X	X	X
Pain relief						
by BM	X	X	X	X	X	X
Bloating	X				X	
Incomplete						
evacuation						
Rectal mucus						
Other Symptoms						
Food reactions		X	X		X	X
Rectal						
bleeding	X					
Abdominal pain						X
Diarrhea						X
Milk reactions					X	

X = Symptom with a loading (i.e., correlation with) the factor of 0.4 or greater; BM = bowel movement. Group 1 data from Taub E, et al., 1995 [17]. Groups 2 and 3 data from Whitehead, et al.1990 [58].

the primary symptoms (excluding bloating) occurred in females, whites, and blacks, while clustering of all four symptoms occurred in males (bloating loaded weakly) [17]. Therefore, the symptoms that withstand assessment to date are discomfort or pain that is relieved by defecation, associated with a change in frequency of stool, or associated with a change in consistency of stool. The word "consistency" is replaced with "form" to conform with the Bristol stool scale (fig. 1, Table 4) [59]. These three symptoms comprise the first part of the Rome I diagnostic criteria.

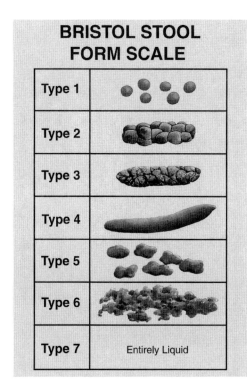

BRISTOL STOOL FORM SCALE

Type 1	
Type 2	
Type 3	
Type 4	
Type 5	
Type 6	
Type 7	Entirely Liquid

Figure 1. The Bristol Stool Form Scale. See Table 4 for standard description for each of the seven types.

Table 4. The Bristol Stool Form Scale

Type	Description
1	Separate hard lumps like nuts (difficult to pass)
2	Sausage shaped but lumpy
3	Like a sausage but with cracks on its surface
4	Like a sausage or snake, smooth and soft
5	Soft blobs with clear-cut edges (passed easily)
6	Fluffy pieces with ragged edges, a mushy stool
7	Watery, no solid pieces, ENTIRELY LIQUID

— Diagnostic Criteria* for IBS

At least 12 weeks or more, which need not be consecutive, in the preceding 12 months of abdominal discomfort or pain that has two out of three features:

(1) Relieved with defecation; *and/or*
(2) Onset associated with a change in frequency of stool; *and/or*
(3) Onset associated with a change in form (appearance) of stool.

Symptoms that Cumulatively Support the
Diagnosis of Irritable Bowel Syndrome

- *Abnormal stool frequency (for research purposes "abnormal" may be defined as greater than 3 bowel movements per day and less than 3 bowel movements per week);*
- *Abnormal stool form (lumpy/hard or loose/watery stool);*
- *Abnormal stool passage (straining, urgency, or feeling of incomplete evacuation);*
- *Passage of mucus;*
- *Bloating or feeling of abdominal distension.*

* In the absence of structural or metabolic abnormalities to explain the symptoms.

— Rationale for Changes in Diagnostic Criteria for Rome II

The 1998 Working Team propose changes to the definition and diagnostic criteria for IBS to reflect new research data, and to improve clarity and internal consistency.

In the definition, the change from "disorder" to "disorders" acknowledges the possibility of several pathophysiologies of IBS. The addition of the term "discomfort" to "pain" allows broader symptom description and is in line with the criteria. "Distension" is deleted since it is no longer a diagnostic criterion. The word "consistency" is replaced by "form," as supported by the above discussion.

In the Diagnostic Criteria, "discomfort" and "pain" are reversed to reflect severity progression. The pain-related criteria are unchanged, a decision supported by factor analyses on non-patients [17,58], and their equal presence in female and male patients [57]. The second part of the 1994 criteria is eliminated because of poor clustering of these non-pain-related symptoms in factor analyses

[17,60], their lesser prevalence in males [57], and duplication of the stool frequency and form symptoms in the pain-related criteria. They are retained as non-essential symptoms, that increase diagnostic accuracy [26,49], and help identify IBS subgroups if desired (Table 5) [51–53,56]. These symptoms are clarified by replacing the term "altered" with "abnormal."

Finally, the requirement that two of the three pain-related criteria be required for the diagnosis of IBS is to insure that altered bowel habit is present. These are three of the four "significant" original Manning criteria that cluster in population studies [17,58], and they occur in the clinic [47,49,54]. The fourth, "distension", is less consistently present [60], and in the clinic, is less common in males [56,57]. These changes are based partly on the results of these factor analyses, which also provide evidence that the IBS is a distinct syndrome. In these studies [17,26,49,54,57,60], subjects were surveyed for groups of symptoms that tend to occur together (cluster or covary) in the same individuals. We considered the degree of correlation or "loading" of each symptom in multiple study groups (Table 3). We also believe that these changes permit greater separation between IBS and functional constipation.

Suggested Way to Subclassify IBS

It should be noted that the Manning and Kruis criteria were derived from clinical data that indicated that they were more likely to be found in patients with IBS than organic abdominal disease. The Rome I Criteria, in contrast, while largely drawn from the Manning and Kruis data, were intended to provide comprehensive clinical definitions of patients with IBS and other functional gastrointestinal disorders in order to better identify clinical syndromes and ensure homogeneity of patients in clinical trials.

If desired, one or more of the symptoms listed in italic type in the Criteria, which are not essential for the diagnosis but are usually present, may be used to identify subgroups of IBS (see below). They add to the doctor's confidence that the intestine is the origin of the abdominal pain. The more of these symptoms that are present, the more confident is the diagnosis [26,49].

We believe that subclassification of IBS into constipation-predominant, diarrhea-predominant and mixed patterns has limited value in understanding the pathophysiology of the disorder [27]. Indeed we believe most patients will be found to alternate if followed long enough. However, when clinical trials require the exclusion of patients with predominant diarrhea or constipation, it is reasonable to use these symptoms as shown in Table 5. An approximate estimate of colonic transit time can also be made by having the patient record the appearance of their stools (e.g., using the Bristol Stool Form Scale) [59].

Table 5. Supportive Symptoms of IBS

(1)	Fewer than three bowel movements a week
(2)	More than three bowel movements a day
(3)	Hard or lumpy stools
(4)	Loose (mushy) or watery stools
(5)	Straining during a bowel movement
(6)	Urgency (having to rush to have a bowel movement)
(7)	Feeling of incomplete bowel movement
(8)	Passing mucus (white material) during a bowel movement
(9)	Abdominal fullness, bloating, or swelling

Diarrhea-predominant: 1 or more of 2, 4, or 6 and none of 1, 3, or 5;
   or: 2 or more of 2, 4, or 6 and one of 1 or 5. (3. Hard or lumpy stools
do not qualify.)

Constipation-predominant: 1 or more of 1, 3, or 5 and none of 2, 4, or 6;
   or: 2 or more of 1, 3, or 5 and one of 2, 4, or 6.

— Clinical Evaluation

Careful interpretation of the pain and stool characteristics is the most important step in recognizing IBS. Pain related in some way to defecation is likely to be a bowel pain, while that associated with exercise, movement, urination, or menstruation may have a different cause. Chaudhary and Truelove retrospectively recorded postprandial symptom exacerbation [61], and many patients report that symptoms follow eating. One group recorded increased sigmoid pressures in response to eating [62]. However, the diagnostic reliability of postprandial symptoms has received little research attention; gastrointestinal reaction to food loaded only weakly in a factor analysis study [58]. Other symptoms that have not been assessed as discriminating for IBS include the "morning rush syndrome," incontinence, and nocturnal pain. Nevertheless, they are frequently reported by IBS patients.

Many women with IBS consult a gynecologist for "pelvic pain" [63–66]. For example, 79% of women outpatients with chronic pelvic pain according to their gynecologists' criteria had IBS [67]. In addition to the symptom overlap, there is a remarkable similarity between the psychosocial factors underlying IBS and the gynecologic patients' disorder [68]. Clearly, a physician's point of view often determines what he/she calls the pain and the subsequent testing and treatment decisions. The common occurrence of dyspareunia or other sexual dysfunction in women with IBS [67,69–71] and sometimes worsening of IBS symptoms during menstruation [72,73] may obscure the diagnosis of IBS, but the association of the pain with defecation and bowel dysfunction defines it as a gastrointestinal, not a gynecological condition.

The patient's use of the terms "diarrhea" and "constipation" may mislead [74]. The stool may be solid even though defecation is frequent [59,74–76]. Conversely, straining to defecate may occur with soft or watery stools. Some patients may feel they are constipated because they have unproductive calls to stool or feelings of incomplete evacuation that prompt them to strain after the stool is passed [77]. These observations make subtypes of IBS problematic (Table 5).

There are often other gastrointestinal, somatic, and psychological symptoms in those patients seen by a specialist. These may include heartburn and other upper gastrointestinal symptoms [70,78,79], fibromyalgia [80–82], headache [83], backache [70], genitourinary symptoms [70,84,85], and psychosocial dysfunction (see below). While these symptoms increase in number as the severity of IBS increases [15,86], they are not essential for the diagnosis since they are infrequent in non-health care seekers [87–89]. Although one group found these "non-colonic" symptoms helped distinguish IBS from organic disease [90], other investigators did not [91]. Obviously, a common disorder such as IBS may coexist with organic gastrointestinal disease [92].

Irritable bowel syndrome should be diagnosed from the history along with absence of symptoms or signs of anatomic disease. These include fever, gastrointestinal bleeding, weight loss, anemia, abdominal mass and other "alarm" symptoms or signs that are not explained by a functional bowel disorder [50, 93]. A physical examination is important to look for other diseases and provide the authority for the physician to reassure the patient. While there are no proven discriminating physical signs of IBS, abdominal tenderness may be present. Abdominal scars are common in those patients who show abnormal illness behaviors. A surgeon may misdiagnose the cause of a patient's IBS pain as a disease predisposing him or her to hospitalization [94], and operation [94–96], especially hysterectomy [13,15]. As many as 47% [97] and 55% [98] of women with IBS have undergone hysterectomy or ovarian surgery. A gastroenterology consultation for gynecologists' patients with "pelvic pain" reduces the hysterectomy rate [99].

A sigmoidoscopy is recommended to rule out inflammation or tumors [100]. Melanosis coli may be found, signaling the likelihood of laxative use or abuse [101]. In addition, mucus, "scybala," or lumpy or ribbon stools may be seen, even though the patient may not have complained about them [59]. Some physicians think the procedure allows detection of hypersensitivity to pain, which is of diagnostic usefulness [102,103]. Reproduction of the pain during sigmoidoscopy may help convince the patient of its source. The symptoms described are not those of microscopic or collagenous colitis, so rectal biopsy is not normally indicated [104]. Nevertheless, only about 10% of primary care physicians ever perform sigmoidoscopy [105,106], and most diagnose IBS with no tests at all [106,107]. In a young person, with typical symptoms and no alarm symptoms, this approach seems realistic.

However, imaging or endoscopy of the large bowel should usually be done in IBS patients referred to specialists. Sigmoidoscopy is often adequate, but colonoscopy or barium enema may be indicated in older patients, atypical symptoms, family history, procedure availability, and other factors as judged by the specialist.

Care should be taken to avoid unnecessary investigations that may be costly and even harmful. Blood may be drawn once for a complete blood cell count and measurement of erythrocyte sedimentation rate or C-reactive protein, but such tests are rarely abnormal in patients identified by symptom criteria [108]. Further testing depends on the individual situation. The physician's decision to test further may be influenced by the age and sex of the patient, the nature and duration of symptoms, the region of practice, costs, and other factors, but common sense must prevail. Tests may include a stool examination for occult blood, leukocytes, or ova and parasites (Giardia). Often, none of these is indicated. Since documentation of lactase deficiency seldom leads to improvement of IBS symptoms [109,110], routine testing for it is unnecessary. Notably, one-third of people who report severe lactose intolerance absorb lactose normally, and lactose malabsorbers can consume eight ounces of milk a day with negligible symptoms [111,112]. Although most physicians would examine for colon neoplasia with barium enema or colonoscopy in selected cases, this is usually unnecessary for IBS patients under 40 or 50 years old who have no family history of colon cancer [113]. Diverticulosis on a barium enema does not change the diagnosis of IBS [114,115] (fig. 2). They often coexist, but are not causally related. Routine abdominal ultrasound examination is not helpful [116]. It is important to try to make the diagnosis and explain it to the patient at the initial visit.

There is no evidence that liability to other diseases or life expectancy are altered by the IBS, but most patients remain symptomatic or experience relapses for many years following diagnosis [28,117–120]. An initial diagnosis of IBS should be a safe one and rarely needs revision over time [117,119,121]. A change in the clinical picture may warrant additional investigation, but the simple persistence of symptoms does not justify suspicion of another diagnosis. Indeed, such persistence is to be expected, and further needless investigation only undermines the patient's confidence in the diagnosis and the physician.

Thus, careful history is the most important diagnostic procedure, and lack of explanatory abnormalities on physical examination lends further support. A confident diagnosis that holds up over time can usually be achieved through limited laboratory and structural evaluations that are appropriate to the patient's age and risk factors for cancer.

— Physiologic Features

Many investigators have sought to identify a unique physiologic abnormality in IBS [122–126]. Abnormalities in large and small gut motility, myoelectric activity, or sensitivity have not proved to be sensitive or specific [127–129]. Observations indicated that the rectosigmoid motility index was increased in constipation and decreased in diarrhea and suggested a sigmoid sphincter action [130,131]. However, this is not noted in all patients, is not

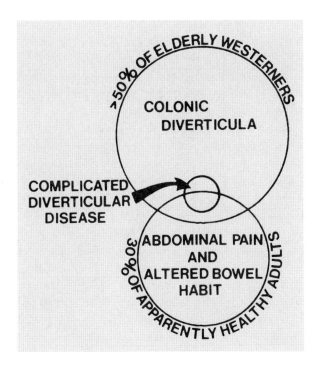

Figure 2. The relationship of colonic diverticula to IBS. Most people with colonic diverticula are unaware of them. However, both IBS and diverticula are very common, the latter especially in the elderly, so it is inevitable that both may occur in many people. The IBS symptoms cannot be blamed on diverticula, nor can diverticula be blamed on IBS. Diverticulitis occurs only in those with diverticula, and some of them also have IBS.

specific for IBS, and is based on data obtained from only the rectosigmoid. A 3-cycle/min colonic myoelectric rhythm was found by two teams of investigators to be more prevalent in IBS patients than in control subjects [132,133]. A third group found this pattern in psychoneurotic patients without IBS [134], and a fourth showed no change in myoelectric pattern or motility when IBS symptoms improved [135]. Using a different technology, French researchers correlated bowel function to fast and slow colon contractions [136]. Colonic transit time measured by scintigraphy has revealed accelerated transit in patients with diarrhea-predominant IBS [137] and delayed transit in constipation [138]. While IBS patients as a group show an exaggerated or altered response in the small and large intestines to various stimuli, which include diet, fatty acids, bile salts, hormones, and physical and psychological stress [139–144], no test has been established as a diagnostic standard. Even the demonstrations in many cases that insufflation of balloons within the small and large intestines of IBS patients can sometimes reproduce their pain [139,145] only shows that the gut could be the site of the pain. Postprandial small bowel dysmotility may be due to gut hypersensitivity [146]. There must, of course, be a motility disturbance in the IBS to the extent that there is true constipation or diarrhea. However, motility observations do not clarify how the symptoms are generated, and they are of little practical value to clinicians.

The inability to demonstrate a precise motility disturbance to explain the symptoms and the apparent hypersensitivity of the irritable bowel to many stimuli raise the possibility that the symptoms might also be due to altered perception. Indeed it is likely that the manner in which gut information is processed in the central nervous system (CNS) may help determine how IBS symptoms are perceived and acted on. For example, urgency, usually associated with loose stools, may be reported by patients with IBS who have normal formed stools. In addition, frequent passage of scybala are often complained of as diarrhea, yet scybala are known to be associated with delayed gut transit [59]. Conversely, some claim to have no defecation for days, yet radio-opaque markers pass within 48 hours (denied defecation). Patient recall for symptoms is less accurate than are daily diaries [76]. Altered perception of such a symptom as pain or bloating is less easy to document (see physiologic data under sections on "functional abdominal bloating" and "functional abdominal pain").

Recent research efforts have addressed the role of visceral hyperalgesia in symptom pathogenesis, including dysfunctions of both peripheral afferent nerves and central processing of afferent information. Altered rectal perception has been found in most IBS patients, and longitudinal evaluations indicated a correlation between changes in perception threshold and symptom severity [147,148]. Repetitive sigmoid stimulation induced rectal hyperalgesia in IBS patients but not in normal controls [149]. The sigmoid is hypersensitive to balloon distension, but not to electrical currents. This suggests there is selective dysfunction of mechanosensitive intestinal pathways and central dysfunction of viscerosomatic referral [150]. Mental activity can also modulate gut perception [151]. Measurements of autonomic function in patients with IBS revealed a cholinergic abnormality in those with predominant constipation, and adrenergic abnormality in patients with predominant diarrhea [152]. Certain personality traits are linked with jejunal sensorimotor dysfunction [146]. Such work suggests that psychosocial factors induce excessive sympathetic response to stress, which in turn leads to small bowel sensorimotor disturbance.

Positron Emission Tomography (PET) was used to evaluate regional CNS response to rectal distension, or the anticipation of rectal distension, in six IBS patients referred to specialists and six control subjects [153]. Irritable bowel syndrome patients (who exhibit visceral hypersensitivity), in contrast to controls, failed to activate the anterior cingulate cortex, an area of the limbic system associated with active opiate binding, but did activate the prefrontal cortex, an area associated with hypervigilance and anxiety. This study suggests that referred IBS patients who have visceral hyperalgesia, may fail to use CNS downregulating mechanisms in response to incoming or anticipated visceral pain. Instead, they may activate an area of the brain that amplifies pain perception. These observations emphasize the importance of an integrative model for IBS which includes biomedical and psychosocial factors [154].

Collins has speculated that mucosal inflammation may play a pathogenetic role in some IBS patients [155]. Cytokines could be released by dietary, infectious, or other factors. Mucosal dysfunction is reflected by ileal sensitivity to bile acids [156] and malabsorption of sugars, such as fructose and sorbitol [157]. Increased lamina propria cellularity has been found in IBS patients, which could alter smooth muscle and enteric nervous system function [155]. IBS frequently dates from an enteric infection, often traveler's diarrhea [61,158,159]. Immune hypersensitivity has been reported [160,161], and preliminary studies reveal increased mast cells in the colonic muscularis mucosa [162] and terminal ileal mucosa [163]. However, careful examination of colon biopsy specimens from patients fulfilling the Rome Criteria for IBS demonstrates no histologic difference from control specimens [164].

The stimulus that generates the experience of pain (nociception) initiates neuronal discharges that must pass through the enteric nervous system (ENS), its vagal and sympathetic connections to the CNS, and the ascending pathways in the spinal cord to centers in the hindbrain and midbrain before reaching consciousness in the cerebral cortex. Along the way, neuronal messages may be altered by synapses with somatic and descending pathways. Thus, the symptoms of pain (or bloating) may be augmented or suppressed by events elsewhere in the body or brain [165].

Painful or pleasurable somatic stimuli, strong emotion, or cognitive experience may thus modify how a visceral sensation is perceived. If an individual has learned as a child to attach great significance to physical symptoms, health care-seeking behavior later in life may be augmented [7,166]. Psychological disturbances may also influence how IBS is perceived. Patients seeing physicians are often suffering from psychological disturbance [89,167].

In summary, potentially important pathophysiological factors have been described throughout the brain-gut axis, including dysmotility, gut hypersensitivity, altered symptom perception, afferent sensory and autonomic nerve dysfunction, altered brain activation, mucosal abnormality, and psychophysiology. The available data do not permit a consensus judgment on the relative importance of these factors, which appear to vary from patient to patient.

— Psychological Features

It is unclear to what extent IBS symptoms represent normal perception of abnormal function or abnormal perception of normal function [168]. Some physiologists theorize that prolonged visceral stimulation by inflammation or other noxious influences may sensitize receptors in the gut with a normally higher threshold [149]. Previously silent nociceptors then trigger central mechanisms that enhance and sustain the symptom even after the stimulation ceases. This postulated mechanism has gained recent experimental support [149], and draws attention to the possible roles of the afferent and central nervous systems in generating IBS symptoms such as pain and bloating. An afferent abnormality may help explain those IBS cases that are apparently triggered by an attack of gastroenteritis [61,158,159]. Despite the presence of visceral hypersensitivity discussed above, IBS patients do not appear to have a lowered somatic pain threshold [169,170].

Most studies indicate that mood and personality disturbances, psychiatric disease, and illness behavior are more common in IBS patients seen by a specialist than in other patients and normal subjects [46,123,125,171–177]. A retrospective study of previously gathered data determined that major depression, panic disorder, and agoraphobia were more common in those with IBS than in others [178]. Other data suggest that psychosocial criteria are of little value in differentiating the IBS from organic disorders [120,179,180]. In two studies of people in the community, those with IBS who did not consult physicians appeared to have psychological and personality profiles similar to those without symptoms [88,89]. In contrast, a New Zealand study found similar neurotic symptoms in health care seekers and non-patients [181]. Other studies have shown that the number of IBS symptoms [11], severity of pain, and health anxiety [182] were

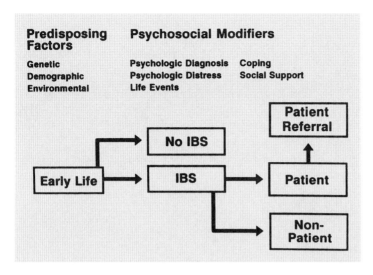

Figure 3. Schema indicating how many factors may interact to produce IBS symptoms, and symptom reporting. (From Drossman and Thompson, 1992[123]. Reprinted with permission)

Table 6. Spectrum of Clinical Features Among Patients with Irritable Bowel Syndrome

	Mild	Moderate	Severe
Estimated prevalence	70%	25%	5%
Clinical setting	Primary	Secondary	Tertiary
Physiologic correlation	+++	++	+
Symptom constancy	0	+	+++
Activity disruption	0	+	+++
Health care use	+	++	+++
Illness behavior	0	+	+++
Psychiatric diagnoses	0	+	+++

0 = generally absent; + = mild; ++ = moderate; +++ = severe. Source: Reproduced with permission from Drossman and Thompson 1992 [123].

major factors in care-seeking. The prevalence of psychological disorders in community samples is much lower than that found in tertiary care centers. Also, it is likely that patients seen in these centers may have more psychological distress than those seen by general practitioners or internists [123] (Table 6). Figure 3 illustrates how these factors may affect disability and health care use.

Stressful stimuli may alter small [141,144] and large [183] gut function. They often cause abdominal pain or bowel habit change in non-consulters, especially women [184]. Stressful life events frequently precede the onset of IBS symptoms, or at least the reporting of them to a physician [185–187]. Multiple lines of evidence support a link between a history of abuse and functional gastrointestinal disorders [188]. Sexual or physical abuse is a frequent, yet often hidden experience in women referred for functional disorders [189]. An abuse history has been found more often in subjects with IBS than in comparison groups in California health maintenance organization examinees [15], Minnesota residents [190], and French patients [191]. There is also a progressive increase in the frequency of abuse history with increasing IBS severity [15,188,189]. The severity of abuse is associated with health status [192,193]. There are associations between abuse and health impact and care seeking; and the number of somatic symptoms [15,189], surgeries [15,189], and physician visits for gastrointestinal symptoms [194]. There is an independent effect of abuse on six measures of health status in female gastroenterology patients [195]. Abuse is also related to health care visits during the subsequent year, but the visits were related to symptoms and disability, not abuse itself [194]. An explanation for the link between abuse and IBS is a tendency for abused patients to use catastrophizing coping strategies and to have a relatively low cognitive standard for judging stimuli as noxious [193,196, 197]; however, the increased pain sensitivity of IBS patients may be independent of abuse [198]. In Australia, abuse is associated with neuroticism and psychological morbidity, but not with IBS when psychological factors were controlled [199].

Therefore a patient's psychological traits, recent exposure to stress, and previous trauma, including abuse, may influence the experience of IBS symptoms and the individual's reaction to them. As with physiological features, these factors may vary among patients. However, interactions between the body and brain play important roles in symptom pathogenesis [200].

— Approach to Treatment

General Measures

We believe that sensible management of the IBS, and indeed of all functional gastrointestinal disorders, depends on a confident diagnosis [48,93, 123]. This can be made with a high degree of accuracy on the first visit using clinical criteria [3]. A confident diagnosis prevents over-investigation and reassures the patient that his or her symptoms are not due to cancer or another serious disease. A careful explanation of the syndrome reassures most patients, and prompt, confident reassurance may be the physician's most important therapeutic tool. Fear of cancer is a major concern for IBS patients in primary care, and one study suggests they are not promptly reassured by their doctors [107]. Repeated or inappropriate tests communicate physician insecurity and breed fear and uncertainty in the patient.

The Patient's Agenda

It is important to consider why the patient is coming now. The reason may be an important clue to management. For example, a recent death in the family may raise fears of serious disease, so treatment should be directed toward convincing the patient that such fears are unfounded. A new diet, medication, or disease may precipitate a visit. Environmental stress, substance abuse, recent life-threatening event, or psychiatric comorbidity may need special attention. There may be some conscious or unconscious benefit from being ill, such as a disability pension or manipulation of a family member. These factors may become more important to the patient than the physical symptoms, and should influence the management plan. One should also assess the patient's quality of life and level of daily functioning. Sometimes, cure is unattainable, and the therapeutic objective should be improving the individual's functioning in society.

A Graded, Multicomponent Approach (Table 6)

Those IBS subjects not seeing physicians appear to be little troubled by their symptoms and require no treatment. In contrast, those seen by specialists in tertiary care centers have the most difficulty and a tendency to depression, anxiety, panic, or other psychosocial disorders. Those in primary or secondary care, although not well studied, likely occupy an intermediate position [107].

Treatment is determined by the type and severity of symptoms as well as psychosocial issues [93,122,123,125,201,202]. In addition to fear of serious disease, careful evaluation of other, frequently unstated, factors is important. The interview should provide the opportunity for the patient to describe his or her symptoms, and the events and life circumstances that may affect the symptoms. Complex psychosocial problems might be lifelong or of recent onset. One should take into account the patient's personality, recent life stress [203–205] (divorce, bereavement, job loss), anxiety, and depression [122,206]. The effect of such stressors must be explored and their role in the genesis of gut symptoms discussed. The patient's reaction to the symptoms may be more important than the symptoms themselves. Indeed, as discussed, psychological factors may alter perception of symptoms. Most patients respond to the psychological support that any sympathetic physician can provide [207]. Dutch patients showed reduced anxiety, fear of cancer, somatic attribution concerning the gastrointestinal tract, and catastrophizing cognitions between the first and last visit in the consulting period for functional abdominal complaints [208]. A strong physician-patient relationship helps control health care utilization. A long-term follow-up study found that notations in the medical record about psychosocial history, precipitating factors, and discussion of diagnosis and treatment with patients were associated with fewer return visits for IBS-related symptoms and fewer hospitalizations [97]. A few patients will require help from psychologists or psychiatrists or need antidepressant or other psychopharmacologic therapy [207,209,210].

The unsatisfied patient is liable to have unnecessary surgery [15,95,98,195, 211], undergo unjustified and hazardous investigation, or take unproven medication, such as those provided by practitioners of alternative medicine [212–214]. In these difficult cases, the primary care physician should provide continuing care. This professional can reinforce the interventions described above and continue to provide emotional support for the patient when these special treatments are completed. Although often helpful, such interventions are seldom curative. The family physician is therefore best positioned to retain medical contact for the patient, guard against overtesting and harmful treatments, and provide the understanding that these patients require.

Diet

Dietary advice may be helpful to some IBS patients. If drugs, lactose, coffee, alcohol, or gas-forming vegetables seem to provoke symptoms, appropriate advice should be provided. However, the poor correlation between reported lactose intolerance and true lactose malabsorption [111], the failure of lactose restriction to improve symptoms [109,110], and the potential denial to the patient of an important source of calcium should be kept in mind. Excess use of artificial sweeteners such as sorbitol or mannitol found in some diet gums and confections should be avoided. Regular meals ingested in quiet surroundings should be encouraged, and potentially dangerous fad diets avoided.

Food intolerance is often suggested as a possible cause of IBS [161,215]. Some successful elimination diets are reported primarily in patients with diarrhea, but the results have not been confirmed [216–218]. An elimination diet (with double-blind identification of provocative foods by nasogastric tube-feeding) is cumbersome and often unrewarding (see category C4). There is no evidence that Candida causes IBS [219,220].

Wheat bran is time-honored therapy, but the high placebo response and methodological difficulties are features of existing clinical trials [202]. However, sufficient doses of bran do improve constipation, hard stools, and straining

[221–225]. The effect is maximized if at least 30 g of fiber is taken daily [226]. Many experience improvement in diarrhea or pain as well, but these may be placebo responses. The principal advantages of bran are its economy and its safety. However, some patients referred to specialists report no improvement or worsening (bran failures) [227,228].

Drugs

Many drugs have been proposed for the treatment of IBS. However, the variety of symptoms, the lack of understanding of the pathophysiology, and the complex interaction of the CNS and ENS and their many receptors, must raise doubts that a single drug could correct IBS. According to Klein [229], clinical trials of IBS treatments published until 1986 all suffer from methodological inadequacies, including unstated [230], unclear, or irrelevant [35] entry criteria; small patient sample [35,231]; too many dropouts; short study periods [230]; or improper use of statistics or study design [231]. All studies are complicated by a placebo response of 40 to 80% [46,229]. To quote Klein [229] "... no single study offers convincing evidence that any therapy is effective in treating the IBS symptom complex."

However, medication may be helpful when diarrhea, constipation, or abdominal pain is the dominant symptom (Table 7). Loperamide [202,232,233] may prevent diarrhea when taken before a meal or an activity that often leads to the symptom. Cholestyramine may theoretically improve diarrhea [234], but controlled trials are lacking. Small clinical trials testing the efficacy of calcium channel blockers such as verapamil [235] have not been encouraging [202].

Constipation may be helped by commercial fiber analogues, such as psyllium and methylcellulose, but they may increase bloating [236]. A preliminary study found calcium polycarbophil to be helpful for constipation with bloating [237]. Cisapride for treatment of constipation-predominant IBS was found to be ineffective [238], and one study supporting its use forbade a high-fiber diet [239]. Lactulose [240,241] or polyethylene glycol [242,243] may be useful in refractory cases, but patient acceptance may be poor, and the diagnosis may not be IBS.

Pain in IBS has been treated by anticholinergics/antispasmodics for half a century without any proven impact, with troublesome side effects, and with disparaging reviews [229,244–246]. New variants still appear [231,247–250,248]. Peppermint oil appears ineffective [247]. Mebeverine, popular in some countries, is said to normalize small bowel motility in IBS [251], and appears useful to some reviewers [202]. A meta-analysis conclusion that seven smooth muscle relaxants and anticholinergics are better than placebo for some IBS symptoms

Table 7. Drugs for a Dominant Symptom in Irritable Bowel Syndrome

Symptom	Drug	Dose
Diarrhea	Loperamide	1–2 tablets when necessary, maximum 6 tablets daily
	Cholestyramine	1 scoop or packet with meals
Constipation	Psyllium	1 Tbsp bid with meals, then adjust
	Methylcellulose	1 Tbsp bid with meals, then adjust
	Calcium Polycarbophil	1g qd to qid
	Lactulose*	1–2 Tbsp bid (may cause bloating)
	70% Sorbitol*	1 Tbsp bid (may cause bloating)
	PEG solution*	250 ml bid
Abdominal pain	Anticholinergic/ Antispasmodic	Take AC, if pain is PC
	Tricyclic antidepressants	For intractable pain

PEG = polyethylene glycol; AC = before meals; PC = after meals.

*Consider a primary diagnosis of constipation if needed.

Note: These drugs are in common use though there is no compelling evidence that these drugs are effective in the treatment of IBS.

[252] should be regarded cautiously. The drugs have disparate activities, and the studies analyzed were among those criticized by Klein [229]. Moreover, this analysis and the literature generally suffer from a significant publication bias as negative trials tend not to be reported.

Pain sometimes responds to tricyclic antidepressant drugs in lower doses than are needed for depression [252–258]. These drugs alter small intestinal motor function [259] and increase orocecal and whole gut transit times [260], but they likely act through analgesic effects on higher centers (see section on Chronic Abdominal Pain for further discussion of antidepressants.). There is no published experience with antidepressant drugs with less anticholinergic side effects, such as trazodone or serotonin reuptake inhibitors, but they are sometimes tried because they have fewer side effects.

Availability of agonists and antagonists for some of the ENS neuroreceptors has led to the testing of new drugs. Opioid agonists of the mu, delta, and kappa receptors have anti-nociceptive effects [261]. A single clinical trial found the kappa agonist fedotozine to be effective [262]. One 5-hydroxytryptamine$_3$ (5-HT$_3$) antagonist, granisetron, reduced rectal hypersensitivity in IBS patients

[263], but another, ondansetron, did not [264,265], nor did it reduce abdominal pain [266]. A multicenter clinical trial found alosetron (5-HT$_3$ antagonist) helpful for relief of pain and diarrhea in female patients with IBS [267]. Somatostatin and its analogues [268] and oxytocin [269] also have visceral antinociceptive effects. Octreotide reduced orocecal transit time in IBS patients [270] and increased colonic visceral sensory thresholds [271], but would be an impractical therapy because of the need to inject it. At publication, alosetron, an A5HT$_3$ antagonist, and other drugs active on 5HT$_3$ and HT$_4$ receptors are the most likely to achieve regulatory approval for IBS in the near future.

Referral for Psychological and Behavioral Treatments

Referral to a psychologist or psychiatrist may be helpful but the physician should maintain control of overall care [272]. There are methodological inadequacies in the reported trials of psychological treatments [265], but some reviewers conclude that such therapy decreases the severity of IBS symptoms [201]. Hypnotherapy [273], biofeedback [274], and psychodynamic therapy [209,275] have their proponents, but are not available in every community. Stress management/relaxation and cognitive behavioral programs [276–282] are under current study [201,283].

C2. Functional Abdominal Bloating

— Definition

Functional abdominal bloating comprises a group of functional bowel disorders which are dominated by a feeling of abdominal fullness or bloating and without sufficient criteria for another functional gastrointestinal disorder.

Borborygmi (audible bowel sounds) and excessive farting (passage of gas per rectum) and visible distension may also be present [284]. While some studies suggest these symptoms are not clearly related to bloating [236], others note a good correlation with the severity of maldigestion and breath hydrogen production [285]. Abdominal bloating was shown by Manning [49] to be one of six factors which discriminated IBS patients from those with organic disease. However, recent studies using factor analysis [179] suggest weak clustering of distension with the three pain-related Manning criteria for IBS in males [17,58] and limited clustering with IBS and constipation [58]. In healthy Dutch and Japanese workers abdominal distension clustered with dyspepsia, and in the Japanese group borborygmi clustered with diarrhea predominant IBS [286]. Factor analysis in Swedish dyspeptic patients referred for esophagogastroduodenoscopy identified an "indigestion syndrome" of borborygmi, eructation, increased flatus, and abdominal distension [287]. These results suggest that functional abdominal bloating may be a separate functional bowel disorder.

Visible distension is often as subjective as the complaint of bloating itself, in that it is seldom observed by the physician.

— Epidemiology

In a community-based Norwegian study of 14,102 residents, 17% complained of bloating and abdominal rumbling without pain [288]. Of 5,430 responders to the US Householder Survey, 30.7% fulfilled the Rome criteria for functional abdominal bloating [4]. This is the only study in which functional abdominal bloating was assessed using these criteria and the only one in which males were affected more frequently than females (34.3% vs. 27.3%). Subjects over 45 years reported to a physician more frequently than did younger subjects (33% versus 28%). Hyams observed similar findings in adolescents [20]. In Danish citizens [289], Minnesota residents [10], British subjects [11], American adolescents [20] and healthy African medical students [37], 5% to 15 % of subjects reported abdominal bloating. A five-year follow-up of Danish subjects demonstrated distension or borborygmi in 4.8% of men and 10.0% of women [14]. A summary of these findings is shown in Table 8.

Table 8. The Prevalence of Bloating in Several Populations

Site	Sample Size	Prevalence Bloating	Associated Symptoms
Tromso, Norway	14,1021	25% M, 30% F	abd. rumbling
		17% M & F	none
USA	5,430	34% M, 27% F	none
		31% M & F	
USA (Minnesota)	1021	13% M & F	none
USA (Minnesota)	328 Elderly	12%	none
Denmark	4851	8% M, 16% F	borborygmi: 11% F; 7% M
UK	1896	15% F, 6% M	none
UK	301	9.3%	borborygmi: 15%

Referred populations, by including patients with health seeking behavior, are likely to have a higher prevalence of bowel symptoms than population-based studies. Sixty-one percent of 699 Scottish dyspeptics reported flatus, 76% to 78% complained of borborygmi and 54% to 57% often felt "blown up" [290]. Similar figures were observed in Mayo Clinic patients, with visible abdominal distension in 36% with non-ulcer dyspepsia, 43% with IBS, 23% with organic bowel disease and 7% of healthy controls [291]. Of gastrointestinal symptoms in 624 diabetic and 648 non-diabetic controls, abdominal distension or flatulence occurred more than once per week in up to 35% of controls and 71% of patients respectively. A significant difference was noted only in males (71% vs. 57% p<0.05) [292]. Korean Gastrointestinal clinic patients described visible distension more frequently in female than male patients (58% vs. 16%; p=0.02) [52], and abdominal bloating occurred more frequently in female than male patients with IBS (42.6% vs. 13.9%; p<0.01) [179]. Among acute psychiatric inpatients whose bowel symptoms predated their psychiatric diagnosis, 39.7% fulfilled the Manning criteria for IBS but only 3 of 31 had sought medical attention for predominant bloating [293].

These studies suggest that functional abdominal bloating occurs in approximately 15% of community-based populations and up to two thirds of referred populations. It appears to be more common in females than males, even in the absence of IBS, but very few studies adequately separate bloating and associated symptoms from IBS and other functional gastrointestinal disorders. Bloating may be more clearly defined in pediatric populations (see Chapter 10). Future studies must ensure appropriate stratification by age and gender. Moreover, prospective cohort studies are needed to determine temporal relationships to other symptoms.

— Diagnostic Criteria

At least 12 weeks, which need not be consecutive, in the preceding 12 months of:

(1) Feeling of abdominal fullness, bloating, or visible distension; *and*
(2) Insufficient criteria for a diagnosis of functional dyspepsia, irritable bowel syndrome, or other functional disorder.

— Rationale for the Bloating Criteria

The term, "bloating" requires definition in order to point out its functional nature and to identify it as a real entity that troubles many people.

Bloating, borborygmi, belching, and farting are part of a spectrum of normal gut function and not necessarily related to one another. Symptoms of functional abdominal bloating may be intermittent but should occur "often." Worsening with dairy or fresh fruits or juices might suggest lactose or fructose intolerance, respectively. Such symptoms warrant appropriate investigations for lactose or fructose intolerance. Patients also should be questioned about the intake of poorly digestible or fermentable food stuffs such as sorbitol, beans or wheat bran. Bloating, fullness or visible distension should be the predominant features but may also occur in other functional gut disorders. Most patients are unable to specify the location of the bloating, but it is generally absent on waking, and tends to increase throughout the day. Patients feel the need to loosen their clothing. Some relate bloating to ingestion of specific foods. The presence of diarrhea, weight loss, or nutritional deficiency should alert the physician to the possibility of malabsorption or maldigestion. Excessive burping or farting may also be complained of, but are not necessarily related to the bloating. Criterion 2 in the 1992 document (symptoms unrelated to obvious maldigestion or other gastrointestinal diseases producing similar symptoms) has been removed by the working team.

— Physiologic Features

Bloating and IBS

A Canadian study of 46 subjects with visible bloating, non-bloated IBS or healthy volunteer controls reported that cases were more likely to have recent weight gain ($p<0.003$), weak abdominal muscles, and increased girth during episodes of distension [294]. In another study, pain and bloating were significantly increased during menses in IBS patients and non-patients but not in healthy controls [295].

Pathogenesis of Bloating

Levitt noted that lactulose, psyllium and methylcellulose produced a sensation of bloating in healthy volunteers, while lactulose also increased flatus and breath hydrogen production [236]. Gas accumulation within the bowel is a putative cause for visible bloating. Chami et al., using a computer digitized radiological technique, observed increased bowel gas in abdominal x-rays of "bloated" IBS patients compared to controls with the increase being more notable on supine than upright films [296]. Computerized tomography has also validated the presence of distension, but not excess gas [297]. Using Argon gas infusion, Lasser showed that postprandial rate and volume of intestinal gas production were normal [298]. Patients with functional dyspepsia [299] or who had a previous vagotomy [300] appeared to experience more bloating after intragastric saline or lipid infusion at lower volumes than controls. A widened gastric antrum and low vagal tone were noted in type I diabetics with autonomic dysfunction and patients with non-ulcer dyspepsia who complained predominantly of postprandial bloating [301]. Galati [302] demonstrated that IBS patients experienced more pain (but not more bloating) with postprandial duodenal gas infusion than sham gas infusion, while motility remained unchanged. Serra et al. noted pooling of infused jejunal gas due to slowing of intestinal transit following intragastric lipid infusion which was associated with visible distension and increased symptoms [303]. Other studies also suggest that bloating is associated with prolonged small bowel and whole gut transit [304, 305]. Using symptoms, transit and anorectal manometry, proctoscopy and defecography, a German study separated 190 patients with chronic constipation into four subgroups: disordered defecation, slow transit, both, or "no finding." Infrequent bowel movements and abdominal bloating occurred more frequently in the slow transit than the other groups [306].

These features suggest that bloating and distension involve perturbation of both motor and sensory responses and may be a consequence of increased gas production or delayed movement of gut contents.

— Psychological Features

Johnsen observed depression, insomnia, difficulty coping and alcohol abuse in patients with frequent bloating and borborygmi in Norway [288]. This was partly explained by social factors such as childhood deprivation more so than by diet. In one community-based study, 'stomach bloating' was observed more frequently with panic (28%) or anxiety disorder (15%) compared to those without a psychiatric disorder (7%) [307]. Although bloating was common (30.7%) in the US Household Survey, only 6.3% of subjects had seen a physician [4]. These subjects visited physicians an average of 0.49 times per year. Employment status and eight days/year missed from work were similar in patients with functional bloating to non-functional bowel disorders respondents. In women with IBS Heaton [75] found a significant temporal correlation between anxiety and depression scores and recording of bloating but not other IBS symptoms. Others have suggested that IBS patients experience more symptoms in relation to hyperventilation, difficulty expressing feelings, anxiety and depression [308].

Compared to healthy subjects, patients with functional abdominal bloating or Crohn's disease had similarly increased anxiety and depression levels [309]. These results suggest that anxiety or depression may be the consequence rather than the cause of these chronic problems. Community-based prospective studies are needed to determine whether functional abdominal bloating is temporally associated with psychosocial morbidity.

— Approach to Treatment

There is no evidence-based therapy for patients with pure functional abdominal bloating. The lack of clinical studies may be partly due to infrequent health seeking behavior, or the limited severity of the symptoms.

The physician should inquire after lactose-containing foods or vegetables such as beans and broccoli that are known to favor flatus production [215], although their exclusion does not guarantee improvement in outcome [110]. Even patients with proven lactase deficiency experience little or no bloating, pain or diarrhea after drinking 250 ml milk [111]. A review of drugs tested in IBS demonstrated no significant benefit for bloating when compared to placebo [310]. However, pain and distension improve together according to some studies. For example, visual analog scale scores for bloating (and pain) were reduced by half from a median of approximately 60 down to 30 (0 to 100) (p<0.02) after 12 half-hour sessions of hypnotherapy in treated versus "waiting list" untreated subjects [273]. A randomized dose-finding study assessing fedotozine, a kappa opiate agonist, in 238 patients with IBS significantly reduced mean and maximal abdominal pain and bloating compared to placebo (p=0.02) [262]. Regrettably, development of this drug has ceased.

Treatment for bloating includes patient education. Bloating is an unexplained nuisance; a harmless manifestation of the hypersensitive gut. Avoidance of foods which induce bloating in some individuals such as a high fat intake or legume vegetables, use of simethicone, an antifoaming agent, have been recommended without supporting evidence. Beano™, an over-the-counter oral solution which digests glucose linkages in complex carbohydrates, reduced episodes of farting, but did not show benefit for bloating or pain [311]. This latter may be due to insufficient statistical power as a result of the study design. Wheat bran and ispaghula are no more effective than placebo for distension, borborygmi, or flatulence, and may worsen symptoms in some patients [227].

C3. Functional Constipation

— Definition

Functional constipation comprises a group of functional disorders which present as persistent difficult, infrequent or seemingly incomplete defecation. Constipation has previously been defined by three methods: (1) symptoms, in descending order of frequency—straining, hard stools or scybala, unproductive calls ("want to but can't"), infrequent stools, incomplete evacuation [74]; (2) parameters of defecation outside the 95th percentile, e.g., <3 bowel movements per week [312,313], daily stool weight <35 g/day) [314], or straining >25% of the time [5,312,315]; and (3) physiological measures such as prolonged whole gut transit or colonic transit, as determined by radio-opaque markers [316,317].

Though none of these definitions is fully satisfactory, the use of symptoms is preferable since constipation becomes a problem only when a patient complains of it. Moreover, physiological measures are difficult to obtain, and symptoms of constipation may occur in the absence of physiological abnormalities. For example, stool frequency does not correlate with colonic transit time [59,76,318–319]. Yet the appearance or form of stool can serve as a measure of transit [59,320] (Table 9).

It is important to understand what the patient means by constipation. Young individuals who were asked to define constipation gave varied and often multiple responses: straining at stool (52%), hard stools (44%), sense of wanting to defecate but can't (34%), infrequent stools (32%), abdominal discomfort (20%), sense of incomplete evacuation (19%), and spending too much time on the toilet (11%) [74]. With this variety of perceptions among lay persons, it is clear that simply asking if a patient is constipated is not satisfactory.

— Epidemiology

Constipation occurs in up to 20% of the population depending on the demographic factors, sampling and definition used [4,5,7–9,76,315,321]. This symptom accounts for 1.2% of physician visits in the United States, and is most frequently treated by primary care physicians [322]. In the survey of US householders, 3% were found to have constipation. It is more common in females, and increases with age in most studies [5,315,322,323]. However, the frequency of stools appears not to change with age [74,324].

Table 9. Constipation: Diagnosis, and Specific Treatment

Pathology	Diagnosis	Specific Treatment
Constipating Drug (opiates, psycho-tropics, anticonvulsants, anticholinergics, dopaminergics, calcium channel blockers, bile acid binders)	history	stop or switch to alternative medication
Endocrine Disorder (pregnancy hypo-thyroidism, hyperparathyroidism, pheochromocytoma)	clinical status, endocrine function test	hormone replacement, operation, etc.
Neurologic Diseases —systemic (e.g., diabetic neuropathy, Parkinson's disease, Shy-Drager-syndrome) —traumatic (e.g., spinal cord lesion)	history, neurologic examination	—no specific treatment —scheduled bowel training, facilitated by suppositories or enemas
Slow Transit due to Neuropathy of Colonic Nerve Plexus	transit time mea-surement, trans-mural colon biopsy	colectomy (laxatives fail) if small bowel motility normal
Megacolon	X-ray	colectomy (laxatives fail)
Pelvic Floor Dyssynergia (anismus)	no confirmatory test available, exclu-sion by proctologic examination, ano-rectal manometry, electromyography, defecography, bal-loon expulsion test	behavioral training, biofeedback training
Short Segment Hirschsprung´s disease	acetyl cholinesterase reaction in rectal biopsy	myotomy of internal anal sphincter
Megarectum	X-ray	regular emptying with enemas and laxatives
Internal Rectal Prolapse, Solitary Rectal Ulcer	proctologic exami-nation, defecography	fiber supplementation, trans-abdominal rectopexy, Delorme procedure
Rectocele with stool retention	proctologic exami-nation, defecography	transanal repair

— Diagnostic Criteria

At least 12 weeks, which need not be consecutive, in the preceding 12 months of two or more of:

(1) Straining >¼ of defecations;

(2) Lumpy or hard stools >¼ of defecations;

(3) Sensation of incomplete evacuation >¼ of defecations;

(4) Sensation of anorectal obstruction/blockage >¼ of defecations;

(5) Manual maneuvers to facilitate >¼ of defecations (e.g., digital evacuation, support of the pelvic floor); and/or

(6) <3 defecations per week.

Loose stools are not present, and there are insufficient criteria for IBS.

— Rationale for the Constipation Criteria

The definitions of constipation usually found in texts are usually based on bowel frequency (e.g., <3 stools/week). However, this ignores the symptoms reported by most patients who consider themselves constipated. These include straining, hard stools, and other symptoms [306,325]. In order to include these the above criteria were developed. They include disorders of transit and defecation (see Chapter 9).

Most patients primarily complaining of constipation also admit to abdominal discomfort [306,325]. However, the constipation of functional constipation is present most of the time with no episodes of diarrhea, while that of IBS is only part of a generally chaotic bowel habit. These criteria may not apply when the patient is taking laxatives. Items 4 and 5 have been added to the 1992 criteria because they do occur in constipated people and since these criteria must embrace those patients who have disordered defecation (see Chapter 9). These two criteria have a sensitivity of only 40 to 50% for disordered defecation and a specificity of 80 to 90% [306,325].

— Clinical Evaluation

For patients who fulfil criteria for functional constipation, investigations may be done to:

(1) exclude medical disorders which may cause constipation, and
(2) identify physiological subgroups in refractory cases which may be responsive to more specific treatments.

The history and physical examination provide the most diagnostic information and will guide the subsequent evaluation.

— Suggested Approach to Constipation

Exclusion of Known Causes of Constipation

From the history, factors that may exacerbate or cause constipation can be identified and eliminated. These include (1) poor general health status [322]; (2) medication use (opiates, psychotropics, anticonvulsants, calcium channel blockers, anticholinergics, dopaminergics, bile acid binders); (3) psychological status (depression [315,326], psychological distress [323]); (4) low fiber diet [315,327]; and (5) medical disease (diabetes, hypothyroidism, porphyria, amyloidosis, pseudoobstruction, hypercalcaemia). The chronicity and nature of the symptoms reported will affect the type of diagnostic studies undertaken. For example, a history of straining with soft stools, or of manual maneuvers suggests anorectal dysfunction. Using a diary and the Bristol Stool Form Scale, a rough estimate of transit time can be obtained [59,76,328] (Table 4 and fig. 1).

One should do a rectal examination to determine the presence of fecal impaction, anal stricture, external or internal rectal prolapse, abnormal perineal descent with straining or rectal mass. Laboratory tests may include complete blood count, serum calcium, and basal TSH. Sigmoidoscopy with barium enema or colonoscopy is required to exclude an obstructing mass in patients >50 yrs with recent onset or change of symptoms, or to identify other colon disease. Other studies may be obtained as clinically indicated.

If the evaluation does not disclose constipation from other disease or medication (see Table 9), the patient may be considered to have functional constipation. However, since it is not justified to apply all tests listed in Table 9 to all patients, a patient with a structural cause such as colonic myenteric neuropathy might be classified as having functional constipation.

Empirical Treatment Trial

If no cause is recognized, a therapeutic trial with fiber supplements is the next step. Only patients with constipation that does not respond to a satisfactory therapeutic trial of fiber supplementation require further diagnostic evaluation to identify physiological subgroups (see below).

Measurement of Colon Transit Time

The measurement of whole gut transit time (as primarily a measure of colonic transit) using radio-opaque markers is inexpensive, simple, and safe. There are several slightly different methods that produce similar results [316,317, 329–333]. A high fiber diet should be eaten during measurement in order to control for one important physiologic determinant of colonic transit which is dietary fiber content. Similar results may be obtained employing a radio-isotope marker such as indium[111] bound to resin microspheres [334]. The radioisotope technique makes frequent observations possible, and more clearly delineates the whole colon. However, radiopaque markers are adequate for screening. The retention of markers in the proximal colon suggests colonic dysfunction, and retention of markers in the rectosigmoid area suggests anorectal dysfunction (e.g., obstructed defecation) [325].

Additional Studies

If the symptoms and marker studies suggest anorectal dysfunction, defecography may detect anatomical etiologies such as intussusception, rectocele with stool retention [335–337]. Rectal manometry, balloon expulsion [338], and electromyography have been used to identify disorders of defecation such as pelvic floor dyssynergia or anismus [339]. The latter diagnosis is supported by a lack of decrease of the anorectal angle upon straining during defecography [340,341] (for further details see Chapter 9).

—   Physiological Data

No adequate physiological studies address the widely believed associations of constipation with long-distance travel and chronic illness. Constipated patients have similar physical activity and drink similar amounts of fluids as controls [342]. There is no evidence that constipation is due to increased colonic water absorption [343]. Acute or chronic physical exercise has probably no major effect on the function of healthy colons [344–346]. However, the appropriate studies have not been done in constipated patients.

The laxative properties of dietary fiber are well known and account for most of the differences in average daily stool weight between communities [347,348]. They also explain most of the variation in stool output within a population having a wide range of fiber intakes [319]. However, low fiber intake is not the main determinant of constipation because (1) within the British population there is little or no relationship between dietary fiber intake and whole gut transit time [349,350]; (2) constipated patients on the average do not eat less fiber than controls [342]; and (3) patients have lower stool weights and longer transit times than controls whether treated with wheat bran or not [351].

Nevertheless, fiber-rich food, and supplements are useful in treating constipation. The laxative action of dietary fiber is complex and not fully understood. Its effects are probably mechanical via distension of the intestine by undigested matter and associated water plus increased bacteria [352,353]. Tactile stimulation of multimodal receptors in the intestinal mucosa by solid particles [354] may explain why coarse bran is more effective than fine bran [355]. More effort is required to expel small stools than those that are large [356]. The net result of a high-fiber diet is larger, softer stools.

Voluntary retention of stools is accompanied by delayed gastric emptying [357], and constipated patients have slowed gastric emptying and small bowel transit [358].

Severe constipation may be due to disturbances in the ENS, its neurotransmitters or receptors, or the CNS-ENS axis. Some patients with severe constipation have morphological changes within the myenteric and submucous plexus in colectomy specimens [359], but this is not the case in functional constipation. The widely held belief that such damage of the myenteric plexus may be due to laxatives is mainly based on a single anecdotal report, and a study in mice that used an ill-defined preparation of anthraquinones and presented no data [360]. Newer evidence in man and rodents is against such damage [361–363]. The "cathartic colon" is a radiologically defined abnormality [364] that has not been observed during recent decades. It was probably caused by toxic laxatives that have since been withdrawn from the market [365].

At least two physiological abnormalities can produce functional constipation: colonic dysfunction with slow transit, and anorectal dysfunction. The rest cannot be explained by current physiological investigations

Delayed or *slow colonic transit* is identified when, despite a high fiber diet radio-opaque markers are cleared abnormally slowly from the colon. In specialized centers these patients may represent one-third of constipated patients [350]. The increased mucosa contact time increases water absorption, resulting in lumpy infrequent stools, straining and a feeling of incomplete evacuation. Some authors restrict the term slow transit constipation to patients with very slow transit that is poorly responsive to all therapeutic measures [366,367].

Anorectal dysfunction describes failure of the anal sphincter or pelvic floor to function normally during defecation, and is discussed in Chapter 9. It can also cause slow transit.

Very few patients with slow transit have a megacolon, and it is unclear whether it is the reason for, or the consequence of, slow transit. The pathogenesis of megarectum is also unknown. It is often associated with fecal soiling. Both conditions may be suspected on plain abdominal x-rays and proved by barium enema. Even in highly specialized practices, clearly defined colonic inertia, anorectal dysfunction, and megacolon constitute a small minority of severely constipated patients.

— Psychological Features

Stool output, altered gut motility, and the reporting of constipation symptoms may be affected by personality, stress levels, and early toilet training [368,369]. Patients reporting severe constipation with normal transit time often have increased psychological distress [323]. Here, the physician's clinical approach may be determined by psychosocial assessment.

Constipation behavior can be learned early in life. A child may learn to contract the sphincters to retain stool and avoid defecation [370]. Drossman [371] proposed that in children the conflict between the gratification of defecation and the parental demand for restraint may contribute to constipation. Some data support the notion that faulty toilet training may produce anorectal disorders such as pelvic floor dyssynergia and encopresis [372]. Deliberate suppression of defecation in volunteers leads not only to reduced stool frequency and weight, but also to increased total and segmental transit time [373]. Suppression of the urge to defecate is common in the population and the urge may not return for several hours in a quarter of subjects [374].

— Approach to Treatment

Rarely, constipation can be cured by treating an endocrine disease or discontinuing a constipating medication. Otherwise, treatments for constipation are based on the severity of the symptoms reported, and the physiological subtype if known. Most patients will evacuate normally with nonspecific treatments [325,350]. Therefore, these should be attempted before extensive evaluation or surgical interventions are considered.

General Measures

Some patients fear that failure to evacuate their bowels for two to three days is harmful. These individuals may be helped by simple reassurance. Other measures such as regular visits to the toilet, increased fluid intake, and physical exercise are recommended, but unproven. Some physicians recommend assumption of the "squat position" on the toilet by raising the feet with a footstool. Abdominal wall massage and electroacupuncture have not been scientifically validated [375]. Laxative use is common and often inappropriate among adults [324].

Fiber Supplementation and Bulk Laxatives

For mild to moderate constipation, a diet containing an increased amount of dietary fiber often improves gut transit, stool frequency, and consistency. The effect of dietary fiber on stool weight is dose dependent [353,376–378], and requires a week to reach a steady state [376]. Patients with chronic constipation or slow transit require more fiber than healthy controls to produce the same increase in stool volume and transit [351]. Slow transit favors more complete bacterial degradation of fiber in the right colon, thus diminishing the effect of fiber on fecal output [379]. Wheat bran, whole grain food products, soluble fiber bulk laxatives (e.g., psyllium products) [380,381], methylcellulose [382], or any combination are suitable fiber therapy.

Compliance with fiber supplementation may be as low as 50% [379,383,384]. Many patients starting fiber complain of flatulence, distension, bloating, poor taste, and are unwilling to continue. If the patient is compliant, fiber treatment may help up to 80%. Those with defecation disorders or slow transit respond much less favorably [350]. Those with severe colonic inertia may not be helped by fiber, since there is decreased smooth muscle contractile activity.

Osmotic Laxatives

Unabsorbed mono- and disaccharides: Lactulose, lactitol, and sorbitol act through their osmotic properties which increase intraluminal bulk and stimulate peristalsis [240,385]. They are rapidly metabolized by colon bacteria to short-chain fatty acids and hence may be considered as very small-molecule soluble dietary fiber [386]. Fifteen to 30 ml twice a day is effective in mild, but not severe constipation. They may produce abdominal cramping and bloating [387]. Sorbitol (where available) is cheaper than lactulose and lactitol and may be as effective [241]. Glycerin, supplied as a 3 g suppository, also acts osmotically. It is absorbed if taken orally.

Saline Laxatives: Incompletely absorbed salts such as magnesium citrate, sodium phosphate, and magesium sulphate produce a net osmotic flux of water into the small intestine and colon [388]. Excessive use of these saline laxatives may lead to electrolyte imbalances, particularly among patients with renal impairment [389].

Other Water Binding Compounds

Four liters of an oral solution containing polyethylene glycol (PEG) was originally used in an isotonic solution to purge the colon for colonoscopy [243,360]. It is available in smaller quantities and has proved to be a very effective laxative in smaller doses for slow transit constipation. It appears to be safe since PEG is not absorbed, has a low sodium content, and does not cause net ion absorption or loss. Calcium polycarbophil has a similar mode of action and effect [380,390].

Stimulant Laxatives

Stimulant laxatives include diphenylmethane derivatives such as phenolphthalein, bisacodyl, and sodium picosulfate; and conjugated anthraquinone derivatives such as cascara sagrada, aloin, and senna [391]. Both groups have a dual action, namely an antiabsorptive-secretagogue and a prokinetic effect [391,392]. Sodium picosulfate (i.e., bisacodyl conjugated with sulfate) and the anthraquinone derivatives are cleaved by bacteria in the colon, where the active (unconjugated) principle may stimulate the enteric nerves. Available over the counter, these agents are the most popular, and the most likely to be abused [393,394]. Melanosis coli is a harmless reversible consequence of prolonged anthraquinone intake [395–398]. The pigment is found only in colon mucosa, and disappears if the anthraquinone is stopped for six months [392].

Prokinetic Agents

Cisapride is a 5-HT_4-agonist that augments the release of acetylcholine but has no antidopaminergic effects [399]. It may be useful in mild to moderate constipation, but is ineffective in severe slow transit [361]. As with any drug, one must be aware of cisapride's potential side effects. There is no evidence that other prokinetic agents such as bethanechol, domperidone, or metoclopramide are effective. Newer 5HT_4-agonists are in development.

Enemas

Enema volume stimulates the rectum to defecate. Tapwater enemas may be necessary for constipation due to disordered defecation or megacolon [400,401].

Specific Treatments

Treatments of the physiological subtypes of constipation are summarized in Table 9, and discussed in Chapter 9. Subtotal colectomy with ileorectal anastomosis has been recommended for patients with severe colonic inertia and normal anorectal function [402,403]. Clinical improvement is reported in 50–100%, but the procedure has many complications including small bowel obstruction in over one-third, diarrhea, incontinence, and recurrence of constipation [404,405]. Therefore, colectomy should be performed only in selected patients with severe documented colonic inertia and normal small bowel motility, for whom all nonsurgical treatments have failed.

C4. Functional Diarrhea

— Definition

Functional diarrhea is continuous or recurrent passage of loose (mushy) or watery stools without abdominal pain.

— Epidemiology

Data on stool form in the general population are available only for Bristol, England. In Bristol, 729 men and 400 women aged 40–69 years who admitted examining their stools were shown the Bristol stool form scale (fig. 1 and Table 4). They chose a liquid stool as the type they commonly passed [76]. Note that in this context liquid means mushy or type 6 on the Bristol stool form scale [59]. Unfortunately, subjects were not asked about completely watery stools (type 7) because the investigators had assumed such stools would rarely if ever be the usual ones of healthy people. Most of these subjects also kept a record of three consecutive defecations including the form of each stool [76]. If functional diarrhea is defined as all these three consecutive stools being liquid on each occasion, then its prevalence in middle-aged Bristol men and women was 4.3% and 2.2%. Functional diarrhea was less common in women under age 50 years (1.7%) than in those of 50 and over (3.1%). Since 50 is the median age of the menopause in Britain, the data suggest the possibility of a hormonal risk factor.

In this same population it was noted that, when the stools were recorded as mushy (type 6), defecation was recorded as being urgent on 80% of occasions, though urgency was rare with more formed stools [75], a finding which would seem to validate a stool form-based definition of diarrhea.

— Diagnostic Criteria

At least 12 weeks, which need not be consecutive, in the preceding 12 months of:
(1) Loose (mushy) or watery stools;
(2) Present > ¾ of the time; *and*
(3) No abdominal pain.

— Rationale for the Diarrhea Criteria

Frequency and urgency are not part of the definition since they are also features of pseudodiarrhea, where solid, broken up or pellety stools are not associated with a shortened gut transit time. Stool frequency is also an unreliable indicator of diarrhea, since it is unrelated to transit time. Stool form, consistency and output more accurately reflect gut transit time [59,76,317–319].

Diarrhea should be distinguished from pseudodiarrhea, which is frequent defecation and urgency with solid stools, a common feature of IBS. As in any diarrhea, urgency of defecation is prominent and there may be fecal incontinence. Therefore, these symptoms are not diagnostic criteria. Stool output—weight or volume—is not mentioned because it is rarely measured outside academic centers and depends on diet. In fact, it varies closely with stool form [319]. Colonic transit time is not mentioned because, though it can be measured [317], it is still cumbersome. The only measure of diarrhea that is both scientifically valid and realistic in everyday practice is stool form or appearance assessed against a standardized scale of descriptors. Two such scales have been published [59,319], but only one—the seven-point Bristol scale [59]—is suitable for use with toilets and has been validated against defecatory symptoms as well as against transit time [75]. On the Bristol scale, liquid stools (i.e., diarrhea) are type 6 (fluffy pieces with ragged edges, mushy) and type 7 (watery, no solid pieces).

— Clinical Evaluation

Compared with the other functional bowel disorders, functional diarrhea is less easy to recognize and some investigation is mandatory. The extent of the work-up is influenced by the history and physical examination but must be limited when there is no clinical evidence of other disease. A history of diarrhea alternating with constipation, i.e., diarrhea punctuated by episodes of two or more successive days without defecations at all, is highly suggestive of a functional cause. It is helpful to ask the patient to keep a record of their defecations including stool form as this quickly detects an alternating pattern as well as pseudodiarrhea or frequent passage of formed stools [59]. The latter can be caused by proctitis and other organic disease of the rectum and so is a strong indication for proctosigmoidoscopy. If done at the initial visit, the physician can explain to the patient without delay that a functional diagnosis is likely.

When inquiry about stool form suggests true diarrhea all patients should have a full blood count and measurement of ESR or C-reactive protein. Serum ferritin and red cell folate serve as screens for malabsorption. When the suspicion of inflammatory bowel disease or malabsorption is strong, there are now sensitive, noninvasive tests—stool fat analysis, gastrointestinal imaging for IBD, and anti-endomysial antibodies for celiac disease. Small bowel biopsy via endoscopy is the most precise diagnostic test for the latter. Other occasionally required tests include a laxative screen of stool and urine, and colonoscopy with multiple biopsies looking for collagenous and microscopic colitis.

Idiopathic bile acid malabsorption is often reported to be common in patients with obscure diarrhea [406–409], although the pathogenesis is uncertain. It might be a form of functional diarrhea in which there is rapid transit through the terminal ileum (where bile acids are chiefly absorbed) because it often responds to antidiarrheal agents as well as to bile acid-binding agents. The response to such an agent can be used as a test for bile acid malabsorption as an alternative to the radioactive bile salt retention test (SeHCAT test). Diarrhea due to other causes such as IBD, post cholecystectomy, and microscopic colitis may also respond to cholestyramine.

Elimination diets searching for specific food intolerances are laborious and the interpretation of the results is controversial. It is extremely difficult to distinguish a physical food intolerance from a psychological food aversion [218, 410]. Multiple blind challenge tests are necessary but are not feasible in clinical practice.

In rare patients with severe watery diarrhea (daily stool weight averaging over 500 g) tests should be done for endocrine causes of diarrhea (VIP, 5-HIAA). In small volume diarrhea such tests are likely to be unrewarding. Those at risk should be tested for the human immunodeficiency virus. One should be mindful that factitious diarrhea due to surreptitious laxative use is a common explanation of the chronic refractory diarrhea seen in academic centers [394]. Alarm symptoms such as weight loss, fever or rectal bleeding warrant testing as determined by the attending physician. Readers are referred to standard gastroenterology texts for a more thorough discussion of the investigation of chronic diarrhea.

— Physiological Features

Intestinal transit-time is the major determinant of fecal output in normal subjects [411]. Rapid transit is present in all patients with true diarrhea and an intact intestine, and is sometimes the primary abnormality [412]. In the case of functional diarrhea it is uncertain whether the primary problem is in the small or large intestine, and also whether it is one of motility or of sensitivity. One study suggested there is a dual abnormality in the colon's reaction to eating —more frequent propagating contractions and fewer nonpropagating ones [413]. This implies a primary colon problem. However, in IBS patients at least, fast colon transit has been linked with fast small bowel transit [305], although in another study the most consistent abnormality was rapid gastric emptying

[414]. When small bowel transit is rapid, the colon is presented with excessive amounts of undigested food products, some of which (short-chain carbohydrates and peptides) are osmotically active, until they have been fermented by bacteria into the rapidly absorbed short-chain fatty acids. With rapid small bowel transit, the colon may also receive excessive amounts of products which have secretory effects in the colon and thus have laxative activity (long-chain fatty acids, dihydroxy bile acids).

Frequency of defecation is not necessarily associated with rapid transit or loose stools [59,318]. The basis of pseudodiarrhea is likely to be rectal hypersensitivity, since the latter is a feature of IBS patients who have a frequent desire to defecate whether or not they have diarrhea [415]. Frequency of defecation is often associated with frequent micturition due to a hypersensitive bladder [84]. Rectal hypersensitivity can be reduced by hypnosis [416], suggesting that psychological factors can be involved in its genesis.

— Psychological Factors

It is common knowledge that acute anxiety induces diarrhea in some people. In surveys of healthy people, many—especially younger women—answer affirmatively when asked whether stress affects their bowel pattern [6,184]. The mechanism is unknown. In the laboratory, emotional stress increases colon motility, but no more so in patients with diarrhea than in normal subjects [417].

There are fewer data to back up the widespread perception that functional diarrhea is related to chronic anxiety or stress. This lack of evidence may exist partly because functional diarrhea is relatively uncommon and under-researched compared with IBS. However, evidence for a link is the finding that patients attending psychiatrists with anxiety and without bowel complaints had faster small and large bowel transit than normal controls (whereas depressed patients tended to have slower transit) [326].

— Approach to Treatment

Functional diarrhea is possibly curable if a cause can be found and be elicited in the patient's psychosocial history, but no data are available to indicate how often this is possible. It makes sense to look for evidence of a stressful lifestyle or situation and to identify anxiety, catastrophic ideation, and undue focusing on the abdomen and bowels. Once these have been dealt with, management is empirical and symptomatic.

A diet history, or diet record, may reveal an unsuspected cause such as excessive intake of fiber, as in vegans, heavy consumption of alcohol or caffeine-containing drinks, high intake of sorbitol in chewing gum or candies, or of fructose in certain fruits and products sweetened with hydrolized corn syrup. If a specific food intolerance has been identified by remission of symptoms on an elimination diet followed by relapse on repeated challenges, the food or drink should of course be excluded. However, some patients find this so difficult or unpleasant they prefer to put up with the diarrhea. The commonest provocative foods for functional diarrhea are probably wheat products, dairy products, citrus fruits, eggs, onions, nuts, caffeine, and alcohol [215]. Patients should be advised that food intolerances often go away and that every 6–12 months they should re-challenge themselves.

When lifestyle measures have failed, cholestyramine is worth a trial [407]. However, it is often poorly tolerated. Simple antidiarrheals are the drugs of first choice, but they too may be of limited value due to side effects. The three most effective antidiarrheals are loperamide, codeine phosphate and diphenoxylate. They are thought to work on opioid receptors and to exert their effects on motility in both the small and large intestine by preventing the release of acetylcholine from cholinergic nerve-endings. Loperamide also has some non-opioid effects, that is, inhibition of calmodulin and calcium channels [418,419]. Patients sometimes give up taking antidiarrheals because with solid stools they develop abdominal discomfort or bloating and/or increased rectal awareness/discomfort. Loperamide seems to have the best ratio of effectiveness to side effects [420]. The dose must be titrated against stool form and frequency. Antidiarrheals are best taken prophylactically, which, when a "morning rush" is the main problem, means taking a dose at bedtime.

—   ## Prognosis

The prognosis of functional diarrhea is poorly documented but spontaneous remissions certainly occur. In one series of 17 cases, chronic diarrhea remitted in 7–31 months, average 15 [421]. Patients can therefore be given a modicum of reassurance.

C5. Unspecified Functional Bowel Disorder

— Diagnostic Criteria

Bowel symptoms in the absence of organic disease that do not fit into the previously defined categories of functional bowel disorders.

Many individual symptoms discussed in the previous sections are very common in the population and in some cases may lead to a medical consultation. When these occur with other symptoms sufficient to satisfy criteria for one of the functional syndromes, classification is straightforward. Otherwise, pending discovery of physiologic markers, these symptoms, or groups of symptoms are best classified as unspecified functional bowel disorder.

D. Functional Abdominal Pain

Functional abdominal pain describes continuous, nearly continuous or frequently recurrent pain localized in the abdomen but poorly related to gut function.

Recent studies indicate that this disorder is more related to central nervous system influences on normal or only slightly disordered bowel function ("abnormal perception of normal gut function"), rather than to disordered motility (abnormal gut function) [422,423].

D1. Functional Abdominal Pain Syndrome (FAPS)

— Definition

Functional abdominal pain syndrome, also called "chronic idiopathic abdominal pain," or "chronic functional abdominal pain," describes pain for at least six months that is poorly related to gut function and is associated with some loss of daily activities.

This disorder is commonly associated with a general tendency to experience and report other unpleasant somatic symptoms. When the pain is persistent over a long period of time, and/or dominates the patient's life and is associated with chronic pain behaviors, there are likely to be associated psychological disturbances [422].

— Epidemiology

Functional Abdominal Pain Syndrome is much less prevalent than IBS or other functional bowel disorders in the community. In the U.S. Householder Study of Functional Gastrointestinal Disorders [4], FAPS was seen in 1.7% (primarily women) of the sample, compared to 9.2% for irritable bowel. This figure may overestimate the true prevalence, since the data were obtained by survey methods. Nevertheless, these individuals missed 11.8 work days from illness (compared to 4.2 days for those without bowel symptoms), and made 7.2 physician visits (compared to 1.9) in the previous year.

Patients with FAPS tend to be seen in referral gastroenterology practices, major medical centers and pain clinics. Lack of recognition of this disorder, and physician efforts to "rule out organic disease," lead to unneeded diagnostic studies and treatments, and patient dissatisfaction. Maxton [424] who followed patients with FAPS over a seven-year period, found they were referred to an average of 5.7 consultants, underwent 6.4 endoscopic or radiological procedures. and had 2.7 major operations, primarily hysterectomy and exploratory laparotomy.

— Diagnostic Criteria

At least six months of:

(1) **Continuous or nearly continuous abdominal pain;** *and*
(2) **No or only occasional relationship of pain with physiological events (e.g., eating, defecation, or menses);** *and*

(3) Some loss of daily functioning; *and*
(4) The pain is not feigned (e.g., malingering); *and*
(5) Insufficient criteria for other functional gastrointestinal disorders that would explain the abdominal pain.

These criteria are derived in part from the DSM-IV [425]. For discussion of, and criteria for, recurrent abdominal pain in children, readers should refer to Chapter 10.

— Clinical Evaluation

For patients meeting diagnostic criteria for FAPS, clinical evaluation usually fails to disclose a specific medical etiology [422], but may incidentally identify other medical conditions that do not fully explain the chronic pain syndrome. A number of clinical and behavioral features may be present which, while not diagnostic [426], can aid in the diagnostic and treatment plan.

Symptom Description

The pain may be described: (1) in emotional or even bizarre terms, e.g., as "nauseating" or "like a knife stabbing" [427]; (2) as constant and not influenced by eating or defecation; (3) as involving a large anatomic area rather than a precise location; (4) as one of several other painful symptoms; and (5) as a continuum of painful experiences beginning in childhood, or recurring.

Pain Behaviors

Pain (or "abnormal" illness) behaviors [428] include: (1) reporting intense symptoms with great emotion and urgency; (2) requesting numerous diagnostic studies or surgery; (3) focusing attention primarily on the illness; (4) relentlessly seeking health care for symptom relief, and to validate the condition as "organic"; (5) ignoring or denying a role for psychosocial contributions; and (6) absolving personal responsibility for self-management, while placing high expectations for relief on the physician.

These behaviors may diminish when the patient is engaged in distracting activities, or is not aware of being observed, but increase when discussing a psychologically distressing issue. In addition, the continued presence of the spouse or parent who takes responsibility for reporting the patient's history, suggests the possibility of family dysfunction that may require counseling to establish the proper level of family involvement to support and improve coping style. Requests for narcotics should alert the clinician to drug-seeking behavior.

Some patients exhibit the clinical features of FAPS, and have a coexistent medical condition (e.g., Crohn's disease, chronic pancreatitis, etc.). Here, the clinician must determine the degree to which CNS versus peripheral nociceptive input from disease contribute to the illness presentation. Typically, when peripheral (visceral) input primarily explains the pain, it is: (1) more recent in onset; (2) intermittent or more variable in intensity; (3) conforming to neuroanatomic pathways; (4) more responsive to antimotility agents and peripherally acting (e.g., NSAIDs) analgesics; and (5) related to events that affect gut function (e.g., eating, defecation, etc.) [429].

Physical Examination

Patients may appear normal or withdrawn, and usually *do not exhibit autonomic arousal* as manifest by tachycardia, diaphoresis, changes in blood pressure and acute anxiety. Their presence suggests a peripheral source for the pain. The *"closed eyes sign"* may be noted during palpation of the abdomen [430]. Patients with FAPS will close their eyes, exhibiting pain behavior, while those with acute abdominal emergencies keep their eyes open in fearful anticipation of their abdomen being touched. Pain behaviors may diminish when the subject is distracted by the use of a stethoscope.

The presence of multiple surgical scars without medical explanation suggest a history of unneeded surgical procedures. *Carnett's test* is usually negative: after the site of maximal abdominal pain is identified, the patient is asked to assume a partial sitting position, to flex the abdominal musculature [431]. A positive test (the pain increases with abdominal muscle flexion) suggests a muscle wall etiology (e.g., cutaneous nerve entrapment, hernia). A negative test suggests either a visceral or CNS contribution to the pain.

— Physiological Data

Pain is a sensory, emotional, and cognitive experience modulated by biological and psychosocial processes [422,423,432]. FAPS appears to be distinct from acute pain conditions, structural gastrointestinal diseases, or functional GI disorders where tissue damage, or altered gut motility or sensitivity lead to pain symptoms based primarily on increased visceral stimulation. Rather, limited, or even normal, regulatory nociceptive stimuli may be associated with chronic or severe pain. In FAPS, afferent input appears to be modified by neural ("gate control") mechanisms via serotoninergic, descending corticofugal pathways (endorphin-mediated analgesic system) [433] that regulate cephalad transmission of pain impulses to the CNS. This permits memory, attention, and other psychological processes to alter the pain experience. There is evidence that the neural circuitry of chronic pain has more contribution from central affective and evaluative levels (medial cortex) than from the lateral (sensory) cortex or from peripheral sensory pathways [423]. Therefore, in the absence of obvious disease, while chronic pain may be attributed to the abdomen, there is little or no peripheral nociceptive input, and cognitive and emotional centers of the brain play a major role.

Chronic abdominal pain, may result from sensitization of peripheral receptors or excitation of spinal or CNS pain regulatory systems (visceral hypersensitivity) [434,435]. Repetitive balloon inflations in the colon can lead to a transient increase in pain intensity in normals [436], and possibly to a greater degree, in patients with IBS [149]. Discrete clustered or prolonged propagated contractions seen in IBS, or recurrent peripheral injury, such as repeated abdominal operations, may sensitize existing receptors or recruit "silent" intestinal nociceptors possibly by releasing pro-inflammatory cytokines [422,423,437]. This could amplify painful afferent activity (hyperalgesia), or even lead to pain from baseline afferent activity (allodynia). Conversely, pre-operative treatment with local or regional anesthesia or non-steroidal analgesics can reduce the severity of postoperative pain [434,435]. These data suggest that the CNS response to peripheral nociceptive input can be up or down regulated by varying visceral input, and chronic stimulation may lead to a chronic pain disorder.

The possible CNS participation in chronic pain is illustrated by the PET experiments (C1). Painful rectal stimuli activated the anterior cingulate gyrus of normal individuals, but not of referred IBS patients, whose prefrontal cortex was activated instead. Perhaps failure of activation of the gyrus permits cortical participation and therefore conscious awareness.

Physiological data tend to distinguish patients with FAPS from those with other functional GI disorders by showing that the CNS, more than altered gut motility or sensitivity, influences the pain experience [422]. This may help explain the strong association of abuse, life stress, poor coping style, and other psychosocial disturbances with increased pain reports among patients with functional GI disorders [195,197,283]. It may also provide the framework for psychopharmacologic (e.g., antidepressants) and behavioral (e.g., cognitive-behavioral treatment) treatments to ameliorate chronic abdominal pain [283]. These associations and their putative neurophysiologic pathways require further research.

— Psychological Data

Any of several psychiatric diagnoses may coexist with FAPS [422]. It is common for patients to have depression or anxiety, or certain personality disorders [438,439]. However, a factitious disorder or malingering is not consistent with this diagnosis. The syndrome is similar to the psychiatric diagnosis of Somatoform Pain Disorder (Pain Disorder Associated with Psychological Factors —307.80) in the DSM-IV, where the symptoms are localized to the abdomen [440]. However, functional gastrointestinal disorders associated with bowel dysfunction (e.g., IBS) should not be included as a somatoform pain disorder. When FAPS coexists with other structural or functional medical conditions, the patient may be classified as "pain disorder associated with a general medical condition" (DSM-IV—307.89). The syndrome may also be seen with other somatoform disorders (e.g., somatization, conversion disorder, hypochondriasis) [425].

Unresolved losses including onset or exacerbation of symptoms after the death of a parent or spouse, personally meaningful surgery (e.g., hysterectomy, ostomy), or an untoward outcome of a pregnancy (abortion, stillbirth) are common in FAPS [441]. A history of sexual and physical abuse is frequent [188,442], and is independent of diagnosis. It predicts poorer health status [195], medical refractoriness, increased diagnostic and therapeutic procedures, and health care visits [188]. Such trauma may increase awareness of bodily sensations, or physiologically lower the visceral pain threshold [423].

Patients may exhibit ineffective coping strategies (e.g., "catastrophizing," or have poor social or family support). These factors are associated with higher pain scores, more psychological distress, and poorer clinical outcomes [443–446]. Their main social support may be provided by the illness (e.g., increased attention from friends, family, and physicians). Despite these observations, patients with FAPS often deny or minimize a role for psychological factors. Perhaps in childhood there was much family attention to illness, rather than to emotional distress [447,448].

— Management

Management of these patients is difficult and depends on establishing an effective physician-patient relationship [422]. The goals of treatment are to limit unnecessary investigations or treatments, to understand what motivates the patient to seek medical treatment, and to provide emotional support and continued care rather than attempt a "cure."

Physician-Patient Relationship

An effective relationship depends upon compassion, acknowledgment of the distress associated with the painful condition, and maintenance of an objective and observant stance [449]. The physician should base diagnostic and treatment decisions on objective data and not overreact through overmedication or unneeded diagnostic studies or treatments [450]. Education involves eliciting the patient's understanding of the condition, addressing any unrealistic concerns, and explaining the nature of the symptoms consistent with the patient's belief system. Patients also need reassurance, since they may fear serious disease or surgery.

General Treatment Approach

After the evaluation is completed, the physician must establish reasonable goals. These may include improved function rather than "cure", and a negotiated treatment plan. He or she must set reasonable limits in time and effort by scheduling brief but regular appointments, and consider concurrent care with a mental health professional. The key is to maintain an ongoing relationship.

Medications

Analgesics (e.g., aspirin, nonsteroidal anti-inflammatory drugs) offer little benefit, because they act peripherally. Narcotics should not be prescribed because of possible addiction and impaired motility and increased pain sensitivity (narcotic bowel syndrome) [451]. Furthermore, their use subordinates the development of treatment strategies to that of providing medication.

Antidepressants

The antidepressants are indicated for chronic pain of various types or for depressive symptoms associated with medical illness. They should be considered for GI patients having "vegetative" signs of depression: poor appetite and weight loss, sleep disturbance, decreased energy and libido, and deterioration in functional status (e.g., inability to work or to maintain usual social or home management activities). They also serve as "central analgesics" to raise perception threshold for abdominal pain or other GI symptoms [256,257,452–454].

The choice of an antidepressant often depends on its side effects. The tricyclic (TCA) antidepressants (e.g., amitriptyline, doxepin, desipramine, nortriptyline) have been the most studied in GI and other medical conditions [283]. In addition to actions on noradrenergic and serotoninergic receptors, they have undesirable antimuscarinic and antihistaminic effects leading to symptoms of orthostatic hypotension, constipation, sicca syndrome, sedation, fluid retention, cardiac arrhythmias, and weight gain. Compared to the selective serotonin inhibitors (see below), these agents require more dose adjustment to achieve clinical efficacy, and have a greater risk of overdose. Amitriptyline and doxepin have strong sedative effects, so they can help promote sleep with a single nighttime dose. However, desiprimine or nortriptyline have less anticholinergic and sedative effects. The TCAs also decrease phase III propagation velocity and increase orocecal transit time [260], and clinically, reduce diarrhea in patients with IBS [256].

Treatment with TCAs should begin with low doses (e.g., 25 mg/day) and be increased as needed. Many studies for functional GI disorders show efficacy at a dose of about half that used to treat major depression. Serum levels of desipramine and nortriptyline show little correlation with clinical effect.

The selective serotonin reuptake inhibitors (SSRI) (e.g., fluoxetine, sertraline, paroxetine, luvoxamine) have not been adequately studied for treatment of patients with GI disorders. They are expensive, but may help reduce painful symptoms and improve general well-being [257]. They may be particularly helpful for patients with coexistent anxiety, panic, or obsessional behaviors [453]. Because these drugs are highly selective for serotoninergic receptors and have little affinity for other neurotransmitter (i.e., antimuscarinic or antihistaminic) receptors, they produce little sedation, orthostatic hypotension, or cardiac effects. They are safer and better tolerated than TCAs, and produce little risk of overdose. Their side effects include nausea, agitation, sleep disturbance (insomnia more often than somnolence), vivid dreams, sexual dysfunction (delayed ejaculation or anorgasmia), night sweats, and possibly weight loss (particularly fluoxetine). Up to 15% of patients using sertraline or fluoxetine will experience diarrhea [453]. In contrast, paroxetine has more antimuscarinic effect than the other SSRIs, and may cause constipation. However, it should be remembered that there are no controlled trials of SSRIs in functional bowel disease, only case reports.

Most patients will benefit from only one morning dose (10–20 mg fluoxetine, 50 mg sertraline, 20 mg paroxetine, 50 mg luvoxamine). Lower doses may be required for the elderly, or patients with liver disease, due to the prolonged half-life of the metabolites. Because of their high affinity for the cytochrome P-450 system (particularly with paroxetine), the SSRIs should be used with caution with TCAs, benzodiazepines, anticonvulsants, antiarrhythmics, or warfarin.

An antidepressant may help when abdominal discomfort causes loss of daily function. The antidepressant should be continued for 6–12 months before tapering. The patient should be informed that the medication is not addicting, and acts as a central analgesic that controls pain in various medical conditions. However, it can also help to treat depressive symptoms induced by the illness [272]. It may take up to several weeks to work, and side effects, if they occur, ameliorate over 1–2 weeks. A poor clinical response may be due to non-compliance, or an inadequate dose [455].

Anxiolytics

The benzodiazepines (e.g., diazepam, lorazepam, alprazolam) are frequently used to treat anxiety. However, the benefit of benzodiazepines must be balanced with the long term risks of sedation, drug and alcohol interactions, habituation, and symptom rebound upon withdrawal. Its value for patients with chronic gastrointestinal disturbances remains to be proven, and these agents may work by decreasing serotonin levels and lowering pain thresholds, as well as by stimulating of gamma-aminobutyric acid (GABA) receptors, which may contribute to depression [456].

Psychological Treatment

Patients may be reluctant to see a psychologist or psychiatrist because they fail to understand the benefits of referral, feel stigmatized for having a possible psychiatric problem, or see referral as a rejection by the physician. Psychologic treatment should be presented, along with ongoing medical care, as a means to help manage pain and reduce the psychological distress from the symptoms.

Based on studies from chronic pain centers [457,458], and of patients with IBS [283], several types of psychological treatments can be considered. However, efficacy studies for patients with FAPS are limited. Cognitive-behavioral treatment identifies maladaptive thoughts, perceptions, and behaviors, which are then used to develop new ways to increase control of the symptoms [459]. Dynamic or interpersonal psychotherapy seeks to reduce psychological distress and physical symptoms that are exacerbated by difficulties in interpersonal relationships [460]. Hypnotherapy has been investigated primarily in irritable bowel syndrome [461], where the focus is on "relaxation of the gut." Stress management attempts to help counteract the physiological effects of stress or anxiety. Finally, referral to pain treatment centers for multidisciplinary treatment programs may be the most efficient method of treating disability from refractory chronic pain [462].

D2. Unspecified Functional Abdominal Pain

— Diagnostic Criteria

This is functional abdominal pain that fails to reach criteria for functional abdominal pain syndrome.

When this diagnosis is made the patient should be kept under review to see whether the full syndrome develops, or whether underlying structural disease declares itself.

Some Topics for Future Research

The Rome Criteria for the functional bowel disorders cannot be frozen in time. In the light of new data their updating should be an ongoing process. Clinical research is essential if there are to be periodic changes that are evidence based. We suggest the following topics around which research may provide the evidence.

(1) Using appropriate methods, validate and test the utility of the funcitonal bowel disorder criteria.

(2) Test the usefulness of criteria in various clinical settings: primary care, referral practice, academic centers, in the population.

(3) Test if the usefulness of the criteria are affected by gender, cultural, or geographic factors.

(4) Determine the usefulness of subgroups in clinical research (studies and trials).

(5) Compare the reliability and effectiveness of prospective diary recording with patients' recall of symptoms.

(6) Perform studies that explore the pathophysiologic basis of symptoms.

(7) Evaluate stool form scales as a means of determining if individuals have diarrhea or constipation.

(8) Explore if abdominal discomfort and pain differ in degree or in nature.

References

1. Thompson WG, Dotevall G, Drossman DA, et al. Irritable bowel syndrome: guidelines for the diagnosis. Gastroenterol Internat 1989;2:92–95.
2. Drossman DA, Richter J, Talley NJ, et al. The Functional Gastrointestinal Disorders: Diagnosis, Pathophysiology, and Treatment. Boston: Little, Brown; 1994.
3. Thompson WG, Creed FH, Drossman DA, et al. Functional bowel disorders and functional abdominal pain. Gastroenterol International 1992;5:75–91.
4. Drossman DA, Li Z, Andruzzi E, et al. U.S. householder survey of functional gastrointestinal disorders: prevalence, sociodemography and health impact. Dig Dis Sci 1993;38:1569–80.
5. Thompson WG, Heaton KW. Functional bowel disorders in apparently health people. Gastroenterol 1980;79:283–88.
6. Drossman DA, Sandler RS, McKee DC, et al. Bowel patterns amongst subjects not seeking health care. Gastroenterology 1982;83:529–34.
7. Whitehead WE, Winget C, Fedoravicius AS, et al. Learned illness behavior in patients with irritable bowel syndrome and peptic ulcer. Dig Dis Sci 1982;27:202–208.
8. Bommelaer G, Rouch M, Dapoigny M, et al. Epidemiologie des troubles fonctionnels dans une population apparement saine. Gastroenterol Clin Biol 1986;10:7–12.
9. Welch GW, Pomare EW. Functional gastrointestinal symptoms in a Wellington community sample. NZ Med J 1990;103:418–20.
10. Talley NJ, Zinsmeister AR, Van Dyke C, et al. Epidemiology of colonic symptoms and the irritable bowel syndrome. Gastroenterology 1991;101:927–34.
11. Heaton KW, O'Donnell LJD, Braddon FEM, et al. Symptoms of irritable bowel syndrome in a British urban community: consulters and nonconsulters. Gastroenterology 1992;102:1962–67.
12. Talley NJ, O'Keefe EA, Zinsmeister AR, et al. I. Prevalence of gastrointestinal symptoms in the elderly: a population-based study. Gastroent 1992;102:895–901.
13. Jones R, Lydiard S. Irritable bowel syndrome in the general population. Brit Med J 1992;304:87–90.
14. Kay L, Jorgensen T, Jensen KH. The epidemiology of irritable bowel syndrome in a random population: prevalence, incidence, natural history and risk factors. J Intern Med 1994;236:23–30.
15. Longstreth GF, Wolde-Tsadik G. Irritable bowel-type symptoms in HMO examinees: prevalence, demographics and clinical correlates. Dig Dis Sci 1993;38:1581–89.
16. Zuckerman MJ, Guerra LG, Drossman DA, et al. Comparison of bowel patterns in Hispanics and non-Hispanic whites. Dig Dis Sci 1995;40:1761–69.
17. Taub E, Cuevas JL, Cook EW, et al. Irritable bowel syndrome defined by factor analysis. Dig Dis Sci 1995;40:2647–55.
18. Talley NJ, et al. Irritable bowel syndrome in a community: symptom subgroups, risk factors and health care utilization. Am J Epidemiol 1995;142:76–83.

19. Talley NJ, Boyce PM, Jones M. Predictors of health care seeking for irritable bowel syndrome: a population based study. Gut 1997;41(3):459–61.
20. Hyams JS, Burke G, Davis PM, et al. Abdominal pain and irritable bowel symptoms in adolescents: a community-based study. J Pediatr 1996;129:220–26.
21. Sullivan SN. Management of the irritable bowel syndrome: a personal view. J Clin Gastroenterol 1983;499–502.
22. Harvey RF, Salih SY, Read AE. Organic and functional disorders in 2000 gastroenterology outpatients. Lancet 1983;1:632–34.
23. Mitchell CM, Drossman DA. Survey of the AGA membership relating to patients with functional gastrointestinal disorders. Gastroenterology 1987;92:1282–83.
24. Ferguson A, Sircus W, Eastwood MA. Frequency of "functional" gastrointestinal disorders. Lancet 1977;2:613–14.
25. Fielding JF. A year in out-patients with the irritable bowel syndrome. Irish J Med Sci 1977;146:162–65.
26. Thompson WG. Gastrointestinal symptoms in the irritable bowel compared with peptic ulcer and inflammatory bowel disease. Gut 1984;25:1089–92.
27. Talley NJ, Weaver AL, Zinsmeister AR, et al. Onset and disappearance of gastrointestinal symptoms and functional gastrointestinal disorders. Am J Epidemiol 1992;136:165–77.
28. Agreus L, Svardsudd K, Nyren O, et al. Irritable bowel syndrome and dyspepsia in the population: overlap and lack of stability over time. Gastroenterology 1995;109: 671–80.
29. Pimparkar BD. Irritable colon syndrome. J Indian Med Assoc 1970;54:95–105.
30. Mendis BLJ, Wijesiriwardena BC, Sheriff JHR, et al. Irritable bowel syndrome. Celon Med J 1982;27:171–81.
31. Mathur A, Tandon BN, Prakkash OM. Irritable colon syndrome. J Indian Med Assoc 1966;46:651–55.
32. Bordie AK. Functional disorders of the colon. J Indian Med Assoc 1972;58:451–56.
33. Kapoor KK, Nigam P, Rastogi CK, et al. Clinical profile of the irritable bowel syndrome. Indian J Gasterenterol 1985;4:15–16.
34. Inoue M. Irritable colon syndrome (Jap). Jap J Clin Med 1992;41:495–504.
35. Mathias JR, Ferguson KL, Clench MH. Debilitating "functional" bowel disease controlled by leuprolide acetate, gonadotropin-releasing hormone (GnRH) analog. Dig Dis Sci 1989;34:761–66.
36. Bi-zhen W, Qi-Ying P. Functional bowel disorders in apparently healthy chinese people. Chinese J Epid 1988;9:345–49.
37. Olubide IO, Olawuya F, Fasanmade AA. A study of irritable bowel syndrome in an African population. Dig Dis Sci 1995;40:983–85.
38. Danivat D, Tankeyoon M, Sriratanaban A. Prevalence of irritable bowel syndrome in a non-Western population. Brit Med J [Clin.Res] 1988;296:1710–12.
39. Segal I, Walker ARP. The irritable bowel syndrome in the black community. S Afr Med J 1984;65:73–74.
40. Everhart JE, Renault PF. Irritable bowel syndrome in office-based practice in the United States. Gastroenterology 1991; 100:998–1005.

41. Talley NJ, Gabriel SE, Harmsen WS, et al. Medical costs in community subjects with irritable bowel syndrome. Gastroenterology 1995;109:1736–41.

42. Sandler RS. Epidemiology of irritable bowel syndrome in the United States. Gastroenterology 1990;99:409–15.

43. Whitehead WE, Burnett CK, Cook EW, et al. Impact of irritable bowel syndrome on quality of life. Dig Dis Sci 1996;41:2248–53.

44. O'Keefe EA, Talley NJ, Zinsmeister AR, et al. Bowel disorders impair functional status and quality of life in the elderly: a population based study. J Gerontol Biol Sci Med Sci 1995;50:184–89.

45. Thompson WG. Irritable bowel syndrome: prevalence, prognosis and consequences. Can Med Assoc J 1986;134:111–13.

46. Thompson WG. Gut Reactions. New York:Plenum;1989.

47. Longstreth GF. Irritable Bowel syndrome: a multibillion-dollar problem. Gastroent 1995;109:2029–42.

48. Longstreth GF. Irritable bowel syndrome: diagnosis in the managed care area. Dig Dis Sci 1997;42:1105–11.

49. Manning AP, Thompson WG, Heaton KW, et al. Towards positive diagnosis of the irritable bowel. Brit Med J 1978;2:653–54.

50. Kruis W, Thieme CH, Weinzierl M, et al. A diagnostic score for the irritable bowel syndrome: its value in the exclusion of organic disease. Gastroenterology 1984;87: 1–7.

51. Rao KP, Gupta S, Agrawal AK, et al. Evaluation of Manning's criteria in the diagnosis of irritable bowel syndrome. J Assoc Physicians India 1993;41:357–58.

52. Jeong H, Lee HR, Yoo BC, et al. Manning criteria in irritable bowel syndrome: its diagnostic significance. Korean J Intern Med 1993;8:34–39.

53. Poynard T, Naveau S, Benoit M, et al. French experience of Manning's criteria in irritable bowel syndrome. Eur J Gastroenterol Hepatol 1992;4:747–52.

54. Talley NJ, Phillips SF, Melton LJ, et al. Diagnostic value of the Manning criteria in irritable bowel syndrome. Gut 1990;31:77–81.

55. Hogston P. Irritable bowel syndrome as a cause of chronic pain in women attending a gynaecology clinic. Brit Med J 1987;294:934–40.

56. Smith RC, Greenbaum DS, Vancouver JB, et al. Gender differences in Manning criteria in the irritable bowel syndrome. Gastroenterology 1991;100:591–95.

57. Thompson WG. Gender differences in irritable bowel symptoms. Eur J Gastroenterol Hepatol 1997;9:299–302.

58. Whitehead WE, Crowell MD, Bosmajian L, et al. Existence of irritable bowel syndrome supported by factor analysis of symptoms in two community samples. Gastroenterology 1990;98:336–40.

59. O'Donnell LJD, Virjee J, Heaton KW. Detection of pseudodiarrhea by simple clinical assessment of intestinal transit rate. Brit Med J 1990;300:439–40.

60. Wise TN, Cooper JN, Ahmed S. The efficacy of group therapy for patients with irritable bowel syndrome. Psychosomatics 1982;23:465–69.

61. Chaudhary NA, Truelove SC. The irritable colon syndrome. Quart J Med 1962; 31:307–22.

62. Sullivan MA, Cohen S, Snape WJ. Colonic myoelectrical activity in irritable bowel syndrome: effect of eating and anticholinergics. New Engl J Med 1978;298 :878–83.

63. Longstreth GF, Preskill DB, Youkeles L. Irritable bowel syndrome in women having diagnostic laparoscopy or hysterectomy. Dig Dis Sci 1990;35:1285–90.

64. Prior A, Wilson K, Whorwell PJ, et al. Irritable bowel syndrome in the gynecological clinic. Dig Dis Sci 1989;34:1820–24.

65. Farquhar CM, Hoghton GB, Beard RW. Pelvic pain: pelvic congestion or the irritable bowel syndrome. Eur J Obstet Gynecol Reprod Biol 1990;37:71–75.

66. Thompson WG. Alternatives to medicine. Can Med Assoc J 1990;142:105–6.

67. Walker EA, Katon WJ, Jemelka R, et al. The prevalence of chronic pelvic pain and irritable bowel syndrome in two university clinics. J Psychosomat Obstet Gynaecol 1990;19 (suppl):65–75.

68. Longstreth GF. Irritable bowel syndrome and chronic pelvic pain. Obstet Gynaecol Surv 1994;49:505–7.

69. Guthrie E, Creed FH. Severe sexual dysfunctioning in women with IBS: comparison with IBD and duodenal ulceration. Brit Med J 1987;295:577–79.

70. Whorwell PJ, McCallum M, Creed FH, et al. Non-colonic features of irritable bowel syndrome. Gut 1986;27:37–40.

71. Crowell MD, Dubin NH, Robinson JC, et al. Functional bowel disorders in women with dysmenorrhoea. Am J Gastroenterol 1994;89:1973–77.

72. Heitkemper MM, Jarrett M. Pattern of gastrointestinal and somatic symptoms across the menstrual cycle. Gastroenterology 1992;102:505–13.

73. Whitehead WE, Cheskin LJ, Heller BR, et al. Evidence for exacerbation of irritable bowel syndrome during menses. Gastroenterology 1990;98:1485–89.

74. Sandler RS, Drossman DA. Bowel habits in young adults not seeking health care. Dig Dis Sci 1987;32:841–45.

75. Heaton KW, Ghosh S, Braddon FEM. How bad are the symptoms and bowel dysfunction of patients with the irritable bowel syndrome? A prospective, controlled study with emphasis on stool form. Gut 1991;32:73–79.

76. Heaton KW, Radvan J, Cripps H, et al. Defecation frequency and timing, and stool form in the general population: a prospective study. Gut 1992;33:818–24.

77. Probert CSJ, Emmett PM, Cripps HA, et al. Evidence for the ambiguity of the word constipation: the role of irritable bowel syndrome. Gut 1994;35:1455–58.

78. Drossman DA. The Functional Gastrointestinal Disorders: Diagnosis, Pathophysiology, and Psychosocial Factors. Philadelphia:WB Saunders;1994.

79. Smart HL, Nicholson DA, Atkinson M. Gastro-oesophageal reflux in the irritable bowel syndrome. Gut 1986;27:1127–31.

80. Triadafilopoulos G, Simms RW, Goldenberg DL. Bowel dysfunction in fibromyalgia syndrome. Dig Dis Sci 1991;36:59–64.

81. Hudson JI, Goldenberg DL, Pope HG, et al. Comorbidity of fibromyalgia with medical and psychiatric disorders. Am J Med 1992;92:363–67.

82. Yunus MB, Masi AT, Aldag JC. A controlled study of primary fibromyalgia syndrome: clinical features and association with other functional syndromes. J Rheumatol 1989;16:62–71.

83. Watson WC, Sullivan SN, Corke M, et al. Globus and headache: common symptoms of the irritable bowel syndrome. Can Med Assoc J 1978;118:387–88.

84. Whorwell PJ, Lupton EW, Eduran D, et al. Bladder smooth muscle dysfunction in patients with irritable bowel syndrome. Gut 1986;27:1014–17.

85. Francis CY. High prevalence of irritable bowel syndrome in patients attending a urological clinic. Dig Dis Sci 1997;42:404–7.

86. Sandler RS, Drossman DA, Nathan HP, et al. Symptom complaints and health care seeking behavior in subjects with bowel dysfunction. Gastroenterology 1984;87:314–18.

87. Dyer NH, Pridie RB. Incidence of hiatus hernia in asymptomatic subjects. Gut 1968;9:696–99.

88. Drossman DA, McKee DC, Sandler RS, et al. Psychosocial factors in the irritable bowel syndrome: a multivariate study of patients and nonpatients with irritable bowel syndrome. Gastroent 1988;95:701–8.

89. Whitehead WE, Bosmajian L, Zonderman AB, et al. Symptoms of psychological distress associated with irritable bowel syndrome: comparison of community and medical clinic samples. Gastroenterology 1988;95:709–14.

90. Maxton DG, Morris J, Whorwell PJ. More accurate diagnosis of irritable bowel syndrome by use of "non-colonic" symptomatology. Gut 1991;32:784–86.

91. Talley NJ, et al. Multisystem complaints in patients with the irritable bowel syndrome and functional dyspepsia. Eur J Gastroenterol Hepatol 1991;3:71–77.

92. Isgar B, Harman M, Kaye MD, et al. Symptoms of irritable bowel syndrome in ulcerative colitis in remission. Gut 1984;24:190–92.

93. Thompson WG. A strategy for management of the irritable bowel. Am J Gastroenterol 1986;81:95–100.

94. Doshi M, Heaton KW. Irritable bowel syndrome in patients discharged from surgical wards with non-specific abdominal pain. Brit J Surg 1994;81:1216–18.

95. Fielding JF. Surgery and the irritable bowel syndrome: the singer as well as the song. J Irish Med 1988;76:33–34.

96. Barton JR. Investigation and surgery in irritable bowel syndrome—a cautionary series. Scot Med J 1994;39:80–81.

97. Owens DM, Nelson DK, Talley NJ. The irritable bowel syndrome: long term prognosis and the patient-physician interaction. Ann Intern Med 1995;122:107–12.

98. Burns DG. The risk of abdominal surgery in irritable bowel syndrome. South Afr Med J 1986;70:91–94.

99. Gambone JC, Reiter RC. Nonsurgical management of chronic pelvic pain. a multidisciplinary approach. Clin Obstet Gynecol 1990;33:205–11.

100. Thompson WG. The irritable bowel syndrome: a strategy for the family physician. Can Fam Med 1993;39.

101. Thompson WG, Tytgat GNJ, van Blankenstein M, Editors.Current Topics in Gastroenterology and Hepatology. New York:Springer-Verlag;1990:236–45.

102. Cullingford GL, Coffee JF, Carr-Locke DL. Irritable bowel syndrome: can the patient's response to colonoscopy help with the diagnosis? Digestion 1992;52:209–13.

103. Kang JY, Gwee KA, Yap I. The colonic air insufflation test indicates a colonic cause of abdominal pain: an aid in the diagnosis of the irritable bowel syndrome. J Clin Gastroenterol 1994;18:19–22.

104. Chobanian AV, Dolecek TA, Dustan HP. National education programs working group report on the management of patients with hypertension and high blood cholesterol. Ann Intern Med 1991;114:224–38.

105. Glaser SR. Utilization of sigmoidoscopy by family physicians in Canada. Can Med Assoc J 1994;150:367–71.

106. Thompson WG, Heaton KW, Smythe GT, et al. Irritable bowel syndrome: the view from general practice. Eur J Gastroenterol Hepatol 1997;9:689–92.

107. Thompson WG, Heaton KW, Smythe GT, et al. Irritable bowel syndrome in general practice: prevalence, characteristics and referral. Gut 2000;46:78–82.

108. Tolliver BA, Herrera JL, DiPalma JA. Evaluation of patients who meet clinical criteria for irritable bowel syndrome. Am J Gastroenterol 1994;89:176–8.

109. Newcomer AD, McGill DB. Irritable bowel syndrome: role of lactase deficiency. Mayo Clin Proc 1983;59:339–41.

110. Tolliver BA, Jackson MS, Jackson KL. Does lactose maldigestion really play a role in the irritable bowel syndrome? J Clin Gastroenterol 1996;23:15–17.

111. Suarez FL, Savaiano DA, Levitt MD. A comparison of symptoms after the consumption of milk or lactose-hydrolyzed milk by people with self-reported severe lactose intolerance. New Engl J Med 1995;333:1–4.

112. Newcomer AD, McGill DB, Thomas PJ, et al. Tolerance of lactose among lactase-deficient American Indians. Gastroent 1978;74:44–6.

113. Treacher DF, Chapman JR, Nolan DJ, et al. Irritable bowel syndrome: Is a barium enema necessary? Clin Radiol 1986;37:87–8.

114. Thompson WG. Do colonic diverticula cause symptoms? Am J Gastroenterol 1986;81:613–14.

115. Sim GPG, Scobie BA. Natural history of diverticulosis of the colon. N Z Med J 1982;95:611–3.

116. Francis CY, Duffy JN, Whorwell PJ, et al. Does routine abdominal ultrasound enhance diagnostic accuracy in irritable bowel syndrome? Am J Gastroenterol 1996;91:1348–50.

117. Holmes KM, Salter RH. Irritable bowel syndrome—a safe diagnosis. Brit Med J 1982;285:1533–34.

118. Mendeloff AI. Thoughts on the epidemiology of diverticular disease. Clinics in Gastroenterology 1986;15:855–77.

119. Svendsen JH, Munck LK, Andersen JR. Irritable bowel syndrome: prognosis and diagnostic safety: a 5-year follow up study. Scand J Gastroenterol 1985;20:415–18.

120. Bleijenberg G, Fennis JFM. Anemnestic and psychological features of functional abdominal complaints: a prospective study. Gut 1989;30:1076–81.

121. Harvey RF, Mauad EC, Brown AM. Prognosis in the irritable bowel syndrome: a five-year prospective study. Lancet 1987;963–65.

122. Camilleri M, Prather CM. The irritable bowel syndrome: mechanisms and a practical approach to management. Ann Intern Med 1992;116:1001–1008.

123. Drossman DA, Thompson WG. Irritable bowel syndrome: a graduated, multi-component treatment approach. Ann Intern Med 1992;116:1009–16.

124. Christensen J. Pathophysiology of the irritable bowel syndrome. Lancet 1992; 340:1444–47.

125. Thompson WG. The irritable bowel syndrome: pathogenesis and management. Lancet 1993;341:1569–72.

126. Kellow JE, Bennett E. Functional disorders of the small intestine. Semin Gastroenterol Dis 1996;7:208–16.

127. Heaton KW. Irritable bowel syndrome. Prescriber's J 1997;37:199–205.

128. Coremans G, Dapoigny M, Muller-Lissner SA, et al. Diagnostic procedures in irritable bowel syndrome. Digestion 1995;56:76–84.

129. McKee DP, Quigley EMM. Intestinal motility in irritable bowel syndrome: is IBS a motility disorder? Part 1: definition of IBS and colon motility. Dig Dis Sci 1993; 38:1761–72.

130. Connell AM. The motility of the pelvic colon: Part II: paradoxical motility in diarrhea and constipation. Gut 1962;3:342–48.

131. Wangel AG, Deller DJ. Intestinal motility in man: III: Mechanisms of constipation and diarrhea with particular reference to the irritable colon syndrome. Gastroenterol 1965;48:69–84.

132. Snape WJ, Carlson GM, Matarazzo SA, et al. Evidence that abnormal myoelectric activity produces colon motor dysfunction in the irritable bowel syndrome. Gastroenterol 1977;72:383–87.

133. Taylor I, Darby C, Hammond P, et al. Is there a myoelectric abnormality in the irritable colon syndrome? Gut 1978;19:391–95.

134. Latimer P, Sarna S, Campbell D, et al. Colonic motor and myoelectric activity: a comparative study of normal subjects, psychoneurotic patients and patients with the irritable bowel syndrome. Gastroenterol 1981;80:893–901.

135. Madhu SV, Vij JC, Bhatnagar OP, et al. Colonic myoelectric activity in irritable bowel syndrome before and after treatment. Indian J Gastroenterol 1993;7:31–33.

136. Bueno L, Fioramonti J, Ruckebusch Y, et al. Evaluation of colonic myoelectrical activity in health and functional disorders. Gut 1980;21:480–85.

137. Vassallo M, Camilleri M, Phillips SF, et al. Transit through the proximal colon influences stool weight in the irritable bowel syndrome. Gastroenterology 1992; 102:102–108.

138. Stivland T, Camilleri M, Vassallo M, et al. Scintographic measurement of regional gut transit in idiopathic constipation. Gastroenterology 1991;101:107–15.

139. Swarbrick ET, Hegarty JE, Bat L, et al. Site of pain from the irritable bowel syndrome. Lancet 1980;2:443–46.

140. Kendall GPN, Thompson DG, Day SJ, et al. Inter and intra individual variation in pressure-volume relations in the rectum of normal subjects and patients with the irritable bowel syndrome. Gut 1990;31:1062–68.

141. Kumar D, Wingate DL. The irritable bowel syndrome: a paraxysmal motor disorder. Lancet 1985;2:973–77.

142. Kellow JE, Phillips SF. Altered small bowel motility in irritable bowel syndrome is correlated with symptoms. Gastroenterology 1987;92:1885–93.

143. Coremans G, Tack J, Vantrappen G, et al. Is the irritable bowel really irritable? Ital J Gastroenterol 1993;23(suppl 1):39–40.

144. Kellow JE, Langeluddecke PM, Eckersley GM, et al. Effects of acute psychologic stress on small-intestinal motility in health and the irritable bowel syndrome. Scand J Gastroenterol 1992;27:53–58.

145. Moriarty KJ, Dawson AM. Functional abdominal pain: further evidence that the whole gut is effected. Brit Med J 1982;1:1602–20.

146. Evans PR, Bennett EJ, Bak T-E, et al. Jejunal sensorimotor dysfunction in irritable bowel syndrome: clinical and psychological features. Gastroenterology 1996; 110:393–404.

147. Mayer EA, Raybould HE. Role of visceral afferent mechanisms in functional bowel disorders. Gastroenterology 1990;99:1688–1704.

148. Mertz H, Naliboff B, Munakata J, et al. Altered rectal perception is a biological marker of patients with irritable bowel syndrome. Gastroenterology 1995;109: 40–52.

149. Munakata J, Naliboff B, Harraf F, et al. Repetitive sigmoid stimulation induces rectal hyperalgesia in patients with irritable bowel syndrome. Gastroenterology 1997;112:55–63.

150. Accarino AM, Azpiroz F, Malagalada J-R. Selective dysfunction of mechanosensitive intestinal afferents in irritable bowel syndrome. Gastroenterology 1995;108: 636–43.

151. Accarino AM, Azpiroz F, Malagalada J-R. Attention and distraction: effects on gut perception. Gastroenterology 1997;113:415–22.

152. Aggarwal A, Cutts TF, Abell TL, et al. Prominent symptoms in irritable bowel syndrome correlate with specific autonomic nervous system abnormalities. Gastroenterology 1994;106:945–50.

153. Silverman DHS, Munakata JA, Ennes H, et al. Regional cerebral activity in normal and pathological perception of visceral pain. Gastroenterology 1997;112:64–72.

154. Drossman DA. Gastrointestinal illness and the biopsychosocial model. J Clin Gastroenterol 1996;22:252–54.

155. Collins SM. Is the irritable gut an inflamed gut? Scand J Gastroenterol 1992;192 (suppl):102–105.

156. Van Tilbrul AJP, de Rooij FWM, van Blankenstein M, et al. Na+ dependent bile acid transport in the ileum: the balance between diarrhea and constipation. Gastroenterology 1990;98:25–32.

157. Rumessen JJ, Goodman-Hayer J. Functional bowel disease, malabsorption and abdominal distress after ingestion of fructose, sorbitol and fructose sorbitol mixture. Gastroenterology 1988;95:694–700.

158. Gwee KA, Graham JC, McKendrick NW, et al. Psychometric scores and persistence of Irritable bowel after infectious diarrhea. Lancet 1996;347:150–53.

159. Neal KR, Hebdon J, Spiller R. Prevalence of gastrointestinal symptoms six months after bacterial gastroenteritis and risk factors for developmant of the irritable bowel syndrome. Brit Med J 1997;314:779–82.

160. Finn R, Smith MA, Youngs GR, et al. Immunological hypersensitivity to environmental antigens in the irritable bowel syndrome. Brit J Clin Pract 1987;41: 1041–43.

161. Jones A, Shorthouse M, McLaughlan P, et al. Food intolerance: a major factor in the pathogenesis of the irritable bowel syndrome. Lancet 1982;2:1115–17.

162. Hiatt RB, Katz L. Mast cells in inflammatory conditions of the gastrointestinal tract. Am J Gastroenterology 1962;37:541–48.

163. Weston AP, Biddle WL, Bhatia PS, et al. Terminal ileal mucosal mast cells in irritable bowel syndrome . Dig Dis Sci 1993;38:1590–95.

164. McIntosh D, Thompson WG, Patel D, et al. Is rectal biopsy necessary in irritable bowel syndrome? Am J Gastroenterol 1992;87:1407–1409.

165. Klein KB. Chronic intractable abdominal pain. Semin Gastroenterol Dis 1990; 1:43–56.

166. Whitehead WE, Crowell MD, Heller BR, et al. Modeling and reinforcement of the sick role during childhood predicts adult illness behaviour. Psychosomat Med 1994;56:541–50.

167. Whitehead WE. Psychosocial aspects of functional gastrointestinal disease. Gastroenterology Clin North Am 1996;25:21–34.

168. Ford MJ. The irritable bowel syndrome. J Psychosomat Med 1986;30:399–410.

169. Cook IJ, van Eeden A, Collins SM. Patients with irritable bowel syndrome have greater pain tolerance than normal subjects. Gastroenterology 1987;93:727–33.

170. Whitehead WE, Holtkotter B, Enck P, et al. Tolerance for rectosigmoid distention in irritable bowel syndrome. Gastroenterology 1990;98:1187–92.

171. Toner BB, Garfinkel PE, Jeejeebhoy KN. Psychological factors in irritable bowel syndrome. Can J Psychiatry 1990;35:158–61.

172. Young SJ, Alpers DH, Norland CC, et al. Psychiatric illness and the irritable bowel syndrome. Practical implications for the primary physician. Gastroenterology 1976;70:162–66.

173. Esler MD, Goulston KJ. Levels of anxiety in colonic disorders. New Engl J Med 1973;288:16–20.

174. Greenbaum DS, Ferguson RK, Kater LA, et al. A controlled therapeutic study of the irritable bowel syndrome. New Engl J Med 1973;288:612–16.

175. Liss JL, Alpers DH, Woodruff RA. Irritable colon syndrome and psychiatric illness. Dis Nerv Sys 1973;34:151–57.

176. Colgan S, Creed F. Psychiatric disorder and illness behaviour in patients with upper abdominal pain. Psychosomat Med 1988;18:887–92.

177. Lydiard RB. Anxiety and the irritable bowel syndrome: psychiatric, medical or both? J Clin Psychiatry 1997;58(suppl 3):51–58.

178. Walker EA, Katon WJ, Jemelka RP, et al. Comorbidity of gastrointestinal complaints, depression, and anxiety in the Epidemiologic Catchment Area (ECA) Study. Am J Med 1993;92:26s–30s.

179. Smith RC, Greenbaum DS, Vancouver JB, et al. Psychosocial factors are associated with health care seeking rather than diagnosis in irritable bowel syndrome. Gastroenterology 1990;98:293–301.

180. Talley NJ, Phillips SF, Bruce B, et al. Relation among personality and symptoms in nonulcer dyspepsia and the irritable bowel syndrome. Gastroenterology 1990;99 (2):327–33.

181. Welch GW, Hillman LC, Pomare EW. Psychoneurotic symptomatology in the irritable bowel syndrome: a study of reporters and non-reporters. Brit Med J 1985; 291:1362–64.

182. Kettell J, Jones R, Lydiard S. Reasons for consultation in irritable bowel syndrome: symptoms and patient characteristics. Brit J Gen Pract 1992;42:459–61.

183. Almy TP, Kern FJr, Tulin M. Alteration in colonic function in man under stress: II. experimental production of sigmoid spasm in healthy persons. Gastroenterology 1949;12:425–36.

184. Longstreth GF. Bowel pattern and anxiety:demographic factors. J Clin Gastroenterol 1993 ;17:128–32.

185. Mendeloff AI, Monk M, Siegel CI, et al. Illness experience and life stresses in patients with irritable colon and with ulcerative colitis: an epidemiologic study of ulcerative colitis and regional enteritis in Baltimore, 1960-1964. New Engl J Med 1970;282:14–17.

186. Ford MJ, Miller PM, Eastwood J, et al. Life events, psychiatric illness and the irritable bowel syndrome. Gut 1987;28:160–65.

187. Hill OW, Blendis L. Physical and psychological evaluation of 'non-organic' abdominal pain. Gut 1967;8:221–29.

188. Drossman DA, Talley NJ, Olden KW, et al. Sexual and physical abuse and gastrointestinal illness: review and recommendations. Ann Intern Med 1995;123: 792–94.

189. Drossman DA, Leserman J, Nachman G, et al. Sexual and physical abuse in women with functional or organic gastrointestinal disorders. Ann Intern Med 1990;113:828–33.

190. Talley NJ, Fett SL, Zinsmeister AR, et al. Gastrointestinal tract symptoms and self-reported abuse: a population-based study. Gastroenterology 1994;107:1040–49.

191. Delvaux M, Denis P, Allemans H.. Sexual and physical abuses are more frequently reported by IBS patients than by patients with organic digestive diseases orcontrols: results of a multicentre inquiry. Eur J Gastroenterol Hepatol 1997; 9:345–52.

192. Springs FE, Friedrich WN. Health risk behaviours and medical sequelae of childhood sexual abuse. Mayo Clin Proc 1992;67:527–32.

193. Scarinci IC, McDonald-Haile J, Bradley LA, et al. Altered pain perception and psychological factors among women with gastrointestinal disorders and history of abuse. Am J Med 1994;97:108–18.

194. Leserman J, Li Z, Drossman DA, et al. Selected symptoms associated with sexual

and physical abuse history among female patients with GI disorders: the impact on subsequent health care visits. Psychol Med 1998;28:417–25.

195. Drossman DA, Li Z, Leserman J, et al. Health status by gastrointestinal diagnosis and abuse history. Gastroenterology 1996;110:999–1007.

196. Drossman DA. Irritable bowel syndrome and sexual/physical abuse history. Eur J Gastroenterol Hepatol 1997;9:327–30.

197. Drossman DA, Li Z, Leserman J, et al. Association of coping pattern and health status among female GI patients after controlling for GI disease type and abuse history: a prospective study. Gastroenterology 1997;112(Abstr):724.

198. Whitehead WE, Crowell MD, Davidoff AL, et al. Pain from rectal distension in women with irritable bowel syndrome: relation to sexual abuse. Dig Dis Sci 1997; 42:796–804.

199. Talley NJ. Is the association between irritable bowel syndrome and abuse explained by neuroticism? Gut 1998;42:47–53.

200. Mayer EA. Does mind-body medicine have a role in gastroenterology. Curr Opin Gastroenterol 1997;13:1–3.

201. Drossman DA, Whitehead WE, Camilleri M, et al. Irritable bowel syndrome: a technical review for guidelines development. Gastroenterology 1997;112:2120–37.

202. Pace F, Coremans G, Dapoigny M, et al. Therapy of irritable bowel syndrome—an overview. Digestion 1995;56:433–42.

203. Craig TK, Brown GW. Goal frustration and life event stress in the aetiology of painful gastrointestinal disorder. J Psychosomat Res 1984;28:411–21.

204. Dumitrascu DL, Baban A. Irritable bowel syndrome complaints following the uprising of December 1989 in Romania. Med and War 1991;7:100–1033.

205. Whitehead WE, Crowell MD, Robinson JC, et al. Effects of stressful life events on bowel symptoms:subjects with irritable bowel symptoms compared with subjects without bowel dysfunction. Gut 1992;33:825–30.

206. Creed FH, Craig T, Farmer RG. Functional abdominal pain, psychiatric illness and life events. Gut 1988;29:235–42.

207. Svedlund J, Sjodin I, Ottosson JO, et al. Controlled study of psychotherapy in irritable bowel syndrome. Lancet 1983;2:589–91.

208. van Dulman AM, Fennis JF, Mokkin K, et al. Doctor dependent changes in complaint-related cognitions and anxiety during medical consultations in functional abdominal complaints. Psychol Med 1995;25:1011–18.

209. Guthrie E, Creed F, Dawson D, Tomenson B. A controlled trial of psychological treatment for the irritable bowel syndrome. Gastroenterology 1991;100:450–57.

210. Creed R, Guthrie E. Psychological treatments of the irritable bowel syndrome. Gut 1989;30:1601–1609.

211. Ryle JA. Chronic spasmodic affections of the colon. Lancet 1928;2:1115–19.

212. Verhoef MJ, Sutherland LR, Brkich L. Use of alternative medicine by patients attending a gastroenterology clinic. Can Med Assoc J 1990;142:121–25.

213. Smart HL, Mayberry JF, Atkinson M. Alternative medicine consultations and remedies in patients with the irritable bowel syndrome. Gut 1986;27:826–28.

214. Zuckerman MJ, Guerra LG, Foland JA, et al. Health care seeking behaviors related to bowel complaints: Hispanics vs non-Hispanics. Dig Dis Sci 1991;41:77–82.

215. Nanda R, James R, Smith H, et al. Food intolerance and the irritable bowel syndrome. Gut 1989;30:1099–1104.

216. Pearson DJ. Pseudo food allergy. Brit Med J 1986;292:221–22.

217. McKee AM, Prior A, Whorwell PJ. Exclusion diets in irritable bowel syndrome: are they worthwhile? J Clin Gastroenterol 1987;9:526–28.

218. Young E, Stoneham MD, Petruckevitch A, et al. A population study of food intolerance. Lancet 1994;343:1127–30.

219. Middleton SJ, Coley A, Hunter JO. The role of candida albicans in the pathogenesis of food-intolerant irritable bowel syndrome. Postgrad Med J 1992;68:453–54.

220. Dismukes WE, Wade JS, Lee JY, et al. A randomized, double-blind trial of nystatin therapy for the candidiasis hypersensivity syndrome. New Engl J Med 1990;323: 1717–23.

221. Manning AP, Heaton KW, Harvey RF, et al. Wheat bran and irritable bowel syndrome. Lancet 1977;2:417–18.

222. Heaton KW. Snape WJ, Editors. Pathogenesis of Functional Bowel Disease. New York:Plenum;1989:79.

223. Cann PA, Read NW, Holdsworth CD. What is the benefit of coarse wheat bran in patients with irritable bowel syndrome? Gut 1984;25:168–73.

224. Lucey MR, Clark ML, Lowndes J, et al. Is bran efficacious in irritable bowel syndrome? a double-blind placebo-controlled crossover study. Gut 1987;28:221–25.

225. Cummings JH, Hill MJ, Jenkins DJA, et al. Changes in fecal composition and colonic function due to cerial fiber. Am J Clin Nutr 1976;29:1468–73.

226. McAllister C, McGrath F, Fielding JF. Altered skin temperature and electromyographic activity in the irritable bowel syndrome. Biomed Pharmacother 1990; 44:399–401.

227. Francis CY, Whorwell PJ. Bran and irritable bowel syndroms: time for reappraisal. Lancet 1994;344:39–40.

228. Snook J, Shepherd AH. Bran supplementation in the treatment of the irritable bowel syndrome. Aliment Pharmacol Ther 1994;8:511–14.

229. Klein KB. Controlled treatment trials in the irritable bowel syndrome: a critique. Gastroenterology 1988;95:232–41.

230. Luttecke K. A trial of trimebutine in spastic colon. J Intern Med Res 1978;6: 86–88.

231. Moshal MG, Herron M. A clinical trial of trimebutine in spastic colon. J Intern Med Res 1979;7:231–34.

232. Cann PA, Read NW, Holdsworth CD, et al. Role of loperamide and placebo in management of irritable bowel syndrome. Dig Dis Sci 1984;29:239–47.

233. Efskind PS, Bernklev T, Vatn MH. A double-blind, placebo-controlled trial with loperamide in irritable bowel syndrome. Scand J Gastroenterol 1996;31:463–68.

234. Oddsson E, Rask-Madsen J, Krag E, et al. A secretory epithelium of the small intestine with increased sensitivity to bile acids in irritable bowel syndrome associated with diarrhea. Scand J Gastroenterol 1978;13:409–16.

235. Krevsky B, Maurer AH, Niewiarowski T, et al. Effect of verapamil on human intestinal transit. Dig Dis Sci 1992;37:919–24.

236. Levitt MD, Furne J, Olsson S. The relation of passage of gas and colonic bloating to colonic gas production. Ann Intern Med 1996;124:422–24.

237. Toskes PP, Connery KL, Ritchey TW. Calcium polycarbophil compared with placebo in irritable bowel syndrome. Aliment Pharmacol Ther 1993;7:87–92.

238. Schultze K. Double blind study of the effects of cisapride on constipation and abdominal discomfort as components of the irritable bowel syndrome. Aliment Pharmacol Ther 1997;11:387–94.

239. Van Outryve M, Milo R, Toussaint J, Van Eeghem PV. "Prokinetic" treatment of constipation-predominant irritable bowel syndrome: A placebo-controlled study of cisapride. J Clin Gastroenterol 1991;13:49–57.

240. Wessalius-DeCasparis A, Braadbaart S, Bergh-Bohekin GE, Mimica M. Treatment of chronic constipation with lactulose syrup: results of a double blind study. Gut 1969;9:84–6.

241. Lederle FA, Busch DL, Mattox KM, West MJ, Aske DM. Cost-effective treatment of constipation in the elderly: a randomized double-blind comparison of sorbitol and lactulose. Am.J Med. 1990;89:597–601.

242. Corazziari E, Badiali D, Habib FI, et el. Small volume isosmotic polyethylene glycol electrolyte balanced solution (PMF-100) in treatment of chronic nonorganic constipation. Dig Dis Sci 1996;41:1636–42.

243. Klauser AG, Muhldorfer BE, Voderholzer WA, Wenzel G, Muller-Lissner SA. Polyethylen glycol 4000 for slow transit constipation. Z Gastroenterologie 1995; 33:5–8.

244. Goulston K. Drug usage in the irritable colon syndrome. Med J Aust 1972;1: 1126–31.

245. Ivey KJ. Are anticholinergics of use in the irritable bowel syndrome? Gastroent 1975;68:1300–7.

246. Camilleri M, Choi M-G. Review Article: Irritable bowel syndrome. Aliment Pharmacol Ther 1997;11:3–15.

247. Dew MJ, Evans BK, Rhodes J. Peppermint oil for the irritable bowel syndrome: a multicentre trial. Brit J Clin Pract 1984;38:394–98.

248. Nash P, Gould SR, Bernardo DE. Peppermint oil does not relieve the pain of irritable bowel syndrome. Brit J Clin Pract 1986;40:292–93.

249. Passaretti S, Guslandi M, Imbimbo BP, et al. Effects of cimetropium bromide on gastrointestinal transit time in patients with irritable bowel syndrome. Aliment Pharmacol Ther 1989;3:267–76.

250. Tasman-Jones C. Mebeverine in patients with the irritable colon syndrome: double blind study. N Z Med J 1973;1:232–35.

251. Evans PR, Bak YT, Kellow JE. Mebeverine alters small bowel motility in irritable bowel syndrome. Aliment Pharmacol Ther 1996;10:787–93.

252. Poynard T, Naveau S, Mory B, et al. Meta-analysis of smooth muscle relaxants in the treatment of irritable bowel syndrome. Aliment Pharmacol Ther 1994;8: 499–510.

253. Lancaster-Smith MJ, Prout BJ, Pinto T, et al. Influence of drug treatment on the irritable bowel syndrome and its interaction with psychoneurotic morbidity. Acta Psychiatr Scand 1982;6632–41.

254. Myren J, Groth H, Larssen SE, et al. The effect of trimipramine in patients with the irritable bowel syndrome. Scand J Gastroenterol 1982;17:871–75.

255. Myren J, Loveland B, Larssen SE, et al. A double-blind study of the effect of trimipramine in patients with the irritable bowel synerome. Scand J Gastroenterol 1984;19:835–43.

256. Greenbaum DS, Mayle JE, Vanegeren LE, et al. The effects of desipramine on IBS compared with atropine and placebo. Dig Dis Sci 1987;32:257–66.

257. Clouse RE. Antidepressants for functional gastrointestinal symptoms. Dig Dis Sci 1994;39:2352–63.

258. Eckardt VF, Lesschafft C, Kanzler G, et al. Disability and health care use in patients with Crohn's disease: a spouse control study. Am J Gastroenterol 1994;89: 2157–62.

259. Gorard DA, Libby GW, Farthing MJ. Effect of a tricyclic antidepressant on small intestinal motility in health and diarrhea-predominant irritable bowel syndrome. Dig Dis Sci 1995;40:86–95.

260. Gorard DA, Libby DW, Farthing MJ. Influence of antidepressants on whole gut and orocecal transit times in health and irritable bowel syndrome. Aliment Pharmacol Ther 1994;8:159–56.

261. Junien J-L, Riviere P. Review article: the hypersensitive gut—peripheral kappa agonists as a new pharmacological approach. Aliment Pharmacol Ther 1995;9: 117–26.

262. Dapoigny M, Abitbol J-L, Fraitag B. Efficacy of peripheral kappa agonist fedotozine versus placebo in treatment of irritable bowel syndrome. Dig Dis Sci 1996;40:2244–48.

263. Prior A, Read NW. Reduction in rectal sensitivity and post prandial motility by granisetron, a 5HT-recepter antagonist, in patients with the irritable bowel syndrome. Aliment Pharmacol Ther 1993;7:175–80.

264. Hammer J, Phillips SF, Talley NJ, et al. Effect of a 5HT$_3$-antagonist (ondansetron) on rectal sensitivity and compliance in health and the irritable bowel syndrome. Aliment Pharmacol Ther 1993;7:543–51.

265. Zighelboim J, Talley NJ, Phillips SF, et al. Visceral perception in irritable bowel syndrome. rectal and gastric responses to distension and serotonin type 3 antagonism. Dig Dis Sci 1995;40:819–27.

266. Maxton DG, Morris J, Whorwell PJ. Selective 5-hydroxytryptamine antagonism: a role for irritable bowel syndrome and functional dyspepsia. Aliment Pharmacol Ther 1996; 10:595–99.

267. Camilleri M, Mayer EA, Drossman DA, et al. Improvement in pain and bowel function in female irritable bowel patients with Alosetron, a 5HT$_3$-receptor antagonist. Aliment Pharmacol Ther 1999;13:1149–59.

268. Hasler WL, Soudah HC, Owyang C. A somatostatin analogue inhibits afferant

pathways mediating perception of rectal distension. Gastroenterology 1993;104: 1390–97.

269. Louvel D, Delvaux M, Felez A, et al. Oxytocin increases thresholds of colonic visceral perception in patients with irritable bowel syndrome. Gut 1996;39:741–47.

270. O'Donnell LJD, Watson AJ, Cameron D, et al. Effect of octreotide on mouth to cecum transit time in healthy subjects and irritable bowel syndrome. Aliment Pharmacol Ther 1990;4:177–82.

271. Bradette M, Delveaux M, Staumont G, et al. J. Octreotide increases thresholds of colonic visceral perception in IBS patients without modifying muscle tone. Dig Dis Sci 1994;39:1171–78.

272. Drossman DA. Diagnosing and treating patients with refractory functional gastrointestinal disorders. Ann Intern Med 1995;123:688–97.

273. Houghton LA, Whorwell PJ. Symptomatology, quality of life and economic features of irritable bowel syndrome—the effect of hypnotherapy. Aliment Pharmacol Ther 1996;10:91–95.

274. Bueno-Miranda F, Cerulli M, Schuster MM, et al. Operant conditioning of colonic motility in irritable bowel syndrome. Gastroenterology 1976;70(abstr): 867.

275. Svedlund J. Psychotherapy in irritable bowel syndrome: a controlled outcome study. Acta Psychiatr Scand 1983;67(suppl):1–86.

276. Shaw G, Srivastava ED, Sadlier M, et al. Stress management for irritable bowel syndrome: a controlled trial. Digestion 1991;50:36–42.

277. Bennett P, Wilkinson S. A comparison of psychological and medical treatment of the irritable bowel syndrome. Brit J Clin Psychol 1985;24:215–16.

278. Lynch PM, Zamble E. A controlled behavioral treatment study of irritable bowel syndrome. Behav Ther 1989;20:509–24.

279. Rumsey N. Heaton KW, Creed F, Goeting NLM, Editors.Current Approaches Towards Confident Management of Iirritable Bowel Syndrome. London: Lyme Regis Printing Company; 1991:33–39.

280. Corney RH, Stanton R, Newell R, et al. Behavioural psychotherapy as a treatment for irritable bowel syndrome. J Psychosomat Res 1991;35:461–69.

281. Blanchard EB, Greene B, Scharff L, et al. Relaxation training as treatment for irritable bowel syndrome. Biofeed Self Reg 1993;3:125–32.

282. Greene B, Blanchard EB. Cognitive therapy for irritable bowel syndrome. J Consult Clin Psychol 1994;62:576–82.

283. Drossman DA, Creed FH, Fava GA, et al. Psychosocial aspects of the functional gastrointestinal disorders. Gastroenterol Internat 1995;8:47–90.

284. Drossman DA, Funch-Jensen P, Janssens J, et al. Identification of subgroups of functional bowel disorders. Gastroenterol Internat 1990;3:159–72.

285. Briet F, Achour L, Flourie B, et al. Symptomatic response to varying levels of fructo-oligosaccharides consumed occasionally or regularly. Eur J Clin Nutr 1995;49:501–507.

286. Schlemper RJ, van der Werf SD, Vandebrouke JP, et al. Peptic ulcer, non-ulcer dys-

pepsia and irritable bowel syndrome in The Netherlands and Japan. Scand J Gastroenterol 1993;200(suppl):33–41.

287. Dimenas E, Glise H, Hallerbach B, et al. Quality of life in patients with upper abdominal symptoms. Scand J Gastroenterol 1993;28:681–87.

288. Johnsen R, Jacobsen BK, Forde OH. Association between symptoms of irritable colon and psychological and social conditions and lifestyle. Brit Med J 1986; 292:1633–35.

289. Kay L, Jorgensen T. Abdominal symptom associations in a longitudinal study. Internat J Epidemiol 1993;22:1093–100.

290. Knill-Jones RP. A formal approach to symptoms of dyspepsia. Clin Gastroenterol 1985;14:517–29.

291. Talley NJ, Phillips SF, Melton LJ, et al. A patient questionnaire to identify bowel disease. Ann Intern Med 1989;111:671–74.

292. Janatuinen EK, Pikkarainen PH, Laakso M, et al. Gastrointestinal symptoms in middle-aged diagetic patients. Scand J Gastroenterol 1993;28:427–32.

293. Dewsnap PA, Gomborone JE, Libby G, et al. The prevalence of symptoms of irritable bowel syndrome among acute psychiatric patients with affective diagnosis. Psychosomat 1996;37:385–89.

294. Sullivan SN. Prospective study of unexplained visible abdominal bloating. N Z Med J 1994;107:428–30.

295. Heitkemper MM, Jarett M, Cain KC, et al. Daily gastrointestinal symptoms in women with and without a diagnosis of IBS. Dig Dis Sci 1995;40:1511–19.

296. Chami TN, Schuster MM, Bohlman M, et al. A simple radiologic method to estimate the quantity of bowel gas. Am J Gastroenterol 1991;86:599–602.

297. Maxton DG, Martin DF, Whorwell PJ, et al. Abdominal distension in female patients with irritable bowel syndrome: exploration of possible mechanisms. Gut 1991;32:662–64.

298. Lasser RB, Levitt MD. The role of intestinal gas in functional abdominal pain. New Engl J Med 1975;293:524–26.

299. Barbera R, Feinie C, Read NW. Abnormal sensitivity to duodenal lipid infusion in patients with functional dyspepsia. Eur J Gastroenterol Hepatol 1995;7:1051–57.

300. Troncon LEA, Thompson DG, Ahlualia NK, et al. Relations between upper abdominal symptoms and gastric distension abnormalities in dysmotility like functional dyspepsia and after vagotomy. Gut 1995;37:17–22.

301. Undeland KA, Hausken T, Svebak S, et al. Wide gastric antrum and low vagal tone in patients with diabetes mellitus type 1 compared to patients with functional dyspepsia and after vagotomy. Dig Dis Sci 1996;41:9–16.

302. Galati JS, McKee DP, Quigley EMM. Response to intraluminal gas in irritable bowel syndrome: motility versus perception. Dig Dis Sci 1995;40:1381–87.

303. Serra J, Azpiroz F, Malagalada J-R, et al. Abdominal symptoms, distension and intestinal gas retention induced by lipids. Gastroenterology 1998;114:A836.

304. Trotman IF, Price CC. Bloated irritable bowel syndrome defined by dynamic 99mtc bran scan. Lancet 1986;2:364–66.

305. Cann PA, Read NW, Brown C, et al. Irritable bowel syndrome: relationship of dis-

orders in the transit of a single solid meal to symptom patterns. Gut 1983;24: 405–11.

306. Koch A, Voderholzer WA, Heinrich CA,et al. Symptoms in chronic constipation. Dis Colon Rectum 1997;40:902–906.

307. Lydiard RB, Greenwald S, Weissman MM, et al. Panic disorder and gastrointestinal symptoms: findings from the NIMH Epidemiologic Catchment Area Project. Am J Psychiatry 1994;151:64–70.

308. Nyhlin H, Ford MJ, Eastwood J, et al. Non-alimentary aspects of the irritable bowel syndrome. J Psychosomat Res 1993;37:155–62.

309. Song JY, Merskey H, Sullivan SN, et al. Anxiety and depression in patients with abdominal bloating. Can J Psychiatry 1993;38:475–79.

310. Fardy J, Sullivan SN. Recent advances in pharmacotherapy: gastrointestinal gas. Can Med Assoc J 1988;139:1137–42.

311. Ganiats TG, Norcross WA, Halverson AL, et al. Does Beano prevent gas? A double-blind, crossover study of oral alpha-galactosidase to treat dietary oligosaccaride intolerance. J Fam Pract 1994;39:441–45.

312. Drossman DA, Sandler RS, McKee DC, et al. Bowel patterns among subjects not seeking health care: use of a questionnaire to identify a population with bowel dysfunction. Gastroenterology 1982;83:529–34.

313. Ruben BD. Public perceptions of digestive health and disease: A survey findings and communications implications. Practical Gastroenterol 1986;10:35–42.

314. Rendtorff RC, Kashgarian M. Stool patterns of healthy adult males. Dis Colon Rectum 1967;10:222–28.

315. Everhart JE, Go VL, Johannes RS, et al. A longitudinal survey of self-reported bowel habits in the United States. Dig Dis Sci 1989;34,8:1153–62.

316. Evans RC, Kamm MA, Hinton JM, et al. The normal range and a simple diagram for recording whole gut transit time. Internat J Colorect Dis 1992;7:15–17.

317. Metcalf AM, Phillips SF, Zinsmeister AR, et al. Simplified assessment of segmental colonic transit. Gastroenterology 1987;92:40–47.

318. Heaton KW, O'Donnell LJD. An office guide to whole gut transit time: patient's recollection of their stool form. J Clin Gastroeterol 1994;19:28–30.

319. Davies GJ, Crowder M, Reid B, et al. Bowel function measurements of individuals with different eating patterns. Gut 1986;27:164–69.

320. Abell TL, Malagelada JR, Lucas AR, et al. Gastric electromechanical and neurohormonal function in anorexia nervosa. Gastroenterology 1987;93:958–65.

321. Sonnenberg A, Koch TR. Physician visits in the United States for constipation: 1958 to 1986. Dig Dis Sci 1989; 34:606–11.

322. Whitehead WE, Drinkwater D, Cheskin LJ, et al. Constipation in the elderly living at home: definition, prevalence and relationship to lifestyle and health status. J Am Geriatr Soc 1989;37:423–29.

323. Wald A, Hinds JP, Caruana BJ. Psychological and physiological characteristics of patients with severe idiopathic constipation. Gastroenterology 1989;97:932–37.

324. Heaton KW, Cripps HA. Straining at stool and laxative taking in an English population. Dig Dis Sci 1993;38:1004–1008.

325. Kuijpers HC. Application of the colorectal laboratory in diagnosis and treatment of functional constipation. Dis Colon.Rectum 1990;33:35–39.

326. Gorard DA, Gamberone JE, Libby GW, et al. Intestinal transit in anxiety and depression. Gut 1996;39:551–55.

327. Lampe JW, Fredstrom SB, et al. Sex differences in colonic function: a randomized trial. Gut 1993;34:531–36.

328. Lewis SJ, Heaton KW. Stool form scale as a useful guide to intestinal transit time. Scand J Gastroenterol 1997; 32:920–24.

329. Arhan P, Devroede G, Jehennin B, et al. Segmental colon transit time. Diseases 1981;26:625–29.

330. Chaussade S, Khyari A, Roche H, et al. Determination of total and segmental transit time in constipated patients. Dig Dis Sci 1989;34:1168–72.

331. Fotherby KJ, Hunter JO. Idiopathic slow-transit constipation: whole gut transit times measured by a new simplified method are not shortened by opiate analgesics. Aliment Pharmacol Ther 198; 1:331–38.

332. Meier R, Beglinger C, Dederding JP, et al. Alters und geschiechtsspezifische normalwerte der dickdarmtransitzeit bei gesunden. Schweiz Med Wochenschr 1992; 122:940–43.

333. Schindlbeck NE, Klauser AG, Muller-Lissner SA. Messung der colon-transitzeit. Z Gastroenterologie 1990;28:399–404.

334. van der Sijp JRM, Kamm MA, Nightingale JMD, et al. Radioisotope determination of regional colonic transit in severe constipation: comparison with radiopaque markers. Gut 1993;34:402–408.

335. Ekberg O, Mahieu PHG, Bartram CI, et al. Defecography:dynamic radiologic imaging in proctology. Gastroenterol Internat 1990;3:63–69.

336. Ting KH, Mangal E, Eibl-Eibesfeldt B, et al. Evaluation of the retained volume at defecography. Dis Colon Rectum 1992;35:762–67.

337. Wald A, Camara BJ, Freimanis MG, et al. Contribution of evacuation proctography and anorectal manometry to the evaluation of adults with constipation and defecatory difficulty. Dig Dis Sci 1990;35:481–87.

338. Barnes PRH, Lennard-Jones JE. Balloon expulsion from the rectum in constipation of different types. Gut 1985;26:1049–52.

339. Preston DM, Lennard-Jones JE. Anismus in chronic constipation. Dig Dis Sci 1985;30(5):413–18.

340. Felt Bersma RJ, Luth WJ, et al. Defecography in patients with anorectal disorders: which findings are clinically relevant. Dis Colon.Rectum 1990;33:277–84.

341. Goei R. Anorectal function in patients with defecation disorders and asymptomatic subjects: evaluation with defecography. Radiology 1990;174:121–23.

342. Klauser AG, Peyeri C, Schindlbeck NE, et al. Nutrition and physical activity in chronic constipation. Eur J Gastroenterol Hepatol 1992;4:227–23.

343. Devroede CH, Sleisenger MH, Fortran JS, Editors. Gastrointestinal Disease: Pathophysiology, Diagnosis, Management. Ed. 4. Philadelphia:Saunders;1989: 331–68.

344. Bingham SA, Cummings JH. Effect of exercise and physical fitness on large intestinal function. Gastroenterology 1989;97:1389–99.

345. Oettle GJ. Effect of moderate exercise on bowel habit. Gut 1991;32:941–44.

346. Coenen C, Wegener M, Wedmann B, et al. Does physical activity influence bowel transit time in healthy young men? Am J Gastroenterol 1992;87:292–95.

347. Burkitt DP, Walker ARP, Painter NS. Effect of dietary fiber on stools and transit times, and its role in the causation of disease. Lancet 1972;2:1408–11.

348. Cummings JH, Bingham SA, Heaton KW, et al. Fecal weight, colon cancer risk, and dietary intake of non-starch polysaccharides (dietary fiber). Gastroenterology 1992;103:1783–89.

349. Eastwood MA, Brydon WG, Baird JD, et al. Fecal weight and composition, serum lipids, and diet among subjects 18 to 80 years not seeking health care. Am J Clin Nutr 1984;40:628–34.

350. Voderholzer WA, Schatke W, Muhldorfer BE, et al. Clinical response to dietary fiber treatment of chronic constipation. Am J Gastroenterol 1997;92:95–98.

351. Muller-Lissner SA. Effect of wheat bran on weight of stool and gastrointestinal transit time: a meta analysis. Brit Med J 1988;296:615–17.

352. Stephen A. Trowell HC, Burkitt DP, et al., Editors. Dietary Fiber, Fiber-depleted Foods and Diseases. London: Academic Press;1985:133–44.

353. Cummings JH. Spiller GA, Editors. Handbook of Dietary Fiber in Human Nutrition. Ed. 1. Boca Raton:CRC Press;1986:211–80.

354. Tomlin J, Read NW. Laxative effects of indigestible plastic particles. Brit Med J 1988;297:1175–76.

355. Brodribb AJM, Groves C. Effect of bran particle size on stool weight. Gut 1978; 19:60–63.

356. Bannister JJ, Davison P, Timms JM, et al. Effect of stool size on defecation. Gut 1987;28:1246–50.

357. Tjeerdsma HC, Smout AJPM, Akkermans LMA. Voluntary suppression of defecation delays gastric emptying. Dig Dis Sci 1993;38:832–36.

358. van der Sijp, Kamm MA, Nightingale JM, et al. Disturbed gastric and small bowel transit in severe idiopathic constipation. Dig Dis Sci 1993;38:837–44.

359. Kirshnamurthy S, Schuffler MD, Rohrmann CA, et al. Severe idiopathic constipation is associated with a distinctive abnormality of the colonic myenteric plexus. Gastroenterology 1985;88:26–34.

360. Einsoff JJ, Howard DA, Marshall JB. A randomized blinded clinical trial of a rapid colonic lavage solution (Golytely^R) compared with standard preparation for colonoscopy and barium enema. Gastroenterology 1983;84:1512–16.

361. Muller-Lissner SA. Adverse effects of laxatives: facts and fictions. Pharmacology 1993;47((suppl 1)):138–45.

362. Riechen EO, Zeitz M, Emde C, et al. The effect of an anthraquinone laxative on colonic nerve tissue: a controlled trial in constipated women. Z Gastroenterologie 1990;28:660–64.

363. Tzavella K, Riepl R, Klauser AG, et al. Decreased substance P levels in rectal biop-

sies from patients with slow transit constipation. Eur J Gastroenterol Hepatol 1996;8(1207):1211–15.

364. Heilbrun N. Roentgen evidence suggesting suggesting enterololitis associated with prolongued cathartic abuse. Radiology 1943;41:486–91.

365. Muller-Lissner SA. Occasional viewpoint: What happened to the cathartic colon? Gut 1997;39:486–89.

366. Kamm MA, Lennard-Jones JE, Thompson DG, et al. Dynamic scanning defines a colonic defect in severe idiopathic constipation. Gut 1988;29:1085–92.

367. Preston DM, Lennard-Jones JE. Severe chronic constipation in young women. Dig Dis Sci 1985;30:413–8.

368. Tucker DM, Sandstead HH, Logan GM Jr, et al. Dietary fiber and personality factors as determinants of stool output. Gastroenterology 1981;81:879–87.

369. Almy TP, Hinkle LE Jr, Berle B, et al. Alterations in colonic function in man under stress: III: experimental production of sigmoid spasm in patients with spastic constipation. Gastroenterology 1949;12:437.

370. Wald A, Chandra A, Chiponis D, et al. Anorectal function and continence mechanisms in childhood encopresis. J Pediatr Gastroenterol Nutr 1986; 5:346–51.

371. Drossman DA, Sleisenger MH, Fordtran JS, et al., Editors. Gastrointestinal Disease: Pathophysiology, Diagnosis, Management. Ed. 6. Philadelphia:W.B. Saunders Co.;1993:69–79.

372. Bellman M. Studies on encopresis. Acta Paediatr Scand 1966;56:1–151.

373. Klauser AG, Voderholzer WA, Heinrich CA, et al. Behavioral modification of colonic function: can constipation be learned? Dig Dis Sci 1990;35:1271–75.

374. Heaton KW, Wood N, Cripps HA, et al. The call to stool and its relationship to constipation: a community study. Eur J Gastroenterol Hepatol 1993;6:145–49.

375. Muller-Lissner SA, Ewe K, Eckardt VF, et al, Editors. Constipation and Anorectal Insufficiency. Boston, London: Kluwer, Dordrecht;1997:130–44.

376. Jenkins DJA, Peterson RD, Thorne MJ, et al. Wheat fiber and laxation: dose response and equilibration time. Am J Gastroenterol 1987;82:1259–63.

377. Kumar A, Kumar N, Vij JC. Optimum dosage of isphagula husk in patients with irritable bowel syndrome: correlation of symptom relief with whole gut transit time and stool weight. Gut 1987;28:150–55.

378. Stephen AM, Wiggens HS, Englyst HN, et al. The effect of age, sex and levels of intake of dietary fiber from wheat on large bowel function in thirty healthy subjects. Brit J Nutr 1986;56:349–61.

379. Edwards CA, Tomlin J, Read NW. Fiber and constipation. Brit J Clin Pract 1988; 42:26–32.

380. Mamtami R, Cimino JA, Cooperman JM. Comparison of total costs of administering calcium polycarbophil in an institutional setting. Clin Ther 1990;12:22–24.

381. Marlett JA, Buk L, Patrow CJ, et al. Comparative laxation of psyllium with and without senna in an ambulatory constipated population. Am J Gastroenterol 1987;82:333–37.

382. Hamilton JW, Wagner J, Burdick DD, et al. Clinical evaluation of methylcellulose as a bulk laxative. Dig Dis Sci 1988;33:993–98.

383. Kruis W, Weinzierl M, Schussler P, et al. Comparison of the therapeutic effect of wheat bran, mebeverine and placebo in patients with the irritable bowel syndrome. Digestion 1986;34:196–201.

384. Read NW, Timms JM, Barfield LJ, et al. Impairment of defecation in young women with severe constipation. Gastroenterology 1986;90:53–60.

385. Bass P, Dennis S. The laxative effectof lactulose in normal andconstipated subjects. J Clin Gastroenterol 1981;3(suppl):23–28.

386. Bown RL, Gibson JF, Sladen GE, et al. Effects of lactulose and other laxatives on ileal and colonic pH as measured by a radiotelemetry device. Gut 1974;15:999–1004.

387. Passmore AP, Wilson-Davies K, Stoker C, et al. Chronic constipation in long-stay elderly patients: a comparison of lactulose and a senna-fiber combination. Brit Med J 1993;303:769–71.

388. Binder HJ, Donowitz M. A new look at laxative action. Gastroenterology 1975; 69:1001–1005.

389. Godding EW. Constipation and allied disorders. Pharmaceutic J 1976;216:1–23.

390. Pimparkar BD, Poustian FF, Roth JLA, et al. Effect of polycarbophil on diarrhea and constipation. Gastroenterology 1962;30:397–404.

391. Brunton LL, Goodman R, Gilman RH, Editors. The Pharmacological Basis of Therapeutics. Ed 8. New York:Pergamon Press;1990:914–32.

392. Thompson WG, Dollery CT, Editors. Drug Therapy: A Clinical Pharmacopoea. Edinburgh:Churchill Livingstone;1991:B85–B87.

393. Bytzer P, Stockholm M, Andersen I, et al. Prevalence of surreptitious laxative abuse in patients with diarrhea of uncertain origin: a cost benefit analysis of a screening procedure. Gut 1989;30:1379–84.

394. Read NW, Krejs GJ, Read MG, et al. Chronic diarrhea of unknown origin. Gastroenterology 1980;78:264–71.

395. Badiali MD, Marsheggiano A, Pallone F, et al. Melanosis of the rectum in patients with chronic constipation. Dis Colon Rectum 1985;28:241–45.

396. Balazs M. Melanosis coli: ultrastructural study of 45 patients. Dis Colon Rectum 1986;28:839–44.

397. Ghadially FN, Parry EW. An electron microscope and histological study of melanosis coli. J Pathol Bacteriol 1966;92:312–17.

398. Speare GS. Melanosis coli: experimental observations on its production and elimination in twenty-three cases. Am J Surg 1951;82:631–37.

399. Schuurkes J. Kamm MA, Lennard-Jones JE, Editors. Gastrointestinal Transit: Physiology and Pharmacology. Bristol: Wright Biomedical; 1991.

400. Thompson WG. The Irritable Gut. Baltimore:University Park Press;1979.

401. Gattuso JM, Kamm MA. Clinical features of idiopathic megarectum and idiopathic megacolon. Gut 1997;41:93–99.

402. Leon SH, Krishnamurthy S, Schuffler MD. Subtotal colectomy for severe idiopathic constipation: a follow up study of 13 patients. Dig Dis Sci 1987;32:1249–54.

403. Gasslander T, Larsson J, Wetterfors J. Experience of surgical treatment for chronic idiopathic constipation. Acta Chir Scand 1987;153:553–55.

404. Vasilevsky CA, Nemer FD, Balcos EG, et al. Is subtotal colectomy a viable option in the management of chronic constipation? Dis Colon Rectum 1988;31(9): 679–81.

405. Kamm MA, Hawley PR, Lennard-Jones JE. Outcome of colectomy for severe idiopathic constipation. Gut 1988;29:969–73.

406. Fromm H, Malavolti M. Bile-acid induced diarrhea. Med Clin North Am 1986; 15:567–82.

407. Williams AJK, Merrick MV, Eastwood MA. Idiopathic bile salt malabsorption: a review of clinical presentation, diagnosis, and response to treatment. Gut 1991; 32:1004–1006.

408. Galatola G, the Italian SeHCAT Multicentre Study Group. The prevalence of bile acid malabsorption in irritable bowel syndrome and the effect of cholestyramine: an uncontrolled open multicentre study. Eur J Gastroenterol Hepatol 1992; 4:533–37.

409. Rudberg U, Nylander B. Radiological bile acid absorption test SeHCAT in patients with diarrhea of unknown cause. Acta Radiologica 1996;37:672–75.

410. Pearson DJ. Food allergy, hypersensitivity and intolerence. J Roy Coll Physicians (Lond) 1985;19:154–62.

411. Cummings JH, Heaton KW, Editors. Dietary Fiber: Current Developments of Importance to Health. London:Libbey; 1978:83–95.

412. Read NW. Diarrhee motrice. Clin Gastroenterol 1986;15:657–86.

413. Bazzocchi G, Ellis J, Villanueva-Meyer J, et al. Effect of eating on colonic motility and transit in patients with functional diarrhea. Gastroenterology 1991;101:1298–1306.

414. Charles F, Phillips SF, Camilleri M, et al. Rapid gastric emptying in patients with functional diarrhea. Mayo Clin Proc 1997;72:323–28.

415. Prior A, Sorial E, Sun W-M, et al. Irritable bowel syndrome: differences between patients who show rectal sensitivity and those who do not. Eur J Gastroenterol Hepatol 1993;5:343–49.

416. Prior A, Colgan SM, Whorwell PJ. Changes in rectal sensitivity after hypnotherapy in patients with irritable bowel syndrome. Gut 1990;31:896–98.

417. Wangel DG, Deller DJ. Intestinal motility in man: III: mechanisms of constipation and diarrhea with particular reference to the irritable bowel. Gastroenterology 1965;48:69–84.

418. Merritt JE, Brown BL, Tomlinson S. Loperamide and calmodulin. J Pharmacol Exp Ther 1982;1984:628–32.

419. Reynolds IJ, Gould RJ, Snyder SH. Loperamide: blockade of calcium channels as a mechanism for antidiarrheal effects. J Pharmacol Exp Ther 1984;23:628–32.

420. Palmer KR, Corbett CL, Holdsworth CD. Double blind cross-over study comparing loperamide, codeine and diphenoxylate in chronic diarrhea. Gastroenterology 1980;79:1272–75.

421. Afzalpurkar RG, Schiller LR, Little KH, et al. The self-limited nature of chronic idiopathic diarrhea. New Engl J Med 1992;327:1849–52.

422. Drossman DA. Chronic functional abdominal pain. Am J Gastroenterol 1996; 91:2270–82.
423. Mayer EA, Gebhart GF. Basic and clinical aspects of visceral analgesia. Gastroenterology 1994;107:271–93.
424. Maxton DG, Whorwell PJ. Use of medical resources and attitudes to health care of patients with chronic abdominal pain. Brit J Med Econ 1992;2:75–79.
425. Diagnostic and Statistical Manual of Mental Disorders—DSM-IV. Ed. 4. Washington, D.C.:American Psychiatric Association;1994.
426. Benjamen S. Psychological treatment of chronic pain: a selection review. Psychsomat Res 1989;33:121–31.
427. Drossman DA. Patients with psychogenic abdominal pain: six years' observation in the medical setting. Am J Psychiatry 1982;139:1549–57.
428. Blackwell B, Gutmann M. McHugh S, Vallis TM, Editors. Illness Behavior: A Multidisciplinary Model. New York:Plenum Press;1986;401–408.
429. Klein KB, Yamada T, Editors. Textbook of Gastroenterology. Philadelphia:J.B. Lippencott;1995:750–71.
430. Gray DWR, Dixon JM, Collin J. The closed eyes sign: an aid to diagnosing nonspecific abdominal pain. Brit Med J 1988;297:837–38.
431. Gallegos NC, Hobsley M. Abdominal wall pain: an alternate diagnosis. Brit J Surg 1990;77:1167–70.
432. Melzack R, Wall P. Melzack R, et al., Editors.The Challenge of Pain. Ed. 2. London:Pelican Books;1988:165–93.
433. Fields HL, Basbaum AI, Wall PD, et al., Editors. Textbook of Pain. New York: Livingston; 1984:142–52.
434. Coderre TJ, Katz J, Vaccarino AL, et al. Contribution of central neuroplasticity to pathological pain. Pain 1993;52:259–85.
435. Mayer EA. Mayer EA, Raybould HE, Editors. Basic and clinical aspects of chronic abdominal pain. New York:Elsevier;1993:3–28.
436. Ness TJ, Metcalf AM, Gebhart GF. A psychophysiological study in humans using phasic colonic distension as a noxious visceral stimulus. Pain 1990;43:377–86.
437. Gebhart GF. Visceral nociception: consequences, modulation and future. Eur J Anaesthesiol 1995;10(suppl):24–27.
438. Engel GL. "Psychogenic" pain and pain-prone patient. Am J Med 1959;26:899–918.
439. Large RG. DSM-III diagnoses in chronic pain: confusion or clarity. J Nerv Ment Dis 1986;174:295–303.
440. Somatoform Disorders. Diagnostic and Statistical Manual of Mental Disorders—DSM-IV. Ed. 4. Washington, D.C.:American Psychiatric Association;1994: 445–69.
441. Hislop IG. Childhood deprivation: an antecedent of the irritable bowel syndrome. Med J Austral 1979;1:372–74.
442. Wurtele SK, Kaplan GM, Keairnes M. Childhood sexual abuse among chronic pain patients. Clin J Pain 1999;6:110–13.

443. Sarason IG, Sarason BR, Potter EH, et al. Life events, social support and illness. Psychosomat Med 1985;47:156–63.

444. Drossman DA, Li Z, Leserman J, et al. Association of coping and health status among female GI patients after controlling for disease type and abuse history. Gastroenterology 1997;112:724A.

445. Jamison RN, Virts KL. The influence of family support on chronic pain. Behav Res Ther 1990;28:283–87.

446. Scarinci IS, McDonald-Haile J, Bradley LA, et al. Altered pain perception and psychosocial features among women with gastrointestinal disorders and a history of abuse: a preliminary model. Am J Med 1994;97:108–18.

447. Drossman DA. Yamada T, Editors. Textbook of Gastroenterology. Philadelphia: J.B. Lippincott Co.;1995:620–37.

448. Toner BB. Cognitive-behavioural treatment of functional somatic syndromes: integrating gender issues. Cog Behav Pract 1994;1:157–78.

449. Zinn W. The empathetic physician. Arch Intern Med 1994;153:306–12.

450. Devaul RA, Faillace LA. Persistent pain and illness insistence: a medical profile of proneness to surgery. Am J Surg 1978;135:828–33.

451. Sandgren JE, McPhee MS, Greengerger NJ. Narcotic bowel syndrome treated with clonidine. Ann Intern Med 1984;101:331–34.

452. Pilowsky I, Barrow CG. A controlled study of psychotherapy and amitriptyline used individually and in combination in the treatment of chronic intractable, 'psychogenic' pain. Pain 1990;40:3–19.

453. Finley PR. Selective serotonin reuptake inhibitors: pharmacologic profiles and potential therapeutic distinctions. Ann Pharmacother 1994;28:1359–69.

454. Eisendrath SJ, Kodama KT. Fluoxetine management of chronic abdominal pain. Psychosomat 1992;33:227–29.

455. Cakkues AL, Popkin MK. Antidepressant treatment of medical-surgical inpatients by nonpsychiatric physicians. Arch Gen Psychiatry 1987;44:157–60.

456. Hendler N. The anatomy and psychopharmacology of chronic pain. J Clin Psychiatry 1982;43:15–21.

457. Peters JL, Large RG. A randomised control trial evaluating in- and outpatient pain management programmes. Pain 1990;41:283–93.

458. Hastings RH, McKay WR. Treatment of benign chronic abdominal pain with neurolytic celiac plexus block. Anesthesiology 1991;75:156–58.

459. Keefe FJ, Dunsmore J, Burnett R. Behavioural and cognitive-behavioural approaches to chronic pain: recent advances and future directions. J Consult Clin Psychol 1992;60:528–36.

460. Guthrie E, Creed F, Dawson D, et al. A randomised controlled trial of psychotherapy in patients with refractory irritable bowel syndrome. Brit J Psychiatry 1993;163:315–21.

461. Whorwell PJ, Prior A, Colgan SM. Hypnotherapy in severe irritable bowel syndrome: further experience. Gut 1987;28:423–25.

462. Kames LD, Rapkin AJ, Naliboff BD, et al. Effectiveness of an interdisciplinary pain management program for the treatment of chronic pelvic pain. Pain 1990; 41(1):41–46.

Chapter 8

E. Functional Disorders of the Biliary Tract and the Pancreas

Enrico Corazziari, Chair,
Eldon A. Shaffer, Co-Chair, *with*
Walter J. Hogan,
Stuart Sherman,
and James Toouli

Introduction

The integrated action of the gallbladder and the sphincter of Oddi (SO) regulates bile flow from the liver through the biliary tract into the duodenum. The SO also plays a relevant role in regulating the flow of pancreatic secretions into the duodenum. Additional factors include hepatic bile and pancreatic secretion rates, gastrointestinal tract motor activity, and the enterohepatic circulation of bile acids. Derangements of integrated function of any of these components may lead to intermittent upper abdominal pain, transient elevations of liver enzymes, common bile duct dilatation, transient elevations of pancreatic enzymes, or episodes of pancreatitis (Table 1).

— Physiologic Features

The gallbladder collects and stores bile during fasting, concentrating it to reduce the volume. Gallbladder evacuation of bile requires smooth muscle contraction. This is coordinated with reduced tone in the sphincter of Oddi.

During fasting in humans about 25% emptying of the gallbladder occurs periodically every 100–120 minutes concomitant with the late phase II of the migrating motor complex (MMC) of the upper gastrointestinal tract [1–3]. Emptying is maximal when phase III of the MMC starts in the antrum; it is mediated by motilin via cholinergic nerves [4–7].

Eating initiates gallbladder contraction through neural (cephalic and local gastroduodenal reflexes) and hormonal (predominantly cholecystokinin, CCK) influences [8–10]. After a meal there is also a net secretion of fluid from the gallbladder mucosa, an event that could facilitate gallbladder emptying [11,12]. Eating causes more than 75% of the gallbladder contents to be discharged into the duodenum. Gallbladder emptying with meals consists of three phases: cephalic, gastric, and intestinal. In the cephalic phase simulated by sham feeding, there is emptying of the gallbladder (up to 30–40% of its fasting contents) [13,14]. In the gastric phase, distension of the stomach wall induces gallbladder contraction, presumably by gastroduodenal (actually enteropylorocholecystic) reflexes. The intestinal phase is hormonal. Gallbladder emptying and filling are not the result of steady phases of contraction and decontraction of the viscus but rather the net effect of minor volume fluctuations with alternating filling and emptying. These minor volume fluctuations are continuously present throughout each of

We thank the following reviewers for their critique of the manuscripts and their suggestions: D. A. Drossman, D. Festi, P. Portincasa, A. Slivka, and J. Svanvik.

Table 1. Functional Gastrointestinal Disorders

A. Esophageal Disorders

A1. Globus	A4. Functional Heartburn
A2. Rumination syndrome	A5. Functional Dysphagia
A3. Functional Chest Pain of Presumed Esophageal Origin	A6. Unspecified Functional Esophageal Disorder

B. Gastroduodenal Disorders

B1. Functional Dyspepsia	B2. Aerophagia
B1a. Ulcer-like Dyspepsia	B3. Functional Vomiting
B1b. Dysmotility-like Dyspepsia	
B1c. Unspecified (nonspecific) Dyspepsia	

C. Bowel Disorders

C1. Irritable Bowel Syndrome	C4. Functional Diarrhea
C2. Functional Abdominal Bloating	C5. Unspecified Functional Bowel Disorder
C3. Functional Constipation	

D. Functional Abdominal Pain

D1. Functional Abdominal Pain Syndrome
D2. Unspecified Functional Abdominal Pain

E. Functional Disorders of the Biliary Tract and the Pancreas

E1. Gallbladder Dysfunction
E2. Sphincter of Oddi Dysfunction

F. Anorectal Disorders

F1. Functional Fecal Incontinence
F2. Functional Anorectal Pain
  F2a. Levator Ani Syndrome
  F2b. Proctalgia Fugax
F3. Pelvic Floor Dyssynergia

G. Functional Pediatric Disorders

G1. Vomiting	G2b. Irritable bowel syndrome
G1a. Infant regurgitation	G2c. Functional abdominal pain
G1b. Infant rumination syndrome	G2d. Abdominal migraine
G1c. Cyclic vomiting syndrome	G2e. Aerophagia
G2. Abdominal pain	G3. Functional diarrhea
G2a. Functional dyspepsia	G4. Disorders of defecation
G2a1. Ulcer-like dyspepsia	G4a. Infant dyschezia
G2a2. Dysmotility-like dyspepsia	G4b. Functional constipation
	G4c. Functional fecal retention
G2a3. Unspecified (nonspecific) dyspepsia	G4d. Functional non-retentive fecal soiling

the major postprandial phases and during the fasting state [15–18]. After a meal, refilling of the gallbladder up to the preprandial volume is a process that takes several hours, but it is reduced to only 60 minutes after CCK blockade [19]. It would appear therefore that meal-induced CCK release delays bile storage in the gallbladder, thus maintaining the hepatic bile flow into the duodenum during the entire phase of gastric emptying.

The meal composition primarily determines the extent to which the gallbladder empties; fat hydrolyzed to long-chain fatty acids makes up the most potent ingredients causing release of CCK-33 [20–22]. Cholecystokinin can initiate gallbladder contraction by a direct effect on smooth muscle, and also via cholinergic nerves [6,8,23–25]. Postprandial levels of CCK probably interact with CCK-A receptors located on cholinergic nerves, rather than being myogenic. Cholecystokinin also interacts with sensory neurons of the vagus, activating vagal afferent pathways [26–28]. Vagal efferent outflow from the brain stem (dorsal motor nucleus) interacts with interneurons in the enteric nervous system. The subsequent release of acetylcholine contracts the gallbladder while vasoactive intestinal peptide (VIP) and nitric oxide relax the sphincter of Oddi [29–32].

Altered gallbladder emptying occurs in several conditions that may or may not be associated with cholesterol gallstone formation (Table 2) [33]. These range from intrinsic disease of the gallbladder in the form of gallstones or obstruction of the biliary tract, and extend to neural and metabolic disorders and drugs. In cholesterol gallstone disease, the basis of decreased contractility is the excessive cholesterol in bile being incorporated into the smooth muscle membrane [34–36]. This impairs transmembrane signaling.

Knowledge concerning the physiology of the human sphincter of Oddi was scarce and primarily qualitative until the introduction of perendoscopic manometry two decades ago. The ability to directly measure the motor activity of the sphincter of Oddi has greatly expanded our understanding of its functions. Sphincter of Oddi manometric studies have defined a basal SO high pressure zone of 8–10 mm with superimposed phasic wave activity [37]. The SO zone provides a pressure gradient between the duct and duodenum which relaxes intermittently to allow flow into the intestine.

Sphincter of Oddi phasic contraction frequency varies in accordance with the fasting cyclical interdigestive migrating motor activity of the duodenum (maximal frequency during phase III) [38], and briefly during digestive periods with meals prior to a prolonged phase of inhibition [39,40]. Phasic contractions may enhance ductal flow in some experimental animals and reduce it in others and in humans [41–43]. It is likely that phasic contractions maintain duct clearance. Basal SO pressure appears to be the primary modulator of fluid outflow from the biliary/pancreatic systems.

Table 2. Causes of Impaired Gallbladder Emptying

1. Primary gallbladder disease

2. Cholesterol gallstones
   —prior to stone formation with microcrystals of cholesterol and after medical dissolution has occurred

3. Cholecystitis
   —acute or chronic, with or without stones

4. Metabolic disorders
   —Obesity, diabetes, pregnancy, VIPoma, sickle hemoglobinopathy

5. Cirrhosis

6. Myotonia dystrophica

7. Denervation

8. Irritable Bowel Syndrome

9. Functional Dyspepsia

10. Deficiency of CCK
    —Celiac disease, fasting/Total Parenteral Nutrition

11. Drugs
    Anticholinergic agents, calcium channel blockers, opioids, ursodeoxycholic acid, octreotide, CCK-A antagonist, nitric oxide donors, sex hormones (progestins)

Cholecystokinin normally inhibits SO phasic and basal motor activity [23,37, 44]. Control mechanisms of SO motor activity have been elucidated from studies performed in animals and on in vitro tissue preparations [23,45,46]. The opossum SO has been studied more thoroughly in recent times. The opossum SO is innervated by intramural cholinergic excitatory nerves and nonadrenergic noncholinergic (NANC) inhibitory nerves [42,46,47]. In animals, the NANC system affects SO relaxation principally through the release of vasoactive intestinal peptide (VIP) and nitric oxide (NO), which act as neurotransmitters at the postganglionic level [30–32]. The human SO also relaxes following topical application of NO to the papilla [48]. Graded infusion of morphine sulfate initially increases phasic SO activity (tachyoddia) and eventually causes tonic contractions [49]. The human SO relaxes following administration of nitroglycerine and glucagon [50,51].

Sphincter of Oddi motor activity is related to gallbladder function via a cholecysto–sphincter of Oddi reflex network, e.g., SO motor activity is inhibited during gallbladder distension [52]. Additionally, there is evidence that gallstones are associated with increased basal SO tone through a similar reflex mechanism [53], and SO response to CCK stimulation is reduced following cholecystectomy [54]. Abnormalities in SO motor activity are generally referred to as SO dysfunction; the term "SO stenosis" is used to indicate a possible structural alteration that is characterized by manometry as an elevated basal SO pressure, as contrasted with "SO dyskinesia," which represents a possible smooth muscle dysfunction [55]. The etiology of SO dysfunction is unknown. A number of possible causes have been suggested and include sphincter damage by the passage of gallstones [56–59], division of the nerves that communicate between the gallbladder and SO, or intrinsic neuromuscular defects.

Bilio-pancreatic Pain

The assumed mechanism for biliary pain is obstruction leading to distension and perhaps inflammation. This might result from incoordination between the gallbladder and either the cystic duct or the sphincter of Oddi due to increased resistance or tone. Occlusion of the cholecystocystic junction may occur with inflammatory edema or torsion of the gallbladder and smooth muscle spasm. The role of inflammation in the production of biliary pain is not clear, but inflammation may stimulate fluid secretion within the gallbladder and thus distend it further and cause pain in the presence of a narrowed or (functionally) obstructed cystic duct [60].

In those patients with demonstrated altered gallbladder emptying in whom histologic abnormalities were found, chronic inflammatory infiltrate, lymphoid aggregates and fibrosis, muscle hypertrophy and cystic duct obstruction, cholesterolosis, and perigallbladder adhesions have been found [61–63]. The severity of these histologic findings does not necessarily correlate with the impairment in gallbladder emptying in those patients [62–65].

If impaired gallbladder emptying is interpreted as being caused by defective smooth muscle contractility, it is difficult to speculate on the mechanism of pain production. Certainly it is not a consistent component of cholesterol gallstone disease since most patients never experience biliary pain despite their intrinsic smooth muscle defect. Could sensory pathways be at fault in biliary symptoms, at least in some individuals? Limited studies have shown that artificially filling the gallbladder reveals that similar distension of the gallbladder elicited pain in symptomatic patients with biliary dysfunction, but not in asymptomatic persons [66]. Thus, it is conceivable that, like other functional disorders of the gastrointestinal tract [67], a lowered threshold of sensitivity may play a role in the pathogenesis of pain in patients with gallbladder dysfunction.

Both SO stenosis and SO dyskinesia may account for obstruction to flow through the SO and may thus induce retention of bile in the biliary tree and pancreatic juice in the pancreatic duct. A distending pressure in the biliary tract and pancreatic duct activates a reflex that reduces SO pressure via intramural nerves [68,69]. It has also been reported that damage of these nerves, similar to that which occurs with cholecystectomy in cats, may cause an impaired outflow of bile into the duodenum [70].

In patients who have had cholecystectomy, or in subjects with an altered SO-gallbladder regulation, SO dysfunction, and the consequent increment in the choledochal [71] or pancreatic duct pressure, may clinically manifest with typical bilio-pancreatic pain. The bilio-pancreatic pain apparently results from the stimulation of the sensory fibers that follows the ductal distension caused by the increased pressure in the ducts.

Although the reservoir function of the gallbladder would counterbalance the intrabiliary pressure increments caused by SO stenosis or dyskinesia, and thus prevent the clinical manifestation [72], symptomatic SO dysfunction has also been observed in patients with a functioning gallbladder.

An increase in the pancreatic ductal pressure is regarded as a possible factor that may induce pancreatic pain via pancreatic ductal distension.

The neural supply to the biliary tract includes vagal efferent nerves (through which CCK acts in a preganglionic fashion) releasing acetylcholine, sympathetic fibers that release norepinephrine, and sensory fibers which contain substance P. There are also other neurotransmitters in the ganglionic plexus.

Sensory fibers may influence the neuronal response, acting via the vagus through central reflexes [73]. Sensory fibers, in response to inflammation and high intraluminal pressure such as that generated by an obstructed gallbladder or common bile duct (CBD), release tachykinins that activate ganglia in the gallbladder; these in turn might further increase gallbladder tone, creating a self-perpetuating cycle. Thus sensory nerves can alter gallbladder contractility [74], and might perpetuate pain, directly or indirectly, by influencing gallbladder tone.

Motor contraction, sensory afferents producing painful sensations, and obstruction/inflammation may all play a role in the perception of biliary-type pain. Increased motility, at least in instances of obstruction, may therefore contribute to the development and maintenance of this pain and referred hyperalgesia [75]. Any injury from a noxious stimulation elicits responses from visceral nociceptors, with transmission proceeding directly to the thalamus and cortex and yielding a perception of pain when the noxious stimulus is very intense or prolonged. When tissue injury and damage ensue, the sensitized nociceptors would exhibit a greater response, which may be heightened by nociceptive neurons in the spinal cord, yielding a more excitable state in the brain. The result might be hyperalgesia, that is, severe pain evolving from mildly painful stimuli

[76]. Ongoing afferent activity then might lead to an overly sensitive CNS. This increased central excitability can persist even after the afferent stimulus ceases. Allodynia then might result; here innocuous stimuli produce pain. The eventual result could be a chronic pain state, perhaps based on neuropathic change. Evidence of visceral hyperalgesia has been reported during duodenal distension in post-cholecystectomy patients with biliary pain [77].

— Definition of Gallbladder and SO Dysfunction

For over a century, motor dysfunction of the gallbladder and SO has been suspected as a major cause for clinical manifestations, but evidence for this has been largely based on indirect and qualitative data. The past two decades have witnessed the development of a number of invasive and noninvasive investigative tools that afford accurate and reproducible recording of motor function. These techniques have made it possible to correlate motility disorders of the gallbladder and SO with a number of clinical presentations attributed to the pancreatobiliary system.

An international panel of clinical investigators has defined functional gastrointestinal disorders as a "variable combination of chronic or recurrent gastrointestinal symptoms not explained by structural or biochemical abnormalities" [78] (Table 1). In the case of functional disorders of the gallbladder and SO, we frequently cannot dissociate purely functional conditions from subtle structural changes. In many instances these merge. In our current state of knowledge, available investigations are not always able to discriminate between purely structural and functional disorders. This difficulty may be due to the following factors.

(1) Ready access to the biliary tract in order to obtain detailed study is hampered by its anatomic position. Any direct method that might be used necessarily interferes with its activity.

(2) The normal histologic details of the biliary tract are not well defined and degrees of histologic variation are commonly found in random autopsy series of normal individuals [79]. Interpretation of subtle histologic abnormalities thus is not standardized.

(3) Identification of microlithiasis as tiny crystals within the biliary tract of patients with recurrent biliary/pancreatic symptoms has suggested a causative role in the pathogenesis of disorders such as sphincter of Oddi stenosis, and in some cases of idiopathic recurrent pancreatitis [80]. Conversely, the loss of SO function, after sphincterotomy, enhances contractility of the gallbladder and in-

hibits gallbladder stone formation [81]. The techniques currently available are not always capable of detecting tiny stones or microcrystals that can engender biliary/pancreatic symptoms and disease.

To date, a definitive cause/effect relationship between such subtle abnormalities and clinical signs has not been substantiated. As a result we have adopted the term "dysfunctional disorders of the gallbladder and SO" to embrace the associated motility disorders without note of potential etiologic factors. These disorders of the gallbladder and SO are referred to as:

(1) Gallbladder dysfunction, and
(2) Sphincter of Oddi dysfunction

Gallbladder and SO dysfunction manifest symptomatically with the same type of pain.

Similar to other functional disorders of the gastrointestinal tract, the clinical symptoms are intermittent. Furthermore, a feature that oftentimes confuses the issue is the observation that even though objective investigation can demonstrate abnormalities, the clinical symptoms may not necessarily coincide temporally with the demonstrated abnormality. A cause-and-effect relationship is often not clear.

Although the diagnosis of SO dysfunction is made in patients submitted to cholecystectomy, SO dysfunction can manifest clinically in the presence of an intact biliary tract with a normal gallbladder in situ, or it can coexist with gallbladder dysfunction.

In these conditions the symptoms of SO and gallbladder dysfunction cannot be differentiated: the diagnosis of SO dysfunction is made after proper investigations have excluded gallbladder abnormalities or after a diseased gallbladder has been removed.

Psychosocial aspects appear to be variably interrelated with functional gastrointestinal disorders [78]. These relationships also occur in patients with functional disorders of the gallbladder and SO, but lack of uniform diagnostic criteria have limited epidemiological studies [82,83].

It is also possible that the syndrome of chronic functional abdominal pain (see chapter 7) manifests itself with clinical characteristics similar to biliary pain. This condition should be suspected in those patients in whom repeated episodes of biliary pain are not associated with any other laboratory, endoscopic, ultrasonographic, radiologic, or scintigraphic findings that support the presence of bilio-pancreatic alterations.

E1. Gallbladder Dysfunction

— Definition

The gallbladder dysfunction that produces biliary-type pain may represent a disorder of gallbladder motility, currently best identified as abnormal gallbladder emptying. Other motor disorders or an impairment of gallbladder filling may exist, but the available methodology does not allow for their definition. The definition does not exclude an overly sensitive gallbladder, but criteria and techniques to assess this are not available. This condition may be associated with histologic changes such as a narrowed cystic duct, muscle hypertrophy, and evidence of chronic inflammation of the gallbladder [61,62].

— Epidemiology

Concepts of biliary pain and gallbladder dysfunction have been defined in gallstone disease, the most common affliction of the biliary system. The symptoms associated with it reveal much about those related to gallbladder dysfunction.

The natural history of gallstones indicates that the majority (70–90%) of people with gallstones do not have symptoms [84,85] and most never go on to develop a complication requiring surgery [86]. Conversely, many patients harboring stones have symptoms, but the relationship to the gallstones is not always clear.

True biliary-type pain appears to be more common in women than men, both in Europeans [84] and Native Americans [87].

Between the extremes of patients with severe biliary symptoms associated with acute cholecystitis and those who are totally asymptomatic ("silent") lies a spectrum of foregut symptoms often attributed to gallstones. Dyspeptic symptoms such as flatulence, heartburn, acid regurgitation, bloating, and belching are not associated with gallstones [88]. The yield from doing ultrasonography of the gallbladder in patients with dyspepsia is low (1–3%), and the findings of gallstones is usually considered incidental [89]. In general there is no clear association between the mere presence of gallstones and upper abdominal pain or discomfort [90]. Neither is there an association with fatty food intolerance [88,91]. Gallstone dyspepsia is a myth, born of the fact that both gallstones and dyspepsia are frequent occurrences. Any overlap is by chance.

The frequency of biliary pain in people without gallstones can be gleaned from these population screening studies performed with ultrasonography: 7.6% of men [84] and 20.7% of women [92] without gallstones have had episodes of biliary pain. However, in another screening study of the general population biliary-type pain without apparent gallstones was lower overall at 2.4% [93].

— Diagnostic Criteria

Episodes of severe steady pain located in the epigastrium and right upper quadrant, and all of the following:

(1)   **Symptom episodes last 30 minutes or more, with pain-free intervals;**

(2)   **Symptoms have occurred on one or more occasions in the previous 12 months;**

(3)   **The pain is steady and interrupts daily activities or requires consultation with a physician;**

(4)   **There is no evidence of structural abnormalities to explain the symptoms; and**

(5)   **There is abnormal gallbladder functioning with regard to emptying.**

The presence of biliary sludge implies gallbladder dysfunction in the form of stasis from impaired emptying but may not necessarily explain the pain. In addition, the pain may be associated with one or more of the following: nausea and vomiting; pain radiating to the back and/or right interscapular region; onset after meals; and/or awakening patients at night. In some persons, these symptoms may be superimposed on a background of low-grade chronic abdominal pain of unknown etiology.

— Rationale for Changes in Diagnostic Criteria

In comparison to the previously published Rome I Diagnostic Criteria, the Rome II Diagnostic Criteria have two major changes. The first refers to the specification of the duration, number of episodes of pain, and the timeframe over which they occur. The second specifies the sole characteristic of organ function in this designation.

Time Criteria

Thirty minutes has been more firmly established in the literature as the minimum duration of a biliary "colic." With regard to chronicity, the committee agreed that even a single pain episode may be so severe as to indicate a need for diagnostic investigation irrespective of the number of the episodes. Furthermore, the frequency of biliary pain may be so irregular that a time window of only three months has been considered too restrictive.

Evidence of Abnormal Functioning

Point 5 has been added to the Criteria to identify abnormal emptying of the gallbladder as the only evidence of abnormal functioning in "Gallbladder Dysfunction."

— Clinical Evaluation

Screening Tests

Laboratory
Tests of liver biochemistries (LFTs) and pancreatic enzymes should be assessed in those patients with the above-mentioned symptomatology. These tests are normal in the presence of gallbladder dysfunction. The findings of abnormal liver function or pancreatic enzyme levels, or both, indicate that other diagnoses should be considered.

To eliminate calculous biliary disease that can produce similar symptoms, the following is recommended.

Ultrasonography
Transabdominal ultrasonographic study of the entire upper abdomen is mandatory in patients with the above symptoms. In the presence of gallbladder dysfunction the biliary tract and pancreas appear normal on ultrasound (US) examination. In particular, gallstones or sludge cannot be demonstrated.

Ultrasound usually detects stones within the gallbladder equal to or greater than 3–5 mm in diameter, but it has a low sensitivity to detection of smaller stones [94]. The ultrasound detection of stones or sludge within the common bile duct is more difficult. Biliary sludge consists of cholesterol microcrystals, bilirubinate, and mucus but cannot be detected by US unless it is greater than 3 mm [95]. Because small echoic precipitates are not always easily detected, microscopic analysis of bile may be necessary [96].

Endoscopic ultrasonography, a technique that is under evaluation, may be more sensitive than traditional transabdominal ultrasonography in detecting microlithiasis (tiny stones < 3 mm) and sludge within the biliary tract [97,98].

Endoscopy

In the presence of normal laboratory and ultrasonographic findings, upper gastrointestinal endoscopy is usually indicated. The diagnosis of gallbladder dysfunction is made in absence of significant abnormality in the esophagus, stomach, and duodenum.

Microscopic Bile Examination

To exclude microlithiasis as a cause for symptoms, a careful microscopic examination of gallbladder bile is recommended.

The detection of microlithiasis and cholesterol microcrystals is best accomplished by a careful examination of gallbladder bile obtained directly at the time of endoscopic retrograde cholangiopancreatography (ERCP) or by aspiration from the duodenum following CCK stimulation, using either exogenous injection (e.g., CCK-8 5 ng/kg i.v. over 10 min) or endogenous stimulation (e.g., 50 ml $Mg\ SO_4$ instilled into the duodenum). The resultant bile should appear deep, golden yellow to dark green-brown. Pale yellow bile from the common duct is not appropriate. This type of bile is inadequate for examination or it does not offer useful information. Even in those patients with cholesterol gallstones or sludge, this hepatic bile often is free of cholesterol microcrystals because bile concentration is insufficient for nucleation to occur. The collected bile should be immediately centrifuged and examined [95]. Two types of deposits may be evident: cholesterol crystals and/or calcium bilirubinate granules. These may be differentiated as follows:

(1) Cholesterol microcrystals are birfringent and rhomboid-shaped, and are best visualized by polarizing microscopy [99]. The presence of cholesterol crystals provides a reasonably high diagnostic accuracy for microlithiasis [100–103] if properly performed.

(2) Bilirubinate granules are red-brown, and can be detected by conventional light microscopy. These precipitates are significant only in freshly analyzed bile.

Tests for Gallbladder Dysfunction

A number of investigations have been used to diagnose gallbladder dysfunction.

Assessment of Cystic Duct Patency

Cystic duct obstruction connotes organic disease. Filling of the gallbladder with radionuclide at cholescintigraphy indicates patency of the cystic duct.

Oral cholecystography historically has been used to demonstrate opacification of the gallbladder, and thus indirectly to assess the patency of the cystic duct. Nonvisualization of the gallbladder is considered evidence of cystic duct obstruction. Patency of the cystic duct can also be evaluated by ultrasound, measuring gallbladder volume reduction after a test meal or other cholecystokinetic stimulus.

Assessment of Gallbladder Emptying by Cholescintigraphy

Cholescintigraphy is performed following the administration of technetium 99m-labeled iminodiacetic acid (IDA) analogs. These compounds have a high affinity for hepatic uptake, are readily excreted into the biliary tract, and are concentrated in the gallbladder. The test has low radiation exposure, equivalent to that of a standard abdominal radiogram.

A region of interest is drawn around the gallbladder, as well as one outside the gallbladder including the liver to determine background counts. Liver counts are subtracted to give the net gallbladder counts. To minimize interference from hepatic bile activity, one should wait 60 minutes after injecting the radionuclide to allow the liver to clear most of it.

The net activity-time curve for the gallbladder is then derived from subsequent serial observations, after either CCK administration or the ingestion of a meal containing fat. Gallbladder emptying is usually expressed as the gallbladder ejection fraction (GBEF), which is the percentage variation of net gallbladder counts following the cholecystokinetic stimulus. A low GBEF has been considered evidence of impaired gallbladder motor function which, in the absence of lithiasis, could identify patients with gallbladder dysfunction.

The most widely used stimulus to contract the gallbladder has been the intravenous infusion of CCK analogs, especially CCK-8. It should be noted that in some countries CCK preparations have not been approved for human use. When CCK is used to stimulate gallbladder contraction, it should be given by slow infusion instead of rapid bolus [104,105]. Administration of CCK over a short period of 2 or 3 minutes produces variable gallbladder evacuation activity [106]. Gallbladder emptying following slow CCK infusion is reproducible in normal volunteers (fig. 1) [61] and patients with gallstones. Cholecystokinin at 20 ng/kg by slow infusion for at least 30 minutes is most useful for assessment of gallbladder emptying, resulting in a GBEF of 70% in normal individuals [61]. Fat meal and variable bolus injections of CCK yield variable results [106].

Reduced emptying can arise from either depressed gallbladder contraction or increased resistance such as an elevated tone in the sphincter of Oddi. Further, several other conditions that do not necessarily present with biliary colic can be associated with reduced gallbladder emptying (Table 2). Although biliary-type pain is rarely elicited with this test, is a reasonable marker of this biliary disorder as cholecystectomy appears beneficial [61,62].

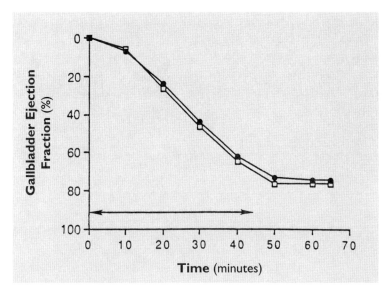

Figure 1. Comparison of the effect of a 45-minute infusion of cholecystokinin (CCK) on 20 normal volunteers on repeated testing. Mean gallbladder ejection fractions (GBEFs) are indicated as solid circles for the first test and as open squares for the repeat test. The arrow indicates the duration of CCK infusion. The GBEF is highly reproducible. Reproduced with permission from Yap L, Wycherley AG, Morphett AD, et al. Gastroenterology 1991;101:786.

Oral Cholecystography

Quantitative evaluation of gallbladder emptying using oral cholecystography is now considered obsolete.

Assessment of Volume Variations

Transabdominal Real-Time Ultrasonography

Unlike cholescintigraphy, this method measures gallbladder volume and provides serial measurements during fasting or following a meal stimulus. Simultaneous measurements with ultrasonography and bolus cholescintigraphy have highlighted the differences of these two methods [18,107]. However, comparison between US and perfusion cholescintigraphy has shown that frequent US gallbladder volume measurements will yield a quantitative estimate of the bile emptied from, and stored in, the gallbladder [17]. In addition, US allows for assessment of residual volume after emptying and of the rate of refilling after gallbladder contraction. Ultrasound may be helpful when radiation should be avoided. Ultrasonographic assessment of gallbladder emptying after slow i.v. infusion of CCK analogs has been performed in lithiasic patients [108] and in patients with acalculous gallbladder dysfunction [109]. In the latter group US showed a high predictive value for postcholecystectomy outcome. One deficiency in the technique is the fact that it is operator-dependent, and the results may not be reproducible among different centers. In conclusion, US assessment of gallbladder emptying has not become the diagnostic standard in gallbladder dysfunction.

Pain Provocation Test

A stimulation test with CCK attempting to duplicate the pain has been historically used as a diagnostic investigation. This test has low sensitivity and specificity in selecting patients with gallbladder dysfunction who respond to therapy [110]. This may relate to problems in the subjective assessment of pain and the use of bolus injections of CCK. The latter can induce intestinal contractions.

— Clinical Evaluation

An algorithm for the diagnostic work-up is shown in figure 2. The following comments elaborate on the diagnostic work-up.

(1) Symptoms consistent with a biliary tract etiology should be evaluated by ultrasound examination of the biliary tract, LFTs, and pancreatic enzyme measurements. If the results are normal, upper gastrointestinal endoscopy is recommended.

(2) If any of these investigations detect abnormalities, appropriate investigation and treatment should follow.

(3) If no abnormal findings are detected, a dynamic cholescintigraphic gallbladder study following CCK analog administration should be performed.

(4) If gallbladder emptying is abnormal (less than 40%) and there is no obvious cause (Table 2), the diagnosis of gallbladder dysfunction is likely; cholecystectomy is the most appropriate treatment.

(5) If gallbladder emptying is normal, bile for microscopic examination to de-

Facing page, Figure 2. Diagnostic work-up in patients with suspected gallbladder dysfunction. Abbreviations: LFTs = liver function tests; US = ultrasound; GB CCK = gallbladder cholecystokinin; GBEF = gallbladder ejection fraction; ERCP = endoscopic retrograde cholangiopancreatography; SO = sphincter of Oddi; ES = endoscopic sphincterotomy; MRCP = magnetic resonance cholangiopancreatography.

Management of Biliary Pain in Patients with Intact Gallbladder

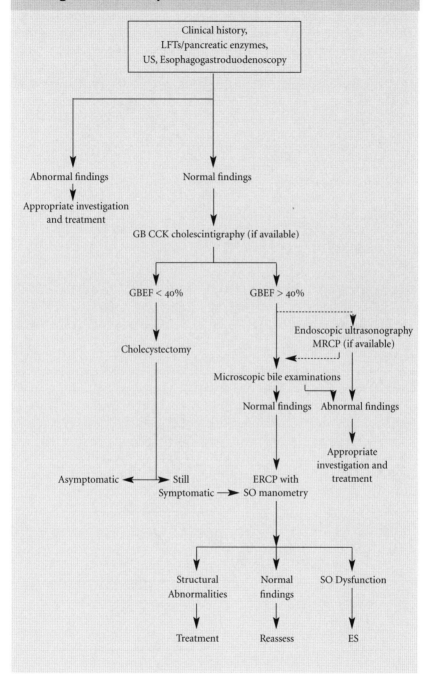

Clinical history,
LFTs/pancreatic enzymes,
US, Esophagogastroduodenoscopy

Abnormal findings
↓
Appropriate investigation
and treatment

Normal findings
↓
GB CCK cholescintigraphy (if available)

GBEF < 40%
↓
Cholecystectomy

GBEF > 40%

Endoscopic ultrasonography
MRCP (if available)

Microscopic bile examinations

Normal findings   Abnormal findings
↓
Appropriate
investigation and
treatment

Asymptomatic ◄─── Still
Symptomatic ──►

ERCP with
SO manometry

Structural
Abnormalities
↓
Treatment

Normal
findings
↓
Reassess

SO Dysfunction
↓
ES

tect cholesterol microcrystals and bilirubinate can be obtained by duodenal drainage, at the time of GI endoscopy or during ERCP. Magnetic resonance cholangiography or endoscopic US, where available, can be performed to detect lithiasis.

(6) If gallbladder emptying is normal, ERCP should be considered. In the absence of common bile duct stones or other abnormalities, SO manometry should also be considered if clinically indicated. Evidence of SO dysfunction is an indication for treatment, which may include sphincterotomy.

As general recommendation we suggest that invasive investigations should be withheld in those patients in whom episodes are infrequent and not accompanied by elevations of LFTs.

— Approach to Treatment

Cholecystectomy retains a role in the treatment of gallbladder dysfunction. Quantitative CCK cholescintigraphy is capable of identifying those with impaired emptying. The challenge is to interpret the subgroup who will benefit from treatment. Some older studies predicated on CCK provocative tests [104, 111] were not well controlled, and the tests, per se, poorly standardized. In addition, favorable outcomes may deteriorate with time after cholecystectomy [112] as one cannot ignore the potential placebo effect of surgery.

Prospective studies are needed in patients with biliary-type pain in whom SO dysfunction has been excluded and standardized gallbladder motility tests have been performed.

Medical therapy might take the form of restoring gallbladder motor function to normal (e.g., use of motility agents) [113]; modifying the composition of bile acids (e.g., use of ursodeoxycholic acid) [114], reducing inflammation (e.g., use of nonsteroidal anti-inflammatory drugs) or visceral hyperalgesia (e.g., use of low dose tricyclic antidepressants).

E2. Sphincter of Oddi Dysfunction

— Definition

SO dysfunction is the term used to define motility abnormalities of the sphincter of Oddi.

— Clinical Presentation

The SO is situated strategically at the duodenal junction of the biliary duct and pancreatic duct. Sphincter of Oddi dysfunction may result in either biliary or pancreatic disorders. Although SO dysfunction may be present in patients with an intact biliary tract, most of the clinical information concerning SO dysfunction refer to post-cholecystectomy patients.

Biliary–Type SO Dysfunction

These patients present with intermittent episodes of biliary-type pain, sometimes accompanied by biochemical features of transient biliary tract obstruction: elevated serum transaminase alkaline phosphatase or conjugated bilirubin.

As indicated in the list below, post-cholecystectomy patients have been arbitrarily classified according to clinical presentation, laboratory results, and ERCP findings [115].

(1) **Biliary-Type I patients** present with pain, elevated liver biochemistries documented on two or more occasions, delayed contrast drainage, and a dilated common bile duct with a corrected diameter equal to or greater than 12 mm at ERCP.

(2) **Biliary-Type II patients** present with pain and only one or two of the previously mentioned criteria.

(3) **Biliary-Type III patients** have only recurrent biliary-type pain and none of the above criteria.

The predictability of SO dysfunction varies among these groups, being highest in Type I and less so in Type III. Conversely, the probability that a syndrome of chronic Functional Abdominal Pain (see chapter 7) manifests as biliary pain is higher in Type III patients, and less likely in Type I. These patients may also present with concurrent psychological difficulties, which should be considered in any decision to undertake invasive investigations.

Pancreatic-Type SO Dysfunction

Pancreatic SO dysfunction is less well classified into types. In its more obvious form (like Biliary-Type I SO dysfunction), it may present with classical pancreatitis with epigastric pain, which often radiates to the back. The pain episode is associated with a significant rise in serum amylase or lipase, yielding the diagnosis of pancreatitis. None of the traditional causes of pancreatitis are found: i.e., the patient does not have associated gallstones, a significant history of alcohol overconsumption, or any of the uncommon causes of pancreatitis. These patients are often labeled as having idiopathic recurrent pancreatitis. In a less obvious form (such as Biliary Type II and III SO Dysfunction), the pain is similar but there might not be elevation of pancreatic enzymes. These patients may also have pancreatic SO dysfunction and respond to sphincterotomy. However, clinical presentation of the pancreatic-type SO dysfunction in the absence of associated laboratory findings may be due to the syndrome of chronic functional abdominal pain (see chapter 7).

— Epidemiology

The prevalence of symptoms suggesting SO dysfunction was noted in 1.5% of postcholecystectomy people in one recent survey on functional gastrointestinal disorders [116]. This survey confirmed that SO dysfunction affects females more frequently than males and indicated a high association with work absenteeism, disability, and health care use [116]. In another study, SO dysfunction was detected in less than 1% of a large consecutive series of cholecystectomized patients, and in 14% of a selected group of patients complaining of postcholecystectomy symptoms [117]. It is possible that the advent of laparoscopic cholecystectomy may affect the prevalence of postcholecystectomy pain, but no data are available. Thirty-three percent of referred symptomatic patients with a dilated common bile duct (indicative of SO stenosis) had abnormal SO manometry (E. Corazziari, personal communication).

The frequency of SO manometric abnormalities differs in subgroups of patients categorized according to clinical history, laboratory results, and ERCP findings. In Biliary-Type I, 65% to 95% of the patients have manometric evidence of biliary SO dysfunction, mainly due to what was thought to be structural alteration (stenosis). In Biliary-Type II, 50% to 63% of the patients have manometric evidence of biliary SO dysfunction. In Biliary-Type III, 12% to 28% of the patients have manometric evidence of biliary SO dysfunction [118,119]. In populations of patients with idiopathic recurrent pancreatitis, manometric evidence of SO dysfunction varies from 39% to 90% [119–122].

Sphincter of Oddi dysfunction can involve abnormalities in either the biliary sphincter, pancreatic sphincter, or both. The true frequency would then depend on whether one or both sphincters were studied. One could be abnormal; the other normal. In a previous study 360 patients were investigated by biliary and pancreatic manometry. Among the 214 patients labeled Type III, 31% had both sphincter pressures elevated; 11%, biliary alone; and 17%, the pancreas alone. Overall, 59% of patients were found to have an abnormal basal sphincter pressure. In the same study, among the 123 patients categorized as Biliary-Type II, pressures in both sphincters were elevated in 32%; in the biliary sphincter alone in 11%; and in the pancreas alone in 22%. Overall, 65% of Type II patients had abnormal results based on sphincter of Oddi manometry [123].

— Diagnostic Criteria

Episodes of severe steady pain located in the epigastrium and right upper quadrant, and all of the following:

(1) **Symptom episodes last 30 minutes or more, with pain-free intervals;**

(2) **Symptoms have occurred on one or more occasions in the previous 12 months;**

(3) **The pain is steady and interrupts daily activities or requires consultation with a physician; *and***

(4) **There is no evidence of structural abnormalities to explain the symptoms.**

In addition the pain may be associated with one or more of the following:

The diagnosis is supported by elevated serum transaminase, alkaline phosphatase, or conjugated bilirubin and/or pancreatic enzymes (amylase/lipase).

Acute recurrent pancreatitis can indicate pancreatic SO dysfunction.

Other clinical features which may be associated with pain episodes are: nausea and vomiting; pain radiating to the back and/or right interscapular regions (biliary) and/or pain partially alleviated by bending forward (pancreatic); onset after meals; and/or awakening patients at night.

Sphincter of Oddi dysfunction may exist in the presence of an intact biliary tract with the gallbladder in situ. As the symptoms of SO or gallbladder dysfunction cannot be readily separated, the diagnosis of SO dysfunction is made commonly following cholecystectomy or less frequently, after proper investigations have excluded gallbladder abnormalities.

— Rationale for Changes in the Diagnostic Criteria

In comparison to the previously published Rome I Diagnostic Criteria, these Rome II Diagnostic Criteria have one major change: the specification of the duration, number of episodes of pain, and the time period when they occur. The committee bases these changes on the following information and clinical observation:

(1) Thirty minutes has been more firmly established in the literature as the minimum duration of a biliary "colic."
(2) Even a single pain episode may be so severe to justify diagnostic investigation, irrespective of the number of the episodes.
(3) The frequency of biliary pain may be so irregular that a time window of only three months has been considered too restrictive.

— Clinical Evaluation

The symptoms of SO dysfunction must be differentiated from organic disease and other more common functional disorders: dyspepsia due to other causes and the irritable bowel symptoms. The only method that can directly assess the motor function of the SO is manometry. This technique is difficult to perform and interpret, is not widely available, and is invasive with potential complications. Further, SO dysfunction is relatively uncommon. Less invasive procedures should therefore be considered first.

Noninvasive Indirect Methods

Serum Biochemistry
Liver Biochemistries
A transient significant elevation of liver enzymes and/or bilirubin stasis, in close temporal relationship to at least two episodes of biliary pain, is suspect for SO dysfunction. Although the diagnostic sensitivity and specificity of abnormal liver biochemistry values are relatively low [124], recent evidence indicates that the finding of abnormal liver biochemistry values in Biliary-Type II patients may predict a favorable response to endoscopic sphincterotomy [125].

Pancreatic Enzymes
A significant elevation of either amylase or lipase in close temporal relationship to pancreatic pain is suggestive of pancreatitis, which may be caused by SO dysfunction.

Pain Provocative Tests
Historically, these tests using morphine(+/− prostigmine) to detect SO dysfunction have had limited sensitivity and specificity [126]. They are no longer recommended.

Ultrasonographic Assessment of Duct Diameter
Ultrasonographic Duct Diameter in the Fasting State
At ultrasound examination, choledochal diameter normally is 6 mm or less [127,128]. A dilated common bile duct may indicate the presence of increased resistance to bile flow at the level of the SO; however, the diagnostic usefulness of this finding is limited since 3% to 4% of asymptomatic cholecystectomized subjects have a dilated common bile duct [117,129]. Likewise, the finding of a dilated pancreatic duct may indicate increased resistance to flow at the level of the SO.

Fatty Meal (Cholecystokinin) Stimulation Test
The fatty meal-induced bile flow caused by the endogenous release of CCK or the administration of CCK analogs may be followed by dilation of the common bile duct in the presence of a partially obstructed bile duct, but not in the absence of obstruction [130,131]. Unlike cholescintigraphy the diagnostic yield has not been satisfactorily identified [132]. It is likely that sensitivity and specificity of the test changes relative to the subgroup of patients. An advantage of fatty meal ultrasound is its use in patients with a functioning gallbladder. Whether or not the test correlates with SO manometry or is a marker for the disorder has not been studied. Its diagnostic usefulness is limited to screening patients with partial common duct obstruction.

Secretin Stimulation Test
Secretin stimulation of pancreatic flow may be followed by dilation of the pancreatic duct [133]. A dilation of the duct that lasts more than 15 minutes after intravenous secretin (1 µg/kg) indicates pancreatic sphincter dysfunction. Such a positive test has been reported to predict a favorable postsurgical outcome in symptomatic patients with SO stenosis [133,134]. Whether or not the test correlates with SO manometry is unknown. In addition, the capability of ultrasonography to identify what is normal and any small changes in pancreatic duct is questionable. In the absence of well structured outcome studies, the diagnostic usefulness of this test remains to be ascertained. Computed tomography and magnetic resonance pancreatography potentially may become alternative techniques to assess the response to this test.

Choledochoscintigraphy

Following cholecystectomy, bile flow into the duodenum is mainly regulated by SO tone. Dysfunction of the sphincter may become apparent when there is a delay in the disappearance of radiopharmaceutical markers of bile from the liver/biliary tract. Early studies employed subjective assessment of the radionuclide disappearance on the sequential scintigraphic images [135, 136]. Subsequently, more accurate quantitation used computer-generated, time-activity curves for the hepatobiliary system.

Several variables have been used, such as time to peak activity [137], slope values [135] and hepatic clearance at predefined time intervals [135–138]. All of these variables, however are affected by the presence of liver disease, do not have satisfactory reproducibility, and their diagnostic sensitivity is controversial [135–138]. Dysfunction of the sphincter becomes manifest by a delay in the disappearance of radiopharmaceutical markers of bile from the biliary tract [138] or a prolonged transit of the radiolabelled bile from the hepatic hilum to the duodenum (choledochoscintigraphy) [139]. Choledochoscintigraphy (figs. 3, 4) is re-

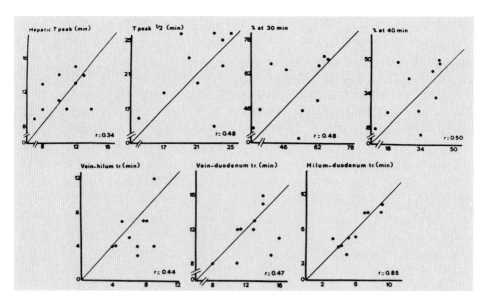

Figure 3. Correlation between values of the most commonly used cholescintigraphic variables derived from two duplicate studies performed at a 2-week interval in 10 asymptomatic cholecystectomized subjects. The solid line is the identity line. Note that only the value of the hepatic hilum-duodenum transit time shows a highly significant correlation between the duplicate studies. Reproduced with permission from Cicala M, Scopinaro F, Corazziari E, et al. Gastroenterology 1991;100:1106.

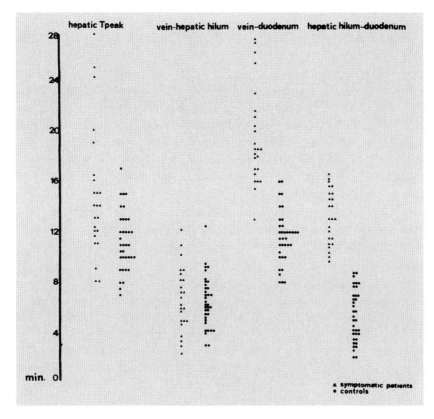

Figure 4. Distribution of the individual data of the four more commonly used cholescintigraphic variables derived from cholecystectomized subjects: asymptomatic controls
(dots) and patients with symptomatic sphincter of Oddi dysfunction (triangles). Data for
the asymptomatic subjects include 10 values derived from duplicate studies. Note that only
the value of hepatic hilum-duodenum transit time discriminates the two groups of subjects. Reproduced with permission from Cicala M, Scopinaro F, Corazziari E, et al. Gastroenterology 1991;100:1106.

producible and significantly correlates with SO basal pressure [140]. A possible
further advance is a scoring system which is closely correlated with SO dysfunction [141]. Specificity is limited in certain instances where there are other causes
of delayed transit of bile from the liver to the duodenum: e.g., pooling of bile
in a dilated choledochus or intrahepatic cholestasis. Choledochoscintigraphy
cannot be used to detect SO dysfunction in patients with a functioning gallbladder because the gallbladder acts as a bile reservoir, thus affecting the transit
of bile from the liver to the duodenum [139,140]. This noninvasive method ap-

pears useful as a screen to select among patients whose symptoms have not responded to cholecystectomy those suitable for SO manometry.

Invasive Indirect Methods

Endoscopic Retrograde Cholangiopancreatography

Certain radiologic features during ERCP—such as a common bile duct
diameter exceeding 12 mm [127] and delayed emptying of contrast media (>45
min)—suggest SO dysfunction. Additionally, pancreatic duct dilatation greater
than 5 mm and delayed emptying of contrast media from the pancreatic duct
(>10 min) can be demonstrated at ERCP in the presence of a dysfunction of the
pancreatic SO [133]. However, these observations are uncontrolled, lack sensitivity and specificity, and are influenced by a number of variables such as pre-
medication, lack of standardization, and the patient's posture.

Invasive Direct Methods

Manometry

Sphincter of Oddi manometry can be performed at endoscopy, at
surgery, or percutaneously [38,142]. It is most commonly done at endoscopy.
Perendoscopic manometry allows measurements to be made in subjects with intact gallbladders in both the biliary and pancreatic tracts of the sphincter, but
recordings are relatively short and may be influenced by drugs used for pre-
medication and by the presence of the endoscope within the duodenum. To
avoid manometric artifacts, proper sedation is necessary to perform intraluminal pressure recordings; drugs that do not interfere with intraluminal pressure
recordings must be used. Intravenous diazepam (5 to 25 mg) has been used
most frequently, but propofol is being increasingly used [143]. Meperidine (at a
dose of less than 1 mg/kg) as an additional analgesia to diazepam does not alter
basal SO pressure but influences phasic activity [144–146]. Anticholinergic
agents should be avoided as they inhibit SO motor activity. If necessary, glucagon
1.0 mg i.v. can be used because its effect, if any [51], on SO motor activity lasts less
than 10 minutes [37].

A three-lumen catheter with an outside diameter of 1.7 mm and distal side
openings is the most widely used SO manometric catheter. Each lumen is continuously perfused with a minimally compliant pneumohydraulic capillary infusion system [147]. Once the distal end of the manometric catheter is deeply inserted into the papilla of Vater, it is withdrawn through the SO by the station
pull-through technique in 1–2 mm increments and then located, with the
recording sensor stationed within the sphincter area to obtain a stable recording

for at least 30 sec. Some authors indicate that a longer period of recording (3–4 min) at each station of the step-by-step pull-through reduces the risks of artifacts [148]. During a pull-through maneuver (i.e., withdrawing a multilumen catheter across the SO), recordings of each port shows, in orderly progression, an increase of the baseline pressure and then a relatively stable plateau, with phasic waves superimposed on it. The sphincter is identified as the zone of (1) elevated resting pressure between the duct, either pancreatic or choledochal, and duodenal pressure with (2) phasic waves superimposed (fig. 5). The variables customarily assessed at SO manometry are basal pressure and amplitude, duration, frequency, and propagation pattern of the phasic waves [149]. Normal reference values for the SO measured at the common bile duct and Wirsung duct are reported in Table 3 [150,151].

Validation studies of SO manometry have shown that interobserver error can be relevant in the absence of a standardized approach to the interpretation of manometric recordings [152]. Observer errors, however, become negligible when interpretation of the tracing follows an agreed-upon standardized approach [153,154]. There is consistency in repeated measures of SO basal pressure over days and even up to a year [148,152]. Phasic contractions vary in relation to the cyclical phases of the duodenal interdigestive motor complex [38] (fig. 6).

Pancreatic enzyme elevation and episodes of pancreatitis can follow manometric evaluation of the SO. Although such enzyme elevations occur as a clinical condition in as many as 61% of patients immediately after endoscopic

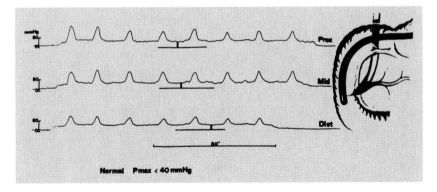

Figure 5. Perendoscopic manometry of the sphincter of Oddi (SO). On the right is shown the perendoscopic cannulation of the papilla of Vater, with the manometric catheter inserted in the choledochus. On the left, the manometric recording from the three sensors, proximal (Prox), middle (Mid), and distal (Dist), positioned within the SO shows phasic activity superimposed on the basal sphincter pressure; duodenal pressure indicated by the solid lines.

Table 3. Pressure Profile of Sphincter of Oddi Measured at Common Bile Duct (CBD) and Pancreatic Duct (PD)

	Normal*		Abnormal**
	CBD	PD	CBD PD
Duct Pressure (mm Hg)	7.4 ± 1.7	8.0 ± 1.6	
Basal Pressure (mm Hg)	16.2 ± 5.8	17.3 ± 5.8	>40mm Hg
	(6–25)	(8–26)	
Phasic Contractions			
Amplitude (mm Hg)	136.5 ± 25.9	127.5 ± 21.5	>350mm Hg
	(82–180)	(90–160)	
Duration (sec)	4.7 ± 0.9	4.8 ± 0.7	
	(3–6)	(4–6)	
Frequency (/min)	5.7 ± 1.4	5.8 ± 1.5	>7/min
	(3–10)	(3–10)	
Propagation Sequence (%)			
Simultaneous	55 (10–100)	53 (10–90)	
Antegrade	34 (0–70)	35 (10–70)	
Retrograde	11 (0–40)	12 (0–40)	> 50%

* Normal values are means ± standard deviations; ranges are given in parentheses.
**Abnormal values for the CBD and the PD are found in references 151 and 121, respectively.

Elevated basal SO pressure indicates either stenosis or spasm of the sphincter. With sphincteric spasm, SO pressure decreases after administering a smooth muscle relaxant. Spasm of the sphincter and the other SO motor alterations indicate a dyskinesia. The distinction between SO stenosis and SO dyskinesia is provided in Table 4.

Reproduced with permission from Guelrud M, Mendoza S, Rossiter G, et al. Dig Dis Sci 1990;35:38. Published by Plenum.

manometry, pancreatitis may develop in as many as 24% of patients. When the pancreatic duct is studied [142,155–157], the incidence of these complications may be reduced if: (1) the manometric recording time is reduced; (2) the pancreatic duct is allowed to drain through a disconnected catheter after the study is complete [158]; and (3) the pancreatic duct is continuously aspirated throughout the manometry [157].

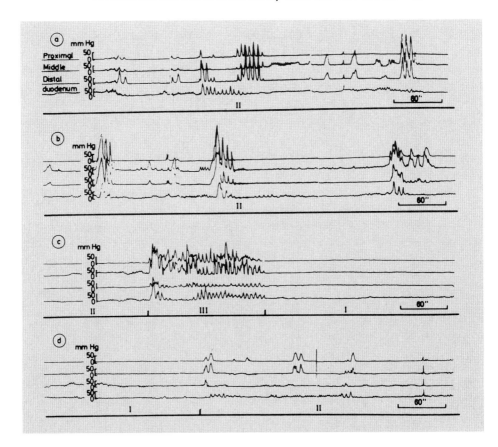

Figure 6. Sphincter of Oddi and duodenal phases of the interdigestive migrating motor complex in a prolonged manometric session (transductal and duodenal manometry). The 35-min continuous recording shows phase II in a, b and d; phase III in c; and phase I in c and d. Reproduced with permission from Torsoli A, Corazziari E, Habib FI, et al. Gut 1986;27:363.

Manometric alterations of the SO include increased basal pressure (fig. 7) [159–161], increased amplitude of phasic waves, paradoxical response to CCK analogs [162,163], increased frequency of phasic waves [151,164], and increased number of retrograde waves [160,163] (Table 4). More than one of these manometric findings may be found in postcholecystectomy patients with no apparent organic alterations [37,151,159].

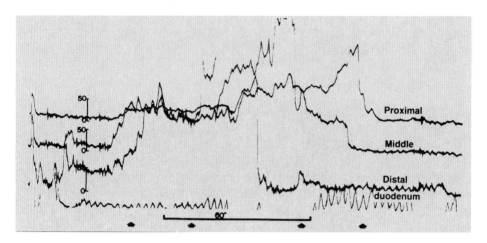

Figure 7. Perendoscopic manometry of the sphincter of Oddi. Manometric recordings from three sensors, proximal, middle, and distal, withdrawn through the pancreatic sphincter. The bottom tracing is the recording from the duodenum. Note the elevated sphincter of Oddi pressure recorded by the three upper sensors.

— Diagnostic Work-up in Patients with Suspected Sphincter of Oddi Dysfunction

As a general recommendation we suggest that invasive investigations should be withheld in those patients in whom episodes are infrequent and not accompanied by elevations of serum LFTs or pancreatic enzymes. Complications from invasive procedures such as ERCP and SO manometry are more frequent in patients with SO dysfunction, and when performed by inexperienced endoscopists. The recommendations presented here apply only to skilled endoscopists, preferably in referral centers.

Post Cholecystectomy Patients

(1) The diagnostic work-up of a patient without a gallbladder for suspected SO dysfunction as a cause of Biliary-Type pain begins with analysis of liver biochemistries and pancreatic enzymes, plus a careful elimination of potential structural causes (fig. 8). This would usually include transabdominal ultrasound and ERCP. Depending upon the available resources, endoscopic ultrasound and nuclear magnetic resonance cholangiography may precede ERCP in specific clinical conditions.

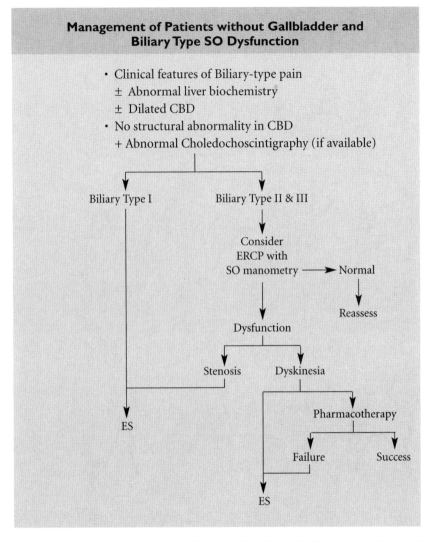

Management of Patients without Gallbladder and Biliary Type SO Dysfunction

- Clinical features of Biliary-type pain
  ± Abnormal liver biochemistry
  ± Dilated CBD
- No structural abnormality in CBD
  + Abnormal Choledochoscintigraphy (if available)

Biliary Type I

Biliary Type II & III

Consider ERCP with SO manometry ——▶ Normal

Reassess

Dysfunction

Stenosis   Dyskinesia

Pharmacotherapy

ES

Failure   Success

ES

Figure 8. Management of patients without a gallbladder and biliary-type sphincter of Oddi dysfunction. Abbreviations: ERCP = endoscopic retrograde cholangiopancreatography; ES = endoscopic sphincterotomy; SO = sphincter of Oddi; CBD = common bile duct.

(2) Choledochoscintigraphy may be a valuable screening before a decision to undertake SO manometry is made.

(3) Patients with Biliary-Type I SO dysfunction may undergo endoscopic sphincterotomy without SO manometry.

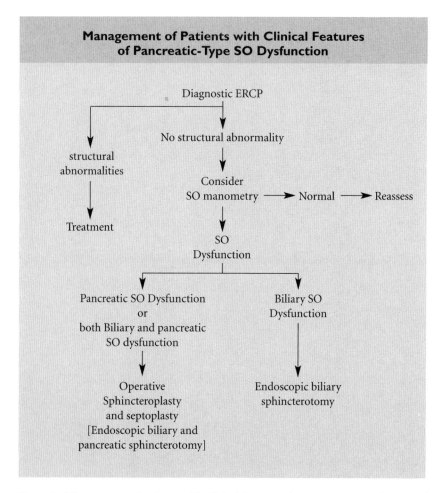

Management of Patients with Clinical Features of Pancreatic-Type SO Dysfunction

Diagnostic ERCP

No structural abnormality

structural
abnormalities

Consider
SO manometry ⟶ Normal ⟶ Reassess

Treatment

SO
Dysfunction

Pancreatic SO Dysfunction
or
both Biliary and pancreatic
SO dysfunction

Biliary SO
Dysfunction

Operative
Sphincteroplasty
and septoplasty
[Endoscopic biliary and
pancreatic sphincterotomy]

Endoscopic biliary
sphincterotomy

Figure 9. Management of patients with clinical features of pancreatic-type sphincter of Oddi dysfunction. Abbreviations: ERCP = endoscopic retrograde cholangiopancreatography; SO = sphincter of Oddi.

(4) Sphincter of Oddi manometry is recommended in Biliary-Type II and should be considered in Biliary-Type III.

(5) If SO manometry is normal, the patient should be reassessed for causes other than SO dysfunction.

(6) If SO stenosis is detected at manometry, treatment is endoscopic sphincterotomy.

(7) If SO dyskinesia is evident, a trial of drug therapy may be in order.

Patients with Gallbladder In Situ

The diagnostic work-up of patients with a gallbladder in situ is part of the same diagnostic algorithm that has initially excluded the presence of a gallbladder dysfunction (fig. 2).

Patients with Clinical Features of Pancreatic-Type Dysfunction

(1) When ERPC demonstrates no structural abnormality, SO manometry of both biliary and pancreatic sphincter is indicated (fig. 9).

(2) When SO manometry reveals pancreatic SO dysfunction alone or with biliary SO dysfunction, the standard therapy is operative sphincteroplasty and pancreatic septoplasty. A combined endoscopic biliary and pancreatic sphincterotomy technique is undergoing investigation in a number of centers.

(3) An endoscopic biliary sphincterotomy should be performed when biliary SO dysfunction is found.

— Approach to Treatment

The therapeutic approach in patients with SO dysfunction is aimed at reducing the resistance caused by the SO to the flow of bile or pancreatic juice.

Table 4. Manometric Criteria of SO Dysfunction

	Stenosis	Dyskinesia
A. Basal SO pressure		
1. Elevation	√	√
2. Response		√
a. Nitrates		√
b. CCK-8		√
B Phasic SO waves		
1. Rapid Rate		√
2. Retrograde Propagation		√
3. High Amplitude		√

Abbreviation: CCK = cholecystokinin.

Pharmacotherapy

Several agents can affect the motor tone of the gallbladder and sphincter of Oddi. Nitroglycerine and butylscopolamine bromide have been used acutely in therapeutic endoscopy allowing extraction of choledochal stones (<8mm diameter) through a relaxed SO without the need for sphincterectomy [50].

Some therapeutic agents have potential, but for most there is limited evidence for their therapeutic usefulness.

Hormones

Although transient reduction of SO motor function has been demonstrated during pharmacologic (bolus) administration of CCK-8 and glucagon [165,51], no long-term studies have been performed in humans during infusion of these hormones to reproduce physiologic values.

Calcium Channel Blockers

Nifedipine at 10–20 mg p.o. decreases the sphincter of Oddi pressure and lessens phasic contractions (amplitude, duration and frequency), both in healthy volunteers and patients with biliary dyskinesia. [166,167]. One controlled clinical trial suggested some benefit for patients with Type II SO dysfunction [168].

Nitrates

Nitrates dilate vascular smooth muscle and have a similar effect on gut smooth muscle, acting through nitric oxide mechanisms. Nitrates decrease sphincteric pressure. Glyceryltrinitrate (1.2 mg sl) decreases SO pressure and enables the endoscopist to obtain higher rates of papillary intubation [169]. In two small studies, isosorbide dinitrate 10 ml tid alleviated the symptoms of SO dysfunction on a short term basis. [170,171].

Botulinum Toxin

Botulinum is a potent inhibitor of acetylcholine release from nerve endings. Recent studies of injecting the sphincter showed relaxed pressure and improved bile flow. This reduction in pressure may be accompanied by symptomatic improvement [172–174]. Further studies are needed, but botulinum toxin may serve as a predictor for a successful result from subsequent sphincter ablation.

Assessment of Medical Therapy

Although medical therapy may be an attractive initial approach in patients with SO dysfunction, several drawbacks exist. First, side effects from calcium channel blockers and nitrates may be seen in up to one-third of patients. Second, smooth muscle relaxants are unlikely to be of any benefit in patients with SO stenosis, and the response is transient in patients with a primary motor abnormality of the SO (i.e., SO dyskinesia). Finally, the long-term outcome of medical therapy has not been reported.

Hydrostatic Balloon Dilatation

In an attempt to be less invasive and possibly to preserve sphincter function, hydrostatic balloon dilatation has been used to treat SO dysfunction [175,176]. Unfortunately, because of the unacceptably high complication rates (primarily pancreatitis), this technique has little role in the management of SO dysfunction.

Sphincterotomy

Division of the sphincter can be accomplished by endoscopic or transduodenal operative approach. Endoscopic sphincterotomy (ES) is the most widely used therapeutic procedure in patients with biliary-type SO dysfunction. Endoscopic sphincterotomy is less expensive and has a lower morbidity than open surgery. For pancreatic SO dysfunction, sphincteroplasty and septectomy are the preferred treatment.

Biliary-Type Sphincter of Oddi Dysfunction

Most studies reporting efficacy of endoscopic therapy in SO dysfunction have been retrospective, except for few randomized trials. In a first study 47 post-cholecystectomy Type II biliary patients were randomized to biliary sphincterotomy versus sham sphincterotomy [115]. Ninety-five percent of patients with an elevated basal sphincter pressure benefited from sphincterotomy. In contrast, only 35% of patients with elevated sphincter pressures improved after sham sphincterotomy. In a second study post-cholecystectomy patients with biliary-type pain were prospectively randomized to endoscopic sphincterotomy or sham following stratification according to SO manometry [177]. Seventy-five percent of patients with elevated SO basal pressure improved at two years following endoscopic sphincterotomy. Forty percent of patients having a sham procedure also improved.

A randomized third study compared endoscopic sphincterotomy and surgical biliary sphincteroplasty with pancreatic septoplasty (with or without cholecystectomy) to sham sphincterotomy for Type II and III biliary patients with manometrically documented SO dysfunction [178]. During a three year follow-up period, 69% of patients who underwent endoscopic or surgical sphincter ablation improved compared to 24% in the sham sphincterotomy group (p= 0.009). There was a trend for Type II patients to benefit more frequently from sphincter ablation than Type III (13/16 [81%] vs. 11/19 [58%] p<0.14) [115].

Pancreatitis is the most common short-term complication of endoscopic sphincterotomy, and its rate is higher when the maneuver is performed for SO dysfunction than for common bile duct stone extraction. This risk is exaggerated in patients without common bile duct dilatation [157,179]. However morbidity has been reported to vary from 5% to >16% in the SO dysfunction group, versus 3% to 10% in the common bile duct stone group. These results clearly indicate that any enthusiasm for sphincter ablation must be balanced against such high complication rates. The risk of pancreatitis after sphincterotomy of the biliary SO is reduced by stenting the pancreatic SO, especially in those patients with elevated pancreatic SO pressure before sphincterotomy. Even in these cases, however, the decision to stent the pancreatic sphincter should be considered carefully [180,181].

Pancreatic-Type Sphincter of Oddi Dysfunction

Ablation of both the biliary and pancreatic sphincter of Oddi has been attempted since treatment with endoscopic biliary sphincterotomy alone usually will not cure patients with idiopathic recurrent pancreatitis and a diagnosis of SO dysfunction. More recently, ablation of the pancreatic sphincter has been performed by the endoscopic route.

Surgical division of the SO is achieved via a transduodenal sphincteroplasty and pancreatic duct septoplasty [182,183]. In all three studies that evaluated this procedure, the operation resulted in greater than 70% improvement in symptoms at one to ten year follow-up. Operative mortality was close to zero. Overall postoperative morbidity was about 30%, and the incidence of pancreatitis was low [183–185].

There are several potential explanations as to why patients with well-documented sphincter of Oddi dysfunction may fail to achieve symptom relief after biliary sphincterotomy is performed. First, the biliary sphincterotomy may have been inadequate, or re-stenosis may have occurred. Although the biliary sphincter is commonly not totally ablated [178], clinically significant biliary re-stenosis occurs relatively infrequently [186]. If no "cutting space" remains in such a patient, balloon dilation to 8–10 mm may suffice, but long-term outcome from such therapy is unknown [187].

Second, the importance of pancreatic sphincter ablation is being increasingly recognized. Severance of the pancreatic sphincter appears necessary to resolve the pancreatitis [188]. In one series, 69 patients with idiopathic pancreatitis due to SO dysfunction underwent either standard biliary sphincterotomy (n=18), biliary sphincterotomy followed by pancreatic sphincterotomy in separate sessions (n=13), or combined pancreatic and biliary sphincterotomy (n=14). Eighty-one percent of patients who underwent pancreatic plus biliary sphincterotomy had resolution of their pancreatitis compared to 28% of patients undergoing biliary sphincterotomy alone (p<0.005). In another study, 25 of 26 patients who failed to respond to biliary sphincterotomy had elevated pancreatic sphincter pressure [189]. Subsequent endoscopic pancreatic sphincterotomy yielded a symptomatic improvement in two-thirds of patients.

Stent Trial as Diagnostic Test
Placement of a pancreatic or biliary stent on a trial basis in hope of achieving pain relief and predicting the response to more definitive therapy (i.e., sphincter ablation) has received only limited application. Pancreatic stent trials, especially in patients with normal pancreatic ducts, are strongly discouraged, as serious ductal and parenchymal injury may occur if stents are left in place for more than a few days [190]. In a biliary stent trial in Type II and III SO dysfunction patients with normal biliary manometry, seven French stents were left in place for at least two months if symptoms resolved and removed sooner if they were judged ineffective. Relief of pain with the stent was predictive of long-term pain relief after biliary sphincterotomy. Unfortunately, 38% of the patients developed pancreatitis (14% were graded severe) following stent placement [191]. Because of this high rate of complications, biliary stent trials are strongly discouraged.

Recommendations for Future Research

Motility disorders of the gallbladder and sphincter of Oddi cause significant clinical symptoms but several aspects of their pathophysiology are still to be clarified.

Future studies should investigate

(1) The potential pathogenetic role of psychosocial conditions and genetic factors on biliary and pancreatic dysfunctions.
(2) The relationship of bilio-pancreatic dysfunction to other functional gastrointestinal disorders.
(3) The relationship of gallbladder dysfunction to lithogenic bile, and the role of lithogenic bile in defining patients with primary gallbladder alteration from those in whom its presence is a secondary effect of SO dysfunction.
(4) The role of the bilio-pancreatic dysfunction in the origin of pain and whether these dysfunctional conditions are associated with visceral hyperalgesia.

A number of noninvasive investigations have been developed which help in the diagnosis of these conditions; however further evaluations are needed to assess the following:

(1) The specific role of cholescintigraphy in the diagnosis and prediction of therapeutic outcome of gallbladder and SO dysfunction.
(2) The role of nuclear magnetic resonance cholangiopancreatography in the visualization and dynamic assessment of the papillary region.

Further studies should also be directed to the therapy of these conditions:

(1) Assessment of pharmacotherapy of the gallbladder and the SO (ranging from prokinetics and relaxants to targeted analgesics).
(2) Improved modes of evaluation of outcome studies.

References

1. Kraglund K, Hjermind J, Jensen FT, et al. Gallbladder emptying and gastrointestinal cyclic motor activity in humans. Scand J Gastroenterol 1984;19:990–94.
2. Toouli J, Bushell M, Stevenson G. Gallbladder emptying in man related to fasting duodenal migrating motor contractions. Austral N Z J Surg 1986;56:147–51.
3. Marzio L, Neri M, Capone F, et al. Gallbladder contraction and its relationship to interdigestive duodenal motor activity in normal human subjects. Dig Dis Sci 1988;33:540–44.
4. Takahashi I, Suzuki T, Aizawa I, et al. Comparison of gallbladder contractions induced by motilin and cholecystokinin in dogs. Gastroenterology 1982;82:419–24.
5. Fiorucci S, Bosso R, Morelli A. Erythromycin stimulates gallbladder emptying and motilin release by atropine-sensitive pathways. Dig Dis Sci 1992;37:1678-84.
6. Suzuki T, Takahashi I, Itoh Z. Motilin and gallbladder: new dimensions in gastrointestinal physiology. Peptides 1981;2(suppl):229–33.
7. Stolk MF, van Erpecum KJ, Smout AJ, et al. Motor cycles with phase III in antrum are associated with high motilin levels and prolonged gallbladder emptying. Am J Physiol 1993;264:G596–G600.
8. Ryan JP. Motility of the gallbladder and biliary tree. In Johnson LR, Editor. Physiology of the Gastrointestinal Tract. New York:Raven Press;1987:695–722.
9. Lilja P, Fagan CJ, Wiener I, et al. Infusion of pure cholecystokinin in humans: correlation between plasma concentrations of cholecystokinin and gallbladder size. Gastroenterology 1982;83:256–61.
10. Wiener I, Inoue K, Fagan CJ, et al. Release of cholecystokinin in man: correlation of blood levels with gallbladder contraction. Ann Surg 1981;194:321–27.
11. Svanvik J, Allen B, Pellegrini C, et al. Variations in concentrating function of the gallbladder in the conscious monkey. Gastroenterology 1984;86:919–25.
12. Igimi H, Yamamoto F, Lee SP. Gallbladder mucosal function: studies in absorption and secretion in humans and in dog gallbladder epithelium. Am J Physiol 1992; 263:69–74.
13. Fisher RS, Rock E, Malmud LS, et al. Gallbladder emptying response to sham feeding in humans. Gastroenterology 1986;90:1854–57.
14. Hopman PM, Jansen JBMJ, Rosenbusch G, et al. Cephalic stimulation of gallbladder contraction in humans: role of cholecystokinin and the cholinergic systems. Digestion 1987;38:197–203.
15. Lanzini A, Jazrawi RP, Northfield TC, et al. Simultaneous quantitative measurements of absolute gallbladder storage and emptying during fasting and eating in humans. Gastroenterology 1987;92:852–61.
16. Pallotta N, Corazziari E, Biliotti D, et al. Gallbladder volume variations after meal ingestion. Am J Gastroenterol 1994;89:2212–16.
17. Pallotta N, Corazziari E, Scopinaro F, et al. Noninvasive estimate of bile flux through the gallbladder in humans. Am J Gastroenterol 1998;93:1877–85.
18. Radberg G, Asztely M, Moonen M, et al. Contraction and evacuation of the gall-

bladder studied simultaneously by ultrasonography and 99mTc-labeled diethyl-iminodiacetic acid scintigraphy. Scand J Gastroenterol 1993;28:709–13.

19. Cicala M, Corazziari E, Diacinti D, et al. The effect of endogenous cholecystokinin on postprandial gallbladder refilling: ultrasonographic study in healthy subjects and in gallstone patients. Dig Dis Sci 1995;40:76–81.

20. Ashkin JR, Lyon DT, Shull SD, et al. Factors affecting delivery of bile to the duodenum in man. Gastroenterology 1976;74:560–65.

21. Liddle RA, Goldfine ID, Rosen MS, et al. Cholecystokinin bioactivity in human plasma: molecular forms, responses to feeding, and relationship to gallbladder contraction. J Clin Invest 1985;75:1144–52.

22. Maton PN, Selden AC, Chadwick VS, et al. Large and small forms of cholecystokinin in human plasma: measurement using high pressure liquid chromatography and radioimmunoassay. Regul Pept 1982;4:251–60.

23. Behar J, Biancani P. Effect of cholecystokinin and the octapeptide of cholecystokinin on the feline sphincter of Oddi and gallbladder. J Clin Invest 1980;66:1231–39.

24. Marzio L, Di Giammarco AM, Neri M, et al. Atropine antagonizes cholecystokinin and cerulein-induced gallbladder evacuation in man: a real-time ultrasonographic study. Am J Gastroenterol 1985;80:1–4.

25. Sturdevant RAL, Stern DH, Resin H, et al. Effect of graded doses of octapeptide of cholecystokinin on gallbladder size in man. Gastroenterology 1973;64:452–56.

26. Mawe GM. The role of cholecystokinin in ganglionic transmission in the guinea-pig gallbladder. J Physiol (Lond) 1991;439:89–102.

27. Gullo L, Bolondi L, Priori P, et al. Inhibitory effect of atropine on cholecystokinin-induced gallbladder contraction in man. Digestion 1984;29:209–13.

28. Takahashi T, May D, Owyan GC. Cholinergic dependence of gallbladder response to cholecystokinin in the guinea pig in vivo Am J Physiol 1991;261:G565–69.

29. Mawe GM, Gokin AP, Wells DG, et al. Actions of cholecystokinin and norepinephine on vagal input to ganglion cells in guinea pig gallbladder. Am J Physiol 1994;267:G1146–51.

30. Wiley JW, O'Dorisio TM, Owyang C, et al. Vasoactive intestinal polypeptide mediates cholecystokinin-induced relaxation of the sphincter of Oddi. J Clin Invest 1988;81:1920–24.

31. Pauletzki JG, Sharkey KA, Davison J, et al. Involvement of L-arginine-nitric oxide pathways in neural relaxation of the sphincter of Oddi. Eur J Pharmacol 1993;232:263–70.

32. Shima Y, Mori M, Harano M, et al. Nitric oxide mediates cerulein-induced relaxation of canine sphincter of Oddi. Dig Dis Sci 1998;43:547–53.

33. Everson GT. Gallbladder function and gallstone disease. Gastroenterol Clin North Am 1991;20:85–110.

34. Behar J, Rhim BY, Thompson W, et al. Inositol triphosphate restores impaired human gallbladder motility associated with cholesterol stones. Gastroenterology 1993;104:563–68.

35. Xu Q-W, Shaffer EA. The potential site of impaired gallbladder contractility in an animal model of cholesterol gallstone disease. Gastroenterology 1996;110:251–57.
36. Yu P, Chen Q, Biancani, et al. Membrane cholesterol alters gallbladder muscle contractility in the prairie dogs. Am J Physiol 1996;270:G56–61.
37. Geenen JE, Hogan WJ, Dodds WJ, et al. Intraluminal pressure recordings from the human sphincter of Oddi. Gastroenterology 1980;78:317–24.
38. Torsoli A, Corazziari E, Habib FI, et al. Frequencies and cyclical pattern of the human sphincter of Oddi phasic activity. Gut 1986;27:363–69.
39. Torsoli A, Corazziari E, Habib FI, et al. Prolonged transductal manometry of the sphincter of Oddi. Ital J Gastroenterol 1985;17:35–37.
40. Worthley CS, Baker RA, Iannos J, et al. Human fasting and postprandial sphincter of Oddi motility. Brit J Surg 1989;76:709–14.
41. Scott RB, Strasberg SM, El-Sharkawy TY, et al. Fasting canine biliary secretion and the sphincter of Oddi. Gastroenterology 1984;87:793–804.
42. Toouli J, Dodds WJ, Honda R, et al. Motor function of the opossum sphincter of Oddi. J Clin Invest 1983;71:208–20.
43. Torsoli A. Physiology of the human sphincter of Oddi. Endoscopy 1988;20:166–70.
44. Toouli J, Hogan WJ, Geenen JE, et al. Action of cholecystokinin octapeptide on sphincter of Oddi basal pressure and phasic activity in humans. Surgery 1982;92:497–503.
45. Wells DG, Talmage EK, Mawe GM, et al. Immunohistochemical identification of neurons in ganglia of the guinea pig sphincter of Oddi. J Comp Neurol 1995;352:106–16.
46. Helm JF, Dodds WJ, Christensen J, et al. Intramural neural control of opossum sphincter of Oddi. Am J Physiol 1989;257:G925–29.
47. Baker RA, Saccone GT, Brookes SJ, et al. Nitric oxide mediates nonadrenergic, noncholinergic neural relaxation in the Australian possum. Gastroenterology 1993;105:1746–53.
48. Slivka A, Chuttani R, Carr-Locke DL, et al. Inhibition of sphincter of Oddi function by the nitric oxide carrier S-nitroso-N-acetylcysteine in rabbits and humans. J Clin Invest 1994;94:1792–98.
49. Helm JF, Venu RP, Geenen JE, et al. Effects of morphine on the human sphincter of Oddi. Gut 1988;29(10):1402–1407.
50. Staritz M, Poralla T, Dormeyer HH, et al. Endoscopic removal of common bile duct stones through the intact papilla after medical sphincter dilatation. Gastroenterology 1985;88:1807–11.
51. Biliotti D, Habib FI, De Masi F, et al. Effect of glucagon on sphincter of Oddi motor activity. Digestion 1989;43:185–89.
52. Thune A, Saccone GT, Scicchitano JP, et al. Distension of the gallbladder inhibits sphinter of Oddi motility in humans. Gut 1991;32:690–93.
53. Cicala M, Habib FI, Fiocca F, et al. Increased sphincter of Oddi basal pressure in patients affected by gallstone disease: a role for biliary stasis and colicky pain. Gastroenterology 1998;114:G2127.

54. Luman W, Williams AJ, Pryde A, et al. Influence of cholecystectomy on sphincter of Oddi motility. Gut 1997;41:371–74.
55. Hogan WJ, Geenen JE. Biliary dyskinesia. Endoscopy 1988;20(suppl 1):179–83.
56. Acosta JM, Kedesma Cl. Gallstone migration as a cause of acute pancreatitis. New Engl J Med 1974;290:484–87.
57. Branch CD, Bailey OT, Zollinger R. Consequences of instrumental dilatation of the papilla of Vater: experimental study. Arch Surg 1939;38:358–71.
58. Manier JW, Cohen WN, Printer KJ. Dysfunction of the sphincter of Oddi in a postcholecystectomy patient. Am J Gastroenterol 1974;62:148–50.
59. Reymolds BM. Immediate effects of instrumental dilatation of the ampulla of Vater: visual and histologic observations in man. Ann Surg 1966;164:271.
60. Jivegard L, Radberg G, Wahlin T, et al. An experimental study on the role of gallbladder mucosal fluid secretion and intraluminal pressure in cholecystitis. Acta Chir Scand 1986;152:605–10.
61. Yap L, Wycherley AG, Morphett AD, et al. Acalculous biliary pain: cholecystectomy alleviates symptoms in patients with abnormal cholescintigraphy. Gastroenterology 1991;101:786–93.
62. Westlake PJ, Hershfield NB, Kelly JK, et al. Chronic right upper quadrant pain without gallstones: does HIDA scan predict outcome after cholecystectomy? Am J Gastroenterol 1990;85:986–90.
63. Hederstrom E, Forsberg L, Herlin P, et al. Fatty meal provocation monitored by ultrasonography: a method to diagnose ambiguous gallbladder disease. Acta Radiol 1988;29:207–10.
64. Pallotta N, Cicala M, Marcheggiano A, et al. Relationship between histopathology and motor function of the gallbladder in gallstone patients. Gastroenterology 1997;112;4:A519.
65. Portincasa P, Di Ciaula A, Baldassarre G, et al. Gallbladder motor function in gallstone patients: sonographic and in vitro studies on the role of gallstones, smooth muscle function and gallbladder wall inflammation. J Hepatol 1994;21:430–40.
66. Caroli J. Etude des dyskinesie biliares (Thesis). Toulouse,France: Imprimerie du Sud;1945.
67. Whitehead WE, Engal BT, Schuster PM. Irritable bowel syndrome: physiological and psychological differences between diarrhea-predominant and constipation-predominant patients. Dig Dis Sci 1980;25:404–11.
68. Thune A, Thornell E, Svanvik J. Reflex regulation of flow resistance in the feline sphincter of Oddi by hydrostatic pressure in the biliary tract. Gastroenterology 1986;91:1364–69.
69. Rolny P, Funch-Jensen P, Kruse A, et al. Effect of cholecystectomy on the relationship between hydrostatic common bile duct pressure and sphincter of Oddi motility. Endoscopy 1991;23:111–13.
70. Thune A, Jivegard L, Conradi N, et al. Cholecystectomy in the cat damages pericholedochal nerves and impairs reflex regulation of the sphincter of Oddi: a mechanism for postcholecystectomy biliary dyskinesia. Acta Chir Scand 1988;154:191–94.

71. Tanaka M, Ikeda S, Nakayama F. Change in bile duct pressure responses after cholecystectomy: loss of gallbladder as a pressure reservoir. Gastroenterology 1984;87:1154–59.

72. Tanaka M, Ikeda S, Matsumoto S, et al. Manometric diagnosis of sphincter of Oddi spasm as a cause of postcholecystectomy pain and the treatment by endoscopic sphincterotomy. Ann Surg 1985;202:712–19.

73. Mawe G. Advances in the neurophysiology of the gallbladder. In: Holle GE, Wood JD, Editors. Advances in the Innervation of the Gastrointestinal Tract. Munich,Germany:Elsevier Science Publishers;1992:181–93.

74. Mawe GM. Tachykinins as mediators of slow Epsps in guinea-pig, gallbladder ganglia: involment of neurokinin-3 receptors. J Physiol (Lond) 1995;485:513–24.

75. Cervero F. Afferent activity evoked by natural stimulation of the biliary system in the ferret. Pain 1982;13:137–51.

76. Cervero F, Laird JM. From acute to chronic pain:mechanisms and hypothesis. Progress in Brain Research 1996;110:3–15.

77. Desautels SG, Slivka A, Hutson WR, et al. Postcholecystectomy pain syndrome: pathophysiology of abdominal pain in Sphincter of Oddi type III. Gastroenterology 1999;116:900–905.

78. Drossman DA, Thompson WG, Talley NJ, et al. Identification of subgroups of functional bowel disorders. Gastroenterol Internat 1990;3:159–72.

79. Grage TB, Lober PH, Imamoglu K, et al. Stenosis of the sphincter of Oddi: a clinopathologic review of 50 cases. Surgery 1960;48:304–17.

80. Lee SP, Nicholls JF, Park HZ, et al. Biliary sludge as a cause of acute pancreatitis. New Engl J Med 1992;326:589–95.

81. Sharma BC, Agarwall DK, Baijal SS, et al. Effect of endoscopic sphincterotomy on gallbladder bile lithogenicity and motility. Gut 1998;42:288–92.

82. Corazziari E, Biondi M. Dysfunctional disorders of the biliary tract. Sem Gastrointest Dis 1996;7:196–207.

83. Abraham HD, Anderson C, Lee D, et al. Somatization disorder in sphincter of Oddi dysfunction. Psychosomat Med 1997;59:553–55.

84. Rome Group for Epidemiology and Prevention of Cholelithiasis (GREPCO). The epidemiology of gallstone disease in Rome, Italy. Part I. Prevalence data in men. Hepatology 1988;8:904–906.

85. Attili AF, Carulli N, Roda E, et al. Epidemiology of gallstone disease in Italy: prevalence data of the multicenter Italian study on cholelithiasis. Am J Epidemiol 1995;141:158–65.

86. Gracie WA, Kansohoff DF. The natural history of silent gallstones: the innocent gallstone is not a myth. New Engl J Med 1982;307:798–800.

87. Sampliner RE, Bennett PH, Comess LJ, et al. Gallbladder disease in Pima Indians: demonstration of high prevalence and early onset. New Engl J Med 1970;283: 1358–64.

88. Kraagg N, Thijs C, Knipschild P. Dyspepsia—how noisy are gallstones? A met-

analysis of epidemiologic studies of biliary pain, dyspeptic symptoms, and food intolerance. Scand J Gastroenterol 1995;30:411–21.

89. Talley NJ, Silverstein MD, Agreus L, et al. Gastroenterological Association Clinical Practice Economics Committee-AGA technical review: evaluation of dyspepsia. Gastroenterology 1998;114:582–95.

90. Jorgensen T. Abdominal symptoms and gallstone disease: an epidemiological investigation. Hepatology 1989;9:856–60.

91. Donaldson RM Jr. Dyspepsia: the broad etiologic spectrum. Hosp Pract (Off Ed) 1987;22(9A):41–9,53.

92. Rome Group for Epidemiology and Prevention of Cholelithiasis (GREPCO). Prevalence of gallstone disease in an Italian adult female population. Am J Epidemiol 1984;119:796–805.

93. Barbara L, Sama C, Morselli Labate AM, et al. A population study on the prevalence of gallstones disease: the Sirmione study. Hepatology 1987;7:913–17.

94. Zeman RK, Gazza BS. Gallbladder imaging. state of the art. Gastroenterol Clin North Am 1991;20:127–56.

95. Lee SP, Maher K, Nicholls JF, et al. Origin and fate of biliary sludge. Gastroenterology 1988;94:170–76.

96. Wilkinson LS, Levin TS, Smith D, et al. Biliary sludge: can ultrasound reliably detect the presence of crystals in bile? Eur J Gastroenterol Hepatol 1996;8:999–1001.

97. Dill JE, Hill S, Callis J, et al. Combined endoscopic ultrasound and stimulated biliary drainage in cholecystitis and microlithiasis: diagnoses and outcomes. Endoscopy 1995;27:424–27.

98. Dahan P, Andant C, Levy P, et al. Prospective evaluation of endoscopic ultrasonography and microscopic examination of duodenal bile in the diagnosis of cholecystolithiasis in 45 patients with normal conventional ultrasonography. Gut 1996;38:277–81.

99. Juniper K, Burson EN. Biliary tract studies II. The significance of biliary crystals. Gastroenterology 1957;32:175–211.

100. Delchier JC, Beufredt P, Preaux AM, et al. The usefulness of microscopic bile examination in patients with suspected microlithiasis: a prospective evaluation. Hepatology 1986;6:118–22.

101. Buscail L, Escourrou J, Delvaux M, et al. Microscopic examination of bile directly collected during endoscopic cannulation of the papilla: utility in suspected microlithiasis. Dig Dis Sci 1992;37:116–20.

102. Gollish SH, Burnstein MJ, Ilson RG, et al. Nucleation of cholesterol monohydrate crystals from hepatic and gall-bladder bile of patients. Gut 1983;24:831–44.

103. Sahlin S, Ahlberg J, Angelin B, et al. Occurrence of cholesterol monohydrate crystals in gallbladder and hepatic bile in man: influence of bile acid treatment. Eur J Clin Invest 1988;18:386–90.

104. Sarva RP, Shreiner DP, Van Thiel D, et al. Gallbladder function: methods of measuring filling and emptying. J Nucl Med 1985;26:140–44.

105. Shaffer EA. Measurement of gallbladder emptying in response to cholecystokinin: the importance of gallbladder emptying in the pathogenesis of cholesterol

gallstone disease and non-surgical therapy of gallstone disease. J Lithotripsy Stone Dis 1991;3:369–80.

106. Fullarton GM, Meek AC, Gray HW, et al. Gallbladder emptying following cholecystokinin and fatty meal in normal subjects. Hepatogastroenterology 1980;37 (Supp II):45–48.

107. Jazrawi RP, Pazzi P, Petroni ML, et al. Postprandial gallbladder motor function: refilling and turnover of bile in health and in cholelithiasis. Gastroenterology 1995;109:502–91.

108. Sharma BC, Agarwal DK, Dhiman RK, et al. Bile lithogenicity and gallbladder emptying in patients with microlithiasis: effect of bile acid therapy. Gastroenterology 1998;115:124–28.

109. Barr RG, Agnesi JN, Schaub CR. Acalculous gallbladder disease: US evaluation after slow-infusion cholecystokinin stimulation in symptomatic and asymptomatic adults. Radiology 1997;204:105–11.

110. Dunn FH, Christensen ED, Reynolds J, et al. Cholecystokinin cholecystography: controlled evaluation in the diagnosis and management of patients with possible acalculous gallbladder disease. JAMA 1974;228:997–1003.

111. Nathan MH, Newman A, Murray DJ, et al. Cholecystokinin cholecystography: four years' evaluation. Am J Roentgenol Rad Ther Nucl Med 1970:110:240–51.

112. Byrne P, Hunter GJ, Vallon A. Cholecystokinin cholecystography: a three year prospective trial. Clin Radiol 1985;36:499–502.

113. Xu QW, Shaffer EA. Cisapride improved gallbladder contractility and bile lipid composition in an animal model of gallstone disease. Gastroenterology 1993;105: 1184–91.

114. Sylwestrowicz TA, Shaffer EA. Gallbladder function during gallstone dissolution: the effect of bile acid therapy in patients with gallstones. Gastroenterology 1988; 95:740–48.

115. Geenen JE. The efficacy of endoscopic sphincterotomy after cholecystectomy in patients with sphincter of Oddi dysfunction. New Engl J Med 1989;320:82–87.

116. Drossman DA, Li Z, Andruzzi E, et al. US householder survey of functional gastrointestinal disorders: prevalence, sociodemography and health impact. Dig Dis Sci 1993;38:1569–80.

117. Bar-Meir S, Halpern Z, Bardan E, et al. Frequency of papillary dysfunction among cholecystectomized patients. Hepatology 1984;4:328–30.

118. Geenen JE, Hogan WJ, Dodds WJ. Sphincter of Oddi. In: Sivak MV, Editor. Gastroenterological Endoscopy. Philadelphia: Saunders;1987:735.

119. Sherman S, Troiano FP, Hawes RH, et al. Frequency of abnormal sphincter of Oddi manometry compared with the clinical suspicion of sphincter of Oddi dysfunction. Am J Gastroenterol 1991;86:586–90.

120. Okazaki K, Yamamoto Y, Nishimori I, et al. Motility of the sphincter of Oddi and pancreatic main ductal pressure in patients with alcoholic, gallstone-associated, and idiopathic chronic pancreatitis. Am J Gastroenterol 1988;83:820–26.

121. Toouli J, Roberts-Thomson IC, Dent J, et al. Sphincter of Oddi motility disorders in patients with idiopathic recurrent pancreatitis. Brit J Surg 1985;72:859–63.

122. Guelrud M, Mendoza S, Viera L. Idiopathic recurrent pancreatitis and hyper-contractile sphincter of Oddi: treatment with endoscopic sphincterotomy and pancreatic duct dilatation. Gastroenterology 1986;90:1443.

123. Eversman D, Sherman S, Bucksot L, et al. Frequency of abnormal biliary and pancreatic basal sphincter pressure at sphincter of Oddi manometry (SOM) in 593 patients. Gastrointest Endoscopy 1997;45:131A.

124. Steinberg WM. Sphincter of Oddi dysfunction: a clinical controversy. Gastroenterology 1988;95:1409–15.

125. Lin OS, Soetikno RM, Young HS. The utility of liver function test abnormalities concomitant with biliary symptoms in predicting a favourable response to endoscopic sphincterotomy in patients with presumed sphincter of Oddi dysfunction. Am J Gastroenterol 1998;93:1833–36.

126. Steinberg WM, Salvato RF, Toskes PP. The morphine-prostigmin provocative test: is it useful for making clinical decisions? Gastroenterology 1980;78:728–31.

127. Dodds WJ. Biliary tract motility and its relationship to clinical disorders. Am J Roentgenol 1990;155:247–58.

128. Hunt DR, Scott AJ. Changes in bile duct diameter after cholecystectomy: 15 year perioperative study. Gastroenterology 1989;97:1485–88.

129. Venu RP, Geenen JE. Diagnosis and treatment of disease of the papilla. Clin Gastroenterol 1986;15:439–56.

130. Aronchick CA, et al. Bile duct pathology, defined by ERCP and sphincter of Oddi manometry, correlates with sincalide aided ultrasonography of the common bile duct. Gastrointest Endoscopy 1986;32:153.

131. Simeone JF, Mueller PR, Ferrucci JT, et al. Sonography of the bile ducts after a fatty meal: an aid in detection of obstruction. Radiology 1982;143:211–15.

132. Cicala M, Pallotta N, Corazziari E, et al. Fatty meal ultrasonography is not reliable in the diagnosis of sphincter of Oddi dysfunction. Gastroenterology 1994;106: A337.

133. Warshaw AL, Simeone J, Schapiro RH, et al. Objective evaluation of ampullary stenosis with ultrasonography and pancreatic stimulation. Am J Surg 1985;149: 65–72.

134. Cavallini G, Rigo L, Bovo P, et al. Abnormal US response of main pancreatic duct after secretin stimulation in patients with acute pancreatitis of different etiology. J Clin Gastroenterol 1994;18:298–303.

135. Lee RG, Gregg JA, Koroshetz AM, et al. Sphincter of Oddi stenosis: diagnosis using hepatobiliary scintigraphy and endoscopic manometry. Radiology 1985; 156:793–96.

136. Zeman RK, Burrell MI, Dobbins J, et al. Postcholecystectomy syndrome: evaluation using biliary scintigraphy and endoscopic retrograde cholangiography. Radiology 1985;156:787–92.

137. Fullarton GM, Allan A, Hildicht T, et al. Quantitative 99mTc-DISIDA scanning and endoscopic biliary manometry in sphincter of Oddi dysfunction. Gut 1988; 29:1397–1401.

138. Shaffer EA, Hershfield NB, Logan K, et al. Cholescintigraphic detection of functional obstruction of the sphincter of Oddi: effect of papillotomy. Gastroenterology 1986;90:728–33.

139. Cicala M, Scopinaro F, Corazziari E, et al. Quantitative cholescintigraphy in the assessment of choledochoduodenal bile flow. Gastroenterology 1991;100:1106–13.

140. Corazziari E, Cicala M, Habib FI, et al. Hepatoduodenal bile transit in cholecystectomized subjects: relationship with sphincter of Oddi function and diagnostic value. Dig Dis Sci 1994;39:1985–93.

141. Sostre S, Spiegler EJ, Camargo EE, et al. A noninvasive test of sphincter of Oddi dysfunction in postcholecystectomy patients: the scintigraphic score. J Nucl Med 1992;33:1216–22.

142. Corazziari E, Torsoli A. Sphincter of Oddi manometry: recording techniques trace interpretation and reproducibility. Gastrointest Endoscopy Clin North Am 1993;3:81–92.

143. Goff JS. Effect of propofol on human sphincter of Oddi. Dig Dis Sci 1995;40: 2364–67.

144. Nebel OT. Manometric evaluation of the papilla of Vater. Gastrointest Endoscopy 1975;21:126–28.

145. Staritz M, Meyer zum Buschenfelde KH. Investigation of the effect of diazepam and other drugs on the sphincter of Oddi motility. Ital J Gastroenterol 1986; 18:14–16.

146. Sherman S, Gottlieb K, Uzer MF, et al. Effects of meperidine on the pancreatic and biliary sphincter. Gastroint Endoscopy 1996;44:239–42.

147. Funch-Jensen P. Sphincter of Oddi motility. Acta Chir Scand 1990;156(suppl 553):1–35.

148. Funch-Jensen P, Kruise A, Ravnsbaek J. Reproducibility and estimation of minimal recording duration in endoscopic sphincter of Oddi manometry. Ital J Gastroenterol 1986;18:37–38.

149. Corazziari E, Biliotti B, and International Club for the Sphincter of Oddi Study Sphincter of Oddi Manometry. Gastroenterol Internat 1989;2:180–84.

150. Guelrud M, Mendoza S, Rossiter G, et al. Sphincter of Oddi manometry in healthy volunteers. Dig Dis Sci 1990;35:38–46.

151. Toouli J, Roberts-Thomson IC, Dent J, et al. Manometric disorders in patients with suspected sphincter of Oddi dysfunction. Gastroenterology 1985;88: 1243–50.

152. Corazziari E, Habib FI, Biliotti D, et al. Reading error and time variability of sphincter of Oddi (SO) recordings. Ital J Gastroenterol 1985;17:339–41.

153. International Club for the Sphincter of Oddi Study. The San Francisco meeting, 1986. Ital J Gastroenterol 1986;18:290.

154. Thune A , Scicchitano J, Roberts-Thomson I, et al. Reproducibility of endoscopic sphincter of Oddi manometry. Dig Dis Sci 1991;36:1401–1405.

155. Gandolfi L, Corazziari E. The International Workshop on sphincter of Oddi manometry: special report. Gastrointest Endoscopy 1986;32:46–8.

156. Caftan EL, et al. Sphincter of Oddi (SO) manometry a survey of methodology, complications, and clinical application. Gastrointest Endoscopy 1988;34:185.

157. Sherman S, Troiano FP, Hawes RH, et al. Sphincter of Oddi manometry decreased risk of clinical pancreatitis with use of a modified aspirating catheter. Gastrointest Endoscopy 1990;36:462–66.

158. Guelrud M. A technique for preventing pancreatitis during sphincter of Oddi manometry using the standard catheter. Gastrointest Endoscopy 1991;37:103–104.

159. De Masi E, Corazziari E, Habib FI, et al. Manometric study of the sphincter of Oddi in patients with and without common bile duct stones. Gut 1984;25:275–78.

160. Bar-Meir S, Geenen JE, Hogan WJ, et al. Biliary and pancreatic duct pressure measured by ERCP manometry in patients with suspected papillary stenosis. Dig Dis Sci 1979;24:209–13.

161. Meshkinpour H, Mollot M, Eckerling GB, et al. Bile duct dyskinesia: clinical and manometric study. Gastroenterology 1984;87:759–62.

162. Hogan WJ, Geenen JE, Dodds WJ, et al. Paradoxical motor response to cholecystokinin (CCK-OP) in patients with suspected sphincter of Oddi dysfunction. Gastroenterology 1982;82:1085.

163. Rolny P, Arleback A, Funch-Jensen P, et al. Paradoxical response of sphincter of Oddi to IV injection of cholecystokinin or ceruletide: manometric findings and results of treatment in biliary dyskinesia. Gut 1986;27:1507–11.

164. Hogan WJ, Geenen JE, Venu R, et al. Abnormally rapid phasic contractions of the human sphincter of Oddi (tachyoddia). Gastroenterology 1983;84:1189.

165. Staritz M. Pharmacology of the Sphincter of Oddi. Endoscopy 1988;20(suppl 1): 171–74.

166. Guelrud M, Mendoza S, Rossiter G, et al. Effect of nifedipine on sphincter of Oddi motor activity: studies in healthy volunteers and patients with biliary dyskinesia. Gastroenterology 1988;95:1050–55.

167. Grace PA, Poston GJ, Williamson RC. Biliary motility. Gut 1990;31:571–82.

168. Sand J, Nordback I, Koskinen M, et al. Nifedipine for suspected type II sphincter of Oddi dyskinesia. Am J Gastroenterol 1993;88:530–35.

169. Kasugai T. Recent advance in the endoscopic cholangiopancreatography. Digestion 1976;13:76–81.

170. Bar-Meir S, Halpern Z, Bardan E. Nitrate therapy in a patient with papillary dysfunction. Gastroenterology 1983;78:94–95.

171. Staritz M, Poralla T, Ewe K, et al. Effect of glyceryl trinitrate on the sphincter of Oddi motility and baseline pressure. Gut 1985;26:194–97.

172. Pasricha PJ, Miskovsky EP, Kalloo AN, et al. Intrasphincteric injection of botulinum toxin for suspected sphincter of Oddi dysfunction. Gut 1994;35:1319–21.

173. Sand J, Nordback I, Arvola P, et al. Effects of botulinum toxin A on the sphincter of Oddi: an in vivo and in vitro study. Gut 1998;42:507–10.

174. Muehldorfer SM, Hahn EG, Ell C. Botulinum toxin injection as a diagnostic tool for verification of sphincter of Oddi dysfunction causing recurrent pancreatitis. Endoscopy 1997;29:120–24.

175. Guelrud M, Siegel JH. Hypertensive pancreatic duct sphincter as a cause of pancreatitis: successful treatment with hydrostatic balloon dilatation. Dig Dis Sci 1984;29:225–31.

176. Bader M, Geenen JE, Hogan WJ. Endoscopic balloon dilatation of the sphincter of Oddi in patients with suspected biliary dyskinesia: results of a prospective randomized trial. Gastrointest Endoscopy 1986;32:158.

177. Toouli J, Roberts-Thomson I, Kellow J, et al. Prospective randomized trial of endoscopic sphincterotomy for treatment of sphincter of Oddi dysfunction. J Gastroenterol Hepatol 1996;11(suppl):A115.

178. Lehman GY, Sherman S. Sphincter of Oddi dysfunction. Internat J Pancreatol 1996;20:11–25.

179. Freeman ML, Nelson DB, Sherman S, et al. Complications of endoscopic biliary sphincterotomy. New Engl J Med 1996;335: 909–18.

180. Tarnasky PR, Palesch YY, Cunningham TC, et al. Pancreatic stenting prevents pancreatitis after biliary sphincterotomy in patients with sphincter of Oddi dysfunction. Gastroenterology 1998;115:1518–24.

181. Hogan WJ. Stenting the pancreas: Is this the solution to post-ERCP pancreatitis? Gastroenterology 1998;115:1591–94.

182. Watanapa P, Williamson RCN. Pancreatic sphincterotomy and sphincteroplasty. Gut 1992;33:865–67.

183. Toouli J, Di Francesco V, Saccone G, et al. Division of the sphincter of Oddi for treatment of dysfunction associated with recurrent pancreatitis. Brit J Surg 1996; 83:1205–10.

184. Moody FG, Becker JM, Potts JR. Transduodenal sphincteroplasty and transampullar septectomy for postcholecystectomy pain. Ann Surg 1983;197:627–36.

185. Bartlett MK, Nardi GL. Treatment of recurrent pancreatitis by transduodenal sphincterotomy and exploration of the pancreatic duct. New Engl J Med 1960; 262:643–48.

186. Manoukian AV, Schmalz MJ, Geenen JE, et al. The incidence of post-sphincterotomy stenosis in group II patients with sphincter of Oddi dysfunction. Gastrointest Endoscopy 1993;39:496–98.

187. Kozarek RA. Balloon dilatation of the sphincter of Oddi. Endoscopy 1988;20: 207–10.

188. Guelrud M, Plaz J, Mendoza S, et al. Endoscopic treatment in type II pancreatic sphincter dysfunction. Gastrointest Endoscopy 1995;41:398.

189. Soffer EE, Johlin FC. Intestinal dysmotility in patients with sphincter of Oddi dysfunction: a reason for failed response to sphincterotomy. Dig Dis Sci 1994;39: 1942–46.

190. Sherman S, Hawes RH, Savides TJ, et al. Stent-induced pancreatic ductal and parenchymal changes: correlation of endoscopic ultrasound with ERCP. Gastrointest Endoscopy 1996;44:276–82.

191. Goff JS. Common bile duct sphincter of Oddi stenting in patients with suspected sphincter dysfunction. Am J Gastroenterol 1995;90:586–89.

Chapter 9

F. Functional
Disorders of the
Anus and Rectum

William E. Whitehead, Chair,
Arnold Wald, Co-Chair, *with*
Nicholas E. Diamant,
Paul Enck,
John H. Pemberton,
and Satish S. C. Rao

Introduction

This chapter will address anorectal symptoms, the etiology of which is currently unknown or is believed to be related to the abnormal functioning of normally innervated and structurally intact muscles, or to psychological causes. This chapter will not deal with anorectal disorders that have a well-established structural basis (e.g., fecal incontinence secondary to obstetrical injury), except where it is necessary to distinguish them from functional anorectal disorders that may produce similar symptoms.

We recognize that the distinction between functional and organic etiologies is arbitrary and may be difficult to make in individual patients for the following reasons. Organic lesions and behavioral adaptations to them may interact. For example, repeated straining to defecate may contribute to rectal prolapse, rectocele, or pudendal nerve injury (organic disorders); and reciprocally, rectal prolapse or rectocele may lead to more straining. Second, the evaluation of the patient may reveal multiple independent findings, some structural and some functional, any of which could contribute to the symptoms but no one of which by itself can explain the symptoms.

We acknowledge also that future research may reveal structural causes for some symptoms currently thought to be functional (e.g., in some patients lactose malabsorption is a cause of abdominal symptoms formerly ascribed to irritable bowel syndrome), or may show that the presumed structural abnormalities are not clinically significant because they are common in asymptomatic individuals (e.g., rectocele is found in up to 80% of healthy females and 13% of healthy males, and internal intussuception is observed in up to 50% of both male and female healthy controls) [1–3].

The functional anorectal disorders are defined primarily on the basis of symptoms [4]. It is recognized that the retrospective reports of symptoms may be unreliable [5,6]. However, the reliability of symptom reports can be improved by clinical judgment based on interviewing the patient, and by symptom diaries. In some instances (e.g., functional fecal incontinence and pelvic floor dyssynergia), supportive evidence from physiological testing and the physical examination may be required, in addition to symptom reports. For each diagnosis there must be no evidence of other structural or metabolic abnormalities to explain the symptoms.

We thank the following reviewers for their critique of the manuscript and their suggestions: Enrico Corazziari, M.D.; Michael Crowell, Ph.D.; James W. Fleshman, M.D.; Hans C. Kuijpers, M.D.; J.E. Lennard-Jones, M.D.; Vera Loening-Baucke, M.D.; Nick Read, M.D.; Robert Sandler, M.D., M.P.H.; Marvin M. Schuster, M.D.; Steven D. Wexner, M.D.

The classification scheme for all functional gastrointestinal disorders is given in Table 1. In this chapter we will define and examine the prevalence of the functional anorectal disorders listed in section F of Table 1. We will summarize what is known about the physiological mechanism of symptoms and the role of psychological traits and stress in their etiology, and we will offer recommendations for diagnostic evaluation. Lastly, we will review and evaluate the efficacy of treatments which have been proposed for these disorders. Readers are also referred to the Working Team Report and practice guidelines on anorectal disorders published by the American Gastroenterological Association (AGA) [7] for a more detailed review of some aspects.

This review and the associated recommendations are based on an authoritative review of the world literature by experts. The authors sought the advice of expert reviewers, listed in the footnote above. The Diagnostic Criteria include minimum duration of symptoms required for diagnosis; these duration criteria were selected arbitrarily so as to avoid including self-limiting conditions while avoiding unnecessary delays in evaluation.

Table 1. Functional Gastrointestinal Disorders

A. Esophageal Disorders

A1. Globus
A2. Rumination syndrome
A3. Functional Chest Pain of Presumed Esophageal Origin

A4. Functional Heartburn
A5. Functional Dysphagia
A6. Unspecified Functional Esophageal Disorder

B. Gastroduodenal Disorders

B1. Functional Dyspepsia
B1a. Ulcer-like Dyspepsia
B1b. Dysmotility-like Dyspepsia
B1c. Unspecified (nonspecific) Dyspepsia

B2. Aerophagia
B3. Functional Vomiting

C. Bowel Disorders

C1. Irritable Bowel Syndrome
C2. Functional Abdominal Bloating
C3. Functional Constipation

C4. Functional Diarrhea
C5. Unspecified Functional Bowel Disorder

D. Functional Abdominal Pain

D1. Functional Abdominal Pain Syndrome
D2. Unspecified Functional Abdominal Pain

E. Functional Disorders of the Biliary Tract and the Pancreas

E1. Gallbladder Dysfunction
E2. Sphincter of Oddi Dysfunction

F. Anorectal Disorders

F1. Functional Fecal Incontinence
F2. Functional Anorectal Pain
F2a. Levator Ani Syndrome
F2b. Proctalgia Fugax
F3. Pelvic Floor Dyssynergia

G. Functional Pediatric Disorders

G1. Vomiting
G1a. Infant regurgitation
G1b. Infant rumination syndrome
G1c. Cyclic vomiting syndrome
G2. Abdominal pain
G2a. Functional dyspepsia
G2a1. Ulcer-like dyspepsia
G2a2. Dysmotility-like dyspepsia
G2a3. Unspecified (nonspecific) dyspepsia

G2b. Irritable bowel syndrome
G2c. Functional abdominal pain
G2d. Abdominal migraine
G2e. Aerophagia
G3. Functional diarrhea
G4. Disorders of defecation
G4a. Infant dyschezia
G4b. Functional constipation
G4c. Functional fecal retention
G4d. Functional non-retentive fecal soiling

FI: Functional Fecal Incontinence

— Definition

Functional fecal incontinence is defined as recurrent uncontrolled passage of fecal material for at least one month in an individual who has no evidence of neurologic or structural etiologies. Clear mucus secretion must be excluded by careful questioning. Uncontrolled passage of flatus without loss of fecal material will not be discussed in this chapter, but may represent an early sign of anal sphincter dysfunction.

The age at which fecal soiling is considered inappropriate (the age of toilet training) varies among cultures from less than one year in Switzerland [8] to four years in Sweden [9–10]. Incontinence should not be considered a medical problem earlier than age four.

Functional fecal incontinence is distinct from fecal incontinence due to neurological injury, seepage from prolapsed rectal mucosa, poor hygiene, and willful soiling. However, neurogenic and anatomic causes of fecal incontinence (e.g., central or peripheral nerve injury) may coexist and interact with functional causes of incontinence (e.g., constipation or diarrhea), as outlined below. When this is suspected, an evaluation directed at identifying all contributing causes of incontinence and assessing which are most amenable to treatment is appropriate. Such an assessment is described in this chapter.

Functional fecal incontinence appears to be more common in children than in adults. However, the childhood version of functional fecal incontinence is dealt with in a separate working team report [11].

— Epidemiology

Published epidemiologic studies have not distinguished between functional fecal incontinence and fecal incontinence due to structural or neurological causes. Nelson and colleagues [12] estimated the prevalence of fecal incontinence in U.S. adults to be 2.2%, based on a random telephone sampling of 2,570 households comprising 6,959 individuals. Incontinence for solid stool was reported by 0.8%, incontinence for liquid stool by 1.2%, and incontinence for flatus by 1.3%. Higher estimates were obtained by Drossman and colleagues [13] in a postal survey of a stratified sample of 5,430 U.S. adults (U.S. Householder Survey): they reported a prevalence of 6.9% for frequent staining of underwear and 0.7% for frequent incontinence of at least two teaspoons of fecal matter (solid and liquid not distinguished).

Similar prevalence estimates have been reported for Europe. In a representative sample of 1,010 French citizens aged 45 and older, 6% reported fecal incontinence more than once per month [14], and in a German study, 5% of respondents reported occasional incontinence, but only 1.5% reported severe incontinence [15]. Differences in prevalence estimates may be related to the definition of incontinence; in the U.S. Householder Survey [13], the incidence of fecal soiling ("a small amount—it stains underwear") in people over age 60 was 9.5%, although the incidence of gross incontinence ("two teaspoons or more") was only 1.3% in this age group. The definition of what constituted incontinence for solids was not given in the French study [14].

Fecal incontinence is more common at the two ends of the life span. It occurs in about 1.5% of children aged seven years [9,16], and in 96% of these children, fecal incontinence consists of functional fecal incontinence associated with fecal impaction [17–18]. The incidence of functional fecal incontinence in children declines with age [9], but the incidence of fecal incontinence from all causes increases again toward the end of the life span [12,13], especially in association with dementia and with being restricted to a wheelchair. In the U.S.

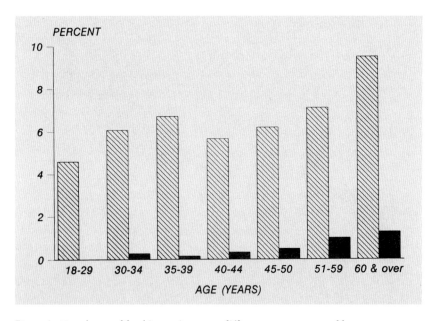

Figure 1. Prevalence of fecal incontinence at different ages as reported by 5,430 community-dwelling US adults. Striped bars show the percent who reported that they often leaked a small amount of stool (stained underwear) in the last 3 months. Solid bars show the percent who reported that they often leaked 2 teaspoons or more of stool in the last 3 months. (Adapted from Drossman D, et al. Dig Dis Sci 1993;38;1569.)

Householder Survey [13], the prevalence of gross fecal incontinence was so low as to be unmeasurable in respondents aged 18 to 29 years but increased steadily up to 1.3% in respondents aged 60 and older (fig. 1). The incidence of fecal incontinence from all causes in the United States and British nursing home populations is estimated to be 30% [19,20] to 39% [21].

In children, functional fecal incontinence occurs four times more frequently in boys than in girls [17]. Among adults with fecal incontinence, women outnumber men in most but not all studies [12–15,22,23].

A risk factor for functional fecal incontinence is retention of stool in the rectum both in fecally incontinent children [17,18] and in incontinent elderly patients [24–26]. A second risk factor is diarrhea. The irritable bowel syndrome (IBS) is also a recognized risk factor; an estimated 23% of patients with irritable bowel syndrome [27] report at least occasional fecal soiling. In addition, 12% of long distance runners [28] with diarrhea experience fecal incontinence. Among the elderly, cognitive, and mobility impairment as well as diarrhea are significant risk factors for functional fecal incontinence [29].

— Diagnostic Criteria

Recurrent uncontrolled passage of fecal material for at least one month, in an individual with a developmental age of at least 4 years, associated with:

(1) Fecal impaction; *or*
(2) Diarrhea; *or*
(3) Nonstructural anal sphincter dysfunction.

It is recognized that functional causes of fecal incontinence such as constipation and diarrhea may overlap with structural abnormalities (e.g., sphincter muscle injury, or afferent or efferent nerve injury). Further investigation (see below) may identify such additional contributing causes of fecal incontinence.

— Rationale for Changes in Diagnostic Criteria

Previously [30], the lower age limit for inferring that the uncontrolled passage of stool constitutes fecal incontinence was three years. This has been increased to four years to bring these Diagnostic Criteria into line with the Diagnostic and Statistical Manual of the American Psychiatric Association [31].

Previously [30], functional fecal incontinence was limited to overflow associated with constipation. However, approximately 20% of patients with diarrhea-predominant irritable bowel syndrome [27], and approximately 12% of people with other types of diarrhea [28], develop fecal incontinence even though they have no evidence of neurological or anatomical defects. Because they satisfied the criteria for functional fecal incontinence except for the absence of constipation, they have been included in the revised criteria.

Previously [30], an elevated threshold for perception of rectal distension was included as a diagnostic criterion. Because elevated sensory thresholds are associated with organic causes of fecal incontinence including spinal cord injury, stroke, and diabetic peripheral neuropathy, this finding was felt to be too nonspecific to serve as a diagnostic criterion for functional fecal incontinence. Consequently, it has been dropped.

Unlike the previous Working Team Report [30], this update explicitly acknowledges that functional causes of fecal incontinence such as constipation and diarrhea may coexist with neurological or anatomical defects. In these cases, the coexistence of organic causes of fecal incontinence with constipation or diarrhea should be recognized because this will affect treatment decisions.

— Clinical Evaluation

The diagnosis of functional fecal incontinence can often be made by history and physical examination. The principal facts to be established are that soiling is associated with altered bowel habits (e.g., constipation or diarrhea) and that the strength of voluntary contraction of the external anal sphincter is adequate. In addition, four alternative causes of soiling must be excluded:

(1) rectal prolapse, in which rectal mucosa extends out of the anus and secretes mucus onto the underclothes (this diagnosis requires physical exam);
(2) mental incompetence due to sedative drug side effects, mental retardation, dementia, or psychosis;
(3) impaired mobility or dexterity making it difficult to reach the toilet; and
(4) willful soiling as a way of soliciting attention, or as an antisocial act.

History

Historical points include the following: the frequency and consistency of bowel movements; the longest period between bowel movements; the frequency, amount and consistency of soiling; and whether incontinence occurs without awareness or is preceded by an urge to defecate. Patients with constipation-related functional fecal incontinence may report occasional passage of large, hard stools, but their incontinence more typically consists in the leakage of small amounts of liquid or pasty stool without awareness. Periods of more than three days between stools and the occurrence of hard or scybalous stools are suggestive of constipation, although more frequent defecation does not exclude significant fecal retention. Inquiry should be made into the surgical and obstetrical history to identify patients who may have anatomical defects as a cause of fecal incontinence. Finally, it should be established whether the patient is retarded or has organic brain syndrome, and whether he or she appears to be soiling to obtain attention or to manipulate parents or care providers; none of these etiologies is consistent with functional fecal incontinence.

Physical Examination

The initial examination should be done without prior enema or laxatives. A characteristic finding in constipation-related fecal incontinence is a large mass of stool in the rectum on digital examination and/or in the colon on abdominal palpation. If the history is suggestive of fecal impaction and if the rectum is empty, physical examination should be supplemented by an abdominal radiograph to assess fecal loading of the large bowel [32]. If the patient is not able to contract the external anal sphincter on command, or if the external anal sphincter gapes open on parting of the buttocks or on traction applied to the anal canal, neurological or anatomical injuries should be suspected. An absent anal wink reflex to a gentle stroking of the perianal region or to perianal pinprick is sometimes observed in patients with a large fecal impaction, but persistence of this finding after disimpaction suggests nerve impairment. The presence of a rectal prolapse can be evaluated by asking the patient to strain as if defecating while sitting on a commode chair.

One can also check for pelvic floor dyssynergia (discussed later in this chapter) during the digital examination by asking the patient to strain as if to defecate. Pelvic floor dyssynergia is suggested by paradoxical contraction of the external anal sphincter and/or the puborectalis, or by poor descent of the perineum during straining. Abnormal findings should be confirmed by objective testing.

In most cases, this brief evaluation will identify patients who have constipation-related or diarrhea-related functional fecal incontinence. If the history and physical examination do not support this diagnosis, or if the patient fails to respond to treatment, further examination by abdominal radiographs, by proctoscopy, and with manometric and electromyographic (EMG) probes may be required.

Proctoscopy

Examination with a rigid anoscope is recommended over flexible sigmoidoscopy to determine whether fissures, inflammation, or mechanical obstruction are contributing causes of fecal soiling.

Manometric and Electromyographic Evaluation

Figure 2 shows the anatomy of the anal canal and rectum and summarizes the physiologic mechanisms responsible for continence and defecation. The manometric evaluation assesses these mechanisms by determining the following:

(1) the threshold volume of rectal distension required to produce each of three sensations: the first sensation of distension, a sustained feeling of urgency to defecate, and the pain threshold or maximum tolerable volume;

(2) rectal compliance as determined by the pressure-volume ratio during stepwise distension;

(3) the amplitude and duration of voluntary contractions of the external anal sphincter;

(4) the presence of an internal anal sphincter inhibitory reflex; and

(5) whether attempts to defecate (straining) are accompanied by increases in intra-abdominal pressure and relaxation of the pelvic floor muscles, which is normal, or by paradoxical contractions of the pelvic floor muscles, which may be abnormal. To accomplish this, a balloon should be positioned in the rectum, and contraction and relaxation of the muscles surrounding the anal canal in response to rectal distension should be monitored by perfused catheters, solid-state pressure transducers, EMG electrodes in the anal canal, or balloons positioned in the anal canal [33–35]. Electromyographic electrodes should not be used alone, but they may provide helpful additional data if used in conjunction with pressure measurements.

Because manometric test protocols are poorly standardized, a recommended test protocol is given below. For additional technical details see the AGA technical review [7].

The threshold for first sensation and the threshold and amplitude of the internal anal sphincter inhibitory reflex are obtained by transiently distending the rectal balloon with varying volumes of air. The normal ranges for first sensation are based on rapid distensions. The order in which the distensions are introduced and the interval between distensions influence the perceptual threshold and the amplitude of the internal anal sphincter inhibitory reflex [36], so it is important

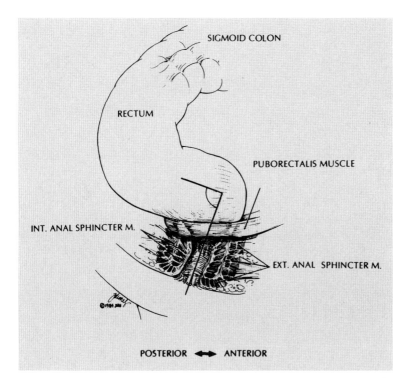

Figure 2. Anatomy of the anal canal and rectum showing the physiologic mechanisms important to continence and defecation. (Reproduced with permission from Whitehead WE, Schuster MM. Gastrointestinal disorders: behavioral and physiological basis for treatment. Orlando, Florida: Academic Press, 1985.)

to standardize the order of presentation. Ideally, rectal distensions should be produced by a pump that provides standardized rates of inflation because rate of inflation influences the perceptual threshold [37]. However, an adequate diagnostic study can be obtained with a hand-held syringe. The range of normal values is highly dependent on the method employed and should be standardized for each laboratory.

The threshold for constant urge to defecate and the maximum tolerable volume are obtained by distending the rectal balloon in a stepwise fashion by adding 50 ml of air (or a smaller fixed volume) every 60 seconds. The patient should be asked about the sense of urgency to defecate at the end of the 60-second trial rather than the beginning because (a) balloon inflation may elicit a reflex contraction of the rectum [38], and (b) approximately 4 seconds is required for the rectum to stretch to accommodate new volumes [39]. The range of normal values must be established for each laboratory. Thresholds may vary with balloon size and configuration. Some authors advocate having the patient contract the sphincter in response to rectal distension and measuring the latency from rectal distension to contraction; this latency may be prolonged in some patients with fecal incontinence [40]. The reader is referred to the AGA technical review on anorectal assessment [7] for a more detailed discussion of the validity and reliability of these measures.

The strength of the external anal sphincter contraction can be tested by instructing the patient to squeeze as strongly as possible as if trying to withhold defecation for 60 seconds. This evaluates both the strength of contraction and the latency for fatigue. When measured by perfused catheter, maximum squeeze pressures decrease with age and are lower in women than men [41]. Normal values for the time-to-fatigue below functionally useful values of anal canal pressure are poorly defined but have been reported to average 45 seconds in normal subjects, and are lower in fecally incontinent patients [42]. This test also provides an indication of whether the patient inappropriately contracts the abdominus rectus muscles, thereby increasing intra-abdominal pressure when trying to withhold a bowel movement.

The ability to increase intra-abdominal pressure during attempts to defecate can be evaluated by monitoring pressure in the rectum, and the ability to relax the pelvic floor can be evaluated by monitoring pressure in the anal canal or EMG activity in the striated pelvic floor muscles (measured with surface electrodes) during straining to defecate a balloon [43]. Figure 3 shows rectal and anal canal pressures during attempts to defecate. Ideally, this test should be done with the patient sitting on a commode chair behind a privacy screen. Sustained contraction of the anal sphincter or failure to relax are abnormal findings, in the opinion of the authors. It is possible that partial (i.e., incomplete) relaxation will also be found to be of pathophysiologic significance [44].

Anorectal manometry has been assessed and found to provide useful information in the evaluation of anorectal disorders [7, 45–46].

Anal Endosonography

Anal endosonography now allows the imaging of both the internal and external anal sphincter and can identify structural defects in either muscle. The procedure is rapid, and less invasive than pelvic CT, MRI, or electromyography. However, the interpretation is very operator dependent. A high frequency (10 MHz) probe provides a better image of the anal canal than a 7.5 MHz probe, but at the expense of a somewhat lower focal range.

Endosonography has been shown to be comparable in sensitivity to EMG mapping of the external anal sphincter [47–50]. In vitro and in vivo dissection studies have confirmed a close correlation between endosonographic images and anatomical structures [51–53].

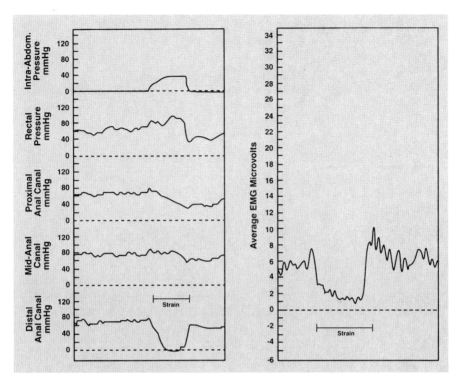

Figure 3. The left panel shows normal anal canal pressure in response to straining to defecate in a patient with colonic inertia type constipation. Top channel shows pressure in a 10-ml air-filled rectal balloon used to detect increases in intra-abdominal pressure during straining. The next four channels show pressures in the anal canal. In the most distal channel, which is in the high pressure zone of the anal canal, straining is associated with a decrease in anal canal pressure, which is the normal response. The right panel, taken from the same patient, shows the averaged EMG recorded from a perineometer type electrode in the anal canal; this patient shows normal reflex inhibition of pelvic floor EMG during straining.

The endosonographic probe is covered by a hard plastic cone which is inserted into the rectum and then slowly withdrawn to image the anal canal along its whole length. The internal anal sphincter muscle is seen as a dark homogeneous ring whereas the external anal sphincter appears with mixed echogenicity, its outer border not clearly distinguishable from perianal tissue. Damage to both muscles appears as an interruption of this specific texture. However, there is more anatomical variation in the external anal sphincter, especially anteriorly. This is clinically important if obstetric damage is not to be over-diagnosed. In women, vaginal as well as anal placement of the probe may be used [54].

Anal endosonography has been used to assess internal and external anal sphincter defects due to trauma (anal stretch, sexual abuse, or delivery) [55,56], and surgery (lateral sphincterotomy) [57], but also with disorders such as progressive systemic sclerosis [58], myotonic dystrophy, and proctalgia fugax [59]. New sphincter defects have been shown to occur in 35% of primiparous women following vaginal deliveries [60]; within the first six months after delivery, ten of 49 women with sphincter defects developed fecal incontinence compared to only one of 78 without sphincter defects.

Vector manometry, which involves recording radial pressures with a multi-lumen catheter, has been advocated by some as a technique for identifying sphincter defects. However, anal endosonography identifies anatomical defects more accurately than vector manometry [61–64]. At present, anal endosonography is superior to conventional MRI techniques with respect to image resolution and defect identification [63], but this may change with the introduction of endo-anal MRI coils [65].

Endo-anal ultrasound provides the best information on structural abnormalities of the anal sphincter muscles. It should be used to exclude suspected structural causes of incontinence.

Neurophysiologic Tests

Additional neurophysiological tests are often performed in patients with fecal incontinence for the purpose of (1) ruling out a specific disease process or (2) better defining the pathophysiological mechanism of the incontinence. The most commonly employed tests are discussed below.

Neurophysiological studies that have been used to evaluate the integrity of the pudendal nerve in patients with fecal incontinence include pudendal nerve terminal motor latencies [66], concentric needle EMG recordings from single motor units in the external anal sphincter or puborectalis muscle [67–71], and surface recordings of EMG activity from the external anal sphincter, which are usually made from electrodes in the anal canal [72,73].

Pudendal Nerve Terminal Motor Latency (PNTML)

PNTML is recorded by stimulating the pudendal nerve transrectally with a glove-mounted electrode and measuring the latency to onset of the anal sphincter EMG response, which is recorded from a second pair of electrodes at the base of the investigator's finger [66,74]. Prolonged conduction time indicates damage to this branch of the pudendal nerve, which may occur as the result of stretch from perineal descent or other trauma. This technique requires some experience and the PNTML can be difficult to assess on both sides; moreover, its clinical value has been questioned in recent studies [68,75,76].

Alternative approaches for assessing the integrity of the motor pathways to the external anal sphincter involve spinal [77] or cortical stimulation with electrical or magnetoelectrical stimulation techniques [78–80]. However, these techniques have so far not been shown to correlate with clinical findings and are regarded as research tools only. Likewise, the recording of cortical evoked potentials from electrical or mechanical stimulation of the rectum [81–83] has been proposed as a method for assessing the sensory innervation of the pelvic floor but has not yet been shown to have clinical value in fecal incontinence [83].

Electromyography

Needle EMG has been used to identify gaps in the external anal sphincter muscle and to detect abnormal spike potentials indicative of pudendal nerve injuries. This has been found to be useful in assessing external anal sphincter damage, which may have occurred as a result of trauma (obstetric, surgical, or other) and in patients who have developmental abnormalities of the anorectum such as congenital imperforate anus. Mapping of the sphincter by needle EMG agrees well with anal ultrasound [47,68] in identifying the area of sphincter injury, but when both are compared with surgical or histological evidence, ultrasound appears to be more sensitive [51]. Thus, ultrasound is less painful and better tolerated than needle EMG for detecting areas of sphincter muscle injury, and it is more accurate because it is less subject to sampling error and can visualize the entire length of the anal canal [47,49].

Surface EMG recordings may be made from metal electrodes mounted on plastic plugs and placed in the lumen of the anal canal, or from perianal skin surface electrodes [72,73]. Intraluminal electrodes are believed to be more accurate because they are closer to the external anal sphincter muscle and less likely to pick up gluteal or other muscles. Of the different types of intraluminal electrodes, longitudinally oriented metal plates (oriented along the long axis of the anal canal) perform better than concentric ring electrodes because they are less likely to lose contact with the muscle. Surface EMG recordings are less invasive than needle EMG recordings, and they are better tolerated by patients. They cannot "map" areas of muscle injury, but may be used to assess the strength of muscle contraction and the occurrence of inappropriate contraction during attempted defecation. Surface EMG is especially useful as a biofeedback signal for pelvic floor retraining to strengthen the external anal sphincter in patients with fecal incontinence or to decrease inappropriate sphincter contractions in pelvic floor dyssynergia.

In summary, recording of PNTML is currently of unproved clinical value. For evaluation of the presence and extent of sphincter muscle trauma, anal endosonography is at least as accurate and is better tolerated by patients than needle EMG. Surface EMG appears to have a role in evaluation of external anal sphincter function and in biofeedback training.

— Physiologic Features

Fecal Impaction

In geriatric patients, constipation associated with a fecaloma is frequently accompanied by functional fecal incontinence [24,25], but the proportion of the incontinent elderly with functional as opposed to structural etiologies for their incontinence is not known.

Impaired Rectal Sensation

Impaired perception of rectal distension has been well documented in both children and adults with functional fecal incontinence [24,84,85]. Impairments in sensory perception are not limited to the rectum: investigators in two laboratories have shown that incontinent patients have decreased ability to detect electrical stimulation of the anal canal as well as decreased ability to sense rectal distension [86,87].

It is often assumed that these changes in sensory threshold are a consequence of fecal impaction, which may alter the tone and viscoelastic properties of the bowel wall. Fecal impaction may also alter afferent nerve pathways [86]. Following effective treatment of constipation, some but not all pediatric patients show improved rectal sensitivity [85,88]. However, adults have not been studied.

Decreased anorectal sensitivity may contribute to incontinence by causing the threshold for reflex inhibition of the internal anal sphincter to occur before the patient perceives the presence of stool in the rectum [40,89–91]. Decreased rectal sensitivity may also exacerbate constipation by decreasing the frequency and intensity of the urge (and hence the motivation) to defecate.

Internal Anal Sphincter Dysfunction

Two types of internal anal sphincter dysfunction have been described in patients with functional fecal incontinence: (1) decreased resting pressure in the internal anal sphincter [92,93], and (2) increased frequency of spontaneous internal anal sphincter relaxation (sampling reflex) [37, 94,95].

Read's group made observations that suggest that decreased resting pressure in the internal anal sphincter is normally not a contributing factor to fecal incontinence in constipated elderly patients [24,25]. When they compared incontinent elderly patients with a fecal impaction at the time they were tested to age-matched healthy control subjects, they saw no differences in basal anal canal pressures. However, the incontinent patients had a decreased ability to sense rectal distension.

An increased frequency of spontaneous relaxation of the internal anal sphincter (sampling reflex) may be more important to the etiology of fecal incontinence than decreased resting pressure [37,95]. Farouk and colleagues [95] described electromechanical dissociation in patients with fecal incontinence, and others report absent activity as well as reduced frequency of slow wave activity [96]. Speakman and colleagues [97] documented reduced sensitivity to noradrenaline and alterations of α-adrenoceptors.

— Psychologic Features

Two research groups [98,99] reported that adult patients with fecal incontinence showed high levels of psychological distress on the SCL-90R [100], and impaired quality of life. It is believed that these findings reflect primarily the consequences of having fecal incontinence rather than being causes of incontinence. Heymen and colleagues [101] found normal Minnesota Multiphasic Personality Inventory (MMPI) profiles in fecally incontinent patients. Patients with functional fecal incontinence have not been compared to those with organic causes of fecal incontinence, nor have patients with diarrhea-associated incontinence been compared to those with constipation-associated incontinence. Psychological symptoms could differ in these subgroups.

— Approach to Treatment

Fecal Impaction

A habit training protocol for functional fecal incontinence associated with fecal impaction was developed for children [18,102]. This begins with an initial catharsis to empty the rectum and distal bowel, and the patient is then required to sit on the toilet for 10 to 15 minutes immediately after a specific meal each day (the choice being determined by prior bowel habits and the family pattern of activity). In one clinic [18], children with functional fecal incontinence received enemas contingent on the absence of a bowel movement for 48 hours, which provided an incentive for them to learn to self-initiate bowel movements as well as preventing fecal impaction. In other programs, patients receive various laxatives routinely for the first several weeks of habit training. Although milk of magnesia, lactulose, or other laxatives or stool softeners may be combined with habit training, laxatives should not be the sole treatment; the awareness that fecal impaction causes fecal incontinence and the sense of self-control that should result from successful treatment with habit training are important to long-term maintenance. In children, habit training resulted in complete continence for approximately 60% of patients and in substantial reductions in the frequency of soiling for another 23%, and results were maintained at follow-up an average of three years later [18]. Patients have usually been offered habit training as a treatment independently of whether their constipation and functional fecal incontinence were associated with colonic inertia or pelvic floor dyssynergia.

Similar habit training protocols have been used successfully in adults and elderly patients [103]. However, for the elderly, Tobin and Brockelhurst [104] recommended a simpler regimen consisting of a daily osmotic laxative (lactulose 10 ml twice daily) plus a weekly enema; they found this regimen to be effective in more than 90% of patients, including those with dementia.

Biofeedback for Pelvic Floor Dyssynergia

Recent studies (see Category F3: Pelvic Floor Dyssynergia) suggest that up to half of patients with functional fecal incontinence have difficulty relaxing the pelvic floor muscles during defecation (pelvic floor dyssynergia) as a contributing cause of constipation and might benefit from specific biofeedback training to relax the pelvic floor. In a number of uncontrolled studies, biofeedback treatment resulted in sustained improvement of constipation and defecation difficulties in adults with dyssynergia [105]. See Section F3 for a more detailed review of these studies. It is recommended, however, that simple habit training be initiated first and that biofeedback training be started only in patients who have failed to respond to habit training and who have objective evidence of pelvic floor dyssynergia.

Diarrhea-Related Functional Fecal Incontinence

Diarrhea-related functional fecal incontinence is treated by controlling diarrhea [106]. This may involve the use of antidiarrheal medications such as loperamide or dicyclomine, or anticholinergics such as hyoscyoamine. In patients with stress-related diarrhea, psychological treatments which help the patient manage stress, e.g., cognitive behavior therapy, progressive muscle relaxation training, interpersonal psychotherapy, or hypnosis, are suggested.

Structural or Neurological Causes of Fecal Incontinence

When fecal incontinence is due to sphincter weakness or impaired ability to perceive rectal distension secondary to neurological or muscle injury, biofeedback training directed at improving sphincter strength and/or perception may be the most effective treatment. These approaches to treatment are reviewed elsewhere [107]. For patients with muscle tears as a primary cause of sphincteric incontinence, surgical approaches to restoration of sphincter integrity or creation of an artificial sphincter may be preferred [108].

F2. Functional Anorectal Pain

Two forms of functional anorectal pain have been described: levator ani syndrome and proctalgia fugax. They are distinguished on the basis of *duration* (hours of constant pain for levator ani syndrome vs. seconds to minutes for proctalgia fugax), *frequency* (constant or frequent pain for levator ani syndrome vs. infrequent pain in proctalgia fugax), and *characteristic quality of pain* (dull pain or urgency in levator ani syndrome vs. sharp pain in proctalgia fugax). Despite these differences, there is a significant overlap in diagnosis [109], and factor analysis studies do not identify separate symptom clusters for these two disorders [110], giving rise to speculation that these are not separate entities but part of the same syndrome. However, there is indirect evidence which suggests that there may be different physiological mechanisms for these two types of pain (striated muscle tension in levator ani syndrome and smooth muscle spasm in proctalgia fugax, see below). Consequently, the historical distinction between these two types of pain will be preserved in this classification system.

F2a. Levator Ani Syndrome

— Definition

The levator ani syndrome is also called levator spasm, puborectalis syndrome, chronic proctalgia, pyriformis syndrome, and pelvic tension myalgia. The pain is often described as a vague, dull ache or pressure sensation high in the rectum. It is often described as worse with sitting than with standing or lying down. Physical examination may reveal overly contracted levator ani muscles and tenderness on palpation of the pelvic floor. For unknown reasons, tenderness is often asymmetric and may be noted on the left more often than on the right side [111].

— Epidemiology

The prevalence of symptoms compatible with levator ani syndrome in the general population is 6.6% [13]. Ages range from 6 to 90 years, but more than half are ages 30–60 years [111]. Prevalence tends to decline after age 45 [13]. It is more common in women (7.4% of all women) than in men (5.7% of all men) [13]. Only 29% consult a physician, but associated disability appears to be significant; in a postal survey of 5,430 adults, those with levator ani syndrome reported missing an average of 17.9 days from work or school in the past year, and 11.5% reported that they were currently too sick to work or go to school [13]. There is no published data on the frequency with which levator ani syndrome is encountered in medical practice.

— Diagnostic Criteria

At least 12 weeks, which need not be consecutive, in the preceding 12 months of:

(1) Chronic or recurrent rectal pain or aching; and

(2) Episodes last 20 minutes or longer; and

(3) Other causes of rectal pain such as ischemia, inflammatory bowel disease, cryptitis, intramuscular abscess, fissure, hemorrhoids, prostatitis, and solitary rectal ulcer have been excluded.

Confidence in the diagnosis is substantially increased if posterior traction on the puborectalis reveals tight levator ani muscles and tenderness or pain. Tenderness may be predominantly left-sided, and massage of this muscle will generally elicit the characteristic discomfort. Two levels of diagnostic classification are proposed: a "highly likely" diagnosis of levator ani syndrome if symptom criteria are satisfied and these physical signs are present, or a "possible" diagnosis if the symptom criteria are met but the physical signs are absent.

It is recognized that symptoms present for less than three months that are otherwise consistent with the diagnosis may warrant clinical diagnosis and treatment, but for research studies, symptoms should be present for at least three months.

— Clinical Evaluation

Diagnosis is based primarily on the presence of characteristic symptoms and physical examination findings (see definition above). Evaluation will usually include sigmoidoscopy and appropriate imaging studies such as defecography, ultrasound, or pelvic CT to exclude alternative diseases.

— Physiologic Features

Levator ani syndrome is hypothesized to result from overly contracted pelvic floor muscles. Treatments claimed to be effective are those that attempt to reduce tension in the striated pelvic floor muscles [109,111–114].

One study [109] suggests that elevated anal canal pressures or EMG levels may constitute a useful quantitative sign for the diagnosis of levator ani syndrome. Grimmaud and colleagues [109] measured anal canal pressures by perfusion manometry and found resting pressures in the anal canal to be elevated in all 12 patients with levator ani syndrome. Moreover, anal canal pressures decreased to normal in association with pain relief when these patients were treated with biofeedback. Elevated anal canal pressures may reflect either increased external anal sphincter contraction or internal anal sphincter tension or both. These observations need to be confirmed in a controlled study with a larger number of patients.

— Psychologic Features

Heymen, Wexner, and Gulledge [101] administered the MMPI to consecutive patients with functional bowel disorders and reported that patients with levator spasm showed significant elevations on the hypochondriasis, depression, and hysteria scales in a pattern seen in chronic pain patients and often referred to as the "neurotic triad." Burnett and colleagues [98] reported that patients with functional rectal pain (levator ani syndrome and proctalgia fugax were combined because of small numbers) had higher scores on the SCL-90R scales [100] for anxiety, depression, obsessive compulsive trait, and somatization. Quality of life as measured by the SF-36 [115] was significantly impaired on the scales for bodily pain, role physical (limitations in ability to work or perform usual physical activities), and social functioning (emotional problems and limitations in social activities), even after correcting for the possible mediating effects of neuroticism.

— Approach to Treatment

A variety of treatments directed at reducing tension in the levator ani muscles have been reported to be effective. These include electrogalvanic stimulation [112,114–116]; biofeedback training [109,114,116–119]; muscle relaxants such as methocarbamol (Robaxin), diazepam, and cyclobenzeprine (Flexeril) [111,120]; digital massage of the levator ani muscles [120–121]; and sitz baths [122].

None of the treatment studies referred to included a control group, and patient selection criteria varied. If the patient's distress or other circumstances require that treatment be undertaken, the only advice that can be offered at present is to do no harm, that is, to select a treatment such as biofeedback which has no significant adverse consequences. Surgery should be avoided.

F2b. Proctalgia Fugax

— Definition

Proctalgia fugax is defined as sudden, severe pain in the anal area lasting several seconds or minutes, and then disappearing completely [123]. Attacks may last from a few seconds to as long as 30 minutes. Only 10% of patients report a duration of more than five minutes. Pain is localized to the anus in 90% of cases [124]. Attacks are infrequent, occurring less than five times per year in 51% of patients [125].

The pain has been described as cramping, gnawing, aching, or stabbing and may range from uncomfortable to unbearable [126]. Thompson [124] found that 49% of patients had to interrupt their normal activities during an attack. The symptoms may awaken the patient from sleep.

— Epidemiology

The prevalence of proctalgia fugax has been difficult to determine because sufferers tend not to report episodes to their physician except in the most severe cases [127]. Estimates of the prevalence range from 8% [13] to 18% [127], with only 17–20% reporting the symptoms to their physicians. There is no clear evidence for a gender difference in prevalence [13,127]. Onset of symptoms is rarely reported before puberty, but cases have been reported in children as young as seven years [124].

Although relatively few patients with proctalgia fugax consult physicians, there is a significant amount of disability associated with the disorder. According to the U.S. Householder Study [13], subjects with proctalgia fugax missed an average of 12.8 days from work or school in the past year, and 8.4% of them reported that they were currently too ill to work or attend school. In this survey, it was not possible to determine whether the reported disability was the result of proctalgia fugax (unlikely) or was associated with other disorders in these patients.

— Diagnostic Criteria

(1) **Recurrent episodes of pain localized to the anus or lower rectum;** *and*
(2) **Episodes last from seconds to minutes;** *and*
(3) **There is no anorectal pain between episodes.**

Symptoms present for less than three months that are otherwise consistent with the diagnosis may warrant clinical diagnosis and treatment. However, for research studies symptoms should be present for at least three months.

— Clinical Evaluation

Diagnosis is based on the presence of characteristic symptoms as described above and exclusion of anorectal and pelvic pathophysiology. Certain urogenital abnormalities may be mistaken for proctalgia fugax. Chronic benign prostatitis may also present with acute bouts of perianal pain.

— Physiologic Features

The short duration and sporadic, infrequent nature of this disorder has made the identification of physiological mechanisms difficult. Several studies suggest that abnormal smooth muscle contractions may be responsible for the pain [59,128,129]. Three studies have reported families in which a hereditary form of proctalgia fugax was found to be associated with hypertrophy of the internal anal sphincter [130–132].

— Psychologic Features

Karras and Angelo [133] reported that attacks of proctalgia fugax are often precipitated by stressful life events or anxiety. Pilling and colleagues [134], using the MMPI and structured psychiatric interviews, found that the majority of patients were perfectionistic, anxious, and/or hypochondriacal. However, there was no control group, and clinical inferences were not based on blind assessments.

As noted previously, Burnett and colleagues [98] compared a combined group of patients with either proctalgia fugax or levator ani or both to a medical control group of patients with other gastrointestinal complaints and found elevations on a variety of psychological scales and impaired quality of life. These data suggest that personality traits and psychological stress may contribute to the development of proctalgia fugax.

— Approach to Treatment

Proctalgia fugax has been described as "harmless, unpleasant, and incurable" [135]. For the majority of patients, the episodes of pain are so brief that remedial treatment is impractical, and they are normally so infrequent that prevention is not feasible. Since the disorder is harmless, treatment will normally consist only of reassurance and explanation. However, a small group of patients have proctalgia fugax on a frequent basis and may require treatment. A recent randomized control trial showed that inhalation of salbutamol (a beta adrenergic agonist) was more effective than placebo for shortening the duration of episodes of proctalgia [136]. Others have recommended the alpha agonist, clonidine [137], amylnitrate, or nitroglycerine.

The psychological findings in patients who consult for proctalgia include anxiety, depression, and a tendency towards hypochondriasis. When these symptoms are present, antidepressant medications, tranquilizers, or psychotherapy may be indicated. However, there are no studies on the outcome of such treatments for proctalgia fugax.

F3. Pelvic Floor Dyssynergia

— Definition

Pelvic floor dyssynergia is defined by paradoxical contraction or failure to relax the pelvic floor muscles during attempts to defecate. It is frequently associated with symptoms of difficult defecation (e.g., straining, feeling of incomplete evacuation, digital facilitation of bowel movements), but physiological evidence that the external anal sphincter or puborectalis muscles fail to relax or paradoxically contract during attempted defecation is required for the diagnosis.

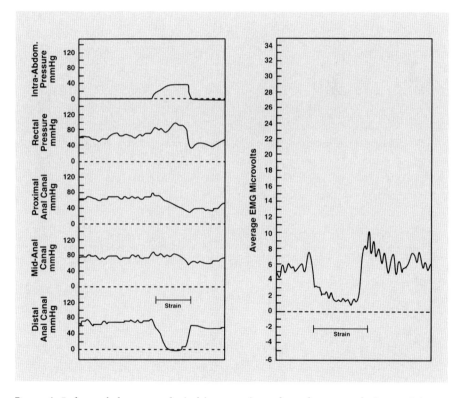

Figure 4. Left panel shows paradoxical increases in anal canal pressure during straining to defecate in a patient with pelvic floor dyssynergia. The top channel shows intra-abdominal pressure recorded from a 10-ml air-filled balloon and reflects normal increases in pressure associated with straining. However, the lower 4 channels all show paradoxical increases in anal canal pressure, which would obstruct defecation, rather than decreases in anal canal pressure which would permit defecation to occur. The right panel, taken from the same patient, shows that these paradoxical increases in anal canal pressure are accompanied by increases in averaged pelvic floor EMG. Compare to figure 3.

Normally, during the act of defecation the puborectalis sling muscle and the external anal sphincter relax to permit defecation. This can be demonstrated by recording EMG activity from the pelvic floor muscles, descent of the perineum, or anal canal pressures during defecation, which can be simulated by having the subject expel water-filled or air-filled balloons [138–140]. Healthy subjects show decreased EMG activity or anal canal pressure when they strain to defecate (fig. 3), but some chronically constipated patients inappropriately contract [138] (fig. 4) or fail to relax the external anal sphincter or puborectalis muscle, or both muscles, which obstructs defecation [141–142].

Preston and Lennard-Jones [138] first described the association of paradoxical contraction of the pelvic floor with constipation, and subsequent investigators confirmed their observations [143]. However, a recent report suggested that the finding of pelvic floor dyssynergia is variable from one occasion of testing to another [144] and is less likely to be seen at home when ambulatory monitors are used to record the response to straining, as compared to laboratory testing. Pelvic floor dyssynergia is also observed in some asymptomatic controls [145].

Other terms have been used interchangeably with pelvic floor dyssynergia. Preston and Lennard-Jones [138] coined the term "anismus," by analogy from "vaginismus," to describe this phenomenon. However, the term anismus implies a psychogenic etiology, which is unproved. The more general term "pelvic floor dyssynergia" is preferable to "anismus" and to terms that refer only to the puborectalis or to the external anal sphincter because the muscle dysfunction can be seen in either one or both of these muscles. At least some patients with pelvic floor dyssynergia also have obstructed micturition [54], as would be expected if there is dyssynergia of the whole pelvic floor. However, pelvic floor dyssynergia is used in this report to refer exclusively to dysfunction of the pelvic floor as it relates to defecation.

— Epidemiology

The prevalence of pelvic floor dyssynergia in the population is unknown because the diagnosis requires laboratory testing (anorectal manometry, pelvic floor EMG, and/or radiological studies). The prevalence of pelvic floor dyssynergia among patients with chronic constipation who have been referred to a tertiary referral center has been reported to be as low as 8% [146] and as high as 74% [147], but more typically 25–50% [139, 148]. As noted above, the prevalence of pelvic floor dyssynergia may have been overestimated due to the high false-positive rates seen in some studies [144]. No information is available on gender differences.

The prevalence of specific symptoms that are frequently associated with and thought to be due to pelvic floor dyssynergia have been reported in several surveys.

(1) *Straining.* Thompson and Heaton [149] found that 10.3% of a sample of British adults reported straining often, Drossman and colleagues [150] found that 17.5% of a large sample of American adults reported straining with more than 25% of bowel movement, and Talley and colleagues [23] reported a frequency of 18.5% for frequent straining. Talley's group analyzed their data separately for males and females and found that women complained of straining more often than men (22.5% vs. 14.5%).

(2) *Feeling of incomplete evacuation after defecation.* Thompson and Heaton [149] found that 10.0% of British adults reported a frequent feeling of incomplete evacuation, and Talley [23] reported an overall frequency of 21.5%, which was nearly identical for males (21.1%) and females (21.7%). In a stratified random sample of 10,018 U.S. adults, Stewart and colleagues [151] reported an overall prevalence of 38% for having a feeling of incomplete evacuation more than 25% of the time; the prevalence was nearly identical in females (39%) and males (37%).

(3) *Digital facilitation of defecation.* Stewart and colleagues [151] reported that 12% of adults acknowledged pressing with fingers on the perineum or in the vagina to facilitate defecation at least 25% of the time. Chaussade and colleagues [152] reported that the prevalence of digital facilitation in medical clinic patients referred for constipation was 68% for patients with right colonic stasis, 28% for patients with left colonic stasis, and 50% for patients with rectosigmoid stasis, as compared to 19% for individuals with normal whole-gut transit time.

(4) *Trouble letting go when attempting to defecate.* Stewart and colleagues [151] reported that 12% of 10,018 randomly selected U.S. adults (15% of females and 11% of males) reported difficulty letting go of a stool on at least 25% of bowel movements. Stewart and colleagues also reported that 19% of their sample of U.S. adults (19% of females and 15% of males) reported blockage of a bowel movement more than 25% of the time.

— Diagnostic Criteria

(1)   The patient must satisfy Diagnostic Criteria for functional constipation in C3*;

(2)   There must be manometric, EMG, or radiologic evidence for inappropriate contraction or failure to relax the pelvic floor muscles during repeated attempts to defecate;

(3)   There must be evidence of adequate propulsive forces during attempts to defecate; *and*

(4)   There must be evidence of incomplete evacuation.

*Diagnostic criteria for functional constipation are twelve weeks or more in the past twelve months of two or more of: (1) straining > ¼ of defecations; (2) lumpy or hard stools > ¼ of defecations; (3) sensation of incomplete evacuation > ¼ of defecations; (4) sensation of anorectal obstruction/blockage > ¼ of defecations; (5) manual maneuvres to facilitate > ¼ of defecations (e.g., digital evacuation, support of the pelvic floor); and (6) less than 3 defecations per week. Loose stools are not present, and there are insufficient criteria for IBS. See reference 204.

— Rationale for Changes in Diagnostic Classification System

The symptoms of difficult defecation, which consist of excessive straining during defecation, a feeling of incomplete evacuation, and pressing around in the anus or in the vagina to facilitate defecation, are frequently associated with pelvic floor dyssynergia. In the previous Working Team Report on functional anorectal disorders [30], these symptoms were used to define an independent diagnostic entity which was called dyschezia, and the diagnosis of pelvic floor dyssynergia could not be made in the absence of at least one of these symptoms. However, subsequent experience suggests that the symptoms of difficult defecation may overlap the symptoms usually attributed to slow colonic transit, rendering unreliable the classification of subtypes of constipation based on symptoms alone [153–154]. (For a differing view, however, see Sandler and colleagues [155] who concluded from a factor analysis of bowel symptoms that symptoms of difficult defecation could be differentiated from symptoms of functional constipation and IBS.) Because this issue is unresolved, in the revised Working Team Reports (cf., Section C4 also), no attempt is made to identify physiological subtypes of constipation based on symptoms, and the criteria for making a diagnosis of pelvic floor dyssynergia depend primarily on physiological findings.

The previous Working Team Report [30] recommended diagnosing pelvic floor dyssynergia on the basis of symptoms of difficult defecation plus manometric, EMG, or radiologic evidence of failure to relax the pelvic floor when attempting to defecate. However, a study by Duthie and Bartolo [144] suggests that these criteria are too nonspecific and that they result in a high false positive rate. More restrictive diagnostic criteria have been recommended which would require the following: (1) puborectalis EMG recruitment of more than 50% when straining; plus (2) evidence of an adequate level of intrarectal pressure during straining (more than 50 cm H_2O); plus (3) inability to defecate at least 40% of contrast during defecography [143,156]. These recommendations seem plausible, but the specific cut-off values recommended are based on observations made in relatively few subjects. The Rome II Working Team therefore recommends augmenting the diagnostic criteria by requiring evidence of adequate propulsive forces and evidence of incomplete evacuation in addition to evidence of paradoxical contraction, but the members felt it would be inappropriate at this point to endorse specific cut-off points for the diagnosis or specific diagnostic tests to determine whether these signs are present. These decisions are left to the investigator.

In the previous working team report [30], a diagnostic category existed for difficult defecation (e.g., straining, feeling of incomplete evacuation, digital facilitation of defecation) which was associated with manometric evidence of internal anal sphincter dysfunction, defined as absent or shallow internal anal sphincter inhibitory reflex or a hypertonic anal canal resting pressure or both in the absence of objective evidence for a structural defect such as aganglionosis. However, this diagnostic category was based on observations made in a single study [156] which was published more than ten years ago and which has not been replicated. A different internal anal sphincter dysfunction was recently described in patients with difficult evacuation, namely, myoelectric ultraslow waves recorded from the anal canal [158]. However, the specificity of this finding for patients with difficult evacuation has not been established. Consequently, the Working Team felt that the category of internal anal sphincter dysfunction should be dropped from the classification system until confirmed by further studies.

Other Mechanisms for Difficult Defecation

The diagnostic criteria given above for pelvic floor dyssynergia attempt to define a specific physiological mechanism for difficult defecation. It is recognized, however, that other types of pelvic floor dysfunction may occur which may give rise to symptoms of difficult defecation. These include, but are not limited to, inadequate propulsive forces (i.e., insufficient increases in intra-abdominal pressure) during attempts to defecate. Further research is needed to determine whether inadequate propulsive force is a distinctly different mechanism for constipation which may require a different approach to treatment.

— Clinical Evaluation

The recommended algorithm for the diagnosis of pelvic floor dyssynergia is given in figure 5. It is recommended that, in the absence of alarm symptoms such as blood in the stools or a sudden change in bowel habits, no physiological investigations be undertaken until the patient has been tried on conservative treatment (e.g., education regarding the normal range of bowel habits,

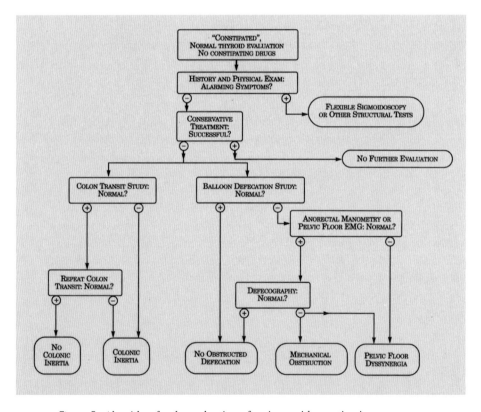

Figure 5. Algorithm for the evaluation of patients with constipation.

increased dietary fiber and liquids, increased exercise, elimination of medications with constipating side effects where possible). Patients who respond to conservative management require no further studies. The physiological investigations considered useful for making a diagnosis of pelvic floor dyssynergia are (1) balloon defecation (simulated defecation), (2) anorectal manometry, (3) defecography, and (4) radio-opaque markers or other colon transit study.

Manometric and EMG Assessment

A protocol for this assessment is given in category F1. Functional Fecal Incontinence. The parts of the examination which are specific to the diagnosis of pelvic floor dyssynergia are (1) measurement of anal canal and rectal pressures during straining to defecate, and (2) measurement of EMG activity from the external anal sphincter during straining to defecate (see figures 3 and 4 for representative tracings).

Simulation of Defecation

It is possible to simulate defecation by introducing lubricated balloons attached to thin catheters into the rectum, filling them with water or air, and asking the patient to defecate them. Additional research is needed to standardize the method of conducting this test with respect to the following:

(1) the position of the patient during straining (lying in bed versus sitting on a toilet chair);
(2) the proportion of trials on which the patient fails to expel the balloon;
(3) the length of time required to expel the balloon;
(4) the intrarectal pressures produced by straining; and
(5) the minimum increase in anal pressure and/or EMG activity that defines a paradoxical contraction.

It is recommended that the patient should sit on a commode chair behind a privacy screen and that changes in balloon pressure be recorded as the patient strains to defecate.

Limited data are available on the normal range of values for this test. Loening-Baucke [159] reported that 10 of 12 asymptomatic adults could defecate 50-ml balloons within one minute, and 11 of 12 could defecate 50-ml balloons within five minutes. Latencies less than 60 sec are considered normal. Peak intra-abdominal pressures associated with defecating these balloons were 61 ±40 mm Hg in healthy adults, and all healthy adults could relax the pelvic floor during defecation.

The balloon defecation test appears to be useful for identifying patients with obstructed defecation, but it does not indicate the cause of obstructed defecation: one cannot distinguish mechanical causes of obstructed defecation from pelvic floor dyssynergia on the basis of the balloon defecation test alone. Many investigators use the balloon defecation test as a screening tool which, if positive, leads to referral for further testing.

Defecography

Defecography is a dynamic radiological technique to evaluate the rectum and pelvic floor during attempted defecation. The technique for performing the test has been described and critically reviewed [160]. Briefly, 150 to 300 ml of barium sulfate mixed with thickening agents to achieve the consistency of soft stool is injected into the rectum, and lateral radiographs (2 images/sec or higher) are taken during resting and straining to defecate. Preferably, video-fluoroscopy should be performed in addition. This test provides information on the presence of structural abnormalities (rectocele, enterocele, intussusception, rectal prolapse, and megarectum) and functional parameters (anorectal angle at rest and during straining, diameter of the anal canal, indentation of the puborectalis, degree of rectal emptying).

The value of defecography has been questioned on several grounds:

(1) Some findings previously thought to be pathologic (e.g., rectoceles, intussuceptions) are now known to be common in asymptomatic control subjects [2,3,161,162];

(2) normal ranges for quantified measures are lacking because such studies have not been performed;

(3) some parameters such as the anorectal angle cannot be measured reliably because of variations in the shape of the rectum [161–166]; and

(4) the test measures only the emptying of liquid or semi-liquid rectal contents, not formed stool.

The principal value of defecography lies in (1) identifying structural causes for obstructed defecation and (2) assessing how well the patient can evacuate the rectum.

Radio-opaque Marker Test of Whole Gut Transit Time

It is recommended that colonic transit studies be performed in all patients who fail to respond to conservative treatment irrespective of whether anorectal manometry or defecography are done and what they show. This recommendation is made because (1) colonic inertia frequently coexists with pelvic floor dyssynergia and (2) these two mechanisms for constipation cannot be reliably distinguished on the basis of symptoms.

The most frequently used technique for measuring whole gut transit time involves having the patient swallow a gelatin capsule containing radio-opaque markers (commercially available capsules contain 24 markers) and taking abdominal radiographs on one or more days thereafter [167,168]. Many investigators prefer the Chaussade-Metcalf technique [169,170] in which patients ingest 20 or 24 markers each day for three days, and obtain an abdominal radiograph on day 4 and day 7. The use of 24 radio-opaque markers per day permits more accurate estimates of whole gut transit time and also allows for estimation of regional transit times. A modification of the Chaussade-Metcalf technique, which involves giving 24 markers each day for five days instead of three days and taking the radiograph 24 hours after the last capsule, has been described [171]. This effectively increases the sensitivity of the technique to prolonged transit times by allowing more time for equilibrium to be established. Information on the regional distribution of markers may prove useful in the diagnosis of pelvic floor dyssynergia when delayed transit is seen to occur only in the descending and sigmoid colon and in the rectum. However, inferences based on segmental transit time should be made cautiously because there appears to be more variability from day to day and from subject to subject in segmental as compared to whole gut transit times [171].

Although it is known that transit times are longer in women than in men [170, 172], separate normal ranges for males and females are not available at this time. Most laboratories treat 67 hours as the upper limit of normal. Values for regional transit time are given by Metcalf and colleagues [170].

Other techniques for measuring whole gut transit time that involve radio-isotopes [173,174], or telemetric capsules [175] have been described. These are less frequently used and appear to have no significant advantage over the relatively inexpensive radio-opaque technique for measurement of colonic transit time [176]. However, scintigraphic techniques provide information on gastric emptying and small bowel transit as well as colonic transit, and they are more sensitive to rapid whole gut transit time than is the radio-opaque marker technique.

— Physiologic Features

The physiologic basis for pelvic floor dyssynergia is implicit in the definition: the symptoms of difficult defecation appear to be caused by contraction or failure to relax the pelvic floor muscles during attempts to defecate.

However, this is not attributable to a neurological lesion since at least two-thirds of patients can learn to relax the external anal sphincter and puborectalis muscles appropriately when provided with biofeedback training [106]. The etiology of this behavioral disorder is discussed below.

Many details of the physiologic mechanism for pelvic floor dyssynergia remain unresolved and complicate the interpretation of diagnostic tests. These include:

(1) The extent to which the external anal sphincter and the puborectalis contract independently of each other is not known. Wald and colleagues [148] found a poor correlation between manometric evidence of sphincter dyssynergia obtained with a balloon probe in the distal anal canal and the results of defecography, and others [156,177] reported poor agreement between EMG evidence for pelvic floor dyssynergia and defecography. This may indicate that these muscle groups can contract independently since a balloon or surface EMG electrodes in the distal anal canal measure primarily from the external anal sphincter whereas defecography measures primarily the puborectalis muscle (anorectal angle, puborectalis indentation). Lebel and Grandmaison [178] showed by needle EMG that dyssynergia can be limited to one of the two muscle groups. This is consistent with the observation that the puborectalis is innervated by the sacral plexus and the pudendal nerve while the external anal sphincter is innervated only by the pudendal nerve [179]. However, one team of investigators [44] found agreement between defecography and anorectal manometry in 78% of patients if failure to relax on manometry was defined as less than a 20% decrease in anal canal pressure.

(2) The contribution that motivation and learning make in these disorders is not known. The voluntary inhibition of defecation [180,181] can be mistaken for pelvic floor dyssynergia; it is unknown how often false-positive diagnoses of dyssynergia result from lack of privacy and the patient's anxiety about the possibility of defecating stool in the situations in which this testing is performed, but many patients who test positive in the laboratory show normal relaxation during straining when they are at home [144].

— Psychologic Features

Pelvic floor dyssynergia may be due to faulty learning as suggested by the fact that the defect may be rapidly reversed with biofeedback training (see below). Some investigators have speculated that the pain associated with attempting to defecate large, hard stools may result in inadvertent learning by children to contract the sphincters in order to avoid or terminate pain during defecation [182–184]. This could result in a spiral of harder stools and further fear of defecation.

Anxiety and/or psychological stress may also contribute to the development of pelvic floor dyssynergia by increasing the level of skeletal muscle tension. Heymen and colleagues [101] found elevations on the MMPI scales for hypochondriasis, depression, and hysteria in these patients; and Burnett and colleagues [98] reported that they had significantly higher scores on the SCL-90R [100] scales for anxiety, depression, hostility, interpersonal sensitivity, obsessive compulsive traits, phobic anxiety, and somatization. Quality of life was also impaired in these patients [98], even after controlling for the mediating effects of neuroticism (a personality trait associated with a generally pessimistic attitude). Patients with symptoms of difficult defecation showed significant impairments in the SF-36 [115] scales for bodily pain, role physical (limitations in ability to work or perform usual physical activities), and general health. Similar studies showing elevated levels of psychological distress in patients with symptoms of difficult defecation were reported by Whitehead [185] and by Emery and colleagues [186]. However, three studies suggest that children with pelvic floor dyssynergia do not have any more behavior problems than children without pelvic floor dyssynergia [187–190].

Leroi and colleagues [191] found a greater incidence of sexual abuse in women with pelvic floor dyssynergia. These authors speculate that following the trauma of sexual abuse, any sensation of rectal fullness may trigger a memory of the original trauma and may lead to an involuntary contraction of the pelvic floor muscles.

Dubois and colleagues [192] developed a quality of life scale which is specific for constipation, and showed that this instrument has good test-retest reliability and that it agrees well with other measures of the impact of constipation on daily living. This scale may be useful as an outcome measure in treatment studies.

— Approach to Treatment

Two types of training have been described for pelvic floor dyssynergia: (1) *biofeedback training* in which sensors in the anal canal or adjacent to the anus are used to monitor and provide feedback to the patient on striated muscle activity [193–195] or anal canal pressures [184,196]; and (2) *simulated defecation* in which the patient practices defecation of a simulated stool consisting of a water-filled balloon; a thick mixture of metamucil or porridge [197]; or a silicone-filled, deformable artificial stool called "fecom" [196]. Simulated defecation was combined with diaphragmatic muscle training by some investigators [196, 198].

Both biofeedback and simulated defecation are reported to be effective. One study [194] found that EMG biofeedback training was more effective than simulated defecation alone. However, two other studies [198,199] found no significant difference between EMG biofeedback and simulated defecation. The two techniques can be combined.

Because 60% of patients with obstructive defecation have impaired rectal sensation, sensory conditioning of the rectum may confer additional benefit [200]. The training methods are similar to those used in treating patients with fecal incontinence.

Many uncontrolled studies of biofeedback for pelvic floor dyssynergia have been previously reviewed [105,106,200], and the systematic review by Enck [105] gives an overall success rate of 67%. Only recent studies involving large series of patients will be reviewed here. Ho, Tan, and Goh [201] found that 90% of patients treated with four sessions of biofeedback reported subjective improvement, and there was a significant increase in the number of spontaneous bowel movements. Similarly, Patankar and colleagues [202] described their experience with EMG biofeedback in 116 chronically constipated patients seen in five centers; 84% of patients reported improvement and the number of spontaneous bowel movements increased from 0.8 to 6.5 per week. Gilliland and colleagues [203] reported data for a series of 194 constipated patients who were treated with biofeedback; 35% achieved complete success defined as three or more spontaneous bowel movements per week, and an additional 13% reported partial success. These authors noted that improvement was related to the number of biofeedback sessions attended by the patient: 63% of those who completed the treatment protocol achieved complete success. Habit training (i.e., scheduled time to attempt defecation each day) was not used in any of these three trials, and stimulant laxatives were discouraged.

Most studies have reported only subjective outcomes. Objective parameters of anorectal function were systematically assessed by Rao and colleagues [196] who reported improved ability to bear down, to coordinate the rectal pushing force with anal relaxation, and to expel a simulated stool. Improvement was maintained for at least 6 months.

Although the results from uncontrolled studies are encouraging, no controlled trials comparing biofeedback to either sham biofeedback or conventional treatment in adults have been reported. Also, there is no data on long-term efficacy or on which component of treatment is most effective. Despite these limitations, biofeedback techniques appear to be effective in 48% [202] to 62% [203] of patients (intent to treat analysis), and biofeedback therapy is therefore regarded as the treatment of choice for this problem in adults.

(1) Multicenter studies of the normal physiology of defecation in large groups of subjects stratified by age, gender, and (in women) by parity are needed. These would (a) help to define the normal ranges for diagnostic tests of fecal incontinence and pelvic floor dyssynergia, and (b) help establish standardized technology for assessment of these conditions.

(2) Studies of the validity of diagnostic criteria for pelvic floor dyssynergia are needed to define cut-off values for changes in anal canal pressure during straining, propulsive forces, percent evacuation of the rectum, and presence of delayed transit in the descending colon. These studies might be approached by defining extreme groups based on clinical assessment and assessing these parameters. Such studies would help to determine whether inadequate propulsive force during attempted defecation is a mechanism for constipation that is separate from pelvic floor dyssynergia and what role rectal contractions play in disordered defecation.

(3) A randomized, blinded study of the efficacy of biofeedback treatment for pelvic floor dyssynergia should be carried out. This study should compare biofeedback to an equally credible (to patients) but ineffective treatment to control for the placebo response.

(4) Studies of the psychological characteristics of patients with levator ani syndrome and proctalgia fugax may help to define the etiology of these disorders and may identify new approaches to treatment. These studies should compare medical clinic patients to individuals in the community who have similar symptoms of rectal pain but who have not consulted physicians.

(5) Studies are needed to determine whether proctalgia fugax and levator ani syndrome are separate disorders. These studies should include detailed symptom reports supplemented by symptom diaries in large groups of patients. A multicenter study is desirable.

(6) A randomized, blinded study comparing the effectiveness of electrogalvanic stimulation, biofeedback, and muscle relaxant drugs for the treatment of levator ani syndrome should be performed. This should be a multicenter study.

References

1. Bartram CI, Turnbull GK, Lennard-Jones JE. Evacuation proctography: an investigation of rectal expulsion in 20 subjects without defecatory disturbance. Gastrointest Radiol 1988;13:72–80.

2. Shorvon PJ, McHugh F, Diamant N, et al. Defecography in normal volunteers: results and implications. Gut 1989;30:1737–49.

3. Berretta O, Chaussade S, Coquet M, et al. Defacographie: description et resultats díune technique simplifie. Presse Med 1990;19:1533–39.

4. Drossman DA, Thompson WG, Talley NJ, et al. Identification of sub-groups of functional gastrointestinal disorders. Gastroenterol Internat 1990;3:159-72.

5. Orr WC, Suluss J, Mellow M. Perceived and actual bowel function in older adults: it's not what it seems. Gastroenterology 1992;102:A571.

6. Ashraf W, Park F, Lof J, et al. An examination of the reliability of reported stool frequency in the diagnosis of idiopathic constipation. Am J Gastroenterol 1996; 91:26–32.

7. Diamant NE, Kamm MA, Wald A, et al. AGA technical review on anorectal testing techniques. Gastroenterology 1999;116:735–60.

8. Largo RH, Stutzle W. Longitudinal study of bowel and bladder control by day and at night in the first six years of life. I. Epidemiology and interactions between bowel and bladder control. Dev Med Child Neurol 1977;19:598–606.

9. Bellman, MM. Studies on encopresis. Acta Paediatr Scand 1966;56(Suppl 170): 1–151.

10. Whiting JS, Child IL. Child Training and Personality. New Haven, Connecticut: Yale University Press; 1953.

11. Hyman PE, Editor. Pediatric Functional Gastrointestinal Disorders. New York: Academy Professional Information Services; in press. A shortened version of this appears as Chapter 10 of this volume.

12. Nelson R, Norton N, Cautley E, et al. Community-based prevalence of anal incontinence. JAMA 1995;274:559–61.

13. Drossman DA, Li Z, Andruzzi E, et al. U.S. Householder survey of functional gastrointestinal disorders: prevalence, sociodemography, and health impact. Dig Dis Sci 1993;38:1569–80.

14. Incontinence fecale: enquete apres de la population generale. Paris: IPSOS Marketing;1989.

15. Enck P, Gabor S, von Ferber L, et al. Haufigkeit der Stuhlinkontinenz und informationsgrad von Hauszrzten und Krankenkassen. Z Gastroenterol 1991;29: 538–40.

16. Schaefer CE. Childhood Encopresis and Enuresis: Causes and Therapy. New York: Van Nostrand Reinhold;1979.

17. Levine MD. Children with encopresis: a descriptive analysis. Pediatrics 1975;56: 412–16.

18. Lowery SP, Srour JW, Whitehead WE, et al. Habit training as treatment of enco-

presis secondary to chronic constipation. J Pediatr Gastroenterol Nutr 1985;4: 397–401.

19. Barrett JA, Brocklehurst JC, Kiff ES, et al. Anal function in geriatric patients with fecal incontinence. Gut 1989;30:1244–51.

20. National Center for Health Statistics. The national nursing home survey: 1977 summary for the US. Health Resources Administration. Washington, DC: US Government Printing Office; 1979; DHEW publication no. (PHS) 79-1794. (Series 3, no. 43).

21. Wisconsin Center for Health Statistics. Profile of Wisconsin Nursing Home Residents, 1992. Madison, Wis: Center for Health Statistics, Division of Health, Dept of Health and Social Services;1994.

22. Johanson JF, Lafferty J. Epidemiology of fecal incontinence: The silent affliction. Am J Gastroenterol 1996;91:33–36.

23. Talley NJ, Zinsmeister AR, van Dyke C, et al. Epidemiology of colonic symptoms and the irritable bowel syndrome. Gastroenterology 1991;101:927–34.

24. Read NW, Abouzekry L. Why do patients with faecal impaction have faecal incontinence? Gut 27:283–87;1986.

25. Read NW, Abouzekry L, Read MG, et al. Anorectal function in elderly patients with fecal impaction. Gastroenterology 1985;89:959–66.

26. Heller BR, Whitehead WE, Johnson LD. Incontinence. J Gerontol Nurs 1989; 15:16–23.

27. Drossman DA, Sandler RS, Broom CM, et al. Urgency and fecal soiling in people with bowel dysfunction. Dig Dis Sci 1986;31:1221–25.

28. Sullivan SN, Wong C. Runner's diarrhea: different patterns and associated factors. J Clin Gastroenterol 1992;14:101–104.

29. Johanson JF, Irizarry F, Doughty A. Risk factors for fecal incontinence in a nursing home population. J Clin Gastroenterol 1997;24:156–60.

30. Whitehead WE, Devroede G, Habib FI, et al. Functional disorders of the anorectum. Gastroenterol Internat 1992;5:92–108.

31. American Psychiatric Association. Diagnostic and Statistical Manual for Mental Disorders. Ed 4. Washington, DC: American Psychiatric Association;1994.

32. Smith RG, Lewis S. The relationship between digital rectal examination and abdominal radiographs in elderly patients. Age and Ageing 1990:19;42-43.

33. Devroede G, Hemond M. Anorectal manometry: small balloon tube. In: Smith LE, Editor. Practical Guide to Anorectal Testing. New York: Igaku-Shoin;1990: 55–64.

34. Meunier PD, Gallaverdin D. Anorectal manometry: the state of the art. Dig Dis Sci 1993;11:252–69.

35. Rao SSC, Sun WM. Current techniques of assessing defecation dynamics. Dig Dis Sci 1997;15:64–77.

36. Arhan P, Devroede G, Persoz B, et al. Response of the anal canal to repeated distention of the rectum. Clin Invest Med 1979;2:83–88.

37. Sun WM, Read NW, Prior A, et al. Sensory and motor responses to rectal disten-

tion vary according to rate and pattern of balloon inflation. Gastroenterology 1990;99:1008–15

38. Whitehead WE, Engel BT, Schuster MM. Irritable bowel syndrome: physiological and psychological differences between diarrhea-predominant and constipation-predominant patients. Dig Dis Sci 1980;25:404–13.

39. Akervall S, Fasth S, Nordgren S, et al. Rectal reservoir and sensory function studied by graded isobaric distention in normal man. Gut 1989;30:496–502.

40. Buser WE, Miner PB Jr. Delayed rectal sensation with fecal incontinence: successful treatment using anorectal manometry. Gastroenterology 1986;91:1186–91.

41. McHugh SM, Diamant NE. Effect of age, gender and parity on anal canal pressures: contribution of impaired anal sphincter function to fecal incontinence. Dig Dis Sci 1987;32:726–36.

42. Chiarioni G, Scattolini C, Bonfante F, et al. Liquid stool incontinence with severe urgency: anorectal function and effective biofeedback treatment. Gut 1993;34:1576–80.

43. Phillips SF, Edwards AW. Some aspects of anal continence and defaecation. Gut 1965;6:396–406.

44. Badiali D, Habib FI, Corazziari E, et al. Manometric and defaecographic patterns of straining. J Gastrointest Motil 1991;3:171.

45. Rao SSC, Patel RS. How useful are manometric tests of anorectal function in the management of defecation disorders? Am J Gastroenterol 1997;92:469–75.

46. Wexner SD, Jorge JM. Colorectal physiological tests: use or abuse of technology? Eur J Surg 1994;160:167–74.

47. Law PJ, Kamm MA, Bartram CI. A comparison between electromyography and anal endosonography in mapping external anal sphincter defects. Dis Colon Rectum 1990,33:370–73.

48. Burnett SJD, Speakman CTM, Kamm MA, et al. Confirmation of endosonographic detection of external anal sphincter defects by simultaneous electromyographic mapping. Brit J Surg 1991;78:448–50.

49. Tjandra JJ, Milsom JW, Schroeder T, et al. Endoluminal ultrasound is preferable to electromyography in mapping anal sphincteric defects. Dis Colon Rectum 1993;36:689–92.

50. Enck P, von Giesen HJ, Schäfer A, et al. Comparison of anal ultraosund with conventional needle electromyography in the evaluation of anal sphincter defects. Am J Gastroenterol 91;1996:2539–43

51. Sultan AH, Kamm MA, Talbot IC, et al. Anal endosonography for identifying external sphincter defects confirmed histologically. Brit J Surg 1994;81:463–65.

52. Sultan AH, Nicholls RJ, Kamm MA, et al. Anal endosonography and correlation with in vitro and in vivo anatomy. Brit J Surg 1993;80:508–11.

53. Eckardt VF, Jung B, Lierse W. Anal endosonography in healthy subjects and patients with idiopathic fecal incontinence. Dis Colon Rectum 37;1994:235–42

54. Thorpe AC, Williams NS, Badenoch DF, et al. Simultaneous dynamic electromyographic protography and cystometrography. Brit J Surg 1993;80:115–20.

55. Speakman CT, Burnett SJ, Kamm M., et al. Sphincter injury after anal dilatation demonstrated by anal endosonography. Brit J Surg 1991;78:1429–30.

56. Engel AF, Kamm MA, Bartram CI. Unwanted anal penetration as a physical cause of faecal incontinence. Eur J Gastroenterol Hepatol 1995;7:65–67.

57. Sultan AH, Kamm MA, Nicholls RJ, et al. Prospective study of the extent of internal anal sphincter division during lateral sphincterotomy. Dis Colon Rectum 1994;37:1031–33.

58. Engel AF, Kamm MA, Talbot IC. Progressive systemic sclerosis of the internal anal sphincter leading to passive faecal incontinence. Gut 1991;35:857–59.

59. Eckardt VF, Dodt O, Kanzler G, et al. Anorectal function and morphology in patients with sporadic proctalgia fugax. Dis Colon Rectum 39;1996:755–62.

60. Sultan AH, Kamm MA, Hudson CN, et al. Anal sphincter disruption during vaginal delivery. New Engl J Med 1993;329:1905–11.

61. Law PJ, Kamm MA, Bartram CI. Anal endosonography in the investigation of faecal incontinence. Brit J Surg 1991;78:312–14.

62. Felt-Bersma P JF, Cuesta MA, Koorevaar M, et al. Anal endosonography: relationship with anal manometry and neurophysiologic tests. Dis Colon Rectum 1992;35:944–49.

63. Schäfer A, Enck P, Fürst G, et al. Anatomy of the anal sphincters: comparison of anal endosonography to magnetic resonance imaging. Dis Colon Rectum 37; 1994:777–81.

64. Engel AF, Kamm MA, Bartram Cl, et al. Relationship of symptoms in faecal incontinence to specific sphincter abnormalities. Internat J Colorectal Dis 1995; 10:152–55.

65. Desouza NM, Kmiot WA, Puni R, et al. High resolution magnetic resonance imaging of the anal sphincter using an internal coil. Gut 1995;37:284–87.

66. Kiff ES, Swash M. Slowed conduction in the pudendal nerves in idiopathic (neurogenic) faecal incontinence. Brit J Surg 1984;71:614–16.

67. Felt-Bersma RJF, Strijers RLM, Janssen JJWM, et al. The external anal sphincter: relationship between anal manometry and anal electromyography and its clinical relevance. Dis Colon Rectum 1989;32:112–16.

68. Cheong DMO, Vaccaro CA, Salanga VD, et al. Electrodiagnostic evaluation of fecal incontinence. Muscle and Nerve 1995;18:612–19.

69. Bartolo DCC, Jarratt JA, Read MG, et al. The role of partial denervation of the puborectalis in idiopathic faecal incontinence. Brit J Surg 1983;70:664–67.

70. Womack NR, Morrison JF, Williams NS. The role of pelvic floor denervation in the aetiology of idiopathic faecal incontinence. Brit J Surg 1986;73:404–407.

71. Rogers J, Levy DM, Henry MM, et al. Pelvic floor neuropathy: a comparative study of diabetes mellitus and idiopathic faecal incontinence. Gut 1988;29:756–61.

72. Pinho M, Hosie K, Bielecki K, et al. Assessment of noninvasive intra-anal electromyography to evaluate sphincter function. Dis Colon Rectum 1991;34:69–71.

73. Sorensen M, Tetzschner T, Rasmussen OO, et al. Relation between electromyography and anal manometry of the external anal sphincter. Gut 1991;32:1031–34.

74. Neill ME, Parks AG, Swash M. Physiological studies of the pelvic floor in idiopathic faecal incontinence and rectal prolapse. Brit J Surg 1981;68:531–36.

75. Vernava AM III, Longo WE, Daniel GL. Pudendal neuropathy and the importance of EMG evaluation of fecal incontinence. Dis Colon Rectum 1993;36:23–27.

76. Wexner SD, Marchetti F, Salanga VD, et al. Neurophysiologic assessment of the anal sphincters. Dis Colon Rectum 1991;34:606–12.

77. Swash M. Anorectal incontinence: electrophysiological tests. Brit J Surgery 1985; 72(suppl):s14–15.

78. Herdmann J, Bielefeldt K, Enck P. Quantification of motor pathways to the pelvic floor in humans. Am J Physiol 1991;260:G720–23.

79. Enck P, Herdmann J, Bergermann K, et al. Up and down the spinal cord: afferent and efferent innervation of the human external anal sphincter. J Gastrointest Motil 1992;4:271–77.

80. Loening-Baucke V, Read NW, et al. Evaluation of the motor and sensory components of the pudendal nerve. Electroenceph Clin Neurophysiol 1994;93:35–41.

81. Frieling T, Enck P, Wienbeck M. Cerebral responses evoked by electrical stimulation of rectosigmoid in normal subjects. Dig Dis Sci 1989;34:202–205.

82. Loening-Baucke V, Anderson RH, Yamada T, et al. Study of the afferent pathways from the rectum with a new distention control device. Neurology 1995;45:1510–16.

83. Speakman CT, Kamm MA, Swash M. Rectal sensory evoked potentials: an assessment of their clinical value. Internat J Colorectal Dis 1993;8:23–28.

84. Meunier P, Louis D, deBeaujeu MJ. Physiologic investigation of primary colonic constipation in children: comparison with the barium enema study. Gastroenterology 1984;87:1351–57.

85. Loening-Baucke VA. Sensitivity of the sigmoid colon and rectum in children treated for chronic constipation. J Ped Gastroenterol Nutr 1984;3:454–59.

86. Miller R, Bartolo DC, Roe A, et al. Anal sensation and the continence mechanism. Dis Colon Rectum 1988;31:433–38.

87. Bielefeldt K, Enck P, Erckenbrecht JF. Sensory and motor function in the maintenance of anal continence. Dis Colon Rectum 1990;33:674–78.

88. De Medici A, Badiali D, Corazziari E, et al. Rectal sensitivity in chronic constipation. Dig Dis Sci 1989;34;747–53.

89. Nixon HH. Megarectum in the child. Proc Roy Soc Med 1967;60:801–803.

90. Whitehead WE, Schuster MM. Gastrointestinal Disorders: Behavioral and Physiological Basis for Treatment. Orlando, Florida:Academic;1985.

91. Hoffman BA, Timmcke AE, Gathright JB, et al. Fecal seepage and soiling: a problem of rectal sensation. Dis Colon Rectum 1995;38:746–48.

92. Verduron A, Devroede G, Bouchoucha M, et al. Megarectum. Dig Dis Sci 1988;33:1164–74.

93. Meunier P, Marechal JM, deBeaujeu MJ. Rectoanal pressures and rectal sensitivity studies in chronic childhood constipation. Gastroenterology 1979;77:330.

94. Kumar D, Waldron DL, Williams NS. Home assessment of anorectal motility

and external sphincter EMG in idiopathic faecal incontinence. Brit J Surg 1989; 76:635–36.

95. Farouk R, Duthie GS, MacGregor AB, et al. Evidence of electromechanical dissociation of the internal anal sphinter in idiopathic fecal incontinence. Dis Colon Rectum 1994;37:595–601.

96. Speakman CTM, Kamm MA. The internal anal sphincter—new insights into faecal incontinence. Gut 1991;32:345–46.

97. Speakman CTM, Hoyle CHV, Kamm MM, et al. Abnormalities of innervation of internal anal sphincter in fecal incontinence. Dig Dis Sci 1993;38:1961–69.

98. Burnett CK, Palsson O, Whitehead WE, et al. Psychological distress and impaired quality of life in patients with functional anorectal disorders. Gastroenterology 1998;114:A729.

99. Crowell MD, Schettler-Duncan VA, Brookhart K, et al. Fecal incontinence: impact on psychosocial function and health-related quality of life. Gastroenterology 1998;114:A738.

100. Derogatis LI. The SCL-90-R. Administration, Scoring, and Procedures Manual. Ed 3. Mineapolis, Minnesota:National Computer Systems, Inc.; 1994.

101. Heymen S, Wexner SD, Gulledge AD. MMPI assessment of patients with functional bowel disorders. Dis Colon Rectum 1993;36:593–96.

102. Young GC. The treatment of childhood encopresis by gastroileal reflex training. Behav Res Ther 1973;11:499–503.

103. Whitehead WE, Burgio KL, Engel BT. Biofeedback treatment of fecal incontinence in geriatric patients. J Am Geriatr Soc 1985;33:320–24.

104. Tobin GW, Brocklehurst JC. Faecal incontinence in residential homes for the elderly: prevalence, aetiology and management. Age and Ageing 1986;15:41–46.

105. Enck P. Biofeedback training in disordered defecation: a critical review. Dig Dis Sci 1993;38:1953–60.

106. Whitehead WE. Functional anorectal disorders. Sem Gastrointest Dis 1996;7: 230–36.

107. Whitehead WE. Behavioral medicine approaches to gastrointestinal disorders. J Consult Clin Psych 1992;60:605–12.

108. Vaizey CJ, Kamm MA, Nicholls RJ. Recent advances in the surgical treatment of faecal incontinence. Brit J Surg 1998;85:596–603.

109. Grimaud JC, Bouvier M, Naudy B, et al. Manometric and radiologic investigations and biofeedback treatment of chronic idiopathic anal pain. Dis Colon Rectum 1991;34:690–95.

110. Palsson OS, Taub E, Cook EC III, et al. Validation of Rome criteria for functional gastrointestinal disorders by factor analysis. Am J Gastroenterol 1996;91: A2000.

111. Grant SR, Salvati EP, Rubin RJ. Levator syndrome: an analysis of 316 cases. Dis Colon Rectum 1975;18:161–63.

112. Sohn N, Weinstein MA, Robbins RD. The levator syndrome and its treatment with high-voltage electrogalvanic stimulation. Am J Surg 1982;144:580–82.

113. Oliver GC, Rubin RJ, Salvati EP, et al. Electrogalvanic stimulation in the treatment of levator syndrome. Dis Colon Rectum 1985;28:662–63.

114. Nicosia JG, Abcarian H. Levator syndrome: a treatment that works. Dis Colon Rectum 1985;28:406–408.

115. Ware JE Jr. SF-36 Health Survey: Manual and Interpretation Guide. Boston:The Health Institute, New England Medical Center;1993.

116. Billingham RP, Isler JT, Friend WG, et al. Treatment of levator syndrome using high-voltage electrogalvanic stimulation. Dis Colon Rectum 1987;30:584–87.

117. Ger GC, Wexner SD, Jorge JM, et al. Evaluation and treatment of chronic intractable rectal pain—a frustrating endeavor. Dis Colon Rectum 1993;36: 139–45.

118. Gilliland R, Heymen JS, Altomare DF, et al. Biofeedback for intractable rectal pain: outcome and predictors of success. Dis Colon Rectum 1997;40:190–96.

119. Heah SM, Ho YH, Tan M, et al. Biofeedback is effective treatment for levator ani syndrome. Dis Colon Rectum 1997;40:187–89.

120. Schuster MM. Rectal pain. In: Bayless T, Editor. Current Therapy in Gastro-enterology and Liver Disease. Ontario, Canada:C.C. Decker;1990:378–79.

121. Thiele GH. Tonic spasm of the levator ani, coccygeus and piriformis muscle: Re-lationship to coccygodynia and pain in the region of the hip and down the leg. Trans Am Proc Soc 1936;37:145–55.

122. Dodi G, Bogoni F, Infantino A, et al. Hot or cold in anal pain? A study of the changes in internal anal sphincter pressue profiles. Dis Colon Rectum 1986;29: 248–51.

123. Thompson WG. Proctalgia fugax. Dig Dis Sci 1981;26:1121–24.

124. Thompson WG. The Irritable Gut. Baltimore:University Park Press;1979.

125. Thompson WG. Proctalgia fugax in patients with the irritable bowel, peptic ulcer, or inflammatory bowel disease. Am J Gastroenterol 1984;79:450–52.

126. Perry WH. Proctalgia fugax: a clinical enigma. South Med J 1988;81:621–23.

127. Thompson WG, Heaton KW. Proctalgia fugax. J Roy Coll Physic (London) 1980; 14:247A–48.

128. Harvey RF. Colonic motility in proctalgia fugax. Lancet 1979;2:713–14.

129. Rao SSC, Hatfield RA. Paroxysmal anal hyperkinesis: a characteristic feature of proctalgia fugax. Gut 1996;39:609–12.

130. Kamm MA, Hoyle CHV, Burleigh DE, et al. Hereditary internal anal sphincter my-opathy causing proctalgia fugax and constipation. Gastroenterology 1991;100: 805–10.

131. Celik AF, Katsinelos P, Read NW, et al. Hereditary proctalgia fugax and constipa-tion: report of a second family. Gut 1995;36:581–84.

132. Guy RJ, Kamm MA, Martin JE. Internal anal sphincter myopathy causing proc-talgia fugax and constipation: further clinical and radiological characterization in a patient. Eur J Gastroenterol Hepatol 1997;9:221–24.

133. Karras JD, Angelo G. Proctalgia fugax: clinical observations and a new diagnostic aid. Dis Colon Rectum 1963;6:130–34.

134. Pilling LF, Swenson WM, Hill JR. The psychologic aspects of proctalgia fugax. Dis Colon Rectum 1972;83:72–76.

135. Douthwaite AH. Proctalgia fugax. Brit Med J 1962;2:164–65.

136. Eckardt VF, Dodt O, Kanzler G, et al. Treatment of proctalgia fugax with salbutamol inhalation. Am J Gastroenterol 1996;91:686–89.

137. Swain R. Oral clonidine for proctalgia fugax. Gut 1987;28:1039–40.

138. Preston DM, Lennard-Jones JE. Anismus in chronic constipation. Dig Dis Sci 1985;30:413–18.

139. Lestar B, Penninck FM, Kerremans RP. Defecometry: a new method for determining the parameters of rectal evacuation. Dis Colon Rectum 1989;32:179–201.

140. Pezim ME, Pemberton JH, Levin KE, et al. Parameters of anorectal and colonic motility in health and in severe constipation. Dis Colon Rectum 1993;36:484–91.

141. Kuijpers HC, Bleijenberg G. The spastic pelvic floor syndrome: a cause of constipation. Dis Colon Rectum 1985;28:669–72.

142. Kuijpers HC, Bleijenberg G, De Moiree H. The spastic pelvic floor syndrome: large bowel outlet obstruction caused by pelvic floor dysfunction: a radiological study. Internat J Colorectal Dis 1986;1:44–48.

143. Roberts JP, Womack NR, Hallan RI, et al. Evidence from dynamic integrated proctography to redefine anismus. Brit J Surg 1992;79:1213–15.

144. Duthie GS, Bartolo DCC. Anismus: the cause of constipation? results of investigation and treatment. World J Surg 1992;16:831–35.

145. Jones PN, Lubowski DZ, Swash M, et al. Is paradoxical contraction of puborectalis muscle of functional importance? Dis Colon Rectum 1987;30:667–70.

146. Surrenti E, Rath DM, Pemberton JH, et al. Audit of constipation in a tertiary referral gastroenterology practice. Am J Gastroenterol 1995;90:1471–75.

147. Kuijpers HC. Application of the colorectal laboratory in diagnosis and treatment of functional constipation. Dis Colon Rectum 1990;33:35–39.

148. Wald A, Caruana BJ, Freimanis MG, et al. Contributions of evacuation proctography and anorectal manometry to the evaluation of adults with constipation and defecatory difficulty. Dig Dis Sci 1990;35:481–87.

149. Thompson WG, Heaton KW. Functional bowel disorders in apparently healthy people. Gastroenterology 1980;79:283–88.

150. Drossman DA, Sandler RS, McKee DC, et al. Bowel patterns among subjects not seeking health care: use of a questionnaire to identify a population with bowel dysfunction. Gastroenterology 1982;83:529–34.

151. Stewart WF, Liberman JN, Sandler RS, et al. Epidemiology of constipation (EPOC) study in the United States: relation of clinical subtypes to sociodemographic features. Am J Gastroenterol 1999;in press.

152. Chaussade S, Khyari A, Roche H, et al. Determination of total and segmental colonic transit time in constipated patients: results in 91 patients with a new simplified method. Dig Dis Sci 1989;34:1168–72.

153. Whitehead WE, Burnett C, Palsson O, et al. Can symptoms distinguish subtypes of constipation? Gastroenterology 1998;114:A859.

154. Probert CSJ, Emmett PM, Cripps HA, et al. Evidence for the ambiguity of the term constipation: the role of irritable bowel syndrome. Gut 1994;35:1455–58.
155. Sandler RS, Stewart WF, Liberman JN, et al. Symptom criteria for constipation subtypes in a U.S. national epidemiological study of constipation. Gastroenterology 1998;114:A831.
156. Miller R, Duthie GS, Bartolo DC, et al. Anismus in patients with normal and slow transit constipation. Brit J Surg 1991;78:690–92.
157. Ducrotte P, Denis P, Galmiche JP, et al. Motricite anorectale dans la constipation idiopathique: etude de 200 patients consecutifs. Gastroenterol Clin Biol 1985;9:10–15.
158. Eckhardt VF, Schmitt T, Bernhard G. Anal ultra slow waves: a smooth muscle phenomenon associated with dyschezia. Dig Dis Sci 1997;42:2439–45.
159. Loening-Baucke V, Metcalf AM, Savage C. Are defecation dynamics important in the pathophysiology of severe idiopathic constipation? Gastroenterology 1988;95:A878.
160. Ekberg O, Mahiew PHG, Bartram CI, et al. Defecography: dynamic radiological imaging in proctology. Gastroenterol Internat 1990;3:93–99;
161. Goei R, van Engelshoven J, Schouten H, et al. Anorectal function: defecographic measurement in asymptomatic subjects. Radiology 1989;173:137–41.
162. Halligan S, Bartram CI, Park HJ, et al. Proctographic features of anismus. Radiology 1995;197:679–82.
163. Penninckx F, Debruyne C, Lestar B, et al. Observer variation in the radiological measurement of the anorectal angle. Internat J Colorectal Dis 1990;5:94–97.
164. Ferrante SL, Perry RE, Schreiman JS,et al. The reproducibility of measuring the anorectal angle in defecography. Dis Colon Rectum 1991;34:51–54.
165. Friemanis MG, Wald A, Caruana B, et al. Evaluation proctography in normal volunteers. Invest Radiol 1991;26:581–85.
166. Mueller-Lissner SA, Bartolo DCC, Christiansen J, et al. Interobserver agreement in defecography in an international study. Z Gastroenterol 1998;36:273–79.
167. Hinton JM, Lennard-Jones JE, Young AC. A new method for studying gut transit times using radio-opaque markers. Gut 1969;24:123–26.
168. Arhan P, Devroede G, Jehannin B, et al. Segmental colonic transit time. Dis Colon Rectum 1981;24:625–29.
169. Chaussade S, Roche H, Khyari A, et al. Mesure du temps de transit colique global et segmentaire; description et validation díune nouvelle technique. Gastroenterol Clin Biol 1986;10:385–89.
170. Metcalf AM, Phillips SF, Zinsmeister AR, et al. Simplified assessment of segmental colonic transit. Gastroenterology 1987;92:40–47.
171. Knowles JB, Whitehead WE, Meyer KB. Reliability of a modified Sitzmark study of whole gut transit time. Gastroenterology 1998;114:A779.
172. Hinds JP, Stoney B, Wald A. Does gender or the menstrual cycle affect colonic transit? Am J Gastroenterol 1989;84:123–26.
173. Proano M, Camilleri M, Phillips SF, et al. Transit of solids through the human

colon: regional quantification in the unprepared bowel. Am J Physiol 1990;258: G856-62.

174. Stiviland T, Camilleri M, Vassallo M, et al. Scintigraphic measurement of regional gut transit in idiopathic constipation. Gastroenterology 1991;101:107–15.

175. Waller SL. Differential measurement of small and large bowel transit times in constipation and diarrhoea: a new approach. Gut 1975;16:372–78.

176. Van der Sijp JRM, Kamm MA, Nightingale MJD, et al. Radioisotope determination of regional colonic transit in severe constipation: comparison with radio opaque markers. Gut 1993;34:402–408.

177. Fink RL, Roberts LJ, Scott M. The role of manometry, electromyography and radiology in the assessment of intractable constipation. Austral N Z J Surg 1991;61: 959–64.

178. Lebel ML, Grandmaison F. Etude electromyographique dynamique du plancher pelvien dans la constipation: importance de la EMG la aiguille. Can J Neurol Sci 1988;15:212.

179. Percy JP, Neill ME, Swash M, et al. Electrophysiological study of motor nerve supply of pelvic floor. Lancet 1981;1:16–17.

180. Klauser AG, Voderholzer WA, Heinrich CA, et al. Behavioural modification of colonic function: can constipation be learned? Dig Dis Sci 1990;35:1271–75.

181. Enck P, Bielefeld K, Legler T, et al. Kann man Verstopfung lernen? Eine experimentelle Untersuchung bei gesunden Probanden. Z Med Psychol 1991;1:31–37.

182. Keren S, Wagner Y, Heldenbert D, et al. Studies of manometric abnormalities of the rectoanal region during defecation in constipated and soiling children: modification through biofeedback therapy. Am J Gastroenterol 1988;83:827–31.

183. Loening-Baucke V. Factors determining outcome in children with chronic constipation and faecal soiling. Gut 1989;30:999–1006.

184. Wald A, Chandra R, Chiponis D, et al. Anorectal function and continence mechanisms in childhood encopresis. J Ped Gastroenterol Nutr 1986;5:346.

185. Whitehead WE. Illness behaviour. In: Kamm, MA, Lennard-Jones JE, Editors. Constipation. Petersfield, UK:Wrightson Biomedical Publishing;1993:95–100.

186. Emery Y, Descos L, Meunier P, et al. Constipation terminale par asynchronisme abdomino-pelvien: analyse des donnees etiologiques, cliniques, manometriques, et des resultats therapeutiques apres reeducation par biofeedback. Gastroenterol Clin Biol 1988;12:6–11.

187. Wald A, Chandra R, Gabel S, et al. Evaluation of biofeedback in childhood encopresis. J Pediatr Gastroenterol Nutr 1987;6:554–58.

188. Loening-Baucke V. Changes in behavioural ratings with treatment of childhood encopresis. Presented at the Ambulatory Pediatric Association meeting, Washington, DC, May 1989.

189. van der Plas RN, Benninga MA, Redekop WK, et al. Randomised trial of biofeedback training for encopresis. Arch Dis Childhood 1996;75:367–74.

190. van der Plas RN, Benninga MA, Buller HA, et al. Biofeedback training in treat-

ment of childhood constipation: a randomized controlled study. Lancet 1996; 348:776–78.

191. Leroi AM, Berkelmans I, Denis P, et al. Anismus as a marker of sexual abuse: consequences of abuse on anorectal motility. Dig Dis Sci 1995;40:1411–16.

192. Dubois DJ, Johnson KI, de la Loge C, et al. Measuring quality-of-life in chronic constipation. Gastroenterology 1998;114:A11.

193. Kawimbe BM, Papachrysostomou M, Binnie NR, et al. Outlet obstruction constipation (anismus) managed by biofeedback. Gut 1991;35:1175–79.

194. Bleijenberg G, Kuijpers HC. Biofeedback treatment of constipation: a comparison of two methods. Am J Gastroenterol 1994;89:1021–26.

195. Cox DJ, Sutphen J, Borowitz S, et al. Simple electromyographic biofeedback treatment for chronic pediatric constipation/encopresis: preliminary report. Biofeedback Self-Regul 1994;19:41–50.

196. Rao SSC, Welcher KD, Pelsang RE. Effects of biofeedback on anorectal function in obstructive defecation. Dig Dis Sci 1997;42:2197–2205.

197. Bleijenberg G, Kuijpers HC. Treatment of the spastic pelvic floor syndrome with biofeedback. Dis Colon Rectum 1987;30:108–11.

198. Koutsomanis D, Lennard-Jones JE, Roy AJ, et al. Controlled randomised trial of visual biofeedback versus muscle training without a visual display for intractable constipation. Gut 1995;37:95–99.

199. Glia A, Gylin M, Gullberg K, et al. Biofeedback retraining in patients with functional constipation and paradoxical puborectalis contraction: comparison of anal manometry and sphincter electromyography for feedback. Dis Colon Rectum 1997;40:889–95.

200. Rao SSC, Enck P, Loening-Baucke V. Biofeedback therapy for defecation disorders. Dig Dis 1997;15(Suppl 1):78–92.

201. Ho YH, Tan M, Goh HS. Clinical and physiologic effects of biofeedback in outlet obstruction constipation. Dis Colon Rectum 1996;39:520–24.

202. Patankar SK, Ferrara A, Levy JR, et al. Biofeedback in colorectal practice: a multicenter, statewide, three-year experience. Dis Colon Rectum 1997;40:827–31.

203. Gilliland R, Heymen JS, Altomare DF, et al. Outcome and predictors of success of biofeedback for constipation. Brit J Surg 1997;84:1123–26.

204. Thompson WG, Longstreth GF, Drossman DA, et al. Functional bowel disorders and functional abdominal pain. Gut 1999;45(suppl 11);1999.

Chapter 10

G. Childhood Functional Gastrointestinal Disorders

Paul E. Hyman, Chair,

Andree Rasquin-Weber, Co-Chair, *with*

David R. Fleisher,

Jeffrey S. Hyams,

Peter J. Milla,

Annamaria Staiano,

and Salvatore Cucchiara

Introduction

Childhood functional gastrointestinal disorders include a variable combination of often age-dependent, chronic or recurrent symptoms not explained by structural or biochemical abnormalities. Functional symptoms during childhood are sometimes accompaniments to normal development (e.g., infant regurgitation), or they may arise from maladaptive behavioral responses to internal or external stimuli (e.g., functional fecal retention often results from painful defecation and/or coercive toilet training). The clinical expression of a childhood functional gastrointestinal disorder depends on an individual's autonomic, affective, and intellectual developmental stage, as well as on concomitant organic and psychological disturbances. Infant regurgitation is a problem for a few months during the first year. Toddler's diarrhea affects infants and toddlers. Most difficult to manage cases of functional fecal retention resolve once a child enters a stage of formal operations thinking. Irritable bowel syndrome and functional dyspepsia are diagnosed only after the child becomes a reliable reporter for pain, some time in the early school years (Table 1).

The decision to seek medical care for a symptom arises from a parent's or caretaker's concern for the child. The caretaker's threshold for concern varies with their own experiences and expectations, coping style, and perception of their child's illness. For this reason, the office visit is not only about the child's symptom, but also about the family's conscious and unconscious fears. The clinician must not only make a diagnosis, but also recognize the impact of the symptom on the family's emotional tone and ability to function. Therefore, any intervention plan must attend to both the child and the family. The success of management depends upon securing a therapeutic alliance with the parents.

Through the first years of life children cannot accurately report symptoms such as nausea or pain. The infant and preschool child cannot discriminate between emotional and physical distress. Therefore, the clinician depends upon the reports and interpretations of the parents, who know their child best, and the observations of the clinician, who is trained to differentiate between health and illness.

Disability from a functional symptom is related to maladaptive coping with the symptom. Childhood functional gastrointestinal disorders are not dangerous when the symptoms and parental concerns are addressed and contained. Conversely, failed diagnosis and inappropriate treatments of functional symptoms may be the cause of needless physical and emotional suffering. In severe cases, well-meaning clinicians inadvertently co-create unnecessarily complex and costly solutions to functional symptoms, prolonging emotional stress and promoting disability.

Table 1. Functional Gastrointestinal Disorders

A. Esophageal Disorders

A1. Globus
A2. Rumination syndrome
A3. Functional Chest Pain of Presumed
Esophageal Origin

A4. Functional Heartburn
A5. Functional Dysphagia
A6. Unspecified Functional Esophageal
Disorder

B. Gastroduodenal Disorders

B1. Functional Dyspepsia
B1a. Ulcer-like Dyspepsia
B1b. Dysmotility-like Dyspepsia
B1c. Unspecified (nonspecific) Dyspepsia

B2. Aerophagia
B3. Functional Vomiting

C. Bowel Disorders

C1. Irritable Bowel Syndrome
C2. Functional Abdominal Bloating
C3. Functional Constipation

C4. Functional Diarrhea
C5. Unspecified Functional Bowel
Disorder

D. Functional Abdominal Pain

D1. Functional Abdominal Pain Syndrome
D2. Unspecified Functional Abdominal Pain

E. Functional Disorders of the Biliary Tract and the Pancreas

E1. Gallbladder Dysfunction
E2. Sphincter of Oddi Dysfunction

F. Anorectal Disorders

F1. Functional Fecal Incontinence
F2. Functional Anorectal Pain
F2a. Levator Ani Syndrome
F2b. Proctalgia Fugax
F3. Pelvic Floor Dyssynergia

G. Functional Pediatric Disorders

G1. Vomiting
G1a. Infant regurgitation
G1b. Infant rumination syndrome
G1c. Cyclic vomiting syndrome
G2. Abdominal pain
G2a. Functional dyspepsia
G2a1. Ulcer-like dyspepsia
G2a2. Dysmotility-like
dyspepsia
G2a3. Unspecified
(nonspecific) dyspepsia

G2b. Irritable bowel syndrome
G2c. Functional abdominal pain
G2d. Abdominal migraine
G2e. Aerophagia
G3. Functional diarrhea
G4. Disorders of defecation
G4a. Infant dyschezia
G4b. Functional constipation
G4c. Functional fecal retention
G4d. Functional non-retentive
fecal soiling

— G I a. Infant Regurgitation

Definition

Regurgitation is the involuntary return of previously swallowed food or secretions into or out of the mouth. Regurgitation is distinguished from vomiting, which is defined by a central nervous system reflex involving both autonomic and skeletal muscles in which gastric contents are forcefully expelled through the mouth because of coordinated movements of the small bowel, stomach, esophagus, and diaphragm. Regurgitation is also different from rumination, in which previously swallowed food is voluntarily returned to the pharynx and mouth, chewed, and swallowed again. Regurgitation, vomiting, and rumination are examples of gastroesophageal reflux. Gastroesophageal reflux refers to movement of gastric contents retrograde and out of the stomach. When gastroesophageal reflux causes or contributes to tissue damage or inflammation (e.g., esophagitis, obstructive apnea, reactive airway disease, pulmonary aspiration, or failure-to-thrive), it is called gastroesophageal reflux disease.

Epidemiology

Daily regurgitation is common in the first year. Regurgitation occurs more than once a day in 67% of healthy 4 month-old infants. Some parents believe regurgitation is a problem, with 24% of all parents complaining during their infant's sixth month [1]. Daily regurgitation decreases with age to 5% of infants 10 to 12 months old. Occasional regurgitation may persist until the third year in a few healthy children.

— Diagnostic Criteria

(1) **Regurgitation 2 or more times per day for 3 or more weeks;**

(2) **There is no retching, hematemesis, aspiration, apnea, failure-to-thrive, or abnormal posturing;**

(3) **The infant must be 1 to 12 months of age and otherwise healthy;** *and*

(4) **There is no evidence of metabolic, gastrointestinal, or central nervous system disease to explain the symptom.**

Neither the forcefulness of the regurgitation nor its outflow through the mouth or nares carries diagnostic relevance.

Choosing a defining duration of regurgitation of three weeks is a departure from other functional gastrointestinal disorders, which most often are defined by symptom durations of three months or more. The Working Team agreed to three weeks because infants come to medical attention more quickly, and symptoms cause more parental anxiety than in older children and adults.

Clinical Evaluation

History and physical examination may provide evidence of disease outside the gastrointestinal tract, including a large number of metabolic, infectious, and neurologic conditions associated with vomiting. Risk factors for the development of gastroesophageal reflux disease include prematurity, developmental delay, and congenital abnormalities of the oropharynx, chest, lungs, central nervous system, or gastrointestinal tract [2]. Physical signs which may indicate a systemic condition associated with chronic regurgitation include eczema (milk allergy), and an abnormal neurological exam. Evidence of failure-to-thrive, hematemesis, occult blood in the stool, anemia, or food refusal should prompt an evaluation for gastroesophageal reflux disease.

If there has not been improvement by 12–18 months of age, a radiographic study to evaluate upper gastrointestinal anatomy should be performed to evaluate for malrotation or another anatomic abnormality responsible for partial bowel obstruction, if it had not been done earlier as part of an evaluation for the possibility of gastroesophageal reflux disease.

Physiologic Features

Infant regurgitation is a transient problem, perhaps in part due to postnatal maturation of upper gastrointestinal motility. In premature infants large volume or high osmolality meals delay gastric emptying by inducing postprandial duodenal hypomotility [3–5]. A full gastric fundus, in turn, predisposes to transient lower esophageal sphincter relaxation. Regurgitation occurs as a consequence of brief lower esophageal sphincter relaxations. Postprandial duodenal motility changes over the first weeks and months of life, to a mature pattern in which meal volume does not affect the rate of emptying, and the duodenum increases motility with larger, more complex meals.

Another factor contributing to regurgitation during infancy is esophageal volume. In the newborn the volume of the esophagus is just a few milliliters. The esophageal volume (V) can be calculated by the formula $V=\pi r^2 h$, where r is the radius and h is the esophageal length (as for a cylinder). As a child grows, the volume increases by both the square of the esophageal radius and its length. Thus, if a newborn esophagus is 10 cm and has a radius of 2.5 mm, then its volume is about 2 ml. If an adult esophagus is 25 cm long and has a radius of 7.5 mm, then its potential volume is 44 ml. Although the length of the newborn esophagus is 40% that of the adult, the infant esophagus volume is only one twentieth of the adult esophageal volume. Refluxed material is likely to go much farther up the esophagus of the infant.

Psychologic Features

Maternal anxiety, infant temperament, and environmental stressors may interact to cause an aberrant maternal-child interaction [6,7]. Infants may regurgitate as one symptom of emotional distress. Feeding problems, such as early satiety, food refusal, and excessive crying may occur with consequent failure-to-thrive [8–10].

Treatment

The natural history of infant regurgitation is one of spontaneous improvement [1]. Therefore, treatment goals are to provide effective reassurance and symptom relief while avoiding complications.

Effective reassurance includes (1) an empathetic, satisfactory response to the stated and unstated fears of the caretakers: *What is wrong with the baby? Is it dangerous? Will it go away? What can we do about it?* and (2) a promise of continuing clinician availability and reassessment [11].

Symptom relief includes adjustments in infant care and medication. Prone positioning reduces reflux and may be of value in diminishing the frequency of vomiting [12]. Thickening the infant formula by adding cereal may be of similar value [13]. Frequent smaller volume feedings to satiety may decrease vomiting. For improving a troubled maternal-child interaction, the clinician prescribes a trial of therapeutic comfort for the mother and child. The steps in providing therapeutic comfort include: (1) relieve the parents' fears about the condition of the infant; (2) aid the parent in identifying sources of physical and emotional distress; make a plan to reduce or eliminate them; and (3) assure clinician availability for follow-up.

Drugs that improve esophageal and gastric motility such as cisapride reduce reflux [14]. Although prescribing drugs for a functional disorder might increase the parents' perception of their child's vulnerability, this effect may be outweighed by symptom resolution. Parents are reminded that, analogous to acetaminophen for fever, the medicine treats a symptom, not a disease.

— G1b. Infant Rumination Syndrome

Definition

Rumination is the voluntary, habitual regurgitation of stomach contents into the mouth for the purpose of self-stimulation [15]. Non-ruminative gastroesophageal reflux may provide a basis in experience for its development [16].

Rumination has three clinical presentations: (1) infant rumination syndrome [17]; (2) rumination in mentally retarded children and adults; and (3) rumination in healthy older children and adults. The latter two presentations are discussed in Chapter 5.

Epidemiology

Infant rumination syndrome is rare. It seems to have been more prevalent earlier in this century, as indicated by Kanner's report of seven cases per thousand admissions to an acute care pediatric hospital [18]. It is five times more prevalent in males than females [19].

— Diagnostic Criteria

(1) At least 3 months of stereotypical behavior beginning with repetitive contractions of the abdominal muscles, diaphragm, and tongue, and culminating in the regurgitation of gastric contents into the mouth, which is either expectorated or rechewed and reswallowed, and 3 or more of the following:
(a) Onset between 3 and 8 months;
(b) Does not respond to management for gastroesophageal reflux disease, anticholinergic drugs, hand restraints, formula changes, and gavage or gastrostomy feedings;
(c) Unaccompanied by signs of nausea or distress and/or
(d) Does not occur during sleep and when the infant is interacting with individuals in the environment.

Clinical Evaluation

Observing the ruminative act is essential for diagnosis. However, such observations require time, patience, and stealth because rumination may cease as soon as the infant notices the observer [15].

No readily available diagnostic test identifies rumination as the etiology of vomiting or regurgitation (antroduodenal manometry identifies rumination in adults and children evaluated at special centers). In the past, the diagnosis of infant rumination depended on the resolution of symptoms with empathic and responsive nurturing [20,21].

Diagnostic efforts should be directed toward the parents as well as the infant because infant rumination syndrome results from malfunction in the infant care giver relationship. Interviews with each parent and the infant and parents together [22] are important.

Physiologic Features

Reversal of the abdominal-thoracic pressure gradient coupled with relaxation of the lower esophageal sphincter mechanism is probably similar in infants and adults who ruminate (see Chapter 5). One of the features that makes infant rumination much more dangerous than adult rumination is the infant's inability to retain enough regurgitated nutrients for nutritional sufficiency. This causes potentially lethal malnutrition, a complication that seldom if ever occurs in older ruminators [17].

Psychologic Features

The emotional and sensory deprivation that prompts rumination may occur in sick infants living in environments that prevent normal handling, e.g., neonatal intensive care units [23]. It may also occur in otherwise healthy infants whose mothers are emotionally unconnected. The mother's behavior may appear to be neglectful or slavishly attentive, but in every case, there is no enjoyment in holding the baby or sensitivity to the infant's needs for comfort and satisfaction [17,24–29]. The aberrant nurturing relationship is one aspect of more pervasive difficulties the parents have with interpersonal relationships. There is often a history of traumatic emotional deprivation during childhood and of marital dysfunction [16, 19–24].

The pathogenesis of infant rumination syndrome can be understood in light of developmental phenomena that emerge at about three months of age [17]. The infant develops a sense of self. The infant learns that the infant and mother are physically separate and have different affective experiences. The awareness of separateness from the need-gratifying mother is the condition that makes possible feelings of helplessness in the infant.

Fortunately, two means of coping also develop at about three months: (1) the infant becomes able to evoke a social response from the mother; and (2) he gains the ability to entertain and satisfy himself by producing interesting noises and activities. If the infant's efforts fail to elicit sufficient tension-relieving responses from the mother, he may resort to more self-stimulation. The concept of rumination as self-stimulating behavior provides both a theoretical basis for its pathogenesis and an effective approach to management [17,25].

Management

Loss of previously swallowed food may cause progressive inanition and death [15,16,25–27,29–31].

Behavioral therapy that employs aversive techniques and positive reinforcement is useful in eliminating rumination in highly motivated adults or children with mental retardation and neurologic handicaps [32]. The use of such measures in infants [33] may be harmful if therapeutic goals are limited to symptom suppression without addressing the infant's unmet needs for mothering and the mother's inability to engage her baby in a mutually satisfying relationship. The most humane, developmentally appropriate and comprehensive management aims at reversing the baby's weight loss by eliminating its need for ruminative behavior. This can be achieved by providing a temporary mother-substitute to hold, comfort, and feed the infant while he or she is awake. The nurturing person should be sufficiently sensitive and observant to know when the infant withdraws into the self-absorbed state that fosters rumination and promptly respond by engaging the baby socially [17,19–22]. Treatment also aims at helping the mother change her feelings toward herself and her infant and to improve her ability to recognize and respond to her infant's physical and emotional needs.

The weight loss and rumination rapidly respond to nurturing that is sensitive and interactive. It may be exacerbated by withdrawal of reciprocal care-giving, and by the noxious stress of the work-up that accompanies "diagnosis by exclusion." After rumination with failure-to-thrive subsides, it usually does not recur, even in families whose overall mental health remains poor [34].

— G I c. Cyclic Vomiting Syndrome

Definition

Cyclic vomiting syndrome (CVS) consists of recurrent, stereotypic episodes of intense nausea and vomiting lasting hours to days which are separated by symptom-free intervals [35]. The frequency of episodes in a series of 71 patients ranged from 1 to 70 per year and averaged 12 per year. Attacks may occur at fairly regular intervals or sporadically. Typically, episodes begin at the same time of day, most commonly during the night or in the morning. The duration of episodes tend to be the same in each patient over months or years [36]. Once vomiting begins, it reaches its highest intensity during the first hours [37]. The frequency of vomiting tends to diminish thereafter, although nausea continues until the episode ends. Episodes usually end as rapidly as they begin and are marked by prompt recovery of well-being, provided the patient has not incurred major deficits of fluids and electrolytes.

Signs and symptoms that may accompany cyclic vomiting include pallor, weakness, increased salivation, abdominal pain, intolerance to noise, light and/ or odors, headache, loose stooling, fever, tachycardia, hypertension, skin blotching, and leukocytosis [38].

Eighty percent of patients can identify circumstances or events that trigger some or most of their attacks. The most common triggers are heightened emotional states, which may be either noxious (e.g., anxiety) or pleasant excitement (e.g., birthdays or vacations), infections (e.g., upper respiratory infection), asthma, or physical exhaustion [36].

Epidemiology

Population-based studies have shown the prevalence of cyclic vomiting syndrome to be 2.3% in Western Australian children [39], and 1.9% in the school children from Aberdeen, Scotland [40]. Cyclic vomiting syndrome affects equal numbers of boys and girls. Onset may occur from infancy to mid-life, but is most common between two and seven years [41]. Migraine, increased susceptibility to motion sickness, and functional bowel disorders are more prevalent in patients with CVS as well as in their families.

— Diagnostic Criteria

(1)   **A history of 3 or more periods of intense, acute nausea and unremitting vomiting lasting hours to days, with intervening symptom-free intervals lasting weeks to months.**

(2)   **There is no metabolic, gastrointestinal, or central nervous system structural or biochemical disease.**

Clinical Evaluation

Patients do not vomit between episodes, but two-thirds of them have symptoms of irritable bowel syndrome, and 11% have migraine headaches. Motion sickness is a problem for about 40% of those affected by CVS. Over half have family histories of irritable bowel syndrome and nearly half have a family history of migraine headache.

The differential diagnosis of CVS includes diseases having similar presentations during at least part of their courses [42]. Brain stem gliomas may infiltrate the vomiting centers and cranial nerves around the medulla causing intermittent vomiting without obstruction of flow of cerebral spinal fluid or signs of increased intracranial pressure. Obstructive uropathy may cause symptoms indistinguishable from cyclic vomiting syndrome [35]. Gastrointestinal causes mimicking cyclic vomiting include peptic disease with pyloric outlet obstruction, recurrent pancreatitis, intermittent small bowel obstruction, chronic intestinal pseudo-obstruction, and the vomiting crises of familial dysautonomia. Endocrine and metabolic conditions to be considered include pheochromocytoma, adrenal insufficiency, diabetes mellitus, ornithine transcarbamylase deficiency, medium-chain acyl coenzyme A dehydrogenase deficiency, proprionic acidemia, isovaleric acidemia (the chronic intermittent form), and porphyria [36, 42].

Physiologic Features

Cyclic vomiting syndrome is a paroxysmal disorder related to the episodic activation of the emetic reflex. The reflex consists of a pre-ejection phase accompanied by autonomic activation (pallor, headache, nausea, drooling, etc.) followed by an ejection phase with repeated retching and vomiting. Cyclic vomiting episodes are accompanied by intense autonomic discharge and release of ACTH, vasopressin, norepinephrine, and prostaglandin E_2 in some or most patients [43,44].

Psychologic Features

A majority of parents in a study (with no control population) described their affected children as having one or more of these personality traits: competitive, perfectionistic, high-achieving, strong-willed, moralistic, caring, and enthusiastic [36].

The natural course of cyclic vomiting syndrome in any individual is unpredictable. Patients and parents feel oppressed and fearful because of the mysterious, uncertain nature of the illness. Depression and anxiety disorders complicate nearly a third of CVS patients [38].

Treatment

There is no standard management for cyclic vomiting syndrome.

Prevention becomes a goal in patients whose episodes are frequent, severe, and prolonged. Prophylactic daily treatment with cyproheptadine, amitriptyline, erythromycin, phenobarbital, or propranolol succeed in reducing the frequency or eliminating episodes in many children [45–48]. Conditions that trigger episodes may be identified and treated.

Aborting episodes is possible in some children with a recognizable prodrome. Prior to the onset of nausea, oral medications such as ondansetron, erythromycin, and ibuprofen may be useful. Early in the episode it may be helpful to begin an oral acid-inhibiting drug agent to protect esophageal mucosa and dental enamel, and lorazepam for its anxiolytic, sedative, and anti-emetic effects.

Patients whose episodes cannot be prevented or interrupted should be sedated until the episodes end because sleep is the only comfort for patients with intractable nausea. Symptoms may be interrupted by titrating intravenous lorazepam until the patient enters restful sleep. In some patients combinations of intravenous ondansetron, granisitron, diphenhydramine, and chlorpromazine may be helpful [49]. Intravenous fluids, electrolytes, and H_2-histamine receptor antagonists are administered until the episode is over. Complications arising during cyclic vomiting episodes include water and electrolyte deficits, hematemesis due to peptic esophagitis and/or Mallory-Weiss tears, deficits in intracellular potassium and magnesium, hypertension, and inappropriate secretion of antidiuretic hormone [49].

Although both are paroxysmal disorders involving interactions between the central nervous system and the gastrointestinal tract, CVS is differentiated from abdominal migraine by the most distressing symptom. In CVS, vomiting is the most distressing symptom, but in abdominal migraine pain is the most distressing symptom.

G2. Abdominal Pain

The Working Team agreed that two well-recognized conditions did not fulfill the necessary criteria to be included as functional gastrointestinal disorders, although they have been useful clinical markers for decades: infant colic and recurrent abdominal pain of childhood.

Infant colic has been defined as crying during the first three months of life for three or more hours per day on three or more days per week in infants who do not suffer from other conditions that may cause crying [61,62,63]. There is no proof that the crying of infant colic is caused by pain in the abdomen or any other part of the infant's body. Nevertheless, parents often assume that the cause of excessive crying is abdominal pain of gastrointestinal origin. There is no evidence that the gastrointestinal tract is involved. We note colic because infants with colic are often referred to pediatric gastroenterologists, but the Working Team achieved consensus to exclude infant colic from the list of childhood functional gastrointestinal disorders.

Forty years ago John Appley's meticulous study of 1000 English schoolchildren set the standard for research on childhood recurrent abdominal pain [53]. The heuristic view of recurrent abdominal pain in the 1950s was based on careful history and observation. Subsequent clinical research in this area utilized Appley's description of recurrent abdominal pain: "three or more bouts of pain severe enough to affect activities over a period of not less than three months" [53].

Despite the Working Team's respect for and familiarity with the term, recurrent abdominal pain of childhood, we reached consensus that this diagnosis may be too vague, and chose not to include it at this time in the listing of childhood functional bowel disorders for several reasons.

Appley's criteria may be too general. Since Appley's publication exceptional scientific advances (e.g., endoscopy, laparoscopy, *H. pylori* as a pathogen) have expanded the ability to diagnose and treat gastrointestinal disease. Also, mental health diagnostic categories for somatization and pain disorders have been clarified. Previous studies of recurrent abdominal pain may have included symptomatic children with unrecognized medical or mental health disorders that were not functional but still met the diagnostic criteria for recurrent abdominal pain of childhood. Appley's description did not anticipate the concept of functional symptoms and symptom-based diagnosis.

Working team members were unanimous in agreeing that the symptoms in school-aged children with chronic or recurrent abdominal pain often meet the Rome Criteria for functional dyspepsia and irritable bowel syndrome. It would seem appropriate to apply the most specific diagnostic category to a symptomatic child, to learn the natural history of functional gastrointestinal disorders with childhood onset, and to consider novel intervention strategies for children who meet the diagnostic criteria for these conditions.

Finally, there is a growing body of evidence to suggest that functional abdominal pain is often associated with visceral hyperalgesia, a lowered threshold for pain related to biochemical changes in the afferent neurons of the enteric and central nervous systems. We use this theory to explain the pathogenesis of pain, thus alleviating guilt and concern that the problem is "psychological."

— G2a. Functional Dyspepsia

Definition

Dyspepsia is defined by a persistent or recurrent pain or discomfort centered in the upper abdomen [54] (see also Chapter 6). Dyspepsia may arise from disease (e.g., gastroesophageal reflux, *Helicobacter pylori* -associated peptic disease, Crohn's disease) or it may be functional. Functional dyspepsia has two presentations, one ulcer-like and the other dysmotility-like, although considerable variation and overlap occur [55]. In ulcer-like dyspepsia, upper abdominal pain is the dominant feature, and it is often relieved by food and by inhibiting gastric acid secretion, and may wake the patient from sleep. In dysmotility-like dyspepsia, pain is not the dominant symptom. Rather, the patient complains of nausea, early satiety, postprandial fullness, retching or vomiting, and a sense of bloating.

Epidemiology

The prevalence of dyspepsia in adolescents is approximately 10% [56].

— Diagnostic Criteria

In children mature enough to provide an accurate pain history, at least 12 weeks, which need not be consecutive, in the preceding 12 months of:

(1) Persistent or recurrent pain or discomfort centered in the upper abdomen (above the umbilicus);

(2) No evidence of organic disease (including at upper endoscopy) that is likely to explain the symptoms; *and*

(3) No evidence that dyspepsia is exclusively relieved by defecation or associated with the onset of a change in stool frequency or stool form (i.e., not irritable bowel).

Functional dyspepsia has not been rigorously defined in a pediatric population. Therefore we have adopted the adult diagnostic criteria for use in children. The concept of subdividing functional dyspepsia based on distinctive features may be useful. These divisions seem especially relevant to those proposing to study functional dyspepsia.

G2a1. Ulcer-like Dyspepsia
Pain centered in the upper abdomen is the predominant (most bothersome) symptom.

G2a2. Dysmotility-like Dyspepsia
An unpleasant or troublesome nonpainful sensation (discomfort) centered in the upper abdomen is the predominant symptom; this sensation may be characterized by early satiety, upper abdominal fullness, bloating, or nausea.

G2a3. Unspecified (Nonspecific) Dyspepsia
Symptomatic patients whose symptoms do not fulfill the criteria for either ulcer-like or dysmotility-like dyspepsia.

Clinical Evaluation

The approach to the child or adolescent with dyspeptic symptoms starts with a detailed history (including dietary, psychological, and social factors), physical examination, and inspection of growth data. Heartburn and regurgitation usually represent gastroesophageal reflux disease. The clinician must inquire about symptoms suggesting organic disease: radiation of the epigastric pain to the back, blood in the stool or emesis, weight loss, persistent vomiting, fever, diarrhea, or dysphagia. Demographic factors such as lower socioeconomic class, family crowding, parents born in Third World countries, and a family history of *Helicobacter pylori* infection should raise suspicion for disease associated with this microorganism [55,57]. Some children may present with persistent dyspepsia following a viral illness. Although the acute viral symptoms such as fever, myalgia, headache, and vomiting abate, these children are left with persistent abdominal discomfort, nausea, and early satiety. These individuals are presumed to be suffering from a post-viral gastroparesis [58].

Failure to respond to an H_2-histamine receptor antagonist or symptom recurrence upon stopping medication should prompt further investigation. The clinician determines whether symptoms are more likely to represent esophagogastroduodenal mucosal disease (esophagitis, gastritis, duodenitis, ulcer) or a disorder of the liver, gallbladder, or pancreas. Upper gastrointestinal endoscopy is warranted for the former. Measuring serum amylase, lipase, and aminotransferase concentrations and an abdominal ultrasound aid in assessing the latter conditions. Controversy exists concerning serologic tests for *H. pylori* in children with recurrent abdominal pain [55,57]. Urea breath tests, while sensitive and specific [59], are currently not readily available. Most clinicians regard endoscopy as the standard for diagnosis of *H. pylori*-associated gastritis and ulcer disease.

Physiologic Features

There are no pediatric data about the physiology of functional dyspepsia as defined by validated symptom-based criteria. Children diagnosed with functional dyspepsia without standardized criteria had abnormalities in antroduodenal manometry [60] and electrogastrography [61].

Psychologic Features

There are no pediatric data.

Treatment

With a normal physical examination including stools without occult blood, normal growth, and the absence of historical factors suggesting medical disease, effective reassurance may be all that is required. Effective reassurance consists of transmitting not only a cognitive message, but also changing the emotional context for the parents from feeling worried to feeling safe [11].

Non-steroidal anti-inflammatory medication or aspirin use may be associated with dyspepsia, and these drugs should be discontinued if possible. Foods aggravating symptoms (e.g., caffeine-containing foods, spicy and fatty foods) should be avoided. Psychological factors which may be contributing to the severity of the problem should be addressed. For mild dyspepsia a therapeutic trial of antacid may improve symptoms. Smaller, more frequent meals that are lower in fat may improve symptoms in those with early satiety.

Treatment for functional dyspepsia is directed toward providing symptomatic relief. No controlled trials exist for medications for functional dyspepsia in children. Histamine receptor antagonists, proton pump inhibitors, sucralfate, and low dose tricyclic antidepressants such as imipramine and amitriptyline have been used. Drugs which increase motility such as cisapride may prove helpful for feelings of early satiety and fullness, while metoclopramide may be helpful for nausea. Anti-nausea medication (phenothiazines, serotonin type-3 antagonists) have been tried.

— G2b. Irritable Bowel Syndrome

Definition

Irritable bowel syndrome comprises a group of functional bowel disorders in which abdominal discomfort or pain is associated with defecation or a change in bowel habit, and with features of disordered defecation [62] (see also Chapter 7).

Epidemiology

Recent population based studies indicate that 6–14% [56] of the adolescent population note symptoms consistent with the irritable bowel syndrome (IBS). In one outpatient pediatric gastroenterology clinic, IBS was the most common cause of recurrent abdominal pain noted over a two year period [63].

— Diagnostic Criteria

In children old enough to provide an accurate pain history, at least 12 weeks, which need not be consecutive, of continuous or recurrent symptoms during the preceding 12 months of:

(1) Abdominal discomfort or pain that has two out of three features:
   (a) Relieved with defecation; *and/or*
   (b) Onset associated with a change in frequency of stool; *and/or*
   (c) Onset associated with a change in form (appearance) of stool.
(2) There are no structural or metabolic abnormalities to explain the symptoms.

Symptoms that Cumulatively Support the
Diagnosis of Irritable Bowel Syndrome:

- *Abnormal stool frequency (for research purposes "abnormal" may be defined as greater than 3 bowel movements per day and less than 3 bowel movements each week);*
- *Abnormal stool form (lumpy/hard or loose/watery stool);*
- *Abnormal stool passage (straining, urgency, or feeling of incomplete evacuation);*
- *Passage of mucus;*
- *Bloating or feeling of abdominal distension.*

Clinical Evaluation

A history that fits the Rome Criteria for a diagnosis of IBS, accompanied by a normal physical examination and normal growth history, are consistent with a diagnosis of childhood IBS. A nutritional history, assessing for adequacy of dietary fiber in those with constipation, as well as ingestion of sugars such as sorbitol and fructose in those with diarrhea, is often useful. Factors alerting the clinician to the possibility of disease include nocturnal pain or diarrhea, weight loss, rectal bleeding, fever, arthritis, delayed puberty, and a family history of inflammatory bowel disease. A limited laboratory screening for disease is frequently reassuring to the clinician, patient, and family for patients with persistent symptoms and may include a complete blood count and erythrocyte sedimentation rate, stool studies for enteric bacterial pathogens and parasites, and breath hydrogen testing or a trial of a milk free diet for lactose malabsorption. During the initial visits, and after establishing rapport with the patient and family, the clinician inquires about the psychosocial history of the patient and family.

Physiologic Features

There are no pediatric data. In adults, motility and sensory abnormalities have been described (see Chapter 7).

Psychologic Features

Anxiety and depression were more prevalent in adolescents with IBS than the control population [56]. Psychological data in childhood are limited to assessments in recurrent abdominal pain [64–71], and so are not directly applicable to childhood irritable bowel syndrome.

Treatment

Once there is a diagnosis of IBS, the treatment goals are to provide effective reassurance, and to reduce or eliminate the symptom. The clinician must educate and reassure the child and family that although IBS causes discomfort it is not serious or life-threatening. The presence or severity of the pain should not be disputed. A review of the current understanding of IBS and the exacerbating effects of stress and anxiety on the problem helps the child and family to understand why the pain occurs. Psychosocial difficulties and triggering events for symptoms should be identified and addressed.

Drug therapy plays an adjunctive role in IBS treatment. Tricyclic antidepressants such as imipramine or amitriptyline in low doses improved symptoms in adults with IBS in controlled, blinded studies [72,73]. These drugs have been used for decades for chronic visceral pain by pain management specialists, but there are only anecdotal reports concerning their use in children with chronic abdominal pain. Amitriptyline has greater sedative and anticholinergic effects than imipramine, and so amitriptyline may be a better choice for children who wake at night with pain, or for children with a diarrheal component to their disorder. Imipramine may be a better choice than amitriptyline for children with a tendency to constipation; at the low doses used for chronic visceral pain, constipation is rarely exacerbated. Anticholinergic medications such as dicyclomine, hyoscine, mebeverine, and octylonium have been used for their antispasmodic properties, but there are no well designed studies confirming efficacy. In those with constipation, increased dietary fiber (recommended daily fiber intake = age (yrs) + 5 grams), milk of magnesia, or mineral oil may be a helpful adjunct.

In patients with intractable symptoms endoscopic evaluation of the colon may be indicated (e.g., colonoscopy and biopsy). If the terminal ileum is not intubated, it may be imaged with small bowel series or white blood cell technetium scan. Irritable Bowel Syndrome may occur concurrently in patients with inflammatory bowel disease.

— G2c. Functional Abdominal Pain

Definition

There are pediatric patients with functional abdominal pain who do not meet the criteria for a diagnosis of IBS or functional dyspepsia. In these children there is no demonstrable organic disease, and there is no recognizable constellation or association of symptoms. The pain does not relate temporally to eating, defecation, menses, or exercise. It may be recurrent or continuous and may affect daily activities. The pain is usually periumbilical and may keep the patient from sleeping or awaken the patient from sleep. It is often associated with school difficulties, and with previously unrecognized learning problems in children and families with expectations for achievement.

The Pediatric Working Team chose to include functional abdominal pain syndrome, the previously defined adult functional gastrointestinal disorder, because we believed that functional abdominal pain syndrome occurs in children and adolescents. The term "functional abdominal pain syndrome" is not related to, and is not meant to substitute for Appley's "recurrent abdominal pain of childhood."

Epidemiology

There are no data.

— Diagnostic Criteria

At least 12 weeks of:

(1) **Continuous or nearly continuous abdominal pain in a school-aged child or adolescent;** *and*

(2) **No or only occasional relationship of pain with physiological events (e.g., eating, menses, or defecation);** *and*

(3) **Some loss of daily functioning;** *and*

(4) **The pain is not feigned (e.g., malingering);** *and*

(5) **Insufficient criteria for other functional gastrointestinal disorders that would explain the abdominal pain.**

Clinical Evaluation

Although abdominal pain is the dominant complaint, there is often a history of headache, lightheadedness, dizziness, nausea (without vomiting), and easy fatigue. Physical examination and growth are normal in children with functional abdominal pain syndrome. Laboratory investigations including urinalysis, erythrocyte sedimentation rate, complete blood count, stool examinations for occult blood, leukocytes, ova and parasites, and blood chemistries are normal. Abdominal ultrasound, breath hydrogen testing, endoscopy, and radiographic tests are normal.

Physiologic Features

There are no data for this entity.

Psychologic Features

Commonly, unrecognized psychological factors, including anxiety and/or depression in the child and family, somatization, and secondary gains for illness behavior are at least partially responsible for the disability associated with this condition. Some children with unidentified learning disabilities may present with abdominal pain, even though they may have a history of high school achievement. There may be associated school phobia, separation anxiety, and maternal-child enmeshment. Sleep disturbances are common.

Treatment

Parents and the affected child often do not accept psychological explanations for the symptoms. Effective reassurance that there is no disease requires not only a convincing explanation for how a symptom occurs in the absence of laboratory abnormalities, but also necessitates a therapeutic alliance between the family and the clinician. Failure to develop a therapeutic alliance guarantees that the family will seek consultations, evaluations, and treatments elsewhere. Each negative test increases the anxiety that something is being missed.

The presence of abdominal pain cannot be disputed. The parents and child anger if they sense that the clinician suspects that the pain is fabricated, "psychogenic," or "all in the head." The child and family are educated about functional pain in the context of other functional disorders. Emphasizing the absence of disease but the presence of sensitive nerves sending pain messages to the brain is a means to introduce the idea that one way to treat the problem is to teach the brain how to decrease the pain signals.

After providing effective reassurance that the condition is understood, and that there is no need for more testing, the clinician promises continuing availability: (1) to guide the child through a period of readjustment and improvement, and (2) to re-evaluate whenever symptoms change or otherwise become worrisome.

Finally, the clinician must provide something for the parents and child to do, so that healthy daily activities resume, healthy sleep patterns re-emerge, and the patient feels in control, even if the pain does not resolve. Physical exercise periods are encouraged. A pain diary describing the intensity and accompanying events, thoughts, and feelings helps the child and parent objectively assess the context in which pain occurs. Tricyclic antidepressants before bedtime may facilitate sleeping, and non-sedating serotonin reuptake inhibitors may be effective in the morning.

In the presence of continued or intractable symptoms, often associated with a disruption of the life of the child and the family, there may be a need for further evaluation for medical disease (e.g., endoscopy) and psychological evaluation. The reluctance to accept psychological testing is managed by presenting the psychologist as one member of a multidisciplinary team that is required to help the child regain function.

— G2d. Abdominal Migraine

Definition

Abdominal migraine is a paroxysmal disorder characterized by the acute onset of incapacitating, non-colicky, mid-line abdominal pain that lasts for hours and is accompanied by pallor and anorexia [74–76]. Associated features include: a family history of migraines, increased susceptibility to motion sickness, prodromal changes in mood and activity, and other accompaniments of migraine episodes, e.g., phonophobia, photophobia, headache, vomiting, and sleepiness. When accompanied by a history of migraine headaches, the diagnosis is straightforward. Rarely, there is no history of headaches, and the diagnosis is presumptive. The affected individual usually has a stereotypical clinical presentation, is well between attacks, and has a family history of migraine headaches. Episodes often begin during the night or early morning. Lethargy commonly signals the end of an attack, and after a period of sleep, the symptoms resolve. Abdominal migraine may be part of the clinical expression of migraine.

Epidemiology

Abdominal migraine affects about 2% of children [75]. It is most prevalent in children 5 to 7 years of age and in twice as many girls and boys. It occurs in adults, although its prevalence is unknown [76].

— Diagnostic Criteria

(1) In the preceding 12 months, 3 or more paroxysmal episodes of intense, acute midline abdominal pain lasting two hours to several days, with intervening symptom-free intervals lasting weeks to months; *and*

(2) Evidence of metabolic, gastrointestinal, and central nervous system structural or biochemical diseases is absent; *and*

(3) **Two of the following features:**
    (a) **Headache during episodes;**
    (b) **Photophobia during episodes;**
    (c) **Family history of migraine;**
    (d) **Headache confined to one side only;**
    (e) **An aura or warning period consisting of either visual symptoms (e.g., blurred or restricted vision), sensory symptoms (e.g., numbness or tingling), or motor symptoms (e.g., slurred speech, inability to speak, paralysis).**

Clinical Evaluation

All organic causes of intermittent severe abdominal pain should be considered, including obstructive uropathy, malrotation and its complications, intermittent bowel obstruction, recurrent pancreatitis, biliary tract disease, intercranial space-occupying lesions, Familial Mediterranean Fever, and metabolic disorders. A favorable response to medications used for prophylaxis of migraine headaches supports the diagnosis of abdominal migraine.

Peptic disease is often considered in the differential diagnosis because of the common presentation of pain beginning at night or in the early morning. However, abdominal migraine patients are entirely well between episodes.

Physiologic Features

The physiologic mechanisms causing the pain of abdominal migraine are unknown.

Psychologic Features

The psychologic features of the disorder are unknown.

Treatment

No treatment regimen for established episodes has been published. Effective prophylaxis of episodes has been reported from the United Kingdom using pizotifen, a serotonin receptor antagonist [77]. This agent is unavailable in the United States. Another anti-serotonergic drug, cyproheptadine, is effective in some patients with migraine headaches and cyclic vomiting syndrome [78] and might be helpful in the prophylaxis of abdominal migraine.

— G2e. Aerophagia

Definition

Aerophagia is a disorder of excessive air swallowing causing progressive abdominal distension. It is associated with repeated audible swallows, anorexia, abdominal pain, excessive flatus, excessive burping, resolving spontaneously each night.

Epidemiology

No data exist on the prevalence of this disorder in childhood.

— Diagnostic Criteria

At least 12 weeks, which need not be consecutive, in the preceding 12 months of two or more of the following signs and symptoms:

(1) Air swallowing;
(2) Abdominal distension due to intraluminal air; and
(3) Repetitive belching and/or increased flatus.

Clinical Evaluation

Partly because it may mimic other entities, partly because the toddler and preschool child does not explain to the parents what is happening, and finally because the child's gulping of air often goes unnoticed by parents, a diagnosis of aerophagia may not be appreciated early in its course [79]. Aerophagia may be confused with gastroesophageal reflux disease because of the noises in the throat noted by the parents and observed by the clinician. Aerophagia may be confused with generalized motility disorders such as chronic intestinal pseudo-obstruction or Hirschsprung's disease because of the associated abdominal distension. There may be a history of chewing gum or drinking excessive amounts of carbonated beverages. A normal physical examination and growth history help to exclude disease. Breath hydrogen testing may be of use, with lactose to test for lactose malabsorption and with lactulose to test for bacterial overgrowth and transit time. It is important to ask about recent stressful life events in the family because anxiety is a frequent cause for excessive swallowing.

Physiologic Features

Air is ingested with every swallow. If swallowing is excessive and persistent, then air fills the gastrointestinal lumen, resulting in excessive flatus, belching, abdominal distension, and pain, presumably a consequence of distension. There are no physiologic studies of aerophagia in children.

Psychologic Features

If stress and anxiety are associated with aerophagia, it makes sense to address the causes of stress, and to treat anxiety while addressing the aerophagia itself.

Treatment

Treatment consists of effective reassurance and an explanation for the symptom for the parents and the child. Often the clinician can help the child become aware of swallows during the visit. Behavioral modification, relaxation and breathing techniques, and other psychotherapies may be helpful for the child in some cases.

— G3. Functional Diarrhea (also called Toddler's Diarrhea, chronic nonspecific diarrhea, irritable colon of childhood)

Definition

Functional diarrhea is defined by the daily painless recurrent passage of three or more large unformed stools for four or more weeks with onset in infancy or pre-school years. There is no evidence for failure-to-thrive if the diet has adequate calories. Parents become aware of a problem when unformed stools containing easily identified pieces of undigested vegetables eaten just a few hours earlier run down or over the diaper. The child appears unperturbed by the loose stools, and the symptom resolves spontaneously by school age.

Epidemiology

Functional diarrhea is the leading cause of chronic diarrhea in an otherwise well child from an industrialized country.

— Diagnostic Criteria

For more than 4 weeks, daily painless, recurrent passage of 3 or more large, unformed stools, in addition to all of these characteristics:

(1) **Onset of symptoms begins between 6 and 36 months of age;** *and*

(2) **Passage of stools occurs during waking hours;** *and*

(3) **There is no failure-to-thrive if caloric intake is adequate.**

Clinical Evaluation

The evaluation of children with chronic diarrhea includes historical queries concerning factors which may cause or exacerbate diarrhea, such as past enteric infections, ingestion of laxatives, prokinetics, antibiotics, or dietary constituents. In toddlers with functional diarrhea, typical stools contain mucus and/or visible indigestible food particles. Often there is a progressive decrease in stool consistency with each bowel movement during the day in infants and toddlers with functional diarrhea. Problems in the diet that may cause diarrhea include overfeeding, excessive fruit juice consumption, excessive carbohydrate ingestion with low fat intake, and food allergy. Excessive sorbitol intake results in diarrhea.

The clinician examines the child, with special attention to height, weight, and signs of malnutrition, diaper rash, and fecal impaction (another cause for chronic loose stools).

Laboratory screening tests include a complete blood count (increased eosinophils suggest allergy, microcytic anemia and thrombocytosis suggest iron deficiency), stool analysis for occult blood and leukocytes, fat globules, and stool collections for ova and parasites. Culture for enteric pathogens and for *Clostridium difficile* toxin may be necessary in selected cases. Although infectious gastroenteritis rarely causes chronic diarrhea, *Giardia lamblia* and *Cryptosporidium* are frequent agents implicated as causing diarrhea in toddlers attending day care centers. If there is growth deceleration or a family history of celiac disease, then screening tests with anti-gliadin and anti-endomysial antibodies are helpful.

In children who fulfill the criteria for functional diarrhea, a malabsorption syndrome would be unexpected. Chronic diarrhea as the sole symptom in a thriving child make cystic fibrosis and celiac disease unlikely. Latent and atypical forms of celiac disease and mild forms of cystic fibrosis with isolated pancreatic involvement are exceptions. If there is deceleration in growth or a family history for either of these two diseases exists, then screening to detect malabsorption (serum iron , ferritin, albumin, immunoglobulins, cholesterol, fat-soluble vitamins) should include more specific tests: sweat chloride and serum anti-endomysial antibodies.

Physiologic Features

Both motility and mucosal factors have been proposed to explain functional diarrhea.

Mucosal Factors

Intestinal transport is not defective in children with functional diarrhea. Water and electrolyte secretion and glucose absorption are normal [80]. Steatorrhea is absent in children with functional diarrhea.

In jejunal biopsies from children with functional diarrhea, activities of the mucosal enzymes Na-K ATPase and adenylate cyclase were elevated [81]. The increase in mucosal enzyme activity was associated with an increase in plasma prostaglandin E_2 and F concentrations [82]. Aspirin reduced plasma prostaglandin concentration and resolved the diarrhea [83]. Loperamide, an opiate agonist, has little effect on prostaglandins, but also reduced stool output. These results are intriguing in view of the normal jejunal secretion in children with functional diarrhea, and because of the action of prostaglandins on cyclase activation and intestinal secretion.

Intestinal Motility

In healthy children and adults, the migrating motor complex—the recurring sequence of three consecutive contraction patterns which cycles through the small bowel during fasting—is interrupted by a meal. A meal normally stimulates a pattern of frequent variable amplitude contractions, some of which mix the luminal contents and others which propagate. In functional diarrhea, food fails to interrupt the migrating motor complex [84]. As soon as phase 3 of the migrating motor complex begins in the stomach, a cluster of high amplitude gastric antral contractions sweep undigested gastric contents through a wide open pylorus, into and through the small bowel, with early arrival to the colon. The failure to induce a postprandial motility pattern results in a kind of colonic dumping, with excess bile salts and incompletely digested food. Sodium and bile acid concentrations are elevated in the extractable water phase of stools from toddlers with functional diarrhea [85].

Psychologic Features

The morbidity associated with functional diarrhea is related to the caloric deprivation caused by the misuse of elimination diets [86]. The misuse of elimination diets may be related to an anxious parent's inability to accept a functional diagnosis for the symptom, or a clinician's attempt to assuage the parent's anxiety.

Wender found a correlation between active temperament and functional diarrhea [87].

Treatment

For the child, no treatment is necessary. For the parents effective reassurance is of paramount importance. A daily diet and defecation diary helps to reassure parents that specific dietary items are not responsible for the symptom. Many families accept effective reassurance readily, and follow-up is unnecessary. For others, it helps to schedule regular visits for monitoring weights and responding to parents' questions. Diet modifications are occasionally effective: increasing daily fiber intake helps to improve stool consistency. Fruit juices containing high fructose and sorbitol are reduced or avoided. Although failure to induce a normal postprandial motor response seems to be the most likely mechanism for functional diarrhea, medications to slow motility are seldom necessary. If chronic diarrhea persists and is troublesome, a trial of loperamide may improve the quality of life.

G4. Disorders of Defecation

The defecation frequency of healthy infants and children varies with age [88]. The normal range is broadest in healthy breast-fed infants. Healthy breast milk-fed infants may defecate as frequently as 12 times per day, or as infrequently as once in 3 or 4 weeks. Firm stools may occur from the first weeks of life in formula-fed infants. Although there is no identifiable enteric neuromuscular disorder, these infants may experience painful defecation, and so have a predisposition towards developing functional fecal retention (see below).

Complaints related to defecatory problems are responsible for 25% of outpatient visits to pediatric gastroenterologists [89].

— G4a. Infant Dyschezia.

Definition

Parents describe infants with dyschezia as straining for many minutes, screaming, crying, turning red or purple in the face with effort. The symptoms persist for 10 to 20 minutes, until there is passage of soft or liquid stool. Stools pass several times daily. The symptoms begin in the first months of life, and resolve spontaneously after a few weeks.

— Diagnostic Criteria

At least 10 minutes of straining and crying before successful passage of soft stools in an otherwise healthy infant less than 6 months of age.

Clinical Evaluation

The examiner performs a history (including diet), physical examination (including rectal examination) to exclude anorectal abnormalities, and charts the infant's growth.

Physiologic Features

Failure to coordinate increased intra-abdominal pressure with relaxation of the pelvic floor results in infant dyschezia. The infant's cries increase intra-abdominal pressure.

Psychologic Features

Defecation requires increasing intra-abdominal pressure and simultaneously relaxing the pelvic floor. Coordination of these two independent events to effect successful defecation may occur by chance, but eventually defecation is learned.

The child's parents require effective reassurance. It is their perception that their child is in pain and that something is wrong with the infant.

Treatment

Parents are reassured by a methodical physical examination completed in their presence. They are happy to accept the explanation that the child needs to learn to relax the pelvic floor at the same time as bearing down. To encourage the infant's defecation learning, the parents are advised to avoid rectal stimulation, which produces artificial sensory experiences which may be noxious.

— G4b. Functional Constipation

Defecation disorder represents the chief complaint in 3% of pediatric outpatient visits and 10 to 25% of pediatric gastroenterology visits. Few reports distinguish between functional constipation and functional fecal retention, so the frequency of functional constipation is unknown [90]. Children with cerebral palsy often develop functional constipation.

— **Diagnostic Criteria**

In infants and children, at least two weeks of:

(1) **Scybalous, pebble-like, hard stools for a majority of stools;** *or*
(2) **Firm stools 2 or less times/week;** *and*
(3) **There is no evidence of structural, endocrine, or meta-bolic disease.**

Clinical Evaluation

In most cases, a thorough history and physical examination are sufficient to diagnose functional constipation. Delayed passage of meconium in a full-term newborn raises the suspicion of Hirschsprung's disease [91]. In a few healthy breast-fed infants there may be weeks between bowel movements but the stools are soft [92]. The transition from breast to formula feedings is often associated with the appearance of functional constipation. However infants on formula feedings and children who pass stools at intervals greater than a week apart and fail to thrive are likely to have an enteric neuromuscular, anatomic, or metabolic disease. Ingestion of medication causing constipation needs to be excluded.

At physical examination inspection of the back and spine and verification of deep tendon and cremasteric reflexes help to exclude occult spinal dysraphism. At least one anorectal examination is performed allowing the physician to evaluate anatomy, tone, and masses. Laboratory and radiologic examinations are not warranted in the absence of poor weight gain, persistent abdominal distension, fever, Down syndrome, bilious vomiting, or any abnormal physical findings mentioned above. Functional constipation is important because it may predispose to the development of functional fecal retention.

Treatment

In infants, fruit juices which contain fructose and sorbitol such as prune and pear increase stool water. Barley, corn syrup, lactulose and sorbitol can also be used, but mineral oils are not recommended [93]. When solid food is introduced, provision of adequate amounts of liquids and fibers is encouraged (age in years + 5 = number of grams of dietary fiber per day).

— G4c. Functional Fecal Retention

Definition

Functional fecal retention (FFR) is the most common cause for constipation and fecal soiling in children. It consists of repetitive attempts to avoid defecation because of fears associated with defecation. The child contracts the pelvic floor in response to the defecatory urge. As a consequence, a fecal mass builds in the rectum. The fecal mass is passed after days, weeks, or even months, during a retentive crisis [94].

Epidemiology

Constipation accounts for 3% of visits to pediatric clinics, and 10–25% of visits to pediatric gastroenterology clinics [95,96]. It is likely that 10% of children will present to a health care provider for constipation at some time. Most problems with chronic constipation are due to functional fecal retention [97].

— Diagnostic Criteria

From infancy to 16 years old, a history of at least 12 weeks of:

(1) Passage of large diameter stools at intervals < 2 times per week; *and*

(2) Retentive posturing, avoiding defecation by purposefully contracting the pelvic floor. As pelvic floor muscles fatigue, the child uses the gluteal muscles, squeezing the buttocks together.

Accompanying symptoms may include fecal soiling, irritability, abdominal cramps, decreased appetite and/or early satiety. The accompanying symptoms disappear immediately following passage of a large stool.

Clinical Evaluation

The history of painful defecation, passage of huge stools at infrequent intervals, and retentive posturing are diagnostic. Onset frequently occurs during one of three periods: (1) in infants with hard stools (often corresponding with the change from breast milk to commercial formula); (2) in toddlers learning toilet behavior, as they attempt to control bowel movements, and find defecation painful; and (3) as school starts, and children attempt to avoid defecation throughout the school day. A physical examination provides reassurance to the clinician and parents that there is no disease. The physical examination includes assessing the size of the rectal fecal mass, which is judged for height above the pelvic brim with bimanual palpation on either side of the rectus sheath. A rectal examination is performed after establishing rapport with patient and family. In functional fecal retention, the initial rectal examination occasionally causes the child to react with acute, intense fear and negative behaviors. An irrational fear of the rectal examination typifies the child with functional fecal retention, and is rarely a problem in children with other complaints, including other defecatory disorders. Some Working Team members believe that when the history is typical for FFR, the perineum should be inspected but a digital rectal examination may be delayed, to facilitate the therapeutic alliance between the child and clinician, until after a treatment trial. Other Working Team members believe that a rectal examination is obligatory on the first visit to evaluate the child for an obstructing mass.

Occult spinal dysraphism (e.g., lipoma of the cauda equina, tethered cord, anterior sacral meningocele) is a cause of retentive or non-retentive fecal soiling. Signs of spinal dysraphism include pelvic floor weakness (patulous anus, involuntary spurt of urine with the Crede maneuver, absence of reflex contraction of the external anal sphincter and pelvic floor with a voluntary cough, urinary incontinence); diminished tactile sensitivity in the sacral dermatomes; asymmetry of the buttocks, calves, or feet; hyperactive or absent Achilles tendon reflexes; abnormal plantar reflexes; pigmentary abnormalities; vascular nevi or sinuses in the lumbo-sacral region; scoliosis suggestive of vertebral malformation; or radiologic abnormalities of the lumbo-sacral spine [98].

Anorectal manometry, anal sphincter ultrasound, or radiography is unnecessary for the routine evaluation of functional fecal retention [99].

Physiologic Features

All the child's symptoms are explained by voluntary efforts to avoid defecation. Pain results from colonic contractions pushing luminal contents against an obstructing fecal mass and closed anal sphincter. Incontinence occurs when stool seeps around the fecal mass, and leaks out when the child relaxes the pelvic floor or anal sphincter, either inadvertently (as in sleep), with fatigue, or with attempts to pass flatus.

Psychologic Features

In most cases fear of painful defecation is the cause for the fecal retention [100]. Occasionally, the fear may be linked to a specific event associated with anxiety or pain, such as an episode of perianal streptococcal disease [101], lichen sclerosus et atrophicus [102], sexual abuse [103], or even a horrifying television show or commercial [104]. When children provide an accurate report of their fears, the fears can be addressed with tact and sensitivity.

Although fear of painful defecation is the initial cause, after several years of FFR affected children often evolve a coping style based on denial. School-aged children insist that they are unaware of a problem. This apparent nonchalance is part of the syndrome as the school-aged child attempts to avoid facing fears about defecation. It is common for the child to deny rectal sensations, an inaccurate statement that is consistent with their choice to feign ignorance of their own fecal soiling.

Toddlers with FFR may attribute the pain associated with defecation to fantastic, living stuff coming out of them. This may be frightening, and create an emotional climate that does not favor toilet learning. Parents may find themselves in a power struggle with their child concerning toilet learning issues.

School-aged children suffering with FFR feel alone and frightened. They have fantasies about their problem, which may include:

(1) They are the only one with this problem.
(2) Their colon might burst, or leak toxic, rotten stuff into them.
(3) They are incurable.
(4) The problem will turn into cancer (*Uncle Jack was constipated and he had cancer!*).

It is possible that some affected children may find the sensations related to withholding stool pleasurable.

Treatment

Education for both parents and child is the first step in treatment, beginning during the initial interview. The child who is frightened and embarrassed appreciates a clinician with a direct approach. The clinician addresses the myths and fears: the child has FFR, the most common cause of childhood constipation, and one of the most common problems in pediatrics. It goes away in time, and it is not dangerous. These statements assuage the child's and family's anxiety, and create an expectation for positive change.

Next, parents need to be helped to understand the child's point of view. For toddlers, toilet training will not proceed smoothly until the child's fear of painful defecation resolves. Parents who are anxious (*"We can not put him into day care until he's potty trained!"*) must understand that coercive toilet training tactics are likely to backfire into an unwinnable struggle for control.

Next, the clinician, child, and parent agree on a plan for evacuating the rectal fecal mass. Some experts favor daily oral mineral oil, which slowly softens the mass until the child chooses to pass it, days or weeks later. In a biopsychosocial model, this developmentally sound, non-intrusive approach returns the control of the child's pelvic floor to the child. Many toddlers with FFR are frightened of any anal manipulation, and find enemas particularly scary. Other experts view the fecal mass as an obstruction, and favor enemas and stimulant laxatives to expedite its expulsion. They argue that early passage of the obstructing mass gives the child immediate relief, and provides the confidence necessary for continuing toilet learning.

For maintenance there are a variety of effective stool softeners, including mineral oil, lactulose, and colonic lavage solutions. Stimulant laxatives should be avoided. Docusate sodium has no role in treating FFR. Although dietary fiber is important for a variety of reasons, fiber supplements are not adequate as a single agent for consistent stool softening. The goal of stool softening is to assure painless defecation for every stool until FFR resolves.

Behavior modification utilizing rewards for successes in toilet learning is often helpful. A child may earn stars for a chart with each successful defecatory effort. Older children may ask for small amounts of money, or special time with a parent, for example.

Another behavior modification technique is to establish a daily routine for sitting on the commode. Sitting on the commode for 10 minutes after eating takes advantage of the gastrocolonic response, the increase in colonic motility following a meal.

— G4d. Non-retentive Fecal Soiling

Definition

Fecal soiling without fecal retention occurs in diarrheal diseases, as the pelvic floor muscles fatigue. Patients may be incontinent of stool because of damaged corticospinal pathways from any cause. Non-retentive fecal soiling occurs after endorectal pull-through surgery, as high amplitude propagating ileal or colonic contractions push luminal contents through the anal sphincter in the absence of a rectosigmoid reservoir. Functional non-retentive soiling may be a manifestation of an emotional disturbance in a school-aged child. Often, soiling episodes have a relationship to the presence of a person (e.g., a parent) or time of day, because the soiling episodes are an impulsive act triggered by unconscious anger. For example, a patient soils daily when his father returns home from work, or at dinnertime, with the family gathered for a meal.

Spock-Bergen syndrome is a rare cause of non-retentive soiling due to delayed acquisition of toilet learning because the parents were excessively fearful of causing emotional trauma to the child during conflict over requirements for more mature behavior [105].

Epidemiology

The incidence and prevalence of functional non-retentive fecal soiling is unknown. One group reported that one-third of children referred for fecal incontinence show no signs of constipation [106]. Most pediatric gastroenterologists estimate that 5–20% of children referred for encopresis have functional non-retentive soiling.

— Diagnostic Criteria

Once a week or more for the preceding 12 weeks, in a child older than 4 years, a history of:

(1) Defecation into places and at times inappropriate to the social context;

(2) In the absence of structural or inflammatory disease; *and*

(3) In the absence of signs of fecal retention (listed in G4c above).

Clinical Evaluation

Most children with non-retentive fecal soiling defecate daily during waking hours, resulting in few complaints of associated constipation. Their episodes of soiling may be small in volume, or consist of a large bowel movement. In contrast to children with functional fecal retention and soiling, children with non-retentive soiling are without masses of stool on physical or X-ray examination.

Physiologic Features

There are no data.

Psychologic Features

The impulse to soil often seems triggered by unconscious anger. The soiling is one of several behaviors (e.g., sloppiness, procrastination, lack of consideration for others) that typifies the child in a passive-aggressive relationship with his parents.

Treatment

There is no need to treat with laxatives or stool softeners. One goal is to help the parent to acknowledge the absence of medical disease and to accept a referral to a mental health professional. The parents are often enraged at a child they interpret as willfully creating an obnoxious symptom. Parents need guidance to understand that soiling is a symptom of emotional upset, not simply bad behavior.

Conclusions and Recommendations for the Future

The child copes with symptoms based not only on genetic predispositions (to sensory stimuli or temperament, for example) and developmental stage, but also from cues and care provided by parents and society. We hypothesize that the keys to understanding the variability in health care utilization for adult functional gastrointestinal disorders may be found, in part, in early childhood experiences and learned behaviors. Early interventions for childhood symptoms may alter the expression of adult functional illness. There are a variety of possible nerve connections, and environmental stimuli influence neuroanatomy and neurochemistry. The goodness of fit between the infant's needs and the response from the environment alter an infant's behavior and the onset of symptoms [107]. Preventing illness might begin by identification and treatment of aberrant relationships in the perinatal period and throughout infancy.

— Recommendations

Functional gastrointestinal disorders other than those mentioned in this chapter occur during childhood, but are defined adequately by the adult criteria. The list of adult functional bowel disorders also found in children and adolescents includes: rumination, functional chest pain, functional heartburn, functional dysphagia, and proctalgia fugax. We did not describe functional biliary disorders because documentation and experience with childhood gallbladder and sphincter of Oddi dysfunction are sketchy at this time.

(1) Validating the diagnostic criteria for the childhood functional gastrointestinal disorders will be an important goal for the next decade. Epidemiologic community-based studies and studies of populations thought to be at risk (e.g., children of patients with functional gastrointestinal disorders, female child abuse victims) are needed to determine the applicability of the diagnostic criteria, which were arrived at by consensus rather than by data analysis.

(2) Clinical trials measuring symptom change as the primary outcome measure will help us to learn which interventions improve outcomes in the childhood functional gastrointestinal disorders.

(3) Definitions and diagnostic criteria for currently unrecognized childhood functional gastrointestinal disorders are needed.

(4) A history of physical, sexual, and/or emotional abuse will be elicited from some children with functional bowel disorders. There is a need for education and training related to the evaluation and treatment of child abuse for all clinicians who care for children with functional gastrointestinal disorders.

(5) The role of childhood functional gastrointestinal disorders on adult functional gastrointestinal disorders should be explored.

References

1. Nelson SP, Chen EH, Syniar GM, et al. Prevalence of symptoms of gastroe-sophageal reflux during infancy. Arch Pediatr Adolesc Med 1997;151:569–72.
2. Vandenplas Y. Gastroesophageal reflux in children. Scand J Gastroenterology 1995;30(suppl 213):31–38.
3. Tawil YA, Berseth CL. Gestational and postnatal maturation of duodenal motor responses to intragastric feeding. J Pediatr 1996;129:374–81.
4. Knapp E, Berseth CL. Immature duodenal motor responses to bolus feedings are associated with delayed gastric emptying in preterm infants. Pediatr Res 1996;39: 313A.
5. Baker JH, Berseth CL. Duodenal motor responses in preterm infants fed formula with varying concentrations and rates of infusion. Pediatr Res 1997;42:618–22.
6. Levy R. Mother-infant relations in the feeding situation. In: Lebenthal E, Editor. Textbook of Gastroenterology and Nutrition in Infancy. New York:Raven Press; 1981:633–44.
7. Lewis M, Lee-Painter S. An interactional approach to the mother-infant dyad. In: Lewis M, Rosenblum LA, Editors. The Effect of the Infant On Its Caregiver. New York:Wiley and Sons;1974:21–48.
8. Ferholt J, Provence S. Diagnosis and treatment of an infant with psychophysio-logical vomiting. Psychoanal Study Child 1976;31:439–59.
9. Fleisher DR. Functional vomiting disorders in infancy: innocent vomiting, ner-vous vomiting, and infant rumination syndrome. J Pediatr 1994;125:s84–s94.
10. Fleisher DR. Comprehensive management of infants with gastro-esophageal reflux and failure to thrive. Curr Prob Pediatr 1995;25:247–53.
11. Fleisher DR. Integration of biomedical and psychosocial management. In: Hyman PE, DiLorenzo C, Editors. In: Pediatric Gastrointestinal Motility Disorders. New York:Academy Professional Information Services;1994:13–31.
12. Orenstein SR, Whittington PF. Positioning for preventing infant gastroesophageal reflux. Pediatr 1982;69:768–72.
13. Orenstein SR, Magill HL, Brooks P. Thickening of infant feedings for therapy of gastroesophageal reflux. J Pediatr 1987;110:181–86.
14. Scott RB, Ferreira C, Smith L, et al. Cisapride in pediatric gastroesophageal reflux. J Pediatr Gastroenterol Nutr 1997;25(5):499–506.
15. Cameron HC. Some forms of habitual vomiting in infancy. Brit Med J 1925;1: 872–76.
16. Hollowell JG, Gardner LI. Rumination and general growth failure in a male fra-ternal twin: association with disturbed family environment. Pediatr 1965;36: 565–71.
17. Fleisher DR. Infant rumination syndrome. Am J Dis Child 1979;133:266–69.
18. Kanner L. Child Psychiatry. Ed. 4. Springfield, IL:Charles C. Thomas;1972:463–64.
19. Mayes SD, Humphrey FJ, Hanford HA, et al. Rumination disorder: differential diagnosis. J Am Acad Child Adolesc Psychiatry 1988;27(3) 300–302.

20. Powell GF, Low JF, Speers MA. Behavior as a diagnostic aid in failure-to-thrive. J Devel Behav Pediatr 1987;8(1):18–24.

21. Singer L. Long-term hospitalization of nonorganic failure-to-thrive infants: patient characteristics and hospital course. J Devel Behav Pediatr 1987;8(1):25–31.

22. Hirschberg L. Clinical interviews with infants and their families. In: Zeanah C, Editor. Handbook of Infant Mental Health. New York:P Guilford Press;1993:173–90.

23. Sheagren TG, Mangurten HH, Brea F, et al. Rumination: a new complication of neonatal intensive care. Pediatr 1980;66(4)551–55.

24. Sauvage D, Leddet I, Hameury L, et al. Infantile rumination: diagnosis and follow-up study of twenty cases. J Am Acad Child Psychiatry 1985;24(2):197–203.

25. Richmond JB, Eddy E, Green M. Rumination: a psychosomatic syndrome of infancy. Pediatr 1958;22:49–54.

26. Stein ML, Rausen AR, Blair A. Psychotherapy of an infant with rumination. JAMA 1959;171:2309–12.

27. Gaddini R, Gaddini E. Rumination in infancy. In: Jessner L, Pavenstedt E, Editors. Dynamic Psychopathology in Childhood. New York:Grune & Stratton Inc.;1959:166–85.

28. Fullerton DT. Infantile rumination. Arch Gen Psychiatry 1963;9:593–600.

29. Menking M, Wagnitz JG, Burton JJ, et al. Rumination: a near-fatal psychiatric disease of infancy. New Engl J Med 1969;280:802–804.

30. Flanagan CH. Rumination in infancy. J Am Acad Child Psychiatry 1977;16:140–49.

31. Clark FH. Rumination. Arch Pediatr 1966;73:12–19.

32. Luckey R, Walson C, Music J. Aversive conditioning as a means of inhibiting vomiting and rumination. Am J Mental Deficiency 1968;73:139–42.

33. Lavigne J, Burns W, Cotter P. Rumination in infancy: recent behavioral approaches. Internat Eating Disorders 1981;1:70–82.

34. Sheinbein M. Treatment of the hospitalized infantile ruminator. Clin Pediatr 1975;14 (8):719–24.

35. Li BUK, Guest Editor. Cyclic vomiting syndrome: proceedings of the international scientific symposium on CVS. J Pediatr Gastroenterol Nutr 1995;21(suppl 1).

36. Fleisher DR, Matar M. The cyclic vomiting syndrome: a report of 71 cases and a literature review. J Pediatr Gastroenterol Nutr 1993;17:361–69.

37. Pfau BT, Li BUK. Differentiating cyclic from chronic vomiting patterns in children: quantitative criteria and diagnostic implications. Pediatr 1996;97:367–68.

38. Fleisher DR. Cyclic vomiting syndrome: a paroxysmal disorder of brain-gut interaction. J Pediatr Gastroenterol Nutr 1997;25(suppl 1):s13–s15.

39. Cullen KJ, MacDonald. The periodic syndrome: its nature and prevalence. Med J Australia 1963;2(5):167–72.

40. Abu-Arefeh I, Russell G. Cyclic vomiting in children: a population based study. J Pediatr Gastroenterol Nutr 1995;21(4):454–58.

41. Fleisher D. The cyclic vomiting syndrome described. J Pediatr Gastroenterol Nutr 1995;21(suppl 1):s1–s5.

42. Forbes D. Differential diagnoses of cyclic vomiting syndrome. J Pediatr Gastro-enterol Nutr 1995;21(suppl 1):s11–s14.

43. Fleisher DR. Cyclic vomiting. In: Hyman PE, DiLorenzo C, Editors. Pediatric Gastrointestinal Motility Disorders. New York:Academy Professional Informa-tion Services;1994:89–103.

44. Sato T, Igarashi N, Minami S, et al. Recurrent attacks of vomiting, hypertension and psychotic depression: a syndrome of periodic catecholamine and prosta-glandin discharge. Acta Endocrinologia (Copenhagen) 1988;117:189–97.

45. Pastricha PJ, Schuster MM, Saudek CD, et al. Cyclic vomiting: association with multiple homeostatic abnormalities and response to ketorolac. Am J Gastro-enterol 1996;91(10):2228–32.

46. Vanderhoof JA, Young R, Kaufman SS, et al. Treatment of cyclic vomiting in childhood with erythromycin. J Pediatr Gastroenterol Nutr 1995;21(suppl 1): s60–s62.

47. Forbes D, Withers G. Prophylactic therapy in cyclic vomiting syndrome. J Pediatr Gastroenterol Nutr 1995;21(suppl 1):s57–s59.

48. Anderson J, Sugerman K, Lockhart JR, et al. Effective prophylactic therapy for cyclic vomiting syndrome in children using amitriplytine or cyproheptadine. Pe-diatr 1997;100:977–81.

49. Gokhale R, Huttenlocher PR, Brady L, et al. Use of barbituates in the treatment of cyclic vomiting during childhood. J Pediatr Gastroenterol Nutr 1997;25:64–67.

50. Wessel MA, Cobb JC, Jackson EB, et al. Paroxysmal fussing in infancy, sometimes called colic. Pediatr 1954;14(5):421–34.

51. Carey WB. "Colic"—Primary excessive crying as an infant-environment interac-tion. Pediatr Clin North Am 1984;31(5):993–1005.

52. Barr RG. Colic and gas. In: Walker WA, Durie PR, Hamilton JR, et al., Editors. Pe-diatric Gastrointestinal Disease. Philadelphia PA:BC Decker;1991:56–61.

53. Apley J, Naish N. Recurrent abdominal pains:a field survey of 1,000 school chil-dren. Arch Dis Child 1958;33:165–70.

54. American Gastrointestinal Association Medical Position Statement: Evaluation of Dyspepsia. Gastroenterology 1998;114:579–81.

55. Graham DY, Malaty HM, Evans DG, et al. Epidemiology of Helicobacter pylori in an asymptomatic population in the United States: effect of age, race, and socio-economic status. Gastroenterology 1991;100:1495–1501.

56. Hyams JS, Burke G, Davis PM, et al. Abdominal pain and irritable bowel syn-drome in adolescents: a community-based study. J Pediatr 1996;129:220–26.

57. Mendall MA, Northfield TC. Transmission of Helicobacter pylori infection. Gut 1995;37:1–3.

58. Sigurdsson L, Flores A, Putnam PE, et al. Postviral gastroparesis: presentation, treatment, and outcome. J Pediatr 1997;131:751–53.

59. Vandenplas Y, Blecker U, Devreker T, et al. Contribution of the 13C-urea breath test to the detection of Helicobacter pylori gastritis in children. Pediatr 1992;90: 608–11

60. DiLorenzo C, Hyman PE, Flores AF, et al. Antroduodenal manometry in children and adults with severe non-ulcer dyspepsia. Scand J Gastroenterol 1994;29:799–806.

61. Cucchiara S, Riezzo G, Minella R, et al. Electrogastrography in non-ulcer dyspepsia. Arch Dis Child 1992;67:613–17.

62. Camilleri M, Prather CM. The irritable bowel syndrome: mechanisms and a practical approach to management. Ann Intern Med 1992;116:1001–1008.

63. Hyams JS, Treem WR, Justinich CJ, et al. Characterization of symptoms in children with recurrent abdominal pain: resemblance to irritable bowel syndrome. J Pediatr Gastroenterol Nutr 1995;20:209–14

64. Scharff L. Recurrent abdominal pain in children: a review of psychological factors and treatment. Clin Psychol Rev 1997;17:145–66.

65. Garber J, Zeman J, Walker LS. Recurrent abdominal pain in children: psychiatric diagnoses and parental psychopathology. J Am Acad Child Adolesc Psychiatry 1990;29:648–56.

66. Wasserman AL, Whitington PF, Rivara FP. Psychogenic basis for abdominal pain in children and adolescents. J Am Acad Child Adolesc Psychiatry 1988;27:179–84.

67. McGrath PJ, Goodman JT, Firestone P, et al. Recurrent abdominal pain: a psychogenic disorder? Arch Dis Child 1983;58:888–90.

68. Walker LS, Greene JW. Children with recurrent abdominal pain and their parents: more somatic complaints, anxiety, and depression than other patient families? J Pediatr Psych 1989; 14:231–43.

69. Walker LS, Garber J, Green JW. Somatization symptoms in pediatric abdominal pain patients: relation to chronicity of abdominal pain and parent somatization. J Abnormal Child Psychol 1991;19:379–94.

70. Hodges K, Kline JJ, Barbero G, et al. Anxiety in children with recurrent abdominal pain and their parents. Psychosomat 1985;26:859–56.

71. Walker LS, Garber J, Green JW. Psychosocial correlates of recurrent childhood pain: a comparison of pediatric patients with recurrent abdominal pain, organic illness, and psychiatric disorders. J Abnorm Psychol 1993;102:248–58.

72. Greenbaum DS, Mayle JE, Vangeren LE, et al. Effects of desipramine on irritable bowel syndrome compred with atropine and placebo. Dig Dis Sci 1987;32:257–66.

73. Pilowsky I, Barroro GG. A controlled study of psychotherapy and amitryptyline used individually in the treatment of chronic intractable psychogenic pain. Pain 1990;40:3–19.

74. Symon DNK, Russell G. Abdominal migraine: a childhood syndrome defined. Cephalagia 1986; 6:223–28.

75. Mortimer MJ, Kay J, Jaron A. Clinical epidemiology of childhood abdominal migraine in an urban general practice. Devel Med Child Neurol 1993;35:243–48.

76. Long DE, Jones SC, Boyd N, et al. Abdominal migraine: a cause of abdominal pain in adults. J Gastroenterol Hepatol 1992;7:210–13.

77. Symon DNK, Russell G. Double blind placebo controlled trial of pizotifen syrup in the treatment of abdominal migraine. Arch Dis Childhood 1995;72:48–50

78. Anderson J, Lockhart J, Sugerman K, et al. Effective prophylactic therapy for

cyclic vomiting syndrome in children using amitriptylene or cyproheptadine. Pediatr 1997;100(6):977–81.

79. Gauderer MWL, Halpin TC, Izant RJ. Pathologic childhood aerophagia: a recognizable clinical entity. J Pediatr Surg 1981;16:301–305.

80. Milla PJ, Atherton DA, Leonard JV, et al. Disordered intestinal functions in glycogen storage disease. J Inher Metab Dis 1978;1:155–57

81. Tripp JH, Muller DPR, Harries JT. Mucosal Na-K ATPase and adenylate cyclase activities in children with toddler diarrhea and postenteritis syndrome. Paediatr Res 1980;14:1382–86.

82. Dodge JA, Hamdi IA, Burns GM, et al. Toddler's diarrhea and prostaglandins. Arch Dis Child 1981;56:705–707

83. Hamdi I, Dodge JA. Toddler diarrhea: observations on the effects of aspirin and loperamide. J Pediatr Gastroenterol Nutr 1985;4:362–65.

84. Fenton TR, Harries JT, Milla PJ. Disordered small intestinal motility: a rational basis for toddler's diarrhea. Gut 1983;24:897–903.

85. Jonas A, Diver Haber A. Stool output and composition in the chronic non-specific diarrhea syndrome. Arch Dis Child 1982;57:35–39.

86. Lloyd-Still JD. Chronic diarrhea of childhood and the misuse of elimination diets. J Pediatr 1979;95:10–13.

87. Wender EH. Chronic non-specific diarrhea: behavioral aspects. Postgrad Med 1977; 62:83–88.

88. Weaver LT. Bowel habit from birth to old age. J Pediatr Gastroenterol Nutr 1988; 7:637–40.

89. Taitz LS, et al. Factors associated with outcome in management of defecation disorders. Arch Dis Child 1986;61:472–77.

90. Molnar D, Taitz LS, Uurwin, et al. Anorectal manometry results in defecation disorders. Arch Dis Child 1983;58:257–61.

91. Swenson O, Sherman JO, Fisher JH. Diagnosis of congenital megacolon: an analysis of 501 patients. J Pediatr Surg 1973;8:587–94.

92. Hyams JS, Treem WR, Etienne NL, et al. Effect of infant formula on stool characteristics of young infants. Pediatr 1995;95:50–54.

93. Fan LL, Graham LM. Radiological cases of the month: lipid pneumonia from mineral oil aspiration. Arch Pediatr Adolesc Med 1994; 148:205–206.

94. Fleisher DR. Diagnosis and treatment of disorders of defecation in children. Pediatr Ann 1976;5:71–101.

95. Levine MD. Children with encopresis: a descriptive analysis. Pediatr 1979;56: 412–16.

96. Loening-Baucke V. Chronic constipation in children. Gastroenterology 1993;105: 1557–64.

97. Loening-Baucke V. Constipation in early childhood: patients characteristics, treatment, and long-term follow-up. Gut 1993;34:1400–404.

98. Anderson FM. Occult spinal dysraphism. Pediatr 1975;55:826–35.

99. Sutphen J, Borowitz S, Ling W, et al. Anorectal manometric examination in encopretic-constipated children. Dis Colon Rectum 1997;40:1051–52.

100. Partin JC, Hamill SK, Fischel JE, et al. Painful defecation and fecal soiling in children. Pediatr 1992;89:1007–1009.

101. Spear M, Rothbaum R, Keating J, et al. Perianal streptococcal cellulitis. J Pediatr 1985;107:557–59.

102. Hurwitz S. Clinical Pediatric Dermatology. Philadelphia:WB Saunders;1993: 671–73.

103. Clayden GS. Anal appearances and child sexual abuse. Lancet 1987;1:620–21.

104. Pilapil VR. A horrifying television commercial that led to constipation. Pediatr 1990;85:592–93.

105. Spock B, Bergen M. Parents fear of conflict in toilet training. Pediatr 1964;34: 112–16.

106. Benninga MA, Buller HA, Heymans HSA, et al. Is encopresis always the result of constipation? Am J Dis Child 1994;71:186–93.

107. Lester BM, Boudykis CFZ, Gracia-Coll CT, et al. Development of outcome as a function of goodness of fit between the infant's cry characteristics and the mother's perception of her infant's cry. Pediatr 1995;95:516–21.

Chapter 11

Design of Treatment Trials for the Functional Gastrointestinal Disorders

Sander J. O. Veldhuyzen van Zanten, Chair,

Nicholas J. Talley, Co-Chair, *with*

Peter Bytzer,

Kenneth B. Klein,

Peter J. Whorwell,

and Alan R. Zinsmeister

Introduction

For many of the functional gastrointestinal disorders there is uncertainty whether truly efficacious treatments are available. Until recently little attention has been paid to the special challenges that design of clinical trials for the functional gastrointestinal disorders pose. An important problem in treatment trials of functional gastrointestinal disorders (FGIDs) is the variation in disease symptomatology and severity, and the possible influence that psychosocial factors may have. No structural or (patho)physiological outcome measures are available for the functional gastrointestinal disorders, making the task of how one determines efficacy of an intervention difficult. In order to establish efficacy of a treatment there must be agreement on what constitutes a clinically meaningful outcome. This has proved especially challenging for the functional gastrointestinal disorders, as there is both a lack of validated outcome measures and lack of consensus on which outcome measures to use.

— Aim of the Working Team

This committee was charged with developing guidelines for the design, conduct, and analysis of treatment trials in the functional gastrointestinal disorders. The guidelines should help researchers with the design of clinical treatment protocols. The guidelines should also enable regulatory agencies, health care providers, and other interested parties to better evaluate the methodologic quality of published studies.

There are few studies which have investigated issues in study design in this area [1,2]. A previous Working Team Report has addressed design issues in the irritable bowel syndrome [3]. Some of the recommendations from that report have been incorporated in this report and expanded upon. We have limited this review to design issues of clinical trials that attempt to evaluate the efficacy of treatment interventions. The report will follow the basic research architecture of randomized clinical trials, i.e., study design, inclusion and exclusion criteria, intervention, outcome measures and their validation, and statistical analyses. In each section recommendations will be made and, where possible, the evidence for the recommendations provided. It is clear, however, that there is an urgent need for empirical data to test these recommendations in clinical trials.

We would like to thank Drs. D. Drossman, J. Everhard, D. Patrick, R. C. Spiller, G. K. Turnbull, and W. E. Whitehead for their helpful suggestions for this manuscript.

— The Study Question

The study design should reflect the main question that the study proposes to investigate.

Although a trial can have several different objectives, the goals of many of the intervention studies in the functional gastrointestinal disorders will fall in one of four categories, listed in Table 1. The patient with irritable bowel syndrome may want a reduction in abdominal pain, the physician less frequent office visits or a more satisfied patient, the third-party payer less use of health care resources, the employer a reduction in sick leave or an increase in productivity, and family members a relative who appears happier and participates more fully in family life. All of these are legitimate endpoints for an intervention. However, a given treatment may not be capable of achieving them all, and it is very unlikely that a single clinical trial could be designed to assess such a multitude of endpoints simultaneously.

Given the current lack of effective therapies most treatment trials will ask the question whether the treatment under study is efficacious, i.e., leads to an improvement in severity or abolition of the symptoms for which the patient sought medical attention. To date no structural, pathophysiological, or functional abnormalities have been found that explain the origin and persistence of the symptoms of the functional gastrointestinal disorders. As a consequence, one has to rely on the subjective reporting of the (most important) symptoms or a global assessment of overall severity of the disease to determine whether an intervention is effective. Depending on the research question it may be reasonable to include other outcome measures. For example, intestinal motility or gut transit time can be measured in an irritable bowel syndrome trial when an agent that affects those parameters is studied. This may help explain why pa-

Table 1. Goals of a Treatment Trial

Reduction in severity or abolition of symptoms

Improvement in functional health status and quality of life

Improved ability to cope with symptoms

Decrease in use of health care resources

Improved ability to carry out normal daily activities and/or decrease in
number of sick leave days

tients' symptoms improve (assuming indeed an improvement in health status took place), or whether the improvement correlates with the other outcome measure(s). As will be discussed, currently pathophysiologic parameters cannot be primary outcome measures of a trial.

The trial must incorporate the principles of best and usual clinical practice as much as possible to ensure that the study results are relevant to the real practice situation.

It is important that investigators keep this important principle in mind while designing the trial. This requirement applies to all components of the study. It requires that all patients should be managed according to normal clinical practice after the diagnosis has first been made. This includes that the patient is given an adequate explanation of the disease and when necessary advice is given about obvious irregularities in the diet and eating habits prior to entering a patient in a trial. It is recognized that trials differ from usual practice in several ways, including use of placebo, use of stringent inclusion and exclusion criteria, frequent follow-up visits with extensive data recording and use of study coordinators. Nevertheless, it is important that standard aspects of diagnosis and management, especially adequate explanation and reassurance about the disease, are not omitted and any intervention be demonstrated to have a benefit over and above standard care.

— Patient Population

In general, it is advisable to include a broad spectrum of patients, as defined by the Rome Criteria.

The functional gastrointestinal disorders are defined by a combination of persistent or recurrent gastrointestinal symptoms that are not explained by structural or biochemical abnormalities. Extra-intestinal symptoms are also reported by patients suffering from these disorders, especially irritable bowel syndrome [4]. These are seen in higher frequency in patients with high health care utilization patterns and are related to psychosocial difficulties, anxiety and somatization disorders [5–7]. Several systematic reviews (meta-analyses) of treatment have shown that the inclusion criteria in trials of functional gastrointestinal disorders were often unclear, making the interpretation of the results difficult [1,2]. Researchers are increasingly adopting the diagnostic criteria of the Rome Working Parties of Functional GI Disorders [8]. The new Rome Diagnostic Criteria itself will require further validation, but this attempt at uniform classification of syndromes and diseases has been a major step forward. Use of similar diagnostic criteria by researchers will make it easier to compare studies.

If investigators want to apply special inclusion criteria, they should be justified.

Specification of inclusion and exclusion criteria is required. Depending on the type of intervention researchers may decide to target enrollment to a special population group, which is more narrowly defined than by the Rome Criteria or other accepted diagnostic criteria. The inclusion and exclusion criteria will involve much more than defining the type of patients that are being studied. It is beyond the scope of this chapter to recommend inclusion and exclusion criteria for all the functional gastrointestinal disorders. The study protocol should specify the criteria that were used to determine patient eligibility.

In general, it is recommended not to subcategorize patients with functional gastrointestinal disorders because of symptom instability.

Subcategorization of patients into subgroups has become more common especially in functional dyspepsia (e.g., ulcer-like or dysmotility-like dyspepsia) and irritable bowel syndrome (diarrhea- or constipation-predominant) [9]. These subgroups have also been used to select patients for treatment trials. In dyspepsia there is evidence for considerable overlap among the subgroups, i.e., patients fulfill the diagnostic criteria for several subgroups at the same time [10,11]. There is evidence that symptoms change over time with patients losing symptoms and acquiring new ones, thereby changing subgroup categories. Because of the noticeable instability of subgroups over time it is preferred that studies include a broad spectrum of patients, as defined by the main Rome Diagnostic Criteria, and changes in subgroup status be carefully measured. This is a change compared to the recommendations in the previous report on design of treatment trials of irritable bowel syndrome patients [3]. Investigators who want to apply special inclusion criteria must recognize that this can introduce a problem with generalizability. If the aim of the study is to target only a certain subgroup, the special reasons for doing so need to be explained. Importantly, the selection criteria need to make clinical sense.

— Overlap Syndromes and Diagnostic Tests

Overlap syndromes can make selection of patients difficult. For some disorders (e.g., dyspepsia), a clear plan is needed to address the ways that overlap between syndromes will be handled. An example is the potential overlap that exists between gastroesophageal reflux disease and functional dyspepsia [12–14]. In practice it may be impossible to completely prevent inclusion of patients with overlap syndromes.

The (minimum) set of investigations that are required of patients to enter studies should be specified, e.g. gastroscopy for functional dyspepsia or flexible sigmoidoscopy / colonoscopy / barium enema for irritable bowel syndrome. As will be discussed below, the timing of required diagnostic tests to meet inclusion criteria of a study may affect the severity of a patient's symptoms. Diagnostic tests should be the same in the different treatment arms of the study. If screening tests or visits are required to determine eligibility, it is useful to summarize basic clinical variables in those screened but not entered in the trial. Such a reject-log will provide useful information about the generalizability of the results.

The patient setting needs to be clearly considered as it may affect outcome.

Patients from primary, secondary, or tertiary level care are likely to have different patterns of response to treatment, e.g., more resistant patients are found in tertiary care. The majority of clinical trials of functional gastrointestinal disorders have been conducted in academic centers or centers with an obvious interest and expertise in particular disorders. For example, in only 8% of functional dyspepsia studies were patients enrolled at the primary care level [2]. Although empirical data is sparse, there likely will be a difference in the severity of symptoms and response to treatment between primary, secondary, and tertiary level patients. Tertiary centers may attract more patients at the severe end of the spectrum in whom it may be more difficult to achieve improvement, or who may truly be "intractable." There is an obvious need for studies carried out in primary care settings. The advantage of such studies will be that their results are likely to be applicable to the "average" patient (i.e., generalizable). In order to facilitate population-based studies, tertiary centers may consider setting up networks with primary care providers for the conduct of studies in which they have an interest.

For multicenter trials patient characteristics need to be measured in detail in order to ensure comparability of patients among centers.

In a single center study the patients are likely more homogeneous, but the disadvantage is that the results may not be generalizable. Most larger clinical trials tend to be multicenter. The advantage of such studies is their generalizability, but their possible disadvantage is patient heterogeneity. The latter may be an even greater problem in multinational studies. To some extent patient heterogeneity in multicenter studies is unavoidable. It is important that information is collected about the setting in which the patients were recruited. This means that for multicenter studies the participating centers need to as homogeneous as possible. For multicenter trials the distribution (average number and range) of included patients per center should be summarized and reported. The ways in which patients are identified for participation, including advertisements, may affect outcome.

— Patient Characteristics

A detailed list of patient characteristics that need to be specified in the protocol is beyond the scope of this chapter. Some of the important patient characteristics that should be measured include: age, gender, race, severity of disease, duration of disease, previous treatments for the condition under study, and coexisting medications. It may also be advisable to measure the presence of psychological distress or a history of mental health problems (e.g., diagnosis of depression, anxiety disorder). To date, most studies have provided little information about duration of disease, previous treatments for the disorder (either use in the past or recent use, or discontinuation of medication prior to enrollment in study), and use of coexisting medications. Some of these medications, e.g., minor tranquilizers, may have relevance for the intervention under study. Investigators should limit enrollment to those who have not participated in similar trials before, as patients who have failed previous experimental interventions may be less likely to respond. This will avoid selection of treatment-resistant patients.

Unique personality profiles have not been identified that help characterize patients with specific functional disorders, and psychological criteria are not part of the diagnostic criteria for any of the FGIDs. Nevertheless, measurement of psychological factors is suggested at least at baseline, as it is possible that such factors may affect the response to treatment (effect modifiers) [12–21]. Several validated instruments are available to assess presence of psychological distress or psychiatric problems. We refer the reader to Chapter 4[18]. For certain disorders it may also be important to collect other clinical information such as abdominal surgeries (irritable bowel syndrome, functional constipation) or cholecystectomy (biliary dyskinesia).

— Architecture of the Trial

A placebo or adequate control group is an essential requirement.

Although certain treatments look promising, such as psychotherapy for irritable bowel syndrome [18] or the use of the proton pump inhibitor omeprazole in functional dyspepsia [22], none of those treatments can be considered the current standard of care. Therefore a placebo control group remains essential. The placebo response can be particularly high in functional gastrointestinal disorders, which can make it more difficult to show superiority of a new treatment over placebo. In functional dyspepsia the placebo response has varied from 13–73% [1], while for irritable bowel syndrome the reported range has been up to 70% [2].

The parallel group design is the study design of choice and should be used in most circumstances.

The randomized clinical trial with parallel group design is now the accepted standard for evaluation of efficacy for the vast majority of treatments [23]. This design aims to provide a comparison between a control and a treatment group that is balanced or evenly distributed on all other (important) factors. Randomization is the most efficient and effective tool to achieve this balance. A strength of the parallel group design is that it is provides a simple means to avoid systematic error or bias, which might influence the comparison of the treatment groups.

Although crossover designs have been popular in treatment trials of certain functional gastrointestinal disorders (33% of functional dyspepsia and 50% of irritable bowel syndrome studies), this design is not recommended. This is an affirmation of the recommendations of a previous Working Team on study design in irritable bowel syndrome (in which two authors participated) [3], and recommendations from previous reviews [1,2]. Importantly, one of the members of this working team who has in the past defended use of crossover studies in certain circumstances also concurred that the parallel group is the design of choice [24].

— Comments About Study Designs

Crossover Design

As studies with crossover design have been popular we will briefly summarize the arguments for our recommendation that they not be used. Recently the N-of-1 design (multiple crossover within the same patient) has also been advocated as being well suited for identification of patients who are treatment responders [25].

The parallel group design makes between-subjects comparisons as opposed to the crossover and N-of-1 design where within-subject comparisons are made. In the N-of-1 design, patients are crossed-over several times and serve as their own controls. Crossover designs have the theoretical advantage that comparisons within rather than between patients need a smaller sample size to achieve a desired power (over parallel group designs) [26–28]. This assumes that within-subject variation is smaller than between-subject variation, but this is not necessarily true.

There are major disadvantages to the crossover design. Two of the baseline assumptions are that patients have symptoms: (1) which remain relatively constant over time, and (2) which return to baseline before crossover to the alternate treatment is begun[26]. A washout period is usually applied to try to achieve the latter. There can be marked variation in the symptoms of functional gastrointestinal disorders over time, which violates the requirement of symptom constancy. A well recognized problem in the two-period, two-treatment crossover trials is that the response in the second period is in part dictated by the response in the first period. This is an order or sequence effect, often referred to in the literature as a period-by-treatment interaction [26,27]. Essential hypertension is an example of a disease in which it is reasonable to expect that patients will go back to baseline during a washout period. A recent meta-analysis examining the use of the prokinetic agent cisapride in functional dyspepsia showed that the studies which used crossover designs found a greater treatment effect than studies using a parallel group design. This suggests that indeed study design may impact on the magnitude of an observed treatment effect [29].

Given the known variability in severity of gastrointestinal symptoms, it is unlikely that a return to baseline takes place in most cases. Furthermore, in many studies of functional gastrointestinal disorders, a continuing improvement in symptoms has been observed in the placebo-treated control groups, thereby creating a period effect [2]. The situation is still more complex if some but not all symptoms show a period-by-treatment interaction. A recent study on H2 receptor blockers in functional dyspepsia showed this phenomenon [30].

If a period-by-treatment interaction is present, the estimator of the treatment effect (based on both periods of the crossover design) is biased and the interpretation of the results is ambiguous. In this situation, it has been recommended that conclusions be based only on the treatment effect that was observed in the first period. By doing this there is a great loss in study power, thereby taking away one of the main advantages of the crossover design—the smaller sample size—over the parallel group design. Others argue that (under certain assumptions) it remains preferable to use the information from both periods. Brown has shown that estimating and adjusting for order effects requires a sample size greater than that needed for parallel group design [31]. Because of the high likelihood of period-by-treatment interactions in functional gastrointestinal disorders, crossover designs should be avoided.

Multiple Crossover and N-of-1 Design

Given the heterogeneity of patients fulfilling the diagnostic criteria for a particular disorder, it is unlikely that a single treatment will work for all patients. Therefore there is a role for methods that help identify true responders to a particular treatment. Parallel group trials convey the average effect of the treatment and do not recognize that there may be a subset of individuals who truly did respond. By using N-of-1 trials—also called single subject trials—subgroups of true responders to treatment may be identified. Multiple crossovers in single subjects (N-of-1 design) have been used in functional dyspepsia, in which they mainly were able to predict response in patients with dominant heartburn, i.e., suffering from gastroesophageal reflux disease [32,33]. Single subject trials have also been applied in the irritable bowel syndrome and in other chronic conditions such as fibromyalgia, obstructive pulmonary disease, rheumatoid arthritis, and ulcerative colitis [34–37].

Two different single subject trial designs have been applied in functional gastrointestinal disorders. The majority of designs have used multiple crossover (MCO) methods, consisting of a randomized sequence of treatment pairs with each pair including one period on active treatment and one period on placebo [32,33,38–42]. In most trials six to eight pairs each of a few days to a few weeks treatment have been used [33,42]. An alternative method (Random Starting Day Trial) was recently developed to allow the testing of drugs with a slower onset of action. In this design all patients receive placebo during a run-in phase and shift to active treatment at a randomized day, both test periods blinded to both patient and investigator [43]. Patients usually rate the outcome measure(s) at the end of each study period.

Provided that strict rules for inclusion criteria, treatment procedures, outcome measures and statistical analysis are met, the results from many individual N-of-1 trials may be combined [44,45], and common characteristics of individual responders to treatment may be detected in a multivariate analysis [33,42, 46]. However, it has been argued that the formal statistical assumptions for these analyses have not been met [47,48].

The MCO design has been able to predict responders to acid-suppressive treatment, although the effect was largely confined to dyspepsia patients who suffered from gastroesophageal reflux disease [32,33]. The ability of an MCO model to correctly predict the treatment response was subsequently confirmed in a study with a conventional parallel group design [41]. The model was also able to predict symptomatic relapse in a subsequent follow-up period on placebo [42,49]. A limitation of the MCO design is that it works best with treatments that are prompt in onset and offset of action. Effective blinding may be more difficult since patients have the opportunity to recognize and compare distinctive features, like side effects, in the active treatment with the placebo directly.

More research in this area is needed, particularly on new designs, validation of outcome, and confirmation of the identification of responders against other more conservative measures. Single subject trials cannot replace conventional group trials, but they may add important information, especially about responder characteristics.

Innovative Study Designs

Given the special methodologic challenges that functional gastrointestinal disorders trials pose, novel designs may be worth developing. One design that might be considered is the double-blind randomized-withdrawal design. This has been successfully used in inflammatory bowel disease [50,51]. In this design all participants are started on active treatment to see whether they improve. If improvement occurs responders are randomized to continue with either placebo or active medication. If the active medication is indeed effective, then those randomized to placebo should have a more frequent relapse of their symptoms than those remaining on active treatment. *In summary,* the randomized, double-blind parallel group design is the preferred study design. The interpretation of the results is straightforward and the analysis is less dependent on assumptions about the natural history of the disease.

Adequate blinding of patients and research personnel administering and monitoring the intervention is essential.

The blinded randomized controlled clinical trial is the gold standard for conducting of treatment studies. Blinding of patients and research personnel is of vital importance due to the subjective nature of the measured responses. For some interventions (psychotherapy, hypnotherapy, sphincterotomy), it may be difficult or impossible to keep patients or investigators blinded. In that case innovative methods need to be used to ensure that the lack of blinding does not invalidate the outcome assessment. One solution is the use of independent assessors who have been kept blinded to the actual intervention, thereby avoiding bias in the recording of outcomes. Use of independent assessors overcomes the problem of blinding because it ensures that the caregivers, who administered the intervention, cannot bias the recording of the outcome measures.

The randomization method needs to be adequate.

Randomization gives the highest likelihood of balancing treatment groups for factors influencing the response [52,53]. For example, diet or stress may modulate symptom endpoints in a clinical trial. Randomization will balance the treatment groups for these and other potential effect modifiers or confounders. A benefit of randomization is that it often balances unknown prognostic factors as well. Another important advantage of randomization, if it is blinded, is prevention of bias of the investigators, which may distort the balance between treatment groups or the interpretation of patient responses during the trial [54]. If one knows that certain patient characteristics are important predictors for a certain outcome, the randomization can be stratified for those factors. This ensures a high likelihood that those prognostic factors will be balanced among the treatment groups. Provided the number of stratification factors is small, such randomization is easy to implement [55].

Randomization requires a process whereby assignment to a particular treatment is equivalent to the flip of a coin. Methods of ensuring true randomization of treatments are well established and are beyond the scope of this chapter. In the review of functional dyspepsia trials it was evident that many studies were vague in their description of the actual randomization process [2]. However, the recently conducted studies were more explicit in their description of randomization, which is likely a reflection of the fact that the procedures for randomization are now well established.

A placebo run-in should be avoided as it may introduce bias.

A placebo run-in phase has been used frequently in functional gastrointestinal disorders trials. For example, in a review of functional dyspepsia it was used in 14 of 52 studies, 12 of which evaluated prokinetic agents [2]. The advantage of a placebo run-in is that it may reduce the high placebo response that is often seen in studies of functional gastrointestinal disorders. The aim is to limit enrollment in the study to patients who have persistent symptoms by excluding those who improved during the placebo run-in period. The expectation is that by eliminating high placebo responders, the chance of detecting a true effect in favor of the active drug under study, if indeed a beneficial effect exists, may be increased. Another proposed benefit of the run-in phase is the elimination of patients with poor compliance.

There are drawbacks in the use of a placebo run-in phase. It is unknown whether the placebo response is sustained after the run-in phase is over. There may be a natural variation in symptoms that coincides with the placebo run-in phase. As time passes this "pseudo"-placebo response may not be sustained, and patients may thereby be eliminated who still might benefit. During the placebo run-in differential dropout may occur; i.e., people who drop out have a different response rate relative to those who stay in the trial. It is also possible that the natural history of the gastrointestinal symptoms differs in placebo responders and non-responders. Indeed one may end up enrolling patients with more resistant symptoms who may in fact be less likely to respond. Finally, it is possible that the placebo response will level off if the trial is of sufficient duration (8–12 weeks). In functional dyspepsia there is some empirical evidence for such an effect [56,57]. Given these potential limitations a placebo run-in period should be avoided.

A period of baseline observation without treatment is recommended.

A placebo run-in period should be distinguished from obtaining baseline observations prior to the start of the intervention. The assessment of the severity of symptoms at baseline is important to document so that patients in the active and comparison group are comparable. The baseline data can also be used for comparison to determine the efficacy of the intervention. The optimal length of time for baseline observation is uncertain and will depend on the type of disorder and type of intervention. The baseline observation can be recorded retrospectively, but ideally is done prospectively. As will be discussed later "spontaneous" improvement may occur during this period. Obviously investigators will want to avoid randomizing patients who are, or become, completely asymptomatic. However, given the known fluctuations in symptoms, patients who have had some improvement should not be excluded, as symptoms will likely persist or may deteriorate again in the future. The study protocol should specify how patients who improved during this baseline observation period are dealt with in the intervention phase. A summary of pertinent clinical variables in patients who entered the observation period but were not randomized should be recorded and reported.

Some study protocols focus only on the question or whether the intervention has resulted in an improvement, irrespective of the baseline situation. Although one can document change (hopefully improvement) that way, measurement of the baseline situation has the benefit of documenting the state (such as severity of the disease) of the patients from which the change takes place.

— Timing of the Intervention

The timing of the intervention should be carefully considered.

Investigators should be aware that there may be spontaneous improvement after recent investigations. Most trials of functional gastrointestinal disorders have shown a varying but often substantial placebo response. The increased medical attention as a result of participating may be one explanation. Reassurance by diagnostic tests, which did not reveal a more serious underlying disease, could also play a role. Usually investigations, such as upper or lower gastrointestinal endoscopy, are required to exclude patients with structural abnormalities. Patients will be reassured by diagnostic tests. As a result, symptoms may improve, which can coincide with the baseline observation period or later during the period that the intervention is administered. It is unclear whether this reassurance effect, if it exists, is long lasting.

Fear of cancer has been shown to be a frequent concern in patients with functional dyspepsia who underwent gastroscopy [58,59]. In keeping with this are the results from a trial by Bytzer et al. in which patients were randomized to direct endoscopy or empiric treatment [60]. Patients were more satisfied in the endoscopy group, and subsequent health care costs were significantly lower in this cohort.

The reassurance effect of diagnostic studies warrants further study. No data is available to provide guidance on the optimal timing of diagnostic studies and the subsequent therapeutic intervention, but it may be worthwhile avoiding testing immediately prior to randomization. To counteract this problem of a "spontaneous" improvement, one may decide to have a longer time interval between the diagnostic tests and start of the study, but the optimal duration is unknown and may vary among disorders. Delaying randomization of patients introduces obvious logistic problems. Alternatively, one may argue that, in the real world, therapy is usually initiated after diagnostic tests have been carried out and patients continue to be symptomatic.

The protocol should define the timing of the diagnostic tests that are part of the entry criteria. If a window period is allowed during which these tests could reasonably be performed (e.g., within the last 6–12 months for colonoscopy in irritable bowel syndrome patients), it is recommended that the timing of these tests in individual patients be considered in the analysis as a possible predictor of therapeutic response.

Whether one is dealing with patients in primary or in specialized care may also affect the placebo response. A higher placebo response might be anticipated following referral to a specialist, simply because patients may have higher expectations of specialists compared to those with their family doctor. Indeed such an effect was recently suggested in a placebo-controlled study of treatment with omeprazole on symptoms of functional dyspepsia when comparing patients recruited in primary care with patients in specialist care [61]. Patients who are referred for evaluation by a specialist may be more concerned about a possibly life-threatening disease than about relief of symptoms [62–68]. A normal investigation ruling out malignancy may thus result in a very large "placebo" effect in this setting, leaving little room for specific treatment-related improvement.

— Duration of Treatment and Follow-up

The duration of treatment and the expected time of response should be specified in the protocol.

The expected time of response may depend on the type of intervention or the type of disorder. The expected time of response may be short if one is testing drugs with a known short-acting effect, e.g., antispasmodic agents for irritable bowel syndrome. In contrast, it may take much longer for psychotherapy or anti-*Helicobacter* therapy to reach the maximum beneficial effect.

Generally a minimum treatment duration of 8–12 weeks is recommended.

Many studies of functional gastrointestinal disorders have been of surprisingly short duration given the chronic nature of these conditions [1,2]. If the treatment being considered is for chronic symptoms (i.e., suppression rather than cure of symptoms), the trial must be long enough to determine whether any response will be sustained. Longer trials also allow for better documentation of emerging side effects that could limit the long-term usefulness of the intervention. In irritable bowel syndrome trials, there is evidence that the response in studies with longer duration has been less than in shorter studies [1]. Given the chronicity of the functional gastrointestinal disorders, we recommend that generally the *minimum duration of treatment* should be *8–12 weeks*. This period was recommended by the working team on study design in irritable bowel syndrome [3], and in an earlier review of irritable bowel syndrome [1]. Although a perceived problem with a 12-week period may be that a patient becomes asymptomatic after, for example, 4 weeks, a study of longer than four weeks duration is advisable nonetheless, given the chronic recurrent nature of functional gastrointestinal disorders. If investigators expect that a response will occur over a very short time period, investigators may decide a shorter duration of treatment is appropriate. For example, in functional dyspepsia, investigators may expect improvement at four weeks, or may feel that the intervention is unlikely to be worthwhile if no response is seen by four weeks. It is recognized that the duration of treatment does depend on the disorder being studied or the question that the study tries to address. It is not unreasonable for studies of short duration to be done first, as one may want to have some evidence of potential efficacy before studies of longer duration are conducted.

Follow-up after treatment is recommended.

Extended follow-up of patients after the intervention should be considered to determine the long-term efficacy of treatment. Given the chronic nature of these conditions, it is surprising how few studies follow up patients after the intervention is stopped [2]. Long follow-up is mainly relevant if the benefit of treatment is expected to last, and thus it may not be necessary for short-acting drugs such as a smooth muscle relaxant.

Once the efficacy of an intervention during short-term treatment (e.g., 8–12 weeks) is documented, it is essential that longer term studies be conducted to document the long-term efficacy of the intervention.

For treatments that are proved to be efficacious during short-term treatment, additional long term studies (the suggested length is 6–12 months) are essential to document the continuous efficacy and safety of the intervention. Some interventions may have long lasting effects (e.g., psychotherapy), whereas others may require continuous treatment (e.g., acid suppression) It may also be appropriate to consider evaluation of "on demand therapy," especially if periods of remission and exacerbations of symptoms are expected to occur.

— The Need for More Natural History Data

Despite the high prevalence of functional gastrointestinal disorders there remains a lack of good data on the natural history of these disorders. Talley et al. have shown that among people with dyspepsia in the general population there is a high turnover with many individuals "losing" the symptoms, or "acquiring" them [69,70]. This turnover of symptoms has obvious implications for recommendations on the optimal duration of trials. Research on the natural history of functional gastrointestinal disorders should be a high priority.

— Adherence to Treatment and Study Protocol

Compliance with treatment should be measured.

Compliance with the intervention should be assessed. Standard methods are available for this and include interviewing the patient, requesting the return of unused medication, and pill counts of returned medications [71–74]. When one is conducting studies of longer duration, compliance may become more of an issue. It may help for documentation of compliance that patients know that, if they forget to take medication on occasion, this does not necessarily constitute non-compliance.

Compliance with the study protocol should be measured.

Documentation that the study protocol is adhered to is important. It is unclear how the study data can best be recorded and how frequently this should be done. A time-efficient way to measure symptoms is to have the patient fill in questionnaires before starting treatment and at regular intervals during followup. Questionnaires can be either self-recorded or filled in while the research assistant or the investigator is present. The protocol should clearly indicate how the data will be recorded and whether the questionnaires will be self-administered. Questionnaires generally provide cross-sectional information during the course of treatment, i.e., the response at a given point in time. Although the answers may reflect how the patient is feeling at the time the questionnaires are filled out, they may not accurately reflect how the patient has been doing in the preceding days or weeks, i.e., recall bias may be introduced. How much of a problem recall bias introduces is unknown. One might argue that in real life patients always tell their physician about their recent experience of symptoms.

— Use of Diary Cards

In many functional gastrointestinal disorders trials diary cards are used to collect data on the patients symptoms. Diary cards can be used alone or in addition to information obtained during regular clinic visits. The use of diary cards has been validated in other diseases [75–77]. Diary cards provide longitudinal information i.e., the response over a period of time. Usually diary cards will not be as comprehensive as questionnaires. Diary cards are filled in by the patients periodically (e.g., daily) throughout the study, or during a specified period in the study, e.g., the seven days preceding a follow-up visit. They theoretically reduce the problem of recall bias and therefore have the potential advantage that the "true state of affairs" is better captured. There are two ways of filling in the cards: either the recording of symptom severity at a fixed point during the day (e.g., before going to sleep) or when the symptoms occur. The first method is the most commonly used. The second method may require several entries each day.

There are potential methodologic problems with the use of diary cards [78]. Patients may forget to fill in the cards on a daily basis and retrospective completion may invalidate their use. It is important that the patient receives clear instructions on the use of the dairy cards, and that the patient is encouraged to comply with the recording. In order to overcome the potential problem of retrospective completion, it may help to allow the patient to forget. This can be achieved either by instructing the patient to leave the cards blank on days on which the patient forgot to fill in the information (i.e., allowing them to forget), or by allowing them to complete the missing information retrospectively. In this way non-completion is not turned into non-compliance. For recording of severity of symptoms, both categorical scales and VAS-scales (see below) can be used on the cards.

Although diary cards may have less chance of introducing recall bias, it is not clear whether they give better insight into the "true state of affairs" than questionnaires administered at regular intervals during treatment. The limitations with diary cards have been addressed with technological innovation, such as through automated daily telephone recording or the use of hand held electronic data collection devices [78,79].

— Outcome Measures

Preamble

The most important outcomes in the treatment of functional gastrointestinal disorders are those that reflect the patient's symptoms. Since individual symptoms can vary from patient to patient and from time to time, a measure of overall change in symptoms should be the primary outcome criterion.

Considerations for Selection and Management of Outcome Measures

The trial's main result should be based on the primary outcome measure.

The most important problem in study design of clinical trials of functional gastrointestinal disorders is the lack of consensus on how to measure outcome, or how to define efficacy of an intervention. Generally accepted validated outcome measures are lacking and as a result there is marked variation in the outcome measures that have been used. The variation in measuring outcome has also made it impossible to compare similar treatments used in different studies. As will be discussed below, the protocol should state a priori what the main objective of the study is and how the primary outcome measure will be assessed.

An assessment that integrates the symptoms of the particular functional gastrointestinal disorder is recommended as the primary outcome measure.

The primary outcome measure(s) should generally focus on the severity of symptoms relevant for the particular disorder and on the impact that the disorder may have on quality of life. Physiologic measurements should not be used as a primary outcome measure. However, as secondary measures, they may help to explain the mechanism of an observed treatment effect. Until recently little attention has been paid to the importance of validated outcome measures. Fortunately, for several functional gastrointestinal disorders there currently are studies ongoing that try to validate primary outcome measures. However, currently no measures for functional gastrointestinal disorders are sufficiently validated to be recommended unequivocally as the primary outcome measure.

As for what the primary outcome measure should consist of, it is this committee's opinion that, *an assessment which integrates the key symptoms of the particular functional gastrointestinal disorder be used as the primary outcome measure*. The symptoms that lead to the diagnosis of a functional gastrointestinal disorder are varied, and interact in complex ways. Thus, there is a strong argument for a primary outcome measure that allows the patient to integrate the contribution of a disparate group of symptoms in a single global clinical rating. Alternatively, the primary outcome measure can be the summary score of a validated disease-specific quality of life questionnaire.

It is preferable that the main assessment of outcome be done by the patient.

An assessment of a patient's response to treatment by the physician has been commonly used as an outcome measure, and in some studies this has been the principal determinant of treatment efficacy [2]. It is doubtful, however, that physician assessment is more accurate or reliable than assessment by the patient, and there may be substantial inter- and intra-individual variation in physician recording of symptom severity. Therefore, physician assessment should not be used as a main outcome measure.

The study protocol should define a priori the definition of a responder or a response, i.e., the change in the outcome measure, which is considered clinically meaningful.

The protocol should give a clear definition of a responder or response. This definition of a responder or response should incorporate the main outcome measure on which the success or failure of the trial depends. Rather than designing the trial to detect a mean change in a score among treatment groups, the committee recommends studies that compare the proportion of patients who achieved the stipulated amount of improvement necessary to be qualified as a responder (e.g., the proportion of patients who become symptom free). Whenever possible, the distribution of changes in the components of the primary outcome measure before and after the intervention should also be reported. This will provide information of the overall magnitude, direction, and variability of the changes that took place over the course of the study.

The study should include measures of change for each of the symptoms that were part of the entry criteria.

Although individual symptoms may not be the primary outcome measure, the study should include measures of change for each of the symptoms that were part of the entry criteria (e.g., the Rome Diagnostic Criteria). Measurement of change should include deterioration and not just improvement. The expectation is that the change (and direction of change) of the cardinal symptoms of a disorder will be similar to the changes that take place for the primary outcome measure. It is possible that one may end up with a study result in which individual symptoms are not better but the primary outcome measures did show definite improvement. The interpretation of such a finding will depend on the clinical context and firm guidelines cannot be given. One explanation might be that patients are coping better with the symptoms. However, concordance between changes in the primary outcome measure and individual symptoms will give the most clear-cut result.

— Definition of Symptoms

Great variation exists in the definitions of common gastrointestinal symptoms, making it difficult to impose strict definitions, particularly since the terminology—and perhaps also the sensations experienced—may vary between cultures and countries. Great care should be taken to be as thorough as possible when eliciting symptoms and describing them. We advise investigators to comply with the definitions of symptoms suggested by the current or previous Rome Working Team [3,8,80]. It is necessary that investigators clearly state the definitions and descriptions that they used to measure symptoms. If investigators, for reasons of preference or culture, decide to measure different symptoms, they should state clearly what was meant by the terms they employed.

It is also important for investigators to decide over what time periods symptoms are reported, i.e., during a clinic visit over what time period (days, weeks or longer) are patients asked to rate the severity of their symptoms. Diary cards and daily automatic recording of symptoms by telephone can overcome the problem of recall but have other problems, which include validity and logistics.

Use of validated outcome measures (instruments) is recommended.

Validation of outcome measures is necessary before they can be accepted for use in clinical trials. As mentioned, the primary outcome measure ideally will focus on the patient's perception of severity of their gastrointestinal symptoms and the impact that the symptoms have on quality of life. In the last decade the importance of assessing the impact of disease on health-related quality of life has received increasing attention and much progress has been made it this area.

Validation of a primary outcome measure or disease-specific quality of life instrument requires that:

(1) it includes symptoms that are relevant and representative of the disorder;

(2) the measure is reproducible, i.e., produces similar results when administered to patients whose health status has not changed;

(3) is able to detect change (responsiveness) in relevant clinical symptoms, assuming a change has taken place; and

(4) a change in outcome measures should reflect a real change in general health status.

Preferably, validation of a new outcome measure is established in a separate study. We refer the reader to several relevant references on this topic [81,82]. The requirement that a change in outcome measures reflects a real change in general health status is important, as an improvement (or deterioration) in symptoms should correlate with a clinically meaningful change in health status. The latter is an especially difficult methodologic problem as no other hard outcome measures for most functional gastrointestinal disorders are available to compare with (or anchor) a new measure. For example, in patients with ulcerative colitis, a change in symptoms can be compared to severity of colonic inflammation. Furthermore, in the absence of interventions with proven therapeutic efficacy, comparison of a new treatment cannot be made to an "old" gold standard treatment with a known effect size. Establishing the four attributes given usually necessitates that a separate study is conducted to demonstrate that the new instruments meet the above requirements. Until recently the need to conduct separate studies to validate outcome measures has been largely ignored as most investigators used outcome measures which were assumed but not proven to be valid.

If validated outcome measures for a particular disorder are either not available or are felt to still have methodologic problems, investigators need to be wary. It is important that the chosen measure makes clinical sense, is rigorous and can be easily replicated by other investigators.

— Measurement of Pain

The previous Working Team report on design of IBS trials discussed measurement of pain [3]. The presence of pain or discomfort is one the key features of many of the functional gastrointestinal disorders and is typically one of the outcome measures in clinical trials. Pain or discomfort is an unpleasant sensation that can be assessed by verbal and non-verbal observation and, in this context, clearly requires the cooperation of the patient. Pain can be considered to have three dimensions; intensity, duration, and frequency. All these aspects of pain can be measured separately. Alternatively, an integrated measure of pain, such as a global assessment of severity of pain, can be used as an outcome measure. Whether such a global assessment indeed incorporates ("weighs") all the relevant aspects of pain, especially in the context of the functional gastointestinal disorders, is unclear. Apart from the above dimensions, one can also measure the impact that pain has on a person's ability to carry out normal daily activities or work.

For measuring pain intensity or overall severity, rating scales are usually used, either ordinal (Likert) scales or VAS scales. Both methods have been shown to be reproducible and sensitive to change [3]. If measurement of pain is chosen as the primary outcome, it is important that the study protocol stipulates how much improvement is considered to be clinically meaningful. The results should be reported as the proportion of patients who reached this endpoint. Multidimensional scales have also been validated for measurement of pain. An example of this is the clinical McGill Pain Questionnaire (MPQ), which assesses three principal dimensions of pain. This includes sensory-discriminative, motivational-affective and cognitive-evaluative aspects of pain. This scale has been extensively used in clinical trials [83]. For a more detailed review of pain measurement we refer to the previous document on the design of clinical trials for irritable bowel syndrome [3].

—   Measurement Scales

A detailed discussion of measurement scales and their properties is beyond the scope of this report [84–91]. The most commonly used scales in trials of the functional gastrointestinal disorders will be briefly discussed. The two most popular scales to assess severity of symptoms are categorical scales (often referred to as Likert Scales) and Visual Analogue Scales (VAS). A categorical scale has several response categories, e.g., a five point scale ranging from 1 = no problem to 5 = a severe problem. A VAS is a horizontal line (usually 10 cm) with endpoints on which the patient must place a mark. The mark can be measured as the severity of the symptom. Categorical scales seem to be more commonly used than VAS-scales, but both scales seem to perform well and the choice therefore depends on the preference of the investigators.

The reproducibility and ability to detect change have been well documented for both categorical and VAS scales in a wide variety of different diseases. The interpretation of a change on categorical scale is easier to conceptualize in clinical terms [92,93]. For example, a two-point improvement on a five point scale may mean going from severe to mild severity of pain. This is easier to understand than, for example, a 3 cm improvement on a 10cm VAS-scale. Categorical scales are also easier to explain to patients, although most patients have no problem with VAS-scales once their use has been explained. Another drawback of the VAS-scale is the need for good hand-eye coordination.

An advantage of the VAS is that it is a continuous scale and, as opposed to the categorical scale, does not rely upon the assumption that individuals perceive the meaning of numerical response categories in the same manner. Statistical analysis of VAS-scales requires fewer underlying assumptions than categorical scales, but in practice this is not a real problem. There have been studies in functional dyspepsia in which VAS-scales were directly compared to categorical scales and the results were very similar [94].

Optimal Number of Categories for Categorical Scales

It is difficult to give stringent guidelines on the optimal number of categories for a categorical scale. The most important property of the scales in clinical trials is their ability to detect change. A separate issue is how much of an improvement is clinically meaningful. For categorical scales, some investigators have stated a preference for seven over four or five point scales. The reason for this is that scales with a higher number of categories are better able to detect smaller changes than scales with a lower number of categories. This may be of importance for the functional gastrointestinal disorders in which patients often do not rate symptoms at the end of the severity scale. This means that if, for example, a four-point scale is used and both ends of the scale are rarely used by patients, the ability of the scale to detect change is reduced to two points.

The definition of a responder, which is recommended as the main outcome measure, must incorporate what is considered by the investigators as a clinically important improvement. At the moment there is no conclusive evidence to strongly recommend an optimal number of categories for categorical scales to measure change induced by the intervention. As meta-analysis becomes more widely applied, reaching an international consensus on the optimal number of categories for categorical scales becomes more helpful as such agreement will allow for comparisons and pooling of the results of different studies. We suggest the use of seven point scales because these are used in many quality of life instruments and because they are able to detect small but potentially relevant differences [95–97].

— Global Outcome Measure and Assessment of Change

As indicated, the clinical trial should be designed around a single predetermined parameter, the primary outcome measure. Examples of how outcome can be measured include a global measure comparing the end-of-study measurement to baseline (e.g., *overall how would you rate the severity of your symptoms?*), or the summary score of a disease-specific questionnaire. Most studies will also evaluate additional parameters.

A global assessment can be considered as a "weighted average" by the patient about the overall impact that the symptoms have had on his or her well-being. Indeed, this parallels usual clinical practice in which one of the first and most important questions the physician asks the patient is, *how are you feeling?* or *how have you been doing since I saw you last?*. The response to these questions involves, at least implicitly, the patient's weighing all aspects of how he or she feels and functions and integrating them into a single overall answer. There are two ways to measure change for a global outcome measure: (1) administer the same rating scale before and periodically during and after treatment and document the amount of change; or (2) use a separate global rating scale of change. Table 2 lists examples of these.

For the first method listed in Table 2, the patient is asked to indicate the overall severity of the functional gastrointestinal disorder's symptoms before and during or after treatment on the same scale. The global rating scale of change is slightly different (example 2 in Table 2). In this situation the patient is only asked whether the symptoms have changed (hopefully improved) compared to the beginning of the study. This can be either done on a single scale or by a combined scale. For the combined scale the patient is asked whether the symptoms have stayed the same, improved or deteriorated. This can be done on a seven point scale as shown in Table 2. As also shown in Table 2, Guyatt et al. have used a variation of this combined scale successfully in the form of a 15 point scale (-7 → 0 → +7) of change in several asthma and heart failure studies [95–97]. Whatever scale is chosen, it is important that they are able to detect both improvement and deterioration.

Another example of global change scales are the "CGI" (clinical global impressions) scales [98]. Clinical global impressions scales were originally developed by the National Institutes of Health about 30 years ago for use in schizophrenia studies, but since then have been widely and successfully validated for use in many therapeutic areas. This score allows the patient (and/or an observer) to integrate the contribution of a disparate group of symptoms in a single global clinical rating. The patient's response involves, at least implicitly, the patient's weighing all aspects of how he/she is feeling and functioning and integrating

Table 2. Examples of Scales to Measure Outcome

1. Seven point Likert scale for measurement of global severity of epigastric pain by the patient. The patient is asked to indicate how much discomfort he/she has in the epigastric region. This same scale can be administered before and after the intervention.

   - 0   No discomfort at all
   - 1   Minor discomfort
   - 2   Mild discomfort
   - 3   Moderate discomfort
   - 4   Moderately severe discomfort
   - 5   Severe discomfort
   - 6   Very severe discomfort

2. Global rating scale of change. The patient is asked how much improvement has been achieved.

   - 0   No improvement at all
   - 1   Minor improvement
   - 2   Mild improvement
   - 3   Moderate amount of improvement
   - 4   Quite a bit of improvement
   - 5   A lot of improvement
   - 6   Great improvement

3. Global seven point rating scale of change incorporating both deterioration and improvement

   - 0   Markedly worse
   - 1   Somewhat worse
   - 2   A little bit worse
   - 3   No change
   - 4   A little better
   - 5   Somewhat better
   - 6   Markedly better

4. Combined scale measuring change. First the patient is asked whether he/she has improved, stayed the same, or deteriorated. If a change has taken place the patient is then asked to rate the amount of change on a seven point Likert scale. This will give a 15 point scale of change, ranging from $-7 \to 0 \to +7$. Only the 7 point scale for deterioration is shown here.

		1	Almost the same, Hardly worse at all
		2	A little worse
1	Worse	3	Somewhat worse
2	About the same	4	Moderately worse
3	Better	5	A good deal worse
		6	A great deal worse
		7	A very great deal worse

them into a single overall answer. Although never formally validated or studied for inter-rater reliability, these scales have high face validity and have the virtue of being simple, brief, and easy to understand across different languages and cultures.

These CGI scales measure two aspects of the disease and the intervention: a) severity of illness and b) global improvement. They are Likert-type scales, with seven descriptors. The "severity of illness" scale ranges from "normal" (=1) to "among the most extremely ill" (=7). The "global improvement" scale goes from "very much improved" (=1) through "no change" (=4) to "very much worse" (=7). The severity-of-illness scale is administered at baseline and periodically during the course of the trial. The global improvement scale, which has the added benefit of "standardizing" the baseline severity of symptoms for each patient, is administered periodically during the study, or in short trials, at the end of the treatment period. There tends to be a high correlation between the severity-of-illness and global-improvement scales, and between-patient and observer ratings.

Determining the Minimal Clinically Important Difference

There is a well-recognized difference between "statistical significance" and "clinical significance" in an outcome measure. For example, in a very large clinical trial of an anti-hypertensive medication, the experimental intervention may lower the systolic blood pressure by a mean of 2 mm Hg more than did placebo. By the appropriate inferential statistical test, this difference could be statistically significant, that is, unlikely to have occurred by chance. However, a difference of only 2 mm Hg would be considered clinically unimportant. As discussed, it is recommended that for the functional gastrointestinal disorders the proportion of patients who are responders are the primary outcome measure. The definition of what is a responder should incorporate the concept of the minimal clinically important difference (MCID) and is based on the difference in symptom severity before and after the intervention. Guyatt et al., using summary scores of disease-specific quality of life questionnaires, have shown (in asthma/chronic obstructive pulmonary disease and heart failure) that a 0.5 change per question (measured on 7-point scale) equates with the MCID [97].

Finally, it must be kept in mind that it is not enough simply to show that an experimental therapy shows a clinically and statistically significant advantage over placebo. At least two other factors must be considered before one could recommend the treatment. First is the safety profile. No matter how effective a treatment proves to be, unless it can be shown to be safe and to have a clinically favorable efficacy/safety ratio, it should not be used in practice. Thus carefully assessing safety in a clinical trial is important. Second, both the efficacy and safety must be put in perspective by an appreciation of the ultimate cost of the treatment. For example, an inexpensive once-a-day tablet that has a modest improvement relative to placebo may be appropriate to employ in treating patients. However, intensive one-to-one psychotherapy that results in the same modest improvement may be too costly to be of practical use.

Use of validated quality of life instruments measuring impact of symptoms on normal daily life is recommended, especially when such instruments have been shown to be able to detect change (responsive).

The outcome assessment of clinical intervention studies, for which no hard outcome measures exist, should aim to capture multidimensional aspects of the disease under study. These may include assessments of how bothersome symptoms are and their frequency, measurement of health-related quality of life, evaluation of functional limitations as a result of the disease (disability), and cost-benefit or cost-effectiveness measures. Utility measures will not be discussed here, but they are becoming more popular since they make it possible to do cost-effectiveness analyses.

Functional gastrointestinal disorders clearly can affect quality of life [99, 100]. Quality of life instruments can be divided in two categories: generic and disease specific [81] (see Chapter 4). Generic instruments are able to assess quality of life in large populations and do not focus on any disorder in particular. Examples of validated generic instruments include the Sickness Impact Profile [101], the Nottingham Health Profile [102], the Rand Corporation Instruments [103], the McMaster Health Index Questionnaire [104], the SF-36 (Short Form of General Health Questionnaire) [105] and the Psychological General Well-being Index (PGWB) [106]. A limitation of the generic instruments is that they do not focus on aspects of health status that are specific and important for the particular disease of interest. Generic instruments therefore may not be truly reflective of a patient's experience.

For many conditions disease-specific quality of life questionnaires have been developed that have been shown to be reproducible and sensitive to change. These questionnaires commonly incorporate several dimensions (disease-related symptoms, general well-being, functional capacity, psychosocial functions) which are relevant for the patient's health-related quality of life [107]. An example is the IBDQ (Inflammatory Bowel Disease Questionnaire) for Crohn's disease [108]. The summary score of this instrument is well accepted as a primary outcome measure in randomized clinical trials [109].

The advantage of disease-specific quality of life instruments is that they focus on the quality of life of the particular disease of interest. Theoretically they should be capable of detecting smaller changes in health status, which are relevant for the patient and which may be missed by the generic instruments. However, this assumption needs to be proven in actual studies. A list of validated outcome measures for all functional gastrointestinal disorders is beyond the scope of this chapter. It is important that agreement is reached about the best existing outcome measures or quality of life instruments for use in clinical trials of functional gastrointestinal disorders. It is possible that some disease specific quality of life instruments will become the primary outcome measure in the future.

As functional dyspepsia and irritable bowel syndrome are so common, we list some of the validated instruments that have become available. For functional dyspepsia there are: the Gastrointestinal Symptoms Rating Scale (GSRS) [110], the DIBS scale [98], the Canadian Dyspepsia score [111], Glasgow Dyspepsia Severity Score [112], and Dyspepsia Symptom Questionnaire (DSQ) [113]. For irritable bowel syndrome there are several recently published quality of life questionnaires [114–16]. Furthermore, an illness severity index [117] for FGIDs and an IBS severity scoring system have been developed [118]. Many of these scales are still in the development phase since for several of them the responsiveness has not been established. As yet there are no data that confirm that these disease-specific quality of life instruments scales are sufficiently "responsive" to detect clinically important change, but the expectation is that they will be. Further validation is required before they can be recommended as main outcome measures. Evidence also needs to be provided that these scales have advantages over the simpler global assessments that were discussed.

Measurement of psychological status is recommended, as this may be an important variable modifying outcome.

In some patients psychological factors have been linked to the syndromes, and these may aggravate symptoms [16–21]. Investigators are likely to measure psychological factors (e.g., anxiety) if interventions are used which can alter psychological status. However, even if the intervention does not specifically target psychological distress we advise measurement of psychological well-being at least at baseline, as it may be a determinant of the success of the intervention. We refer the reader to Chapter 4, which reviews a large number of suitable instruments [18].

Physiological parameters should not be used as primary outcome measures, but may be used as secondary outcome measures to help explain the therapeutic effect of the intervention.

Depending on the intervention investigators may want to assess change in certain other objective clinical outcome measures. For example, in irritable bowel syndrome, interventions that can alter transit time, motility, and visceral sensitivity may be studied. Clearly the investigators will want to know whether their intervention alter these parameters, as this would provide support for the presumed physiological basis of the treatment's effect. However, treatment that "normalizes" such parameters, without improving symptoms, is unlikely to be of value to the patient. Therefore although relevant, these outcome measures cannot be the primary ones. An example of a potentially attractive secondary outcome measure for IBS is the Bristol stool scale [119]. This seven-point scale of stool form has been shown to be scored differently by irritable bowel syndrome patients compared to normal controls [119]. It is possible that improvement in this stool scale will correlate with clinical improvement, but until this has been shown, this stool scale cannot be a primary outcome measure.

— Frequency of Data Recording

Recording of symptoms at regular intervals is recommended, as it will allow for documentation of treatment response over time.

A successful treatment would be expected to demonstrate a gradual and sustained improvement from baseline and not to show extensive fluctuations over the course of the study. Thus data on fluctuations should be summarized and reported. The study results will be much stronger if an improvement is seen comparing the end of study data to baseline, along with demonstration of a gradual and sustained response over the course of the study. For most treatments it may take some time before the maximum effect is achieved. This can be documented by regular measurement of symptoms. Investigators must decide on the optimal frequency of data recording, and whether it is done by use of diary cards, regular clinic visits, phone follow-up, questionnaires, or appropriate combinations of these. New technology such as use of electronic data collection by touch-tone telephone is becoming more widely available [79]. Such systems can either dial patients on a regular basis or the patients can call in to electronically record the severity of their symptoms. The acceptance rate of these systems is high, and as data are collected on an ongoing basis, this should minimize problems with recall bias or retrospective completion.

An a priori specification of the time interval over which a responder or response occurs should be included. This should usually be towards the end of the treatment trial.

Investigators should not only specify their definition of a responder at the start of the trial but also indicate the time interval over which they expect the effect to occur. In many instances this will be towards the end of the intervention, but sometimes the final effect of the treatment, e.g., with psychotherapy, may occur later.

— Statistical Analysis and Data Reporting

In reporting the results of the study investigators should adhere to the CONSORT statement on reporting of clinical trials.

The CONSORT statement has made explicit recommendations about the necessity of a detailed flowchart which clearly describes how patients progressed through the study [120–122]. Requirements are: a description of the number of enrolled patients; a log of eligible patients who were not randomized and the reasons why; the number of patients who received active or control treatment; the number of patients who completed the study; the number of withdrawals by treatment group, when they occurred and the reasons why; and the number of patients who were lost to follow-up and when this occurred. It is recommended that the CONSORT guidelines be followed in reporting all trial results.

The main result of the study must be based on evaluation of the primary outcome measure that is stated in the protocol before the study begins.

The main analysis should focus on the chosen primary outcome measure on which the overall conclusion of the study is based. This should determine whether the study has a positive or a negative result. Although the main outcome often will be reported as a comparison between the end-of-treatment result and baseline, it is also important that data are provided on how patients changed throughout the course of the study. A result in which patients are classified as responders some of the time and as failures at other times is far less convincing than results in which patients have a sustained response after the intervention is started.

The main analysis will depend on the definition of the primary outcome measure.

A detailed discussion of data analysis cannot be provided as the type of statistical analysis will depend on the study design and definition of primary outcome measure(s). The statistical analysis should be primarily based on an intention-to-treat (ITT) analysis [123,124]. Many studies also report a per-protocol (all patients who followed the protocol) or an all-patients-treated (all patients who received treatment following randomization) analysis. These analyses may provide insight into how a treatment might work under optimal conditions, but generally cannot replace the ITT analysis. The study report should clearly state the numbers of patients for both the ITT and per protocol or all-patients-treated analysis and how they were arrived at. The number of patients who were lost to follow-up needs to be stated, and when each occurred. For all outcome measures the results should state the estimated effect of the intervention (difference between active and placebo treatment) and a 95 % confidence interval [123,125, 126]. The results should be stated in absolute numbers. It is not sufficient to list just percentages (not 20%, but 10/50, 20%).

The effect of potential-effect modifiers such as gender, age, duration, or severity of disease and presence of psychological stress can be assessed using a logistic regression analysis where the binary dependent variable represents the a priori specified definition of a responder. The CONSORT statement makes recommendations about key elements of statistical reporting, and investigators should adhere to them.

Analysis of Secondary Outcome Measures

It is recommended that changes be reported for each of the symptoms that are part of the entry criteria. Most likely the different symptoms of a functional gastrointestinal disorder are not independent of each other, and hence they may tend to respond in a similar fashion. Reporting on secondary outcome measures will help support (or refute) the direction and magnitude of the effect of the intervention on the primary outcome measure. For example, if the primary outcome measures showed improvement, it is likely that some of the cardinal symptoms of the disease will also show amelioration.

Analysis of these secondary outcome measures may suffer from the problem of multiple comparisons [127,128]. Multiple comparisons are probably the reason that many treatment trials of functional gastrointestinal disorders came to the conclusion that the intervention was superior to placebo. One approach to overcome this problem is to adjust by using, for example, the Bonferroni correction [129]. This correction divides the P-value (usually set at 0.05) by the number of comparisons of outcome measures. Such corrections have generally not been used in the analysis of functional gastrointestinal disorders. It has been argued that the Bonferroni corrections may be too conservative [129]. It also increases the likelihood of type II errors, so that truly important differences are deemed non-significant. Because of the potential problem of multiple comparisons, it is recommended that secondary outcome measures are mainly analyzed with descriptive rather than inferential statistics. If investigators specify a priori a small number of key symptoms as important outcome measures, correction for multiple comparisons of each specified outcome measure is not necessarily required.

The sample size calculation should be based on the expected behavior of the primary outcome measure.

The protocol should clearly specify what assumptions the sample size calculation was based on [130]. The sample size should be based, a priori, on what is considered to be the clinically important difference in the proportion of responders between active treatment and placebo. It is straightforward to specify the necessary sample sizes for simple endpoints, such as the proportion of patients with a positive response. The study must have sufficient power to detect a clinically important difference in the proportion of responders [131–134]. The smaller the difference that is felt to be meaningful, the larger the number of patients that must be enrolled in the study to avoid a Type II error. Often a power of 80% is used (beta error or type II error of 20%) and alpha (type I) error of 5% using a two-sided test. An allowance for dropouts should also be made in determining the appropriate sample size, but efforts should be made to keep the dropout rate below 10–20%. When dealing with dropouts in studies of longer duration, it is reasonable to use the last observation of the patient while in the study in order not to lose all the information gathered from this individual. The number and timing of the dropouts should be reported.

Interim Analysis

There is no compelling reason to incorporate specific interim analyses for the functional gastrointestinal disorders since they are not life threatening. Therefore, it is generally inappropriate to perform interim analyses to determine efficacy of an intervention. Such analyses should be distinguished from monitoring because of safety. Unplanned preliminary analyses should be avoided since premature presentation of results may affect the further conduct of the trial.

— Ethical Issues

It is unethical to change the primary outcome measure(s) in the analysis phase of the study.

There is an understandable desire to have positive results come out of well-designed and well-conducted studies. The main results of a trial must be presented according to the predetermined primary outcome measure(s). It is misleading if the originally stated primary outcome measures are exchanged for other outcome measures that turned out in favor of the active treatment. A secondary analysis of data may lead to the discovery of positive results that were not part of the original hypotheses that the study was designed to answer [130]. Such data should be considered as hypothesis-generating rather than hypothesis testing. The positive results of such secondary analyses should be further tested in subsequent studies to determine whether they are indeed true.

Adherence to the study goals is strengthened if there are independent advisors for the trial, which is one function of data and safety monitoring committees.

It is unethical to withhold publishing the results of a completed trial.

Investigators have an ethical obligation to publish the results of all completed studies regardless of whether the results were positive or negative. The only exception to this is a study that turned out to have a fatal flaw in design that was discovered after the trial was completed. For treatment trials of functional gastrointestinal disorders there is a concern that negative studies have not always been published. This may skew the interpretation of the efficacy of treatments. Now that there is a concerted effort underway to review systematically the entire medical literature through the Cochrane collaboration it is all the more important that all relevant studies are published [135]. To help facilitate this process several major medical journals recently have allowed for an amnesty of previously unpublished studies. This also means that journal editors have an obligation to publish methodologically sound studies with negative results.

Recommendations for Future Research and Conclusions

The following areas were identified as priorities for future research on study design.

(1) Development of validated outcome measures and disease-specific quality of life instruments for functional gastrointestinal disorders. As discussed, there is an urgent need for better validated outcome measures that can be used in treatment trials of functional gastrointestinal disorders. There also is a need to develop innovative methods to determine what amount of clinical improvement is clinically relevant, i.e., determination of the minimal clinically important difference (MCID).

(2) Studies on the associations between physiological and psychological measures and symptom outcome are needed. At the moment there are no physiologic parameters available suitable for use as primary outcome measures in treatment trials of functional gastrointestinal disorders. More basic research is necessary to help unravel the pathophysiologic substrate(s). Adding physiologic measures into new clinical trials is encouraged, especially in those instances where it may help explain the origin of symptoms or the therapeutic effect of an intervention.

(3) Studies on the natural history of the functional gastrointestinal disorders are needed. Studies are also needed to investigate the natural fluctuation of symptoms in order to help identify the optimal duration of trials. Despite the high prevalence of these disorders, there are surprisingly few data on the natural history. The natural fluctuation in symptom severity poses special problems for study design. Such data will be necessary to make firm recommendations on optimal duration of new trials.

(4) Studies on the effect of recent diagnostic tests on treatment response are required. The reassurance effect of diagnostic studies is a possible contributing explanation for the "spontaneous" improvement that is observed in many treatment trials. The exact magnitude and frequency of this phenomenon is unclear. It is also uncertain whether this reassurance effect is sustained over time and what the predictors of a long-term beneficial response are. Studies should also investigate whether certain diagnostic tests, if used for reassurance early in the disease, predict a favorable response over time.

(5) Studies on the placebo response in functional gastrointestinal disorders, including studies of the patient-doctor relationship as an explanation for different response rates, are needed. The large placebo response observed in some

treatment trials of functional gastrointestinal disorders make it difficult to demonstrate superiority of new interventions. This substantial placebo response is poorly understood and may have many etiologies. These include recent diagnostic tests, which provide reassurance that no serious disease is present, increased medical attention as a result of participation in a clinical trial, and possibly certain characteristics of the patient-doctor relationship. All of these aspects deserve further study.

(6) Identification of patient characteristics that predict the response to treatment are needed. It is clear that in many but not all patients psychosocial stress factors may be present. Such factors may be important determinants of how patients will fare over time. Studies are required that will help to explain why some patients do well long term with their functional gastrointestinal disorders and others continue to do poorly.

(7) Studies on potential differences in disease severity and treatment response in primary care vs. secondary or tertiary care are required. Although there is a belief that there are important differences in disease severity and treatment response in patients at the primary versus secondary or tertiary care level, there are very few studies that have addressed this issue in detail.

— Conclusion

Until recently many treatment trials of functional gastrointestinal disorders suffered from important weaknesses in study design and/or analysis. Fortunately, this problem has been increasingly recognized and the more recent studies have paid greater attention to these issues. Methodologically sound clinical trials are possible in the functional gastrointestinal disorders. Clearly, further research is needed on the challenging design issues of such trials, but adherence to the recommendations discussed in this report should result in improved quality of studies. A summary of the recommendations is given in Table 3.

A major methodological problem that has not been resolved is the lack of validated outcome measures. Progress in this area is being made as several outcome measures for dyspepsia and irritable bowel syndrome have recently been developed or are being tested. At the moment, however, there is no generally accepted outcome measure, and all current instruments require more validation. It would also be helpful if agreement could be reached on the best scales to include in outcome measures; as this agreement would allow for comparisons among studies and possible statistical pooling of the result in the future.

It is important that the newly developed disease-specific outcome tools continue to be tested in various populations using appropriate study designs to determine which instruments perform optimally. It will be important that investigators, representatives of regulatory and funding agencies, and patients reach consensus on the best outcome measures for future studies. For this level of formal agreement to take place, regular exchanges of data and consensus meetings on design issues, in which all stakeholders participate, are encouraged.

Treatment trials of functional gastrointestinal disorders pose special methodologic challenges but it is this committee's belief that they can be overcome. It is hoped that the recommendations in this chapter will help this process. Clearly there remains a need for further empiric data on which to base evaluations of study design in this field.

Table 3. Summary of Recommendations
___

1. Goal of the Study
   1. The study design should reflect the main question that the study proposes to investigate.
   2. The trial must incorporate the principles of best and usual clinical practice as much as possible to ensure that the study results are relevant to the real practice situation.

2. Patient Population
   1. In general, it is advisable to include a broad spectrum of patients, as defined by the Rome Criteria.
   2. If investigators want to apply special inclusion criteria, they should be justified.
   3. In general, it is recommended not to subcategorize patients with functional gastrointestinal disorders because of symptom instability.
   4. The patient setting needs to be clearly considered as it may affect outcome.
   5. For multicenter trials patient characteristics need to be measured in detail in order to ensure comparability of patients among centers.

3. Architecture of the Trial
   1. A placebo or adequate control group is an essential requirement.
   2. The parallel group design is the study design of choice and should be used in most circumstances.
   3. Adequate blinding of patients and research personnel administering and monitoring the intervention is essential.
   4. The randomization method needs to be adequate.
   5. A placebo run-in period should be avoided as it may introduce bias.
   6. A period of baseline observation without treatment is recommended.

4. Timing of Intervention

1. The timing of the intervention should be carefully considered.

5. Duration of Treatment and Follow-up

1. The duration of treatment and the expected time of response should be specified in the protocol.
2. Generally a minimum treatment duration of 8–12 weeks is recommended.
3. Follow-up after treatment is recommended.
4. Once the efficacy of an intervention during short-term (e.g., 8–12) weeks is documented, it is essential that longer-term studies be conducted to document the long-term efficacy of the intervention.

6. Adherence to Treatment and Study Protocol

1. Compliance with treatment should be measured.
2. Compliance with the study protocol should be measured.

7. Outcome Measures

Preamble: The most important outcomes in the treatment of functional gastrointestinal disorders are those that reflect the patient's symptoms. Since individual symptoms can vary from patient to patient and from time to time, a measure of overall change in symptoms should be the primary outcome criterion.

1. The trial's main result should be based on the primary outcome measure.
2. An assessment that integrates the symptoms of the particular functional gastrointestinal disorder is recommended as the primary outcome measure.
3. It is preferable that the main assessment of outcome be done by the patient.
4. The study protocol should define a priori the definition of a responder or a response, i.e., the change in the outcome measure that is considered clinically meaningful.
5. The study should include measures of change for each of the symptoms that were part of the entry criteria.
6. Use of validated outcome measures (instruments) is recommended.
7. Use of validated quality of life instruments measuring impact of symptoms on normal daily life is recommended, especially when such instruments have been shown to be able to detect change (responsive).
8. Measurement of psychological status is recommended, as this may be an important variable modifying outcome.
9. Physiological parameters should not be used as primary outcome measures, but may be used as secondary outcome measures to help explain the therapeutic effect of the intervention.

Currently no measures for the functional gastrointestinal disorders are sufficiently validated to be recommended unequivocally as the primary outcome measure.

Table 3. Summary of Recommendations *(cont'd)*

8. Frequency of Data Recording

   1. Recording of symptoms at regular intervals is recommended, as it will allow for documentation of treatment response over time.
   2. An a priori specification of the time interval over which a responder or response occurs should be included.

9. Statistical Analysis and Data Recording

   1. In reporting the results of the study investigators should adhere to the CONSORT statement on reporting of clinical trials.
   2. The main result of the study must be based on evaluation of the primary outcome measure that is stated in the protocol before the study begins.
   3. The main analysis will depend on the definition of the primary outcome measure.
   4. The sample size calculation should be based on the expected behavior of the primary outcome measure.

10. Ethical Issues

   1. It is unethical to change the primary outcome measures in the analysis phase.
   2. It is unethical to withhold publishing the results of a completed trial.

11. Recommendations for Future Research

   1. Development of validated outcome measures and disease-specific quality of life instruments for functional gastrointestinal disorders.
   2. Studies on the associations between physiological and psychological measures and symptom outcome are needed.
   3. Studies on the natural history of the functional gastrointestinal disorders are needed. Studies are also needed to investigate the natural fluctuation of symptoms in order to help identify the optimal duration of trials.
   4. Studies on the effect of recent diagnostic tests on treatment response are required.
   5. Studies on the placebo response in functional gastrointestinal disorders, including studies of the patient-doctor relationship as an explanation for different response rates, are needed.
   6. Identification of patient characteristics that predict the response to treatment are needed.
   7. Studies on potential differences in disease severity and treatment response in primary care versus secondary or tertiary care are required.

References

1. Klein KB. Controlled treatment trials in the irritable bowel syndrome: a critique. Gastroenterology 1988;95:232–41.
2. Veldhuyzen van Zanten SJO, Cleary C, Talley NJ, et al. Drug treatment of functional dyspepsia: a systematic analysis of trial methodology with recommendations for design of future trials. Am J Gastroenterol 1996;91:660–71.
3. Talley NJ, Nyren O, Drossman DA, et al. The irritable bowel syndrome: toward optimal design of controlled treatment trials. Gastroenterol Internat 1993;6:189–211.
4. Maxton DG, Morris J, Whorwell PJ. More accurate diagnosis of irritable bowel syndrome by the use of 'non-colonic' symptomatology. Gut 1991;32:784–86.
5. Sandler RS, Drossman D.A. et al. Symptom complaints and health care seeking behavior in subjects with bowel dysfunction. Gastroenterology 1984;87:314–18.
6. Katon W, Von Korff M, Lin E, et al. Distressed high utilizers of medical care: DSM-IIIR diagnoses and treatment needs. Gen Hosp Psychiatry 1990;12:355–62.
7. Lin E, Katon W, Von Korff M, et al. Frustrating patients: physician and patient perspectives among distressed high utilizers. J Gen Intern Med 1991;6:241–46.
8. Drossman DA, Richter JE, Talley NJ, et al. Editors. The Functional Gastrointestinal Disorders: Diagnosis, Pathophysiology, and Treatment—A Multinational Consensus. McLean,VA:Degnon & Associates;1994.
9. Drossman DA, Thompson G, Talley NJ, et al. Identification of subgroups of functional gastrointestinal disorders. Gastroenterol Internat 1990;3:159–72.
10. Talley NJ, Zinsmeister AR, Schleck CD, et al. Dyspepsia and dyspepsia subgroups: a population-based study. Gastroenterology 1992;102:1259–68.
11. Talley NJ, Weaver AL, Tesmer DL, et al. Lack of discriminant value of dyspepsia subgroups in patients referred for upper endoscopy. Gastroenterology 1993;105: 1378–86.
12. Johannessen T, Petersen H, Kleveland PM, et al. The predictive value of history in dyspepsia. Scand J Gastroenterol 1990;25:689–97.
13. Small PK, Loudon MA, Waldron B, et al. Importance of reflux symptoms in functional dyspepsia. Gut 1995;36:189–92.
14. Klauser A, Voderholzer WA, Knesewitsch PA, et al. What is behind dyspepsia. Dig Dis Sci 1993;38:147–54.
15. Drossman DA. Illness behaviour in the irritable bowel syndrome. Gastroenterology Internat 1991;4:77–81.
16. Drossman DA, McKee DC, Sandler RS, et al. Psychosocial factors in the irritable bowel syndrome. A multivariate study of patients and nonpatients with irritable bowel syndrome. Gastroenterology 1988;95:701–708.
17. Whitehead WE, Bosmajian L, Zonderman AB, et al. Symptoms of psychologic distress associated with irritable bowel syndrome: comparison of community and medical clinic samples. Gastroenterology 1988;95:709–14.
18. Drossman DA, Creed FH, Olden KW, et al. Psychosocial aspects of the functional gastrointestinal disorders. In: Drossman DA, Corazziari, Talley NJ, et al., Editors. Rome II: The Functional Gastrointestinal Disorders: Diagnosis, Pathophysiology

and Treatment—A Multinational Consensus. Ed. 2. McLean,VA:Degnon Assoc.; 2000(in press).

19. Heaton KW, O'Donnell LJD, Braddon FEM, et al. Symptoms of irritable bowel syndrome in a British urban community: consulters and non-consulters. Gastroenterology 1992;102:1962–67.

20. Whitehead WE, Engel BT, Schuster MM. Irritable bowel syndrome: physiological and psychological differences between diarrhea-predominant and constipation-predominant patients. Dig Dis Sci 1980; 25:404–13.

21. Hahn BA, Kirchdoerfer LJ, Fullerton S, et al. Patient-perceived severity of irritable bowel syndrome in relation to symptoms, health resource utilization and quality of life. Aliment Pharmacol Ther 1997;11:553–59.

22. Talley NJ, Meineche-Schmidt V, Pare P, et al. Efficacy of omeprazole in functional dyspepsia: double-blind, randomised placebo-controlled trials with omeprazole (the Bond and Opera studies). Aliment Pharmacol Ther 1998;12:1055–65.

23. Lavori PW, Louis TA, Bailar III JC, et al. Designs for experiments—parallel comparisons of treatment. New Engl J Med 1983;309:1291–98.

24. Maxton DG, Morris JA, Whorwell PJ. Improving clinical trials in irritable bowel syndrome: some practical aspects. Eur J Gastroenterol Hepatol 1992;4:337–41.

25. Guyatt GH, Keller JL, Jaeschke R, et al. The n-of-1 randomized controlled trial: clinical usefulness: our three-year experience. Ann Intern Med 1990;112:293–99.

26. Hills M, Armitage P. The two-period cross-over clinical trial. Brit J Clin Pharmacol 1979;8:7–20.

27. Louis TA, Lavori PW, Bailar III JC, et al. Crossover and self-controlled designs in clinical research. New Engl J Med 1984;310:24–31.

28. Woods JR, Williams JG, Tavel M. The two-period crossover design in medical research. Ann Intern Med 1989;110:560–66.

29. Veldhuyzen van Zanten SJO, Jones M, Talley NJ. Cisapride for treatment of non-ulcer dyspepsia: a meta-analysis of randomized controlled trials. Gastroenterology 1998;114(suppl 4):A323(G1322).

30. Jebbink HJA, Smout AJPM, van Berge-Henegouwen GP. Pathophysiology and treatment of functional dyspepsia. Scand J Gastroenterol 1993;28(suppl 200): 8–14.

31. Brown BW. The crossover experiment for clinical trials. Biometrics 1980;36: 69–79.

32. Johannessen T, Fjosne U, Kleveland P, et al. Cimetidine responders in non-ulcer dyspepsia. Scand J Gastroenterol 1988;23:327–36.

33. Johannessen T, Kristensen P, Petersen H, et al. The symptomatic effect of 1-day treatment periods with cimetidine in dyspepsia: combined results from randomized, controlled, single-subject trials. Scand J Gastroenterol 1991;26:974–80.

34. Jaeschke R, Guyatt GH, Keller J, et al. Interpreting changes in Quality-of-Life score in N of 1 randomized trials. Control Clin Trials 1991;12:226s–33s.

35. Guyatt G, Sackett D, Adachi J, et al. A clinician's guide for conducting randomized trials in individual patients. Can Med Assoc J 1988;139:497–503.

36. Mahon J, Laupacis A, Donner A, et al. Randomised study of n of 1 trials versus standard practice. Brit Med J 1996;312:1069–74.

37. Lashner BA, Hanauer SB, Silverstein MD. Testing nicotine gum for ulcerative colitis patients: experience with single-patient trials. Dig Dis Sci 1990;35:827–32

38. Kleveland PM, Larsen S, Sandvik L, et al. The effect of cimetidine in non-ulcer dyspepsia: experience with a multi-cross-over model. Scand J Gastroenterol 1985;20:19–24.

39. Farup PG, Wetterhus S, Osnes M, et al. Ranitidine effectively relieves symptoms in a subset of patients with functional dyspepsia. Scand J Gastroenterol 1997;32: 755–59.

40. Farup PG, Larsen S, Ulshagen K, et al. Ranitidine for non-ulcer dyspepsia: a clinical study of the symptomatic effect of ranitidine and a classification and characterization of the responders to treatment. Scand J Gastroenterol 1991;26:1209–16.

41. Farup PG, Hovde Ø, Breder O. Are frequent short gastro-oesophageal reflux episodes the cause of symptoms in patients with non-ulcer dyspepsia responding to treatment with ranitidine? Scand J Gastroenterol 1995;30:829–32.

42. Johannessen T. Controlled trials in single subjects. Brit Med J 1991;303:173–74.

43. Bytzer P, Hansen JM, The Danish Dyspepsia Study Group. Response to acid suppression in dyspepsia: identifying responders with a random starting day trial. Gastroenterology 1997;112:A81.

44. Johannessen T, Fosstvedt D, Petersen H. Combined single subject trials. Scand J Prim Health Care 1991;9:23–27.

45. Zucker DR, Schmid CH, McIntosh MW, et al. Combining single patient (N-of-1) trials to estimate population treatment effects and to evaluate individual patient responses to treatment. J Clin Epidemiol 1997;50:401–410.

46. Spiegelhalter DJ. Statistical issues in studies of individual response. Scand J Gastroenterology 1988;23(suppl 147):40–45.

47. Lewis JA. Controlled trials in single subjects: limitations of use. Brit Med J 1991; 303:175–76.

48. Senn S. Suspended judgment. N-of-1 trials. Control Clin Trials 1993;14:1–5.

49. Larsen S, Farup P, Flaten O, et al. The multi-crossover model for classifying patients as responders to a given treatment. Scand J Gastroenterol 1991;26:763–70.

50. O'Donoghue DP, Dawson AM, Powell-Tuck Brown RL, et al. Double blind withdrawal trial of azathioprine as maintenance treatment for Crohn's disease. Lancet 1978;2:955–57.

51. Hawthorne AB, Logan RFA, Hawkey CJ, et al. Randomized controlled trial of azathioprine withdrawal in ulcerative colitis. Brit Med J 1992;305:20–22.

52. Altman DG. Randomisation. Brit Med J 1991;302:1481–82.

53. Altman DG. Comparability of randomised groups. The Statistician 1985;34:125–36.

54. Schulz KF, Chalmers I, Hayes RJ, et al. Empirical evidence of bias. JAMA 1995; 273:408–12.

55. Therneau TM. How many stratification factors are "too many" to use in a randomization plan? Control Clin Trials 1993;14:98–108.

56. Rösch W. Efficacy of cisapride in the treatment of epigastric pain and concomitant symptoms in non-ulcer dyspepsia. Scand J Gastroenterol 1989;24(s165): 54–58.

57. Rösch W. Cisapride in non-ulcer dyspepsia: results of a placebo-controlled trial. Scand J Gastroenterol 1987;22:161–64.

58. Christie J, Shepherd V, Codling BW, et al. Gastric cancer below the age of 55: implications for screening patients with uncomplicated dyspepsia. Gut 1997;41:513–.

59. Talley NJ, Silverstein MC, Agreus L, et al. AGA Technical Review: evaluation of dyspepsia. Gastroenterology 1998;114:582–95.

60. Bytzer P, Hansen JM, Schaffalitzky de Muckadell OB. Empirical H2-blocker therapy or prompt endoscopy in management of dyspepsia. Lancet 1994;343;811–816.

61. Talley NJ, Meineche-Schmidt V, Pare P, et al. Efficacy of omeprazole in functional dyspepsia: double-blind, randomised placebo-controlled trials with omeprazole (the Bond and Opeca studies). Aliment Pharmacol Ther 1998;12:1055–65.

62. Drossman DA, McKee DC, Sandler RS, et al. Psychosocial factors in the irritable bowel syndrome: a multivariate study of patients and nonpatients with irritable bowel syndrome. Gastroenterology 1988;95:701–708.

63. Whitehead WE, Bosmajian S, Zonderman AB, et al. Symptoms of psychologic distress associated with irritable bowel syndrome: comparison of community and medical clinic samples. Gastroenterology 1988;95:709–14.

64. Lydeard S, Jones R. Factors affecting the decision to consult with dyspepsia: comparison of consulters and non-consulters. J Roy Coll Gen Pract 1989;39:495–98.

65. Johannessen T, Petersen H, Kleveland PM, et al. The predictive value of history in dypepsia. Scand J Gastroenterol 1990;25:689–97.

66. Drossman DA. Illness behaviour in the irritable bowel syndrome. Gastroenterology Internat 1991;4:77–81.

67. Campbell SM, Roland MO. Why do people consult the doctor? Fam Pract 1996; 13:75–83.

68. Talley NJ. Predictors of health care seeking for irritable bowel syndrome: a population based study. Gut 1997;41:394–98.

69. Talley NJ, Weaver AL, Zinsmeister AR, et al. Onset and Disappearance of gastrointestinal symptoms and functional gastrointestinal disorders. Am J Epidemiol 1992;136:165–77.

70. Talley NJ, McNeil D, Hayden A, et al. Prognosis of chronic unexplained dyspepsia: a prospective study of potential predictor variables in patients with endoscopically diagnosed nonulcer dyspepsia. Gastroenterology 1987; 92:1060–66.

71. Haynes RB, Taylor DW, Sackett DL, Editors. Compliance in Health Care. Baltimore:Johns Hopkins University Press;1979.

72. Eraker SA, Kirscht JP, Becker MH. Understanding and improving patients compliance. Ann Intern Med 1984;100:258–68.

73. Anonymous. Patient compliance in therapeutic trials. Lancet 1991;337:823–24.

74. Feinstein AR. Intent-to-treat policy for analyzing randomized trials: statistical distortions and neglected clinical challenges. In: Cramer JA, Spilker B, Editors. Pa-

tient Compliance in Medical Practice and Clinical Trials. New York:Raven Press; 1991:359–70.

75. Hyland ME, Crocker GR. Validation of an asthma quality of life diary in a clinical trial. Thorax 1995;50:724–30.

76. Russell EB, Lee AJ, Garraway WM, et al. Use of a 7-day diary for urinary symptom recording. Eur Urol 1994;26:227–32.

77. Geddes DM, Dones L, Hill E, *et al.* Quality of life during chemotherapy for small cell lung cancer: assessment and use of a daily diary card in a randomized trial. Eur J Cancer 1990;26:484–92.

78. Sandha GS, Hunt RH, Veldhuyzen van Zanten SJO. A systematic overview of the use of diary cards, quality of life questionnaires and psychometric tests in the treatment trials of *Helicobactor pylori* positive and negative non-ulcer dyspepsia. Scand J Gastroenterol 1999;34:244–49.

79. Harding JP, Hamm LR, Ehsanullah RSB, et al. Use of a novel electronic data collection system in multicenter studies of irritable bowel syndrome. Aliment Pharmacol Ther 1997;11:1073–76.

80. Thompson WG, Creed F, Drossman DA, et al. Functional bowel disease and functional abdominal pain. Gastroenterol Internat 1992;5:75–91.

81. Guyatt GH, Veldhuyzen van Zanten SJO, Feeney DH, et al. Measuring quality of life in clinical trials: a taxonomy and review. Can Med J Assoc 1989;140:1441–88.

82. Guyatt GH, Feeney DH, Patrick DL. Measuring health-related quality of life. Ann Intern Med 1993;118:622–29.

83. Melzack R. The McGill Pain Questionnaire: major properties and scoring methods. Pain 1975;1:277–99.

84. Miller GA. The magical number of seven plus or minus two: some limits on our capacity for processing information. Psychol Rev 1956;63:81–87.

85. MacKenzie CR, Charlson ME. Standards for the use of ordinal scales in clinical trials. Brit Med J1986;292:40–43.

86. Reading AE. Comparisons of pain rating scales. J Psychosomat Res 1980;24: 119–24.

87. Kerns RD, Finn P, Haythornthwaite J. Self-monitored pain intensity: psychometric properties and clinical utility. J Behav Med 1988;11:71–82.

88. Guyatt GH, Walter S, Norman G. Measuring change over time: assessing the usefulness of evaluative instruments. J Chron Dis 1987;40:171–78.

89. Huskisson EC. Measurement of pain. Lancet 1974;ii:1127–31.

90. Ohnaus EE, Adler R. Methodological problems in the measurement of pain: a comparison between the verbal rating scale and the visual analogue scale. Pain 1975;1:379–84.

91. Guyatt GH, Townsend M, Keller JL, et al. Should study subjects see their previous responses: data from a randomized control trial. J Clin Epidemiol 1989;42: 913–20.

92. Guyatt GH, Townsend M, Berman LB, et al. A comparison of Likert and visual analogue scales for measuring change in function. J Chron Dis 1987;40:1129–33.

93. Jaeschke R, Singer J, Guyatt GH. A comparison of seven-point and visual analogue scales. Control Clin Trials 1990;11:43–51.

94. Sjoden PO, Bates S, Nyren O. Continuous self-recording of epigastric pain with two rating scales: compliance, authenticity, reliability, and sensitivity. J Behav Assess 1983;314:339–43.

95. Guyatt GH, Townsend M, Keller J, et al. Measuring functional status in chronic lung disease: conclusions from a randomized control trial. Respir Med 1989;83: 293–97.

96. Juniper EF, Guyatt GH, Willan A, et al. Determining a minimal important change in a disease-specific quality of life questionnaire. J Clin Epidemiol 1994; 47:81–87.

97. Jaeschke R, Singer J, Guyatt GH. Measurement of health status: ascetaining the minimal clinically important difference. Control Clin Trials 1989;10:407–15.

98. National Institute of Mental Health. CGI: Clinical Global Impressions. In: Guy W, Editor. ECDEU Assessment for Psychopharmacology. Rev. ed. Rockville,MD: NIMH;1976:217–22.

99. Whitehead WE, Burnett CK, Cook III EW, et al. Impact of irritable bowel syndrome on quality of life. Dig Dis Sci 1996;41:2248–53.

100. Talley NJ, Weaver AL, Zinsmeister AR. Impact of functional dyspepsia on quality of life. Dig Dis Sci 1995;40:584–89.

101. Gergner M, Bobbitt RA, Carter WB. The Sickness Impact Profile: development and final revision of a health status seasure. Med Care 1981;19:787–805.

102. Hunt SM, McKenna SP, McEwen J, et al: A quantitative approach to perceived health status: a validation study. J Epidemiol Commun Health 1980;34:281–86.

103. Ware JE, Brook RH, Davies-Avery A, et al: Conceptualization and measurement of health for adults in the health insurance study. In: Model of Health and Methodology, Vol. 1. Santa Monica CA:The Rand Corporation;1980.

104. Sackett DL, Chambers LW, MacPherson AS, et al: The development and application of indicies of health: general methods and a summary of results. Am J Public Health 1997;67:423–28.

105. Stewart AL, Hays RD, Ware JE. The MOS short-form general health survey. Med Care 1988;26:724–34.

106. Dimenas E, Glise H, Hallerback B, et al. Quality of life in patients with upper gastrointestinal symptoms: an improved evaluation of treatment regimens? Scan J Gastroenterol 1993;28:681–87.

107. Guyatt GH, Bombardier C, Tugwell P. Measuring disease specific quality of life in clinical trials. Can Med Assoc J 1986;134:889–95.

108. Guyatt G, Mitchell A, Irvine EJ, et al. A new measure of health status for clinical trials in inflammatory bowel disease. Gastroenterology 1989;96:804–10.

109. Irvine EJ, Feagan B, Rochon J, et al., for the Canadian Crohn's Relapse Prevention Trial. Quality of life: a valid and reliable measure of therapeutic efficacy in the treatment of inflammatory bowel disease. Gastroenterology 1994;106:287–96.

110. Dimenas E, Glise H, Ballerback B, et al. Well-being and gastrointestinal symptoms

among patients referred to endoscopy due to suspected duodenal ulcer. Scand J Gastroenterol 1995;30:1046–52.

111. Veldhuyzen van Zanten SJO, Tytgat KMAJ, Pollak PT, et al. Can severity of symptoms be used as outcome measures in trials of non-ulcer dyspepsia and *Helicobacter pylori*. J Clin Epidemiol 1993;46:273–79.

112. El-Omar EM, Banerjee S, Wirz A, et al. The Glasgow Dyspepsia Severity Score: a tool for the global measurement of dyspepsia. Eur J Gastroenterol Hepat 1996; 8:967–71.

113. Wiklund I, Junghard O, Grace E, et al. Quality of life in reflux and dyspepsia: psychometric documentation of a new disease-specific questionnaire (QUALRAD). Eur J Surg 1998;583(suppl):41–49.

114. Houghton LA, HeymanDJ, Whorwell PJ. Symptomatology, quality of Life and economic features of irritable bowel syndrome: the effect of hypnotherapy. Aliment Pharmacol Ther. 1996;10:91–95.

115. Hahn BA, Kirchdoerfer LJ, Fullerton S, et al. Evaluation of a new quality of life questionnaire for patients with irritable bowel syndrome. Aliment Pharmacol Ther 1997;11:547–52.

116. Patrick DL, Drossman DA, Frederick IO, et al. Quality of life in persons with irritable bowel syndrome: development and validation of a new measure. Dig Dis Sci 1998;43:400–11.

117. Drossman DA, Li Z, Toner BB, et al. Functional bowel disorders: a multicenter comparison of health status and development of illness severity index. Dig Dis Sci 1995;40:986–95.

118. Francis CY, Morris J, Whorwell PJ. The irritable bowel severity scoring system: a simple method of monitoring irritable bowel syndrome and its progress. Aliment Pharmacol Ther 1997;11:395–402.

119. Heaton KW, Ghosh S, Braddon FEM. How bad are the symptoms and bowel dysfunction of patients with irritable bowel syndrome? A prospective controlled study with emphasis on stool form. Gut 1991;31:73–79.

120. Altman DG. Better reporting of randomized controlled trials: the CONSORT statement. JAMA 1996;276:637–39 .

121. Beg, Cho M, Eastwood S, et al. Improving the quality of reporting of randomized controlled trials: the CONSORT statement. Brit Med J 1996;313:570–71.

122. Altman DG. Better reporting of randomised controlled trials: the CONSORT statement: *Authors must provide enough information for readers to know how the trial was prepared*. Brit Med J 1996;313:570–71.

123. DerSimonian R, Charette LJ, McPhee B, et al. Reporting on methods in clinical trials. New Engl J Med 1982;306:1332–37.

124. Gore SM, Jones G, Thompson SG. *The Lancet's* statistical review process: areas for improvement by authors. Lancet 1992;340:100–102.

125. Simon R. Confidence intervals for reporting results of clinical trials. Ann Intern Med 1986;105:429–35.

126. Guyatt G, Jaeschke R, Heddle N, et al. Basic statistics for clinicians: 2. Interpreting

study results: confidence intervals. Can Med Assoc J 1995;152:169–73.

127. Oxman AD, Guyatt GH. A consumer's guide to subgroup analyses. Ann Intern Med 1992;116:78–84.

128. Smith DG, Clemens J, Crede W, et al. Impact of multiple comparisons in randomized clinical trials. Am J Med 1987;83:545–50.

129. Perneger T. What is wrong with Bonferroni adjustments? Brit Med J 1998;316: 1236–38.

130. Campbell MJ, Julious SA, Altman DG. Estimating sample sizes for binary, ordered categorical, and continuous outcomes in two group comparisons. Brit Med J 1995;311:1145–48.

131. Reed JF, Slaichert W. Statistical proof in inconclusive 'negative' trials. Arch Intern Med 1981;141:1307–10.

132. Freiman JA, Chalmers TC, Smith H, et al. The importance of beta, the type II error and sample size in the design and interpretation of the randomized control trial. New Engl J Med 1978;299:690–94.

133. Detsky AS, Sackett DL. When was a 'negative' clinical trial big enough? How many patients you needed depends on what you found. Arch Intern Med 1985; 145:709–12.

134. Makuch RW, Johnson MF. Some issues in the design and interpretation of 'negative' clinical studies. Arch Intern Med 1986;146:986–89.

135. Bero L, Rennie D. The Cochrane collaboration: preparing, maintaining and disseminating systematic reviews of the effects of health care. JAMA 1995;274: 1935–38.

Chapter 12

Definition of a Responder in Clinical Trials for Functional Gastrointestinal Disorders: Report on a Symposium

William E. Whitehead, Chair, *with*
the Organizing Committee:
Enrico Corazziari,
Robert Prizont,
John R. Senior,
W. Grant Thompson,
and Sander J. O. Veldhuyzen van Zanten

623

Introduction

On September 10 and 11, 1998, approximately 125 participants met at a symposium in Vienna, Austria, with the goal of determining whether a consensus could be developed on the definition of responders in clinical trials in the functional gastrointestinal disorders. Present at this meeting were representatives of the United States Food and Drug Administration (Robert Prizont, M.D. and John Senior, M.D.), a representative of the Japanese International Motility Society (Kei Matsueda, M.D., Ph.D.), academic investigators from around the world, and representatives of several pharmaceutical companies currently engaged in the development of therapeutic compounds for the functional gastrointestinal disorders. The discussion centered primarily on irritable bowel syndrome (IBS), the functional gastrointestinal disorder for which there is the largest development program underway. However, the discussion also addressed the measurement of outcomes in functional constipation.

This conference was sponsored by the Multinational Working Teams to Develop Diagnostic Criteria for Functional Gastrointestinal Disorders (MWT), also known as Rome II. Over a two-year period, the executive committee of the MWT held a series of informal meetings with representatives of the Food and Drug Administration, and on one occasion, with a representative of the European Agency for the Evaluation of Medicinal Products. During these meetings, representatives of the regulatory groups indicated that there was a need for a more broad-based consensus on the best ways of defining responders in clinical trials. The MWT organized this conference to meet this need.

Drs. Robert Prizont and John Senior participated as individual scientists. Their views do not represent the official policy of the FDA. A detailed summary of this conference is available on request.

This conference was unique in several respects. It is the first time representatives of the regulatory agencies, the academic community, and the pharmaceutical research teams have met together with the goal of developing a consensus on outcome measurement. It also represents a milestone in the willingness of different pharmaceutical companies to share data from actual clinical trials for the purpose of developing outcome measures that could be used by all of them. The degree of consensus achieved at this initial meeting was modest. However, this represents the first step in a process that is expected to lead to a broad-based consensus on these issues.

The conference was organized as a multi-stage process. First, representatives of the FDA and of Japanese International Motility Society presented position papers; Dr. Drossman described the history of the MWT; and Dr. Sander Van Zanten presented the provisional recommendations of the MWT, which dealt with the design of clinical trials. Following this, academic investigators described their views on the measurement of outcomes. The representatives of six pharmaceutical companies then presented data. These companies were asked to select clinical trials completed by their companies in which at least one outcome measure had been found to be significantly different between drug and placebo groups, and to compare the different outcome measures used in these trials on a common scale, making it possible to compare their relative efficacy and the magnitude of the placebo response. These presentations were followed by an open discussion whose purpose was to assess the degree of consensus among the participants and to summarize their recommendations for measurement. Following the conference, these recommendations, together with a summary of the presentations at the conference, were circulated to the participants and to other members of the scientific community for comment. After this review process was completed, the recommendations were forwarded to the regulatory agencies and to the companies that participated in the conference.

Consensus Recommendations

The participants were not able to reach a consensus on a single approach to the measurement of outcomes in clinical trials. However, the following points of agreement were reached:

(1) Evaluation should be based on patient reports rather than ratings by investigator/clinicians.

(2) Efficacy evaluation should be based on the percentage of subjects meeting a predefined criterion of clinical significance rather than on the statistical significance of differences between groups or between periods of observation.

(3) Outcome measures based on self-reported relief of symptoms appear to be promising because they are easily understood by patients and have face validity. However, such measures often have dichotomous response scales (e.g., yes or no), and there is evidence that dichotomous scales are associated with lower statistical power (greater error of measurement) than continuous measures or ordinal-scaled measures with more than five steps.

(4) Global ratings of symptom severity or symptom change in which the patient is asked to integrate his/her experience, or summated indices such as validated questionnaires, appear to be as good as specific symptom measures.

(5) Retrospective ratings of "usual" symptom severity are generally good approximations of daily diary averages over brief periods such as one month or less.

(6) Visual Analog Scales (VAS) and numerical scales have been criticized because (a) approximately 10% of patients find them difficult to comprehend, and (b) it has been difficult to define clinically significant change or group differences. However, simultaneous use of VAS or numerical rating scales of intensity, change, or relief can greatly complement and help in the interpretation of dichotomous or categorically-scaled primary outcome measures. When VAS and numerical scales are used, patients should be carefully instructed.

(7) Quality of life scales, symptom severity indices, and psychological or cognitive measures cannot be recommended as primary outcome measures at this time because they have not been sufficiently validated in the context of drug evaluation.

(8) Placebo run-ins are not recommended because they may interfere with the assessment of treatment effects, but baseline periods of measurement without treatment are acceptable.

(9) Psychological measures are recommended at baseline because they may be useful as covariates in the interpretation of differential treatment responses.

(10) Physiological investigations are encouraged because they advance our understanding of the disorder and the mechanism of therapeutic benefit, but they are not recommended for primary outcome measures.

(11) Multinational treatment trials require attention to linguistic and cultural translation of outcome measures, and they require full disclosure of the methods used to develop and validate transcultural instruments.

Chapter 13

The Road
to Rome

W. Grant Thompson

Medical diagnosis generally requires observed anatomical or physiological abnormalities. Description of the illness and criteria for its diagnosis follow naturally. Recognized symptoms can then be attributed to the observation, and a diagnosis predictably follows. In the case of the functional disorders, such a process is impossible. Since there are no observed defects, we only know of the existence of these disorders through the words of our patients. Hence there can be no animal model. Parrots may talk, but are not likely to discuss their bowels. The need to define these disorders of unknown pathology represents a major paradigm shift, a substantial change in thinking for doctors whose training concentrates on basic science and palpable "evidence." Since more than half of gut disorders encountered by gastroenterologists and primary care doctors are functional, we must face the reality that scientific evidence to explain these disorders does not exist, and develop alternate methods to identify them.

For too long, functional diseases have been described by what they are not, rather than as real entities. Yet they are real enough to our patients. Not only does this exclusive approach fail to provide the patient with the dignity of a diagnosis, but it also generates needless tests and consultations. The fruitless pursuit of an anatomical cause renders functional disorders "diagnoses of exclusion." Their very numbers and cost demand a more positive approach.

There are many references to gut dysfunction in the ancient and early European literature. However, the first credible English language descriptions of irritable bowel syndrome (IBS) appeared in the early nineteenth century. One such description in 1818 drew attention to the three cardinal symptoms of IBS; abdominal pain, "derangement of . . . digestion" and "flatulence" [1]. A few years later, Howship described a "spasmodic stricture" of the colon reflecting the enduring, but still unsubstantiated belief that functional gut disorders are somehow the product of gut spasm [2]. Mid-century brought more sophisticated treatises (and very unsophisticated cures such as purging and "electro galvanism"). In 1849, Cumming asks incredulously: "the bowels are at one time constipated and at another lax in the same person . . . how the disease has two such different symptoms I do not propose to explain" [3]. Were Dr. Cumming to return to a modern consensus meeting, he would discover that this enigma remains unexplained! Cumming's treatise contained one other comment in line with modern thinking about IBS. "One can tell, without more minute examination what the nature of the complaint is." The authors of this book agree with Cumming's notion of a positive diagnosis, even though many doctors persist in recognizing IBS and the other functional gut disorders only after the patient has undergone extensive investigation.

Medicine's understanding of the IBS progressed little during the next 120 years. Indeed, it may have lost ground! In Edwardian times, functional disorders were considered diseases of the wealthy. In fact, only the affluent could afford to be the patients of the Harley Street doctors who published their observations in the medical literature [4]. Through the writings of Metchnikoff and Arbuthnot Lane, constipation became associated with uncleanness [5]. The quaint notion of "autointoxication" resulting from colon contents prompted an urge to purge that persists to this day. In the 1920s and 1930s pejorative descriptors such as "psychogenic," "neurogenic," and "The Abdominal Woman" [6] did little to help patients with functional gut disorders. Proctalgia fugax was long thought to be a disease of young professional males, because only doctors had the temerity to describe their symptoms in letters to the editor of the *Lancet*. [7]. Use of terms such as "spastic colitis" and "hyperacidity" inferred etiologies that do not exist for these disorders [5].

The first systematic attempt to bring discipline to this area was a 1962 retrospective review of IBS patients seen at Oxford by Chaudhary and Truelove [8]. From this experience, the authors were able to report many of the features that we recognize as those of the IBS (or the "irritable colon syndrome" as they termed it). They even separated IBS from what we now call functional diarrhea, and noted that one-quarter of their patients' complaints began with an enteric infection. Their report ushered in a new era, and scientific publications on functional disorders increased rapidly thereafter (fig. 1).

The first attempt to classify all the functional gastrointestinal disorders appears in the index of my book, *The Irritable Gut*, published in 1979 [9]. In 1978, led by Ken Heaton, Adrian Manning and I reported results obtained by questionnaire administered to Bristol outpatients with abdominal pain and disordered bowel habit [10]. The 6 out of 15 symptoms we found more common in the IBS than organic gut disease (as determined by a chart review a year later) are now known as the Manning Criteria (see Chapter 7). In 1984, Kruis and his colleagues from Germany reported a similar study [11]. Their report recalls the three cardinal IBS symptoms of pain, bowel dysfunction, and flatulence mentioned by Powell in 1818. If all three were present, IBS was highly likely. Kruis et al. stressed chronicity and other symptoms as well, but their major contribution was to quantitate the alarm symptoms that should alert the physician to organic disease. These two discriminant function studies, in addition to epidemiologic data provided by Drossman [12] and Whitehead [13], are the basis of the Rome Criteria.

The inspiration for the Rome Criteria followed the 12th International Congress

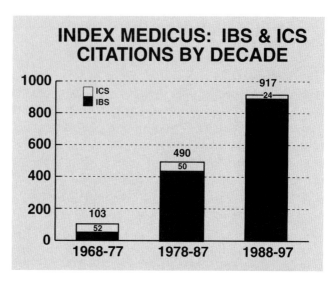

Figure 1. Results of a Medline literature search for irritable bowel syndrome (IBS) and irritable colon syndrome (ICS) by decade, for the 30 years ending with 1997. Note the rapid rise in publications, and the relative decline in the use of the term irritable colon.

of Gastroenterology held in Lisbon in 1984. I chaired one of the earliest international symposia on the IBS, and my panel and the organizers of the Congress were astonished that despite untranslated presentations in three languages, the attendees far outstripped the capacity of the assigned room. One of the panel members was Professor Aldo Torsoli, an organizer of the next international congress to be held four years later in Rome. Over coffee in Portugal, we discussed the need for guidelines for the diagnosis and study of IBS. A working team was set up to produce such guidelines for the next congress.

Delighted at the opportunity to chair this working team, I corresponded with Doug Drossman (USA), Ken Heaton (UK), Gerhard Dotteval (Sweden), and Wolfgang Kruis (Germany) for two years. In 1987, we met in Rome to debate a draft proposal and reach consensus on definitions. The penultimate draft was sent to 16 noted colleagues in seven countries. Their comments and suggestions were considered by the working team, and the first Rome Criteria were presented at the 13th Congress in Rome in 1988. They were published the following year [14].

Following that Rome meeting, Dr. Doug Drossman, who was a member of the Rome Working Team, was invited by Professor Torsoli and Dr. Enrico Corazziari to set up another committee to look at subgroups of IBS. As a result of their discussions, the project was expanded to include all the functional gastrointestinal disorders. This working team, which included most of the editors of this book, met in Rome to classify the functional gastrointestinal disorders into 21 entities in five anatomical regions of the gut [15].

Having achieved generous sponsorship, Doug Drossman organized a succession of working teams that further developed these criteria in the five anatomical regions (esophageal [16], gastroduodenal [17], biliary [18], and anorectal [19]) and discussed topics related to functional gut disorders. In 1994, their collective work was updated and published in *The Functional Gastrointestinal Disorders: Diagnosis, Pathophysiology and Treatment—A Multinational Consensus* [20].

While this work is now known as Rome I, it includes the second rendition of the Rome IBS criteria. The new functional bowel working team published some revisions to the 1988 IBS criteria in 1992. Pain became a requisite for the diagnosis, and duration parameters were added [21].

The Rome Criteria have generated much energy and controversy. They are imperfect. Validation studies are difficult and rare. Those interested in the condition possess disparate viewpoints: epidemiologists, primary care physicians, consultants, researchers, psychologists, physiologists, third party payers, and of course, the patients themselves. Nevertheless, the criteria have gained such currency that they are the basis for entry into most research studies of functional gut disorders and have compelled an accurate description of entered patients in the remainder. They are the industry standard for entry into clinical drug trials, although they are sometimes modified to suit the characteristics of the product to be tested. They have given these disorders, particularly IBS, a profile. Patients can now be reassured they suffer from a legitimate disorder, not symptoms rendered imaginary by a negative test. The criteria have created a language with which the above-mentioned groups can communicate. The coming together of such disparate constituencies in a common effort is a major achievement, due in no small way to this systematic recognition of the functional gut disorders.

This book culminates a new four-year effort to update the Rome Criteria and, like Rome I, owes much to the energy and drive of Doug Drossman. The mechanics of this process are described elsewhere, but more than Rome I, the Rome II process is generously supported by industry, and has attracted the interest and participation of many people in several disciplines from around the world. There can be no better testimony to the stature that the Rome criteria have achieved. However, this book is not the end, or even the beginning of the end. It is, at best, the end of the beginning of what promises to be an ongoing process that may last as long as knowledge of the pathophysiology of functional gut disorders eludes us. Meanwhile, here is a great need to generate data that will sharpen the criteria and validate their use. Discussions have begun for Rome III.

References

1. Powell R. On certain painfull afflictions of the intestinal canal. Med Trans Royal Coll Phys 1818;6:106–17.
2. Howship J. Practical remarks on the discrimination and successful treatment of spasmodic stricture of the colon. London:Burgess and Hill;1830.
3. Cumming W. Electro-galvanism in a peculiar affliction of the mucous membrane of the bowels. Lond Med Gazette 1849;NS9:969–73.
4. Hale-White W. Colitis. Lancet 1895;1:537.
5. Thompson WG. Gut Reactions. New York:Plenum;1989.
6. Hutchison R. Lectures on Dyspepsia. 2nd ed. London:Edward Arnold;1927.
7. Thompson WG. Proctalgia fugax. Dig Dis Sci 1981;26:1121–24.
8. Chaudhary NA, Truelove SC. The irritable colon syndrome. Quart J Med 1962;31:307–22.
9. Thompson WG. The Irritable Gut. Baltimore:University Park Press;1979.
10. Manning AP, Thompson WG, Heaton KW, et al. Towards positive diagnosis of the irritable bowel. Brit Med J 1978;2:653–54.
11. Kruis W, Thieme CH, Weinzierl M, et al. A diagnostic score for the irritable bowel syndrome: its value in the exclusion of organic disease. Gastroenterology 1984;87:1–7.
12. Drossman DA, Sandler RS, Mckee DC, et al. Bowel patterns among subjects not seeking health care: use of a questionnaire to identify a population with bowel dysfunction. Gastroenterology 1982;83:529–34.
13. Whitehead WE, Winget C, Fedoravicius AS, et al. Learned illness behavior in patients with irritable bowel syndrome and peptic ulcer. Dig Dis Sci 1982;27:202–208.
14. Thompson WG, Dotevall G, Drossman DA, et al. Irritable bowel syndrome: guidelines for the diagnosis. Gastroenterol Internat 1989;2:92–95.
15. Drossman DA, Funch-Jensen P, Janssens J, et al. Identification of subgroups of functional bowel disorders. Gastroenterol Internat 1990;3:159–72.
16. Richter JE, Baldi F, Clouse RE, et al. Functional Oesophageal Disorders. Gastroenterol Internat 1992;5:3–17.
17. Talley NJ, Colin-Jones D, Koch KL, et al. Functional dyspepsia: a classification with guidelines for diagnosis and management. Gastroenterol Internat 1991;4:145–60.
18. Corazziari E, Funch-Jensen P, Hogan W, et al. Working team report: functional disorders of the biliary tract. Gastroenterol Internat 1993;6:129–44.
19. Whitehead WE, Devroede G, Habib FI, et al. Functional disorders of the anus and rectum. Gastroenterol Internat 1992;5:92–108.
20. Drossman DA; Richter J; Talley NJ, et al., Editors. The Functional Gastrointestinal

Disorders: Diagnosis, Pathophysiology, and Treatment—A Multinational Consensus. McLean VA: Degnon Assoc; 1994.

21. Thompson WG, Creed FH, Drossman DA, et al. Functional bowel disorders and functional abdominal pain. Gastroenterol Internat 1992;5:75–91.

Glossary

Prepared by
W. Grant Thompson
and the Working
Team Members

abdominal distension: sensation that the abdomen is swollen, bloated, or full. May be visible to the patient or to an observer.

abuse: threats or actions of an emotional, sexual, or physical nature in which a power differential exists between the perpetrator and the victim.

achalasia: failure of the lower esophageal sphincter to relax.

action potential: sometimes called "spike potential." A short-lasting, all-or-none change in membrane potential of a nerve or muscle cell that arises when a graded membrane depolarization passes a threshold; usually becomes a propagated nerve or muscle cell impulse.

adherence (also called compliance): execution by a subject or patient of therapeutic instructions, i.e., use of medication.

aerophagia: ingestion of air. *See* Mueller maneuver.

afferent nerve (afferents): nerve fibers (usually sensory) carrying impulses from an organ or tissue toward the central nervous system or the information-processing centers of the enteric nervous system.

aganglionosis: congenital absence of ganglionic cells in the enteric nervous system in a segment of bowel. This may affect the anal canal and is the pathophysiological basis for Hirschprung's disease.

alarm symptoms: symptoms such as fever, bleeding, anemia, weight loss, or physical findings such as an abdominal mass that cannot be explained by functional gastrointestinal disorders.

allodynia: a form of visceral hypersensitivity where there is an abnormal pain response to an innocuous or non-noxious visceral afferent signal.

anemia: reduced blood hemoglobin or red cell concentration.

antidepressant: a class of drugs, the primary effect of which is to correct neurotransmitter imbalance in the central nervous system occurring in a major depression. Antidepressants tend to be useful in the functional GI disorders both to treat concomitant anxiety and depression and to reduce pain.

anal fissure: crack in the skin or mucosa in or adjacent to the anal canal, causing symptoms of stinging or itching during defecation.

anal wink reflex/perianal wink reflex: a reflex contraction of the external anal sphincter, which can be elicited by gentle stroking of the perianal skin.

anismus: synonym for pelvic floor dyssynergia.

anorexia: lack or loss of appetite for food.

anoscopy: examination of the anus and lower rectum with a rigid, side-viewing cone or tube.

anorectal angle: the (approximately) 90 degree angle between the rectum and the anal canal. This angle becomes more obtuse during defecation and more acute when holding back stool. The angle is formed by the contraction of the puborectalis muscle.

antipsychotic: a drug which acts mainly via dopaminergic pathways in the central nervous system to decrease symptoms of psychosis, such as delusions (including somatic delusions), hallucinations, and severe agitation.

antral dysrhythmia: abnormality of electrical rhythm in the gastric antrum (bradygastria/tachygastria) analogous to cardiac arrhythmia.

anxiety: a subjective sense of feeling worried, often accompanied by bodily symptoms, including for example palpitations, breathlessness, abdominal churning. Occasionally amounts to panic.

anxiety disorder: excessive anxiety and worry which cannot be controlled, and is persistent with a range of symptoms. Mild forms include phobias; more severe forms include panic disorder.

anxiolytic: a drug which can decrease, via action on the central nervous system, the symptoms of acute or chronic anxiety, including panic disorder, obsessive-compulsive disorder, phobia, or generalized anxiety.

area postrema: brain stem region outside the blood-brain barrier believed to be an emetic (vomiting) trigger zone.

Auerbach's plexus: ganglionated plexus of the enteric nervous system situated between the longitudinal and circular muscle coats of the muscularis externa of the digestive tract. May be referred to as the myenteric plexus.

axons: fibers that carry impulses away from the perikaryon of a nerve cell.

barostat: device for maintaining a constant pressure, enabling (1) assessment of gut intraluminal tone, by measuring volume changes that reflect variations in gut tone; (2) assessment of gut sensitivity by determining perception in response to isobaric distension of a specific gut region.

behavior: acts, activities, responses to actions, movements, processes, operations, etc.; in short, any measurable response of an organism.

behavioral: any variable that can assess a person's activity, especially that which can be externally observed.

belch: retrograde expulsion of gas or air (usually ingested) from the upper gut.

benzodiazepine: a class of drugs which acts on the cerebral cortex and ascending reticular activating system (ARAS) to facilitate the effect of the inhibitor peptide gamma amino butyric acid (GABA), which in turn decreases central nervous system irritability and promotes smooth muscle relaxation, sleep, lessened arousal (decreased anxiety). Benzodiazepines are useful in the functional GI disorders to decrease the symptoms of panic disorder, phobias, and generalized anxiety if they are present.

biliary sphincter of Oddi dysfunction: motility abnormalities of the sphincter of Oddi, which include sphincter of Oddi dyskinesia.

biliary type pain (I, II, III): classification of patients with biliary-type pain despite cholecystectomy according to clinical presentation, laboratory results, and ERCP findings.

biofeedback: the use of electronic or mechanical devices to provide visual and/or auditory information (feedback) on a biological process for the purpose of teaching an individual to control the biological process.

biogenic amines: group of chemical substances that include the neurotransmitters, 5-hydroxytryptamine and norepinephrine.

biomedical model: the model of illness and disease in Western medical education and research. It has two assumptions: (1) reductionism—that all conditions can be linearly reduced to a single etiology, and (2) dualism—where illness and disease are dichotomized either to an "organic" disorder having an objectively defined etiology, or a "functional" disorder, with no specific etiology or pathophysiology. The biomedical model is not sufficient to explain the functional GI disorders.

biopsychosocial model: a model that proposes that illness and disease result from simultaneously interacting systems at the cellular, tissue, organismal, interpersonal, and environmental level. It incorporates the biologic aspects of the disorder with the unique psychosocial features of the individual, and helps explain the variability in symptom expression among individuals having the same biologic condition.

bipolar depression: an affective disorder in which the patient experiences both depressive and manic episodes.

blind: in clinical trials, subject or observer is unaware of the treatment (drug vs. placebo) that an individual subject is given.

bloating: abdominal distension or fullness that may be felt and/or may be visible. (*See* abdominal distension).

bloating in the upper abdomen: a feeling of tightness located in the upper abdomen; it should be distinguished from visible abdominal distension.

borborygmi: audible bowel sounds.

brain-gut axis: the bi-directional connections between the brain (CNS), autonomic nervous system and gut (enteric nervous system) that serve various physiological functions. Visceral afferent fibers project to somatotypic, emotional, and cognitive centers of the CNS producing a variety of interpretations to the stimuli based on prior learning and one's cognitive and emotional state. In turn, the CNS can inhibit or facilitate afferent nociceptive signals, motility, secretory function, or inflammation.

Bristol stool form scale: a 7-point descriptor scale of stool form ranging from watery to hard and lumpy. The scale correlates with whole gut transit time. (See chapter 7, table 4 and fig. 1).

bulking agents: macromolecular substances which increase stool bulk and soften feces by water binding. They may be of plant origin (e.g., bran, plantago) or synthetic (e.g., polyethylene glycol). They cannot be split by the enzymes of the human gut, but may be partially digested by the colon flora.

burp: retrograde expulsion of gas or air (usually ingested) from the upper gut.

Carnette's test: abdominal tenderness increases with abdominal muscle flexion indicating a muscle wall etiology (e.g., cutaneous nerve entrapment, a hernia or a radicular source), or central hypervigilance. If the tenderness is reduced with abdominal muscle flexion, the pain is usually visceral.

catagorical scale (Likert Scale): a scale with several response categories (usually 5 or 7), ranging from nil to very severe (e.g., "no pain" and "very severe pain").

catastrophizing : a type of unhelpful thinking. Catastrophic thoughts tend to dwell on the worst possible outcome of any situation in which there is a possibility of an unpleasant outcome (e.g., a person embarking on an airplane dwells on the possibility of the airplane crashing).

Chagas' disease: neuropathic degeneration of autonomic neurons resulting from autoimmune attack in patients infected with the blood-borne parasite *Trypanosoma cruzi*.

cholecystokinin (CCK): a messenger peptide in the digestive tract that may be released as a hormone from entero-endocrine cells or as a neurotransmitter from enteric neurons.

choledochoscintigraphy: quantitative scintigraphic measurement of the time for bile transit from the hepatic-hilum to the duodenum in patients who have undergone cholecystectomy.

cholescintigraphy: quantitative scintigraphic measurement of gallbladder emptying after i.v. infusion of CCK-8.

closed eyes sign: physical finding often seen in chronic abdominal pain syndrome. The patient will close his/her eyes when the abdomen is palpated, thereby communicating chronic pain behavior. In contrast, patients with acute visceral pain are hypervigilant and will usually keep their eyes open.

coding: physiological term for the translation or representation of a message by one of a set of signals.

cognitions: beliefs, attitudes, expectations, and other mental events.

cognitive behavioral therapy: several approaches or sets of techniques drawn from a large pool of cognitive and behavioral strategies. The theme that unifies these approaches in functional GI disorders centers on an exploration of how certain cognitions and behaviors affect gut symptoms and associated psychosocial distress.

colic: cramps; pain that waxes and wanes over periods of minutes.

compliance: the capability of a region of the gut to adapt to an increased intraluminal volume.

compliance: *see* adherence.

contractile activity: muscular activity of the gut wall, either of short duration (phasic contractions) or more sustained activity (tonic contractions).

control: a subject in an experiment (in this context, a therapeutic trial) who does not receive the treatment under study and thus serves as a comparison to subjects who receive active treatment; also, controlled trial, control group, etc.

coping: behaviors or mental activities that manage (i.e., master, tolerate, minimize) environmental and internal stressors that threaten to tax or exceed a person's resources. It may be adaptive (e.g., problem-focused) or maladaptive (emotion-focused, "catastrophizing") in terms of health status. Therefore, coping is a mediating psychosocial factor in illness that may positively or negatively affect health outcome.

cortical evoked potentials: electrical manifestation of cerebral responses to sensory stimuli recorded by electrodes placed on the scalp.

crossover design: a therapeutic trial containing at least two random-ordered treatment periods for each individual; one for the active treatment, the other for the placebo.

dendrites: fibers that receive synaptic inputs and transmit electrical signals toward the perikaryon of a nerve cell.

depression: a feeling of pessimism, sadness, tearfulness, and/or irritability.

depressive disorders: depression accompanied by reduced activities, appetite, sleep pattern, feelings of fatigue or loss of energy, guilt, worthlessness. Suicidal ideas occur in severe forms.

defecography: radiographic assessment of the shape of the rectum during attempted defecation. A mixture of barium sulfate and a thickening agent is inserted into the rectum prior to attempted defecation.

depolarization: a change in electrical potential in the direction of a more positive potential across the membrane of cells. In excitable cells, depolarization to a threshold potential triggers an action potential.

descending corticifugal pathways: often associated with "down-regulation" of incoming afferent signals. It is part of a homeostatic system whereby higher brain centers can inhibit signals going cephalad from the dorsal horn. It is the efferent limb of the "gate control system."

diabetic peripheral neuropathy: peripheral nerve injury resulting from diabetes.

dietary fiber: naturally occurring bulking agents mostly of plant origin (cell wall constituents).

discomfort: (upper abdomen) a subjective, unpleasant sensation or feeling that is not interpreted as pain according to the patient and which, if fully assessed, can include any of the following: nausea, fullness, bloating, and early satiety.

disinhibitory motor disease: disordered gastrointestinal motility resulting from neuropathic degeneration of enteric inhibitory motor neurons.

dissociation: the usual integration of consciousness, memory, and perception of the environment is disrupted. This may lead to a number of symptoms including loss of memory, apparent loss of identity, and numerous unexplained bizarre bodily symptoms.

distension: *see* abdominal distension.

dorsal root ganglion: location of cell bodies of spinal afferent neurons.

dorsal vagal complex: combined structures of dorsal vagal motor nucleus, nucleus tractus solitarius, and area postrema in the medulla oblongata (brain stem).

dorsal vagal motor nucleus: location in the medulla oblongata (brain stem) of cell bodies of vagal efferent (motor) fibers to the digestive tract, excluding parts of the esophagus.

double blind: neither subjects nor observers are aware of treatment received by an individual in a therapeutic trial.

dualism: a concept first proposed by Descartes, which separates mind and body. Cartesian dualism (the biomedical model) is the dominant model of illness in Western society and is challenged by the biopsychosocial model.

dyschezia: difficult defecation, defined by straining, a feeling of incomplete evacuation, and/or digital facilitation of defecation (pressing around the anus or inside the vagina).

dyspepsia: pain or discomfort centered in the upper abdomen.

dysphagia: a sensation of abnormal bolus transit through the esophageal body.

early satiety: a feeling that the stomach is overfilled soon after starting to eat. The sensation is out of proportion to the size of the meal being eaten, so that the meal cannot be finished.

effector systems: the musculature, secretory epithelium, and blood/lymphatic vasculature in the digestive tract.

efferent nerve (efferents): nerve fibers carrying impulses away from the central nervous system which cause a muscle or gland to contract, or which modifies its contraction (inhibitory efferent nerves).

electrical syncytium: a tissue (e.g., gastrointestinal and cardiac muscle) in which the cells are electrically coupled one to another at cell-to-cell appositions that do not include cytoplasmic continuity. Accounts for three-dimensional spread of excitation in excitable tissues.

electrical slow waves: omnipresent form of electrical activity (rhythmic depolarization and repolarization) in gastrointestinal muscle cells.

electrogalvanic stimulation: transrectal low frequency electrical stimulation, used to treat rectal pain by relaxing skeletal muscles in the pelvic floor.

electrogastrography: the recording of gastric electrical activity from surface electrodes positioned on the abdominal wall.

electromyographic (EMG): refers to recordings of the electrical potentials generated by muscle cells when they contract.

emotion: a state usually caused by an event of importance to the person. It typically includes: (a) a conscious mental state with recognizable quality of feeling that is directed toward some object; (b) a bodily perturbation of some kind; (c) recognizable expressions of the face, tone of voice and gesture; (d) a readiness toward certain kinds of action.

emotion-focused coping: a method in which the individual seeks to manage the distressing emotions evoked by the situation or condition (e.g., praying or denial).

endosonography: use of reflected sound waves to image tissues. Anal endosonography is done by placing the transducer/probe into the anal canal and imaging the internal and external anal sphincters.

enmeshment: a dysfunctional interaction style occurring usually in families where individuals have difficulty in establishing boundaries in behavior (i.e., separation).

enteric minibrain: used in reference to the brain-like functions of the enteric nervous system.

enteric nervous system: the autonomic nervous system situated within the walls of the digestive tract and involved with independent integrative neural control of digestive functions.

enterocele: descent of loops of small intestine into the pelvis, that bulge into the vagina during straining. An enterocele may cause pain and/or obstructed defecation.

etiology: cause.

excitable cells: cells such as neurons and muscle with membranes capable of giving rise to action potentials and propagated impulses.

external anal sphincter: a ring of skeletal muscle surrounding the anal canal which can be voluntarily contracted to postpone defecation.

face validity: the degree to which an item in a questionnaire makes clinical sense.

factor analysis: a statistical method to reduce a large number of intercorrelated symptoms or variables that have been measured in a group of subjects to a smaller number of underlying dimensions which are relatively independent.

fecal impaction: larger than normal, firm mass of stool in the rectum or colon which is difficult for the patient to evacuate. This may contribute to fecal incontinence (overflow).

fecaloma: mass of hard stool in the rectum, fecal impaction.

fart: *v.*, to pass gas per rectum. *n.*, the act, sound, odor of gas passing per rectum; there are no synonyms.

farting: passing gas from the bowel via the anus.

fever: body temperature in excess of 37 degrees C.

flatulence: usually a euphemism for farting, but may embrace gasiness, bloating, even belching. Therefore, is of little value.

flatus: gas (wind) passed per anum.

fullness: an unpleasant sensation like the persistence of food in the stomach; this may or may not occur post-prandially (slow digestion).

functional abdominal bloating: a group of functional bowel disorders which are dominated by a feeling of abdominal fullness or bloating and without sufficient criteria for another functional gastrointestinal disorder.

functional abdominal pain: continuous, nearly continuous or frequently recurrent pain localized in the abdomen but poorly related to gut function.

functional abdominal pain syndrome (FAPS): pain for at least six months, that is poorly related to gut function and is associated with some loss of daily activities. Also called "chronic idiopathic abdominal pain" or "chronic functional abdominal pain."

functional bowel disorder (FBD): a functional gastrointestinal disorder with symptoms attributable to the mid or lower gastrointestinal tract.

functional chest pain: of presumed esophageal origin and characterized by episodes of unexplained chest pain that is usually midline and of visceral quality.

functional constipation: a group of functional disorders which present as persistent difficult, infrequent, or seemingly incomplete defecation.

functional diarrhea: daily or frequently recurrent passage of loose (mushy) or watery stools without abdominal pain or intervening constipation.

functional dysphagia: dysphagia where there is no structural abnormality, pathological reflux, or pathology-based motility disturbance to explain the symptom. However, dysphagia usually has a structural cause.

functional fecal incontinence: recurrent uncontrolled passage of fecal material for at least one month in an individual with a developmental age of at least 4 years who has no evidence of neurological or structural etiologies for incontinence.

functional heartburn: episodic retrosternal burning in the absence of pathologic gastroesophageal reflux, pathology-based motility disorders, or structural explanations.

functional outlet obstruction: inability or difficulty to void the rectum due to pelvic floor dyssynergia, internal prolapse, or enterocele that become apparent only upon straining.

gallbladder dysfunction: an unexplained disorder of gallbladder motility.

ganglia: a grouping of nerve cell bodies situated outside the central nervous system.

ganglionated plexus: an array of ganglia and interganglionic fiber tracts forming parts of the enteric nervous system.

gas: known as *wind* in the U.K. In the context of this book, gas refers to the gases in or escaping from the gut.

gastroesophageal reflux: the retrograde flow of gastric contents into the esophagus (GER).

gastrointestinal motility: the organized application of forces of muscle contraction that results in movement or nonmovement of intraluminal contents.

generalizability: the degree to which the data from a sample of patients in a treatment trial is applicable to other populations.

global outcome measure: response of subject or observer usually to a single general question about the subject's well-being, or degree of suffering from the illness under study.

globus (globus pharyngis, globus pharyngeus): a sensation of something stuck or of a lump or tightness in the throat. "Globus hystericus" is an obsolete term.

gut hypersensitivity: ambiguous term referring to both conscious perception of gut stimuli, and to afferent input within gastrointestinal sensory pathways, whether related to perception or reflex responses.

halitosis: foul (unpleasant) breath odor.

health beliefs (health concerns): cognitive theories of patients' beliefs about the causes of illness, and worries that they may have a disease.

health-related quality of life (HRQOL): the impact that illness has on quality of life, including the individual's perception of his/her illness.

heartburn: episodic retrosternal burning. Also, pyrosis.

hemoglobin: the oxygen-carrying protein in red cells.

holism: : from the Greek *holos,* or whole, was proposed by Plato, Aristotle, and Hippocrates in ancient Greece. It postulates that mind and body are inseparable, so the study of medical disease must take into account the whole person rather than merely the diseased part. This concept fell into disfavor after Descartes proposed the separation between mind (*res cogitans*) and body (*res extensa*) (*see* dualism).

5-hydroxytryptamine (5-HT): an important neurotransmitter in both central and peripheral digestive neurophysiology.

hyperalgesia: a form of visceral hypersensitivity where there is an increased pain response to a noxious stimulus.

hyperpolarization: a change in electrical potential in the direction of a more negative potential across the membrane of cells.

hypervigilance: an intensified version of being vigilant or paying attention to/or focusing on specific things. A person who is hypervigilant may be constantly scanning the environment or his/her body for signs of impending disaster or personal harm. Such hypervigilance may severely limit one's ability to focus on specific tasks or to engage in reflective thinking. Because the person uses up a large part of his/her cognitive capacity by scanning for threatening stimuli, the amount available for attending to other demands may be severely restricted. For example, a person with a functional GI disorder may be hypervigilant in looking for the bodily sensations that reinforce his/her fear of serious disease, such as cancer.

hypnotherapy: the use of hypnosis to improve psychological and/or physical symptoms. Hypnosis renders patients more responsive to suggestions for symptom improvement.

hypnosis: a state of focused attention and heightened suggestibility which can be induced in a variety of ways. During this state, patients are responsive to suggestions for symptom improvement.

hypochondriasis: fear of disease (disease phobia) combined with the conviction that one has a disease, in the absence of objective evidence that one is present.

illness behavior: a conduct or behavior in response to an individual's perceptions of being ill or not well. Examples of "illness behavior" may include visits to the doctor, taking time off work, staying in bed, and taking medications.

inclusion criteria: demographic, disease, symptom, or other information that qualifies a subject for entry into a clinical trial, e.g., the Rome or Manning criteria.

incontinence (fecal): leakage of stool (fecal soiling).

inhibitory junction potential: membrane hyperpolarization leading to decreased excitability in gastrointestinal muscles. Evoked by the release and action of inhibitory neurotransmitters from enteric motor neurons.

integration: organization of individual digestive effector systems into the harmonious function of the whole organ.

intention-to-treat analysis: analysis of data from subjects in a therapeutic trial on the basis of their selection for the trial and randomization into a treatment arm. Subjects are included whether or not they complete the treatment protocol.

interganglionic fiber tracts: bundles of nerve fibers connecting adjacent ganglia of the enteric nervous system.

interneuron: an internuncial neuron that is neither sensory nor motor. Connects neurons with neurons.

inter-rater reliability: the degree to which two observers agree, usually about a clinical outcome.

interstitial cells of Cajal: specialized cells of mesodermal origin believed to be the pacemaker cells for intestinal electrical slow waves.

imperforate anus: congenital malformation in which the colon does not open at the anus but ends in a blind sack.

indigestion: abdominal (usually) discomfort or pain. A vague term that has little meaning to physicians. It is not used in this volume.

innervated: the structure referred to is supplied with intact nerves.

internal anal sphincter: smooth muscle sphincter surrounding the anal canal, which provides a passive barrier to leakage of liquid and gas from the rectum.

interpersonal therapy: a form of psychotherapy in which the therapist identifies aspects of the relationship between the patient and therapist which mirror difficulties in relationships outside of the therapy.

intussuception: telescoping of any part of the intestine or rectum.

irritable bowel syndrome (IBS): functional bowel disorders in which abdominal discomfort or pain is associated with defecation or a change in bowel habit, and with features of disordered defecation.

Kruis criteria: symptom criteria for irritable bowel syndrome (See chapter 7, table 2).

laxative: a compound which increases fecal water content. The primary mechanism is the inhibition of colonic water absorption or stimulation of active or passive colonic water secretion. Some laxatives are also prokinetics.

laxative abuse: laxative ingestion without proper indication or at higher than necessary doses.

levator ani syndrome: chronic or recurring dull aching pain in the rectum or anal canal, with episodes lasting 30 minutes or longer, in the absence of organic etiologies.

life stress: stressful events which are part of life but occur rarely, e.g., bereavement, divorce, severe financial loss, severe illness in a family member, serious accident, etc.

Likert scale: *see* categorical scale.

Manning criteria: symptom criteria for the irritable bowel syndrome (See chapter 7, table 2).

manometric: refers to pressure measurements (in this context, within the gut lumen).

mechanical obstruction: any physical obstacle to the caudal movement of intestinal contents, including tumors, scar tissue, or volvulus (kinking). Mechanical obstruction is distinguished from a functional obstruction, which is due to absent or abnormal contractions of the intestine.

meta-analysis: an analysis of the sum of data from two or more clinical trials that assumes that the patients entered in the trials, the conditions of the studies, the treatments applied, and the outcome measures are discreet and identical. These conditions are seldom met in trials of functional disorders; the patients are heterogeneous, the entry criteria vary, treatment schedules are seldom the same, and the outcome measures may be indistinct.

metioresm: archaic. flatulent dyspepsia with gas in the alimentary canal.

migrating motor complex (MMC): an organized, distinct, cyclically recurring and distally propagating sequence of contractile activity occurring in the small intestine during the fasting state; it may be associated with similar activities in the stomach and proximal colon.

morning rush syndrome: urgent diarrhea upon arising.

motility: movements within the intestinal tract, encompassing the phenomena of contractile activity, myoelectrical activity, tone, compliance, wall tension, and transit within the gastrointestinal tract.

motor neuron: a nerve cell that sends an axon to a muscle, or any effector.

Mueller maneuver: deep inspiration against a closed glottis.

myenteric plexus: ganglionated plexus of the enteric nervous system situated between the longitudinal and circular muscle coats of the muscularis externa of the digestive tract; also Auerbach's plexus.

myogenic: originating in muscle tissue.

myopathic pseudo-obstruction: pathologic failure of propulsion in the gastrointestinal tract related to muscular degeneration and weakened contractility.

nausea: queasiness or sick sensation; a feeling of the need to vomit.

neural networks: aggregates of interconnected neurons that produce a range of behaviors associated with the central and enteric nervous systems.

neurogastroenterology: a subdiscipline of gastroenterology that encompasses all basic and clinical aspects of nervous system involvement in normal and disordered digestive functions and sensations.

neuropathic pseudo-obstruction: pathologic failure of propulsion in the gastrointestinal tract related to enteric neuropathy and loss of nervous control mechanisms.

neuropil: a tangle of fine nerve fibers (dendrites and arborizations of axons) and their endings.

neuroticism: a personality trait characterized by a predisposition to experience anxiety, depression, anger, and a sense of hopelessness and helplessness about the future (negative affect).

neurotransmitter: substance released from nerve cells at synapses that amounts to a chemical signal from one neuron to another or from motor neurons to effectors.

nitric oxide: a putative inhibitory neurotransmitter released by enteric motor neurons to gastrointestinal muscles.

nodose ganglion: location of cell bodies of vagal afferent neurons.

n-of-one study: a series of treatment periods employing a variety of treatments including placebo in random fashion in an individual to determine the best treatment for that individual, i.e., multiple crossovers in a single subject.

non-patients: for the purpose of this publication, those who have never sought health care for their functional gastrointestinal disorder.

nonspecific thalamocortical projection: a sensory pathway from the periphery to the cerebral cortex that involves multiple synaptic connections in the brain stem and thalamus.

nucleus ambiguus: located in the medulla oblongata (brain stem) of cell bodies of vagal efferent (motor) fibers.

nucleus rapine obscurus: a group of neurons in the brain stem that send projections to form synapses with neurons in the dorsal vagal complex.

nucleus tractus solitarius; located in medulla oblongata, contains cell bodies of second order neurons in vagal afferent sensory pathway.

obsessive-compulsive disorder: illness characterized by recurrent, intrusive thoughts and compulsive, stereotyped repetitive behaviors or cognitions. The person may fear that some potential danger has been left unchecked or that they are about to perform an act that is harmful to themselves or others. Behaviors such as hand washing, or counting, may be conducted to forestall the imagined danger. Functioning is impaired because patients are so focused on obsessive thoughts and compulsive rituals that they ignore many daily concerns. The obsessions or compulsions may seem irrational to the patient, but when they attempt to resist them, they experience increased anxiety that can be relieved only by returning to compulsive behaviors and preoccupations.

odynophagia: painful passage of food through the esophagus. Painful swallowing.

outcome measure: measure of a clinical feature (symptom or sign) at the end of a therapeutic trial, that when compared to baseline or placebo indicates the degree of improvement induced by the treatment under study.

pain: a subjective, unpleasant sensation; some patients may feel that tissue damage is occurring. Other symptoms may be extremely bothersome without being interpreted by the patient as pain. Pain should be distinguished from discomfort but that is not always possible.

pancreatic sphincter of Oddi dysfunction: motility abnormalities of the sphincter of Oddi that involve the pancreatic duct.

paradoxic sphincter contraction: contraction of the external anal sphincter and/ or the puborectalis muscle upon straining, impeding stool passage. Causes are painful anal disorders (fissures, perianal thrombosis, abscess) or pelvic floor dyssynergia.

paraneoplastic syndrome: neuropathic degeneration of autonomic neurons resulting from autoimmune attack in patients e.g., with small cell carcinoma of the lung.

parasympathetic: division of the autonomic nervous system with its outflow from the central nervous system in certain cranial and sacral nerves. The ganglia are in or near the innervated viscera.

patients: (in this publication) people with symptoms of functional gastrointestinal disease (FGID) who have ever sought health care for them. They can be subdivided as follows:
incident cases: Those who have sought health care for FGID for the first time in the past year.
prevalent cases: Those who have ever sought health care for FGID.
(Incidence and prevalence are only meaningful when referring to population-based studies.)

pattern generator: interneuronal neural networks that generate rhythmic or repetitive behavior patterns of effector system behavior.

pelvic floor dyssynergia (also anismus, spastic pelvic floor syndrome): chronic disorder of defecation, due to functional outlet obstruction by paradoxic puborectalis muscle and/or external anal sphincter contraction.

pelvic pain: a term used by gynecologists to describe pain in the lower abdomen. It is not clear where the pelvis begins and the abdomen ends. For clarity, and to avoid suggesting etiology, "lower abdominal pain" is preferred.

pelvic tension myalgia: synonym for levator ani syndrome.

per protocol analysis: analysis of data from subjects in a therapeutic trial on the basis of their completion of the treatment protocol. Opposite of "intention to treat."

personality disorder: an enduring pattern of inner experience and behavior that deviates markedly from the expectations of the individual's culture. It is persistent, starts in adolescence, is stable over time, and is not amenable to psychiatric treatment.

phasic contraction: a contraction that is not long maintained (transitory) in contrast to a tonic contraction.

phobia: an anxiety disorder characterized by: (a) persistent fear of a specific situation out of proportion to the reality of the danger; (b) compelling desire to avoid and escape the situation; (c) recognition that fear is unreasonably excessive; (d) not due to any other disorder.

physician-patient relationship (physician-patient interaction): ideally understood in terms of interpersonal behaviors that enhance or diminish mutual communication, satisfaction, and trust. In particular, physician behaviors may enhance or diminish mutual communication, satisfaction, and trust. Positive physician behaviors are characterized by empathy, respect, and positive regard.

placebo: (Latin; I will please.) defies definition. A dummy or inert treatment. In clinical trials serves as a comparison to the treatment being tested. Also a "harmless" nostrum thought to benefit or satisfy the patient.

placebo response: theoretically can only be accurately measured in a randomized, controlled double-blind therapeutic trial that includes an active treatment arm (the treatment under study), a placebo arm, and a "no treatment" arm. The response to no treatment is a function of the natural history of the illness to which the treatment is addressed; any further improvement in those receiving placebo is the "placebo effect," and any improvement over placebo in those receiving the treatment is the therapeutic effect. In practice, there is seldom a "no-treatment" arm, and the natural history and placebo effect are lumped as the "placebo response."

placebo run-in: a run-in period during which a placebo is administered to all subjects to determine the placebo response and sometimes to eliminate "placebo responders". This is no longer recommended for clinical trials of FGIDs, and placebo responders probably cannot be eliminated in this way.

postprandial: after meals.

power propulsion: an intestinal motility pattern associated with defense and pathologic conditions. Rapid propulsion of luminal contents over extended lengths of intestine.

presynaptic inhibitory receptors: receptors on axons that suppress the release of neurotransmitters at neural synapses and neuroeffector junctions.

primary care: first contact medical care provided to patients without referral, as by a general practitioner, family doctor. In North America this may include some care provided by internists, pediatricians, and gynecologists.

primary outcome measure: that which is crucial to judging the benefit of a treatment in a clinical trial.

problem-based coping: a method in which the individual tries to deal directly with situational stressors by changing the stressor or oneself. (e.g., by seeking social support, reappraising the stressor, etc.). In general, problem-focused coping is used in situations appraised by patients to be changeable or adaptable, and is an appropriate coping method for chronic illness.

proctalgia fugax: fleeting (less than 30 minutes duration) sharp pains in the rectum or anal canal, in the absence of known organic etiology.

progressive muscle relaxation: voluntary relaxation through systematically tensing and relaxing different muscle groups.

prokinetic: drug that acts on enteric nerve endings to enhance propulsion of contents through the gut. May act by direct muscle stimulation, release of motor neurotransmitters, or blockade of inhibitory neurotransmitters.

pseudodiarrhea: frequent and/or urgent defecations with stools of normal or firm/lumpy form.

pseudo-obstruction: unsatisfiable urges to defecate associated with normal or even loose stools and/or straining to pass such stools. Also, pathologic failure of propulsion in the gastrointestinal tract in the absence of mechanical obstruction.

psychiatric diagnosis: a diagnosis of one of the psychiatric disorders (now standardized in DSM-IV and WHO International Classification of Diseases).

psychodynamic therapy: the application of psychological theories derived from the works of Freud and others. The theories base current problems on past difficulties in relationships, especially with parents.

psychological: pertaining to psychology and any/all of its manifestations. Psychology is that branch of science which deals with the mind and mental processes especially in relationship to human and animal behavior.

psychological distress: symptoms of anxiety or depression not amounting to anxiety or depressive disorders.

psychological state: A temporary or changeable phenomenon, for example, anxiety.

psychological traits: personality characteristics or an internal predisposition to respond in a particular way.

psychologist: specialist with a doctorate (Ph.D. degree) in one or more branches of psychology, who is licensed to practice and/or certified to teach in one of these specialties.

psychoneuroendocrinology: the study of the inter-relationship between environmental stress and neuroendocrine functions.

psychoneuroimmunology: the study of the influence of environmental stress on immune cellular function, and susceptibility to disease.

psychopharmacology: the study of drugs to treat symptoms of psychiatric disease.

psychophysiology: the study of the interactions between psychological factors (e.g., anxiety, stress) and physiological factors (e.g., muscle tension, cardiovascular arousal).

psychosocial: psychological and social difficulties (which often occur together).

psychosomatic: describes medical diseases believed to be caused by a pre-existent biologic susceptibility and disease-specific psychologic characteristics. Ulcerative colitis and peptic ulcer disease were two examples. Often misused as "psychogenic," the term is seldom employed today.

psychotherapist: an individual who engages in behavioral treatment of emotional distress, using various modalities, including hypnosis, relaxation training as well as traditional talk therapy.

puborectalis muscle: a sling muscle which anchors to the symphysis pubis anteriorly and loops around the rectum to form the anorectal angle. This muscle is important to continence for stool.

pudendal nerve terminal motor latency: time between electrical stimulation of pudendal nerve with electrodes on the tip of a gloved finger, and the contraction of the external anal sphincter. This is used as a measure of the integrity of the pudendal nerve.

pyrexia: fever.

pyriformis syndrome: synonym for levator ani syndrome.

pyrosis: heartburn.

quality of life: a person's perception that they are able to meet their needs in self-care, physical activities, work and social interactions, and psychological well-being.

radiograph: x-ray image.

randomization: selection of subjects for study (epidemiologic or therapeutic) on a random basis. In a therapeutic trial, treatment groups are selected in a random manner that ensures that there is no bias between groups with respect to demographic or other characteristics.

recall bias: the extent to which the presence or absence and degree of a symptom is influenced by memory.

receptor (membrane): membrane surface proteins with unique conformations for specific binding of chemical signal substances capable of triggering changes in the cell's behavior.

rectal prolapse: protrusion of the mucosal lining of the rectum through the anus.

rectocele: weakness in the tissues surrounding the rectum which permits it to bulge abnormally. The most common rectocele is one affecting the rectovaginal septum in women.

reflex: a neuronal event occurring beyond volition. In neurophysiology, a relatively simple behavioral response of an effector produced by influx of sensory afferent impulses to a neural center and its reflection as efferent impulses back to the periphery and the effector (e.g., muscle). The neural center may consist of interneurons. The simplest reflex circuit consists only of sensory and motor neurons.

regurgitation: retrograde flow of stomach contents into the throat or mouth.

reliability: degree to which an instrument such as a questionnaire or scale can be trusted to provide consistent information over time.

responder: a subject who responds to a treatment or placebo in a therapeutic trial as judged by a predetermined outcome measure.

Rome criteria: lists of symptoms amongst which a specified minimum number allows a diagnosis of a functional gastrointestinal disorder.

rumination: a regurgitation of recently ingested food into the mouth with subsequent remastication and reswallowing or spitting out. The regurgitation is effortless, unassociated with abdominal discomfort, heartburn, or nausea, and sometimes seems to be a voluntary pleasurable experience.

run-in period: a short period, often 2 weeks, at the beginning of a therapeutic trial during which baseline data is collected, eligibility and compliance tested, and previous treatments are eliminated or standardized.

scintigraphic techniques: the use of radioisotopes, either ingested with food or released from swallowed capsules, (in this case) to measure transit times through different regions of the gastrointestinal tract.

scybala: fecal material formed into small balls resembling the stools of a rabbit, sheep, or deer.

scyballous: describes feces as scybala.

secondary care: consultant care provided by specialists to whom a patient is referred by a primary care physician.

secondary outcome measure: that which may support the benefit of a therapeutic measure in a clinical trial, but that is neither crucial, nor by itself sufficient to deem the treatment a success.

self esteem: a personality trait where an individual is able to evaluate his/her abilities, achievements and value in society in a way that promotes confidence and personal satisfaction.

sensory neuron: a neuron that conducts impulses arising in a sense organ or at sensory nerve endings.

sensory receptor: a cell or part of a cell specialized functioning to convert environmental stimuli into nerve impulses or some response which in turn evokes nerve impulses. Most sensory receptor cells are nerve cells, but some non-nervous cells can be receptors (e.g., intestinal entero-endocrine cells). One method of classifying receptors is by the form of adequate stimulus. Chemoreceptors, osmoreceptors, mechanoreceptors are normally stimulated by chemicals, osmotic pressure differences and mechanical events, respectively.

silent nociceptor: an unresponsive afferent that becomes responsive to mechanical stimulation during inflammatory states.

sitzmark test: test of whole gut transit time. Ingested small radio-opaque markers are followed through the gastrointestinal tract.

slow wave: membrane electrical potential which waxes and wanes in a rhythmic fashion. The slow wave determines the timing of a contraction but is not enough to produce a contraction in the absence of a burst of spike potentials triggered by the release of a neurotransmitter.

somatization: the behavior of reporting physical symptoms which are not associated with any known pathophysiological process, or which are excessive when compared to known pathophysiology.

specific thalamocortical projection: a sensory pathway from the periphery to the cerebral cortex that involves only two synaptic connections.

sphincter of Oddi dysfunction: unexplained motility abnormalities of the sphincter of Oddi.

sphincter of Oddi dyskinesia: functional abnormalities of the sphincter of Oddi presenting at manometry as reversible elevated basal pressure or abnormal phasic contractions.

sphincter of Oddi stenosis: structural abnormality of the sphincter of Oddi presenting as elevated basal pressure which does not decrease after administrating a smooth muscle relaxant.

stress: may be environmental stress or the feeling of being stressed. Also, any external or internal stimulus or sequence of stimuli that tend to disrupt homeostasis. Stress is damaging when mechanisms of homeostatic adjustment fail.

submucous plexus: a ganglionated plexus of the enteric nervous system situated between the mucosa and circular muscle coat of the small and large intestine. Consists of an inner ganglionated plexus called Meissner's plexus and an outer ganglionated plexus called Schabadasch's plexus.

sympathetic: division of the autonomic nervous system with its outflow from the central nervous system in the thoracolumbar segments of the spinal cord and having its ganglia on either side of the spinal cord, grouped in three nerve plexes (celiac, superior and inferior mesenteric) in the abdomen.

synapse: a functional (noncytoplasmic) connection between neurons consisting of a presynaptic site of chemical transmitter release and a postsynaptic site of action of the released transmitter.

synthase: an enzyme that catalyzes synthesis of neurotransmitters in the enteric nervous system.

tenesmus: painful urge to defecate.

tertiary care: best used to describe the care provided in a highly specialized center such as brain surgery, cardiac surgery, transplants, etc.; often loosely used to describe a University referral center and includes much that is secondary, or even primary care.

test-retest: application of a questionnaire twice under similar conditions to determine that the data are constant. If the interval is too short, the test-retest data may be influenced by memory; if too long, the results may be confounded by a change in the respondent.

thyrotropin-releasing hormone: a hormone in the hypothalamic-pituitary axis that also functions as a neurotransmitter at synapses in the dorsal vagal complex in the brain stem.

tonic contraction: a degree of tension, firmness or maintained contraction in a muscle, in contrast to a phasic contraction.

transit time: the time taken for food or other material to traverse a specified region of the gut.

type 1 error: the data falsely indicate a benefit of a treatment in a clinical trial.

type 2 error: the data are insufficient to show a true benefit of a treatment in a clinical trial. Usually the sample size is too small.

unspecified functional abdominal pain: functional abdominal pain which does not meet criteria for FAPS.

unspecified functional bowel disorder: functional bowel symptoms that do not meet criteria for the previously defined categories.

vago-vagal reflex: a reflex for which both afferent and efferent fibers are contained in the vagus nerves.

validation: of an outcome measure, questionnaire item or disease specific quality of life instrument requires that: (1) it includes symptoms that are relevant and representative of the disorder; (2) the measure is reproducible, i.e. produces similar results when administered to subjects whose health status has not changed; (3) is able to detect change (responsiveness) in relevant clinical symptoms assuming a change took place; and (4) a change in outcome measures should reflect a real change in general health status.

validity: the degree to which a test, questionnaire item, data item is sound or true, and applicable to a defined population.

VAS: see visual analogue scale.

vasoactive intestinal peptide: a putative inhibitory neurotransmitter released by enteric motor neurons to gastrointestinal muscles.

visceral hyperalgesia: gut hypersensitivity. The appreciation or exaggeration of gut symptoms with stimuli (such as balloon distension of the gut) that would ordinarily not be noticed, or considered noxious.

visceral hypersensitivity: gut hypersensitivity. A condition in which the individual's responses to visceral afferent signals are amplified or increased. The appreciation of unpleasant gut symptoms elicited by stimuli (such as balloon distension of the gut) that would ordinarily not be noticed or considered noxious.

viscoelastic: compliance of a hollow visceral organ (when used in gastroenterology).

visual analogue scale (VAS): a horizontal line usually 10 cms in length with points at each end such as "no pain" and "most severe pain" between which a subject marks the degree of his experience of the severity of a symptom.

vomit: ejection of stomach contents through the mouth.

wall tension: the force acting on the gut wall resulting from the interaction between intraluminal content and the action of the muscle and elastic tissue of the gut wall.

washout period: in a crossover study, a period of no treatment is inserted between treatments to ensure that no drug effect carries over from one treatment period to the next.

whole gut transit time: time required for transit from mouth to anus.

wind: in the context of this book, refers to gases in or from the gut. Known as *gas* in the U.S. and Canada.

withdrawal design: a therapeutic trial design in which the subjects are established on a treatment and then the treatment is withdrawn. Usually a placebo is blindly and randomly substituted in half the sample. The continued treatment group may then be compared to the control group, who have discontinued treatment.

Diagnostic Criteria for Functional Gastrointestinal Disorders

A. Functional Esophageal Disorders

The diagnosis of a Functional Esophageal Disorder always presumes the absence of a structural or biochemical explanation for the symptoms.

A1. Globus
     At least 12 weeks, which need not be consecutive, in the preceding 12 months of:

1. The persistent or intermittent sensation of a lump or foreign body in the throat;
2. Occurrence of the sensation between meals;
3. Absence of dysphagia and odynophagia; *and*
4. Absence of pathologic gastroesophageal reflux, achalasia, or other motility disorder with a recognized pathologic basis (e.g., scleroderma of the esophagus).

A2. Rumination Syndrome
     At least 12 weeks, which need not be consecutive, in the preceding 12 months of:

1. Persistent or recurrent regurgitation of recently ingested food into the mouth with subsequent remastication and swallowing or spitting it out;
2. Absence of nausea and vomiting;
3. Cessation of the process when the regurgitated material becomes acidic; *and*
4. Absence of pathologic gastroesophageal reflux, achalasia, or other motility disorder with a recognized pathologic basis as the primary disorder.

A3. Functional Chest Pain of Presumed Esophageal Origin
     At least 12 weeks, which need not be consecutive, within the preceding 12 months of:

1. Midline chest pain or discomfort that is not of burning quality; *and*
2. Absence of pathologic gastroesophageal reflux, achalasia, or other motility disorder with a recognized pathologic basis.

A4. Functional Heartburn
     At least 12 weeks, which need not be consecutive, in the preceding 12 months of:

1. Burning retrosternal discomfort or pain; *and*
2. Absence of pathologic gastroesophageal reflux, achalasia, or other motility disorder with a recognized pathologic basis.

A5. Functional Dysphagia
     At least 12 weeks, which need not be consecutive, in the preceding 12 months of:

1. Sense of solid and/or liquid foods sticking, lodging, or passing abnormally through the esophagus; *and*

2. Absence of pathologic gastroesophageal reflux, achalasia, or other motility disorder with a recognized pathologic basis.

A6. Unspecified Functional Esophageal Disorder
At least 12 weeks, which need not be consecutive, in the preceding 12 months of:
1. Unexplained symptoms attributed to the esophagus that do not fit into the previously described categories; *and*
2. Absence of pathologic gastroesophageal reflux, achalasia, or other motility disorder with a recognized pathologic basis.

B. Functional Gastroduodenal Disorders

The diagnosis of a Functional Gastroduodenal Disorder always presumes the absence of a structural or biochemical explanation for the symptoms.

B1. Functional Dyspepsia
At least 12 weeks, which need not be consecutive, in the preceding 12 months of:
1. Persistent or recurrent symptoms (pain or discomfort centered in the upper abdomen);
2. No evidence of organic disease (including at upper endoscopy) that is likely to explain the symptoms; *and*
3. No evidence that dyspepsia is exclusively relieved by defecation or associated with the onset of a change in stool frequency or stool form (i.e., not irritable bowel).

B1a. Ulcer-like Dyspepsia
Pain centered in the upper abdomen is the predominant (most bothersome) symptom.

B1b. Dysmotility-like Dyspepsia
An unpleasant or troublesome nonpainful sensation (discomfort) centered in the upper abdomen is the predominant symptom; this sensation may be characterized by or associated with upper abdominal fullness, early satiety, bloating, or nausea.

B1c. Unspecified (Nonspecific) Dyspepsia
Symptomatic patients whose symptoms do not fulfill the criteria for ulcer-like or dysmotility-like dyspepsia.

B2. Aerophagia
At least 12 weeks, which need not be consecutive, in the preceding 12 months of:
1. Air swallowing that is objectively observed; *and*
2. Troublesome repetitive belching.

B3. Functional Vomiting
At least 12 weeks, which need not be consecutive, in the preceding 12 months of:

1. Frequent episodes of vomiting, occurring on at least three separate days in a week over three months;
2. Absence of criteria for an eating disorder, rumination, or major psychiatric disease according to DSM-IV;
3. Absence of self-induced and medication-induced vomiting; *and*
4. Absence of abnormalities in the gut or central nervous system, and metabolic diseases to explain the recurrent vomiting.

C. Functional Bowel Disorders

The diagnosis of a Functional Bowel Disorder always presumes the absence of a structural or biochemical explanation for the symptoms.

C1. Irritable Bowel Syndrome
At least 12 weeks, which need not be consecutive, in the preceding 12 months of abdominal discomfort or pain that has two out of three features:

1. Relieved with defecation; *and/or*
2. Onset associated with a change in frequency of stool; *and/or*
3. Onset associated with a change in form (appearance) of stool.

Symptoms that Cumulatively Support the Diagnosis of Irritable Bowel Syndrome
- *Abnormal stool frequency (for research purposes "abnormal" may be defined as greater than 3 bowel movements per day and less than 3 bowel movements per week);*
- *Abnormal stool form (lumpy/hard or loose/watery stool);*
- *Abnormal stool passage (straining, urgency, or feeling of incomplete evacuation);*
- *Passage of mucus;*
- *Bloating or feeling of abdominal distension.*

C2. Functional Abdominal Bloating
At least 12 weeks, which need not be consecutive, in the preceding 12 months of:

1. Feeling of abdominal fullness, bloating, or visible distension; *and*
2. Insufficient criteria for a diagnosis of functional dyspepsia, irritable bowel syndrome, or other functional disorder.

C3. Functional Constipation
At least 12 weeks, which need not be consecutive, in the preceding 12 months of two or more of:

1. Straining > ¼ of defecations;
2. Lumpy or hard stools > ¼ of defecations;

3. Sensation of incomplete evacuation > ¼ of defecations;
4. Sensation of anorectal obstruction/blockage > ¼ of defecations;
5. Manual maneuvers to facilitate > ¼ of defecations (e.g., digital evacuation, support of the pelvic floor); *and/or*
6. < 3 defecations per week.

Loose stools are not present, and there are insufficient criteria for IBS.

C4. Functional Diarrhea

At least 12 weeks, which need not be consecutive, in the preceding 12 months of:

1. Loose (mushy) or watery stools
2. Present > ¾ of the time; *and*
3. No abdominal pain.

C5. Unspecified Functional Bowel Disorder

Bowel symptoms in the absence of organic disease that do not fit into the previously defined categories of functional bowel disorders.

D. Functional Abdominal Pain

The diagnosis of Functional Abdominal Pain always presumes the absence of a structural or biochemical explanation for the symptoms.

D1. Functional Abdominal Pain Syndrome

At least 6 months of:

1. Continuous or nearly continuous abdominal pain; *and*
2. No or only occasional relationship of pain with physiological events (e.g., eating, defecation, or menses); *and*
3. Some loss of daily functioning; *and*
4. The pain is not feigned (e.g., malingering), *and*
5. Insufficient criteria for other functional gastrointestinal disorders that would explain the abdominal pain.

D2. Unspecified Functional Abdominal Pain

This is functional abdominal pain that fails to reach criteria for functional abdominal pain syndrome.

E. Functional Disorders of the Biliary Tract and the Pancreas

The diagnosis of a Functional Disorder of the Biliary Tract and Pancreas always presumes the absence of a structural or biochemical explanation for the symptoms.

E1. Gallbladder Dysfunction

Episodes of severe steady pain located in the epigastrium and right upper quadrant, and all of the following:

1. Symptom episodes last 30 minutes or more, with pain-free intervals;
2. Symptoms have occurred on one or more occasions in the previous 12 months;
3. The pain is steady and interrupts daily activities or requires consultation with a physician;
4. There is no evidence of structural abnormalities to explain the symptoms; *and*
5. There is abnormal gallbladder functioning with regard to emptying.

E2. Sphincter of Oddi Dysfunction

Episodes of severe steady pain located in the epigastrium and right upper quadrant, and all of the following:

1. Symptom episodes last 30 minutes or more, with pain-free intervals;
2. Symptoms have occurred on one or more occasions in the previous 12 months;
3. The pain is steady and interrupts daily activities or requires consultation with a physician; *and*
4. There is no evidence of structural abnormalities to explain the symptoms.

F. Functional Disorders of the Anus and Rectum

The diagnosis of a Functional Disorder of the Anus and Rectum always presumes the absence of a structural or biochemical explanation for the symptoms.

F1. Functional Fecal Incontinence

Recurrent uncontrolled passage of fecal material for at least one month, in an individual with a developmental age of at least 4 years, associated with:

1. Fecal impaction; *or*
2. Diarrhea; *or*
3. Nonstructural anal sphincter dysfunction.

F2. Functional Anorectal Pain

F2a. Levator Ani Syndrome

At least 12 weeks, which need not be consecutive, in the preceding 12 months of:

1. Chronic or recurrent rectal pain or aching;
2. Episodes last 20 minutes or longer; *and*
3. Other causes of rectal pain such as ischemia, inflammatory bowel disease, cryptitis, intramuscular abscess, fissure, hemorrhoids, prostatitis, and solitary rectal ulcer have been excluded.

F2b. Proctalgia Fugax
1. Recurrent episodes of pain localized to the anus or lower rectum;
2. Episodes last from seconds to minutes; *and*
3. There is no anorectal pain between episodes.

F3. Pelvic Floor Dyssynergia
1. The patient must satisfy diagnostic criteria for functional constipation in Diagnostic Criteria C3;
2. There must be manometric, EMG, or radiologic evidence for inappropriate contraction or failure to relax the pelvic floor muscles during repeated attempts to defecate;
3. There must be evidence of adequate propulsive forces during attempts to defecate, *and*
4. There must be evidence of incomplete evacuation.

G. Childhood Functional Gastrointestinal Disorders

The diagnosis of a Childhood Functional Gastrointestinal Disorder always presumes the absence of a structural or biochemical explanation for the symptoms.

G1. Vomiting

G1a. Infant Regurgitation
1. Regurgitation 2 or more times per day for 3 or more weeks;
2. There is no retching, hematemesis, aspiration, apnea, failure-to-thrive, or abnormal posturing;
3. The infant must be 1 to 12 months of age and otherwise healthy; *and*
4. There is no evidence of metabolic, gastrointestinal, or central nervous system disease to explain the symptom.

G1b. Infant Rumination Syndrome
1. At least 3 months of stereotypical behavior beginning with repetitive contractions of the abdominal muscles, diaphragm, and tongue, and culminating in regurgitation of gastric contents into the mouth, which is either expectorated or rechewed and reswallowed, and 3 or more of the following:
   a. Onset between 3 and 8 months of age;
   b. Does not respond to management for gastroesophageal reflux disease, anticholinergic drugs, hand restraints, formula changes, and gavage or gastrostomy feedings;
   c. Unaccompanied by signs of nausea or distress; *and/or*
   d. Does not occur during sleep and when the infant is interacting with individuals in the environment.

G1c. Cyclic Vomiting Syndrome

1. A history of 3 or more periods of intense, acute nausea, and unremitting vomiting lasting hours to days, with intervening symptom-free intervals lasting weeks to months.
2. There is no metabolic, gastrointestinal, or central nervous system structural or biochemical disease.

G2. Abdominal Pain

G2a. Functional Dyspepsia

In children mature enough to provide an accurate pain history, at least 12 weeks, which need not be consecutive, in the preceding 12 months of:

1. Persistent or recurrent pain or discomfort centered in the upper abdomen (above the umbilicus);
2. No evidence of organic disease (including at upper endoscopy) that is likely to explain the symptoms; *and*
3. No evidence that dyspepsia is exclusively relieved by defecation or associated with onset of a change in stool frequency or stool form (i.e., not irritable bowel).

G2a1. Ulcer-like Dyspepsia
Pain centered in the upper abdomen is the predominant (most bothersome) symptom.

G2a2. Dysmotility-like Dyspepsia
An unpleasant or troublesome nonpainful sensation (discomfort) centered in the upper abdomen is the predominant symptom; this sensation may be characterized by early satiety, upper abdominal fullness, bloating, or nausea.

G2a3. Unspecified (Nonspecific) Dyspepsia
Symptomatic patients whose symptoms do not fulfill the criteria for either ulcer-like or dysmotility-like dyspepsia.

G2b. Irritable Bowel Syndrome

In children old enough to provide an accurate pain history, at least 12 weeks, which need not be consecutive, of continuous or recurrent symptoms during the preceding 12 months of:

1. Abdominal discomfort or pain that has two out of three features:
   a. Relieved with defecation; *and/or*
   b. Onset associated with a change in frequency of stool; *and/or*
   c. Onset associated with a change in form (appearance) of stool.

2. There are no structural or metabolic abnormalities to explain the symptoms.

Symptoms that Cumulatively Support the Diagnosis of Irritable Bowel Syndrome

- *Abnormal stool frequency (for research purposes "abnormal" may be defined as greater than 3 bowel movements per day and less than 3 bowel movements per week);*
- *Abnormal stool form (lumpy/hard or loose/watery stool);*
- *Abnormal stool passage (straining, urgency, or feeling of incomplete evacuation);*
- *Passage of mucus;*
- *Bloating or feeling of abdominal distension.*

G2c. Functional Abdominal Pain

At least 12 weeks of:

1. Continuous or nearly continuous abdominal pain in a school-aged child or adolescent; *and*
2. No or only occasional relationship of pain with physiological events (e.g., eating, menses, defecation); *and*
3. Some loss of daily functioning; *and*
4. The pain is not feigned (e.g., malingering); *and*
5. Insufficient criteria for other functional gastrointestinal disorders that would explain the abdominal pain.

G2d. Abdominal Migraine

1. In the preceding 12 months, 3 or more paroxysmal episodes of intense, acute midline abdominal pain lasting 2 hours to several days, with intervening symptom-free intervals of weeks to months; *and*
2. Evidence of metabolic, gastrointestinal, and central nervous system structural or biochemical diseases is absent; *and*
3. Two of the following features:
   a. Headache during episodes;
   b. Photophobia during episodes;
   c. Family history of migraine;
   d. Headache confined to one side only; *and*
   e. An aura or warning period consisting of either visual symptoms (e.g., blurred or restricted vision) or sensory symptoms (e.g., numbness or tingling), or motor symptoms (e.g., slurred speech, inability to speak, paralysis).

G2e. Aerophagia

At least 12 weeks, which need not be consecutive, in the preceding 12 months of two or more of the following signs and symptoms:

1. Air swallowing;
2. Abdominal distension due to intraluminal air; *and*
3. Repetitive belching and/or increased flatus.

G3. Functional Diarrhea (also called Toddler's Diarrhea, chronic nonspecific diarrhea, irritable colon of childhood)

For more than 4 weeks, daily painless, recurrent passage of 3 or more large, unformed stools, in addition to all these characteristics:

1. Onset of symptoms begins between 6 and 36 months of age;
2. Passage of stools occurs during waking hours; *and*
3. There is no failure-to-thrive if caloric intake is adequate.

G4. Disorders of Defecation

G4a. Infant dyschezia

At least 10 minutes of straining and crying before successful passage of soft stools in an otherwise healthy infant less than 6 months of age.

G4b. Functional Constipation

In infants and children, at least 2 weeks of:

1. Scybalous, pebble-like, hard stools for a majority of stools; *or*
2. Firm stools 2 or less times/week; *and*
3. There is no evidence of structural, endocrine, or metabolic disease.

G4c. Functional Fecal Retention

From infancy to 16 years old, a history of at least 12 weeks of:

1. Passage of large diameter stools at intervals < 2 times per week; *and*
2. Retentive posturing, avoiding defecation by purposefully contracting the pelvic floor. As pelvic floor muscles fatigue, the child uses gluteal muscles, squeezing the buttocks together.

Accompanying symptoms may include fecal soiling, irritability, abdominal cramps, decreased appetite and/or early satiety. The accompanying symptoms disappear immediately following passage of a large stool.

G4d. Functional Non-retentive Fecal Soiling

Once a week or more for the preceding 12 weeks, in a child older than 4 years, a history of:

1. Defecation into places and at times inappropriate to the social context;
2. In the absence of structural or inflammatory disease; *and*
3. In the absence of signs of fecal retention (listed in G4c above).

Research Diagnostic Questions for Functional Gastrointestinal Disorders

Rome II Modular Questionnaire: Investigator and Respondent Forms

Investigator Version

— Information for Investigator

This questionnaire has been developed primarily for clinical investigation or clinical practice, though it may also be used in epidemiologic surveys. It is an updated version of the original US Householder's survey published in 1993 using Rome I criteria. This questionnaire contains the Rome II diagnostic criteria.

To make a diagnosis, the questionnaire criteria must be fulfilled as indicated in the coding form. The clinician or investigator must also determine that structural disease(s) that would explain these symptoms are excluded.

Note that the Rome criteria require that symptoms be present for at least 12 weeks (at least one day in that week) over the past year. However, the committee accepts that for survey purposes, symptoms might only be present in the previous three months. This questionnaire allows only for symptoms being present for at least 3 months.

ROME II Modular Questionnaire:
Investigator Form

Question	Answer

Esophageal Disorders

Globus

1. In the last 3 months, did you *often** get the feeling of a lump in your throat when you were *not* swallowing? $\square_0$ No or rarely   ⟶   Skip to question 3. $\square_1$ Yes

2. When you are eating or drinking, is it difficult to swallow, or does it hurt to swallow? $\square_0$ No or rarely $\square_1$ Yes

Rumination Syndrome

3. In the last 3 months, did you *often** bring up food, chew it again, and either spit it out or re-swallow it? $\square_0$ No or rarely   ⟶   Skip to question 6. $\square_1$ Yes

4. At these times, did you vomit or feel sick to your stomach? $\square_0$ No or rarely $\square_1$ Yes

5. Do you stop bringing up food when the food turns sour (acidic)? $\square_0$ No or rarely $\square_1$ Yes

Functional Chest Pain of Presumed Esophageal Origin

6. In the last 3 months, did you *often** have pain in the middle of your chest (that is not due to angina or a heart attack)? $\square_0$ No or rarely   ⟶   Skip to question 8. $\square_1$ Yes

7. Did this chest pain occur when it felt like food got stuck going down? $\square_0$ No or rarely $\square_1$ Yes

Functional Heartburn

8. In the last 3 months, did you *often** have heartburn, a burning pain or discomfort in your chest? $\square_0$ No or rarely $\square_1$ Yes

Functional Dysphagia

9. In the last 3 months, did you *often** have difficulty after swallowing (solid or liquids sticking in your chest, or passing down abnormally)? $\square_0$ No or rarely $\square_1$ Yes

* *Often* means that the symptoms were present during at least 3 weeks (at least one day in each week) in the last 3 months.

Rome II Modular Questionnaire: Investigator Form

Question	Answer

Gastroduodenal Disorders

Functional Dyspepsia

10. In the last 3 months, did you *often**
have discomfort or pain centered in
your upper abdomen (above your
belly button, or the pit of your
stomach)?

$\square_0$ No or rarely ⟶ Skip to
$\square_1$ Yes   question 15.

11. Check your best description of this
symptom, or the one that bothers
you more . . .

$\square_1$ *pain* in your upper
abdomen or
stomach ⟶ Skip to
$\square_2$ *discomfort* (that is   question 13.
not painful) in your
upper abdomen or
stomach

12. If you have discomfort, which of the
following describe your discomfort?
(*check all that apply*)

$\square_1$ nausea
$\square_2$ bloating (a sensation
of upper abdominal
swelling)
$\square_3$ feeling full after eating very little
$\square_4$ none of the above

13. Does your upper abdominal discomfort or pain usually get better or stop
after you have a bowel movement?

$\square_0$ No or rarely
$\square_1$ Yes

14a. When the upper abdominal discomfort or pain starts, do you usually
have a change in your usual number
of bowel movements (either more or
fewer)?

$\square_0$ No or rarely
$\square_1$ Yes

14b. When the upper abdominal discomfort or pain starts, do you usually
have either softer or harder stools
than usual?

$\square_0$ No or rarely
$\square_1$ Yes

* *Often* means that the symptoms were present during at least 3 weeks (at least one day
in each week) in the last 3 months.

Rome II Modular Questionnaire: Investigator Form

Question	Answer

Aerophagia

15. In the last 3 months, did you *often** burp or belch?
$\square_0$ No or rarely   ➤ Skip to question 17.
$\square_1$ Yes

16. Did you swallow air to help you belch?
$\square_0$ No or rarely
$\square_1$ Yes

Functional Vomiting

17. In the last 3 months, did you have frequent episodes of vomiting (on at least 3 separate days in each week)?
$\square_0$ No or rarely   ➤ Skip to question 20.
$\square_1$ Yes

18. During these episodes, did you make yourself vomit?
$\square_0$ No or rarely   ➤ Skip to question 20.
$\square_1$ Yes

19. Were you vomiting because of a medication you were taking or another medical condition that you had?
$\square_0$ No or rarely
$\square_1$ Yes

Bowel Disorders

Irritable Bowel Syndrome/
Functional Abdominal Bloating/
Functional Constipation

20. In the last 3 months, did you *often** have discomfort or pain in your abdomen?
$\square_0$ No or rarely   ➤ Skip to question 24.
$\square_1$ Yes

21. Does your discomfort or pain get better or stop after you have a bowel movement?
$\square_0$ No or rarely
$\square_1$ Yes

22. When the discomfort or pain starts, do you have a change in your usual number of bowel movements (either more or fewer)?
$\square_0$ No or rarely
$\square_1$ Yes

23. When the discomfort or pain starts, do you have either softer or harder stools than usual?
$\square_0$ No or rarely
$\square_1$ Yes

see question 24 on the next page

---

* *Often* means that the symptoms were present during at least 3 weeks (at least one day in each week) in the last 3 months.

Question	Answer
24. Have you had any of the following symptoms at least one-fourth (¼) of the time (occasions or days) in the last 3 months? (*check all that apply*)	❑₁ Fewer than three bowel movements a week (0–2)
	❑₂ More than three bowel movements a day (4 or more)
	❑₃ Hard or lumpy stools
	❑₄ Loose, mushy or watery stools
	❑₅ Straining during a bowel movement
	❑₆ Having to rush to the toilet to have a bowel movement
	❑₇ Feeling of incomplete emptying after a bowel movement
	❑₈ Passing mucus (slime) during a bowel movement
	❑₉ Abdominal fullness, bloating or swelling
	❑₁₀ A sensation that the stool cannot be passed (i.e., blocked) when having a bowel movement
	❑₁₁ A need to press on or around your bottom or vagina to try to remove stool in order to complete the bowel movement

* *Often* means that the symptoms were present during at least 3 weeks (at least one day in each week) in the last 3 months.

Rome II Modular Questionnaire: Investigator Form

Question	Answer

Functional Diarrhea

25. In the last 3 months, did you have loose, mushy, or watery stools, during more than three quarters ($3/4$) of your bowel movements?

☐$_0$ No or rarely
☐$_1$ Yes

Functional Abdominal Pain

26. In the last 6 months, did you have pain in your abdomen all the time (continuously) or most of the time (nearly continuously)? *(If you are female, this should not be related to your menstrual cycle or period)*

☐$_0$ No ⟶ Skip to question 28.
☐$_1$ Yes

27. Has this pain limited or restricted your ability to work or go to social events?

☐$_0$ No or rarely
☐$_1$ Yes

Biliary Disorders

28. In the last year, did you have any severe steady pain in the middle or right side of your upper abdomen?

☐$_0$ No or rarely ⟶ Skip to question 33.
☐$_1$ Yes

29. Did the pain last 30 minutes or more?

☐$_0$ No or rarely
☐$_1$ Yes

30. Did the pain keep you from your usual daily activities, or cause you to see a doctor?

☐$_0$ No or rarely
☐$_1$ Yes

31. Have you had your gallbladder removed?

☐$_0$ No ⟶ Skip to question 33.
☐$_1$ Yes

32. Did you have any severe or steady pain in the middle or right side of your upper abdomen since your gallbladder was removed?

☐$_0$ No or rarely
☐$_1$ Yes

* *Often* means that the symptoms were present during at least 3 weeks (at least one day in each week) in the last 3 months.

Question	Answer

Anorectal Disorders

Functional Incontinence

33. In the last year, when you had consti- $\Box_0$ No $\longrightarrow$ Skip to
pation or diarrhea, did you acciden- $\Box_1$ Yes question 35.
tally leak or pass stool for more than
one occasion in a month?

34. How much stool did you accidentally $\Box_1$ A small amount (it
lose? Would you say . . . stains underwear)
  $\Box_2$ A moderate or large
  amount (2 teaspoons
  or more)

Functional Anorectal Pain

35. In the last year, did you have more $\Box_0$ No $\longrightarrow$ Skip to
than one episode of aching pain or $\Box_1$ Yes question 38.
pressure in the anal canal or rectum?

Levator Ani Syndrome/Proctalgia Fugax

36. Did this pain occur frequently or $\Box_0$ No
continuously in the last 3 months? $\Box_1$ Yes

37. Which of the following 2 statements $\Box_1$ Lasts from seconds to
better describes the aching, pain, or minutes and disap-
pressure that you had in the anal pears completely
canal or rectum? $\Box_2$ Lasts more than 20
  minutes and up to
  several days or longer

---

* *Often* means that the symptoms were present during at least 3 weeks (at least one day
in each week) in the last 3 months.

Question	Answer

Pelvic Floor Dyssynergia

38. In the last 3 months, when you were having bowel movements, did you. . . (*check all that apply*)

$\Box_1$ Feel as if you had to strain to pass your stool on at least one quarter of the time

$\Box_2$ Feel as if you were unable to empty the rectum at least one quarter of the time

$\Box_3$ Have difficulty relaxing or letting go to allow the stool to come out at least one quarter of the time

$\Box_4$ None of the above

End of Questionnaire

Please read this first ...

Instructions

The purpose of this survey is to learn more about the health problems that people sometimes have with the stomach and intestines. The questionnaire will take about 15 minutes to complete. Your participation is voluntary, and you may refuse to answer any of the questions in the survey.

To answer each question, place a check mark inside the box directly to the left of the correct answer. You may find that you have not had some or any of the symptoms that we'll ask you about. When this happens, you will be instructed to skip over the questions that do not apply to you. *Please be careful to follow the skip instructions.* They are typed next to the response for "No or rarely". See the example below.

Question	Answer	
3. In the last 3 months, did you *often** bring up food, chew it again, and either spit it out or re-swallow it?	$\square_0$ No or rarely ⟶ $\square_1$ Yes	Skip to question 6.

The questions will ask if you have the different symptoms *often*. By often, we mean that symptoms were present during at least 3 weeks (at least once a week) in the last 3 months. *Please keep this in mind as you answer the questions.*

If you are not sure about an answer, or you can't remember the answer to a question, just answer as best you can. It is easy to miss questions, so please check that you haven't left any out as you go.

Thank You!

Rome II Modular Questionnaire: Respondent Form

Question	Answer

Esophageal Symptoms

1. In the last 3 months, did you *often** get the feeling of a lump in your throat when you were *not* swallowing?
   $\square_0$ No or rarely   → Skip to question 3.
   $\square_1$ Yes

2. When you are eating or drinking, is it difficult to swallow, or does it hurt to swallow?
   $\square_0$ No or rarely
   $\square_1$ Yes

3. In the last 3 months, did you *often** bring up food, chew it again, and either spit it out or re-swallow it?
   $\square_0$ No or rarely   → Skip to question 6.
   $\square_1$ Yes

4. At these times, did you vomit or feel sick to your stomach?
   $\square_0$ No or rarely
   $\square_1$ Yes

5. Do you stop bringing up food when the food turns sour (acidic)?
   $\square_0$ No or rarely
   $\square_1$ Yes

6. In the last 3 months, did you *often** have pain in the middle of your chest (that is not due to angina or a heart attack)?
   $\square_0$ No or rarely   → Skip to question 8.
   $\square_1$ Yes

7. Did this chest pain occur when it felt like food got stuck going down?
   $\square_0$ No or rarely
   $\square_1$ Yes

8. In the last 3 months, did you *often** have heartburn, a burning pain or discomfort in your chest (that is not due to angina or a heart attack)?
   $\square_0$ No or rarely
   $\square_1$ Yes

9. In the last 3 months, did you *often** have difficulty after swallowing (solid or liquids sticking in your chest, or passing down abnormally)?
   $\square_0$ No or rarely
   $\square_1$ Yes

* *Often* means that the symptoms were present during at least 3 weeks (at least one day in each week) in the last 3 months.

Rome II Modular Questionnaire: Respondent Form

Question	Answer

Gastroduodenal Symptoms

10. In the last 3 months, did you *often** have discomfort or pain centered in your upper abdomen (above your belly button, or the pit of your stomach)?

$\square_0$ No or rarely ⟶ Skip to question 15.
$\square_1$ Yes

11. Check your best description of this symptom, or the one that bothers you more . . .

$\square_1$ *pain* in your upper abdomen or stomach ⟶ Skip to question 13.
$\square_2$ *discomfort* (that is not painful) in your upper abdomen or stomach

12. If you have discomfort, which of the following describe your discomfort? (*check all that apply*)

$\square_1$ nausea
$\square_2$ bloating (a sensation of upper abdominal swelling)
$\square_3$ feeling full after eating very little
$\square_4$ none of the above

13. Does your upper abdominal discomfort or pain usually get better or stop after you have a bowel movement?

$\square_0$ No or rarely
$\square_1$ Yes

14a. When the upper abdominal discomfort or pain starts, do you usually have a change in your usual number of bowel movements (either more or fewer)?

$\square_0$ No or rarely
$\square_1$ Yes

14b. When the upper abdominal discomfort or pain starts, do you usually have either softer or harder stools than usual?

$\square_0$ No or rarely
$\square_1$ Yes

* *Often* means that the symptoms were present during at least 3 weeks (at least one day in each week) in the last 3 months.

Rome II Modular Questionnaire: Respondent Form

Question	Answer	
15. In the last 3 months, did you *often** burp or belch?	$\square_0$ No or rarely $\square_1$ Yes	→ Skip to question 17.
16. Did you swallow air to help you belch?	$\square_0$ No or rarely $\square_1$ Yes	
17. In the last 3 months, did you have frequent episodes of vomiting (on at least 3 separate days in each week)?	$\square_0$ No or rarely $\square_1$ Yes	→ Skip to question 20.
18. During these episodes, did you make yourself vomit?	$\square_0$ No or rarely $\square_1$ Yes	→ Skip to question 20.
19. Were you vomiting because of a medication you were taking or another medical condition that you had?	$\square_0$ No or rarely $\square_1$ Yes	

Bowel Symptoms

20. In the last 3 months, did you *often* have discomfort or pain in your abdomen?	$\square_0$ No or rarely $\square_1$ Yes	→ Skip to question 24.
21. Does your discomfort or pain get better or stop after you have a bowel movement?	$\square_0$ No or rarely $\square_1$ Yes	
22. When the discomfort or pain starts, do you have a change in your usual number of bowel movements (either more or fewer)?	$\square_0$ No or rarely $\square_1$ Yes	
23. When the discomfort or pain starts, do you have either softer or harder stools than usual?	$\square_0$ No or rarely $\square_1$ Yes	

see question 24 on the next page

* *Often* means that the symptoms were present during at least 3 weeks (at least one day in each week) in the last 3 months.

681

Question	Answer
24. Have you had any of the following symptoms at least one-fourth (¼) of the time (occasions or days) in the last 3 months? (*check all that apply*)	❏₁ Fewer than three bowel movements a week (0–2) ❏₂ More than three bowel movements a day (4 or more) ❏₃ Hard or lumpy stools ❏₄ Loose, mushy or watery stools ❏₅ Straining during a bowel movement ❏₆ Having to rush to the toilet to have a bowel movement ❏₇ Feeling of incomplete emptying after a bowel movement ❏₈ Passing mucus (slime) during a bowel movement ❏₉ Abdominal fullness, bloating or swelling ❏₁₀ A sensation that the stool cannot be passed (i.e., blocked) when having a bowel movement ❏₁₁ A need to press on or around your bottom or vagina to try to remove stool in order to complete the bowel movement

* *Often* means that the symptoms were present during at least 3 weeks (at least one day in each week) in the last 3 months.

Rome II Modular Questionnaire: Respondent Form

Question	Answer	
25. In the last 3 months, did you have loose, mushy, or watery stools, during more than three quarters (¾) of your bowel movements?	$\square_0$ No $\square_1$ Yes	
Abdominal Pain Symptoms		
26. In the last 6 months, did you have pain in your abdomen all the time (continuously) or most of the time (nearly continuously)? *(If you are female, this should not be related to your menstrual cycle or period)*	$\square_0$ No → $\square_1$ Yes	Skip to question 28.
27. Has this pain limited or restricted your ability to work or go to social events?	$\square_0$ No or rarely $\square_1$ Yes	
Biliary Symptoms		
28. In the last year, did you have any severe steady pain in the middle or right side of your upper abdomen?	$\square_0$ No or rarely → $\square_1$ Yes	Skip to question 33.
29. Did the pain last 30 minutes or more?	$\square_0$ No or rarely $\square_1$ Yes	
30. Did the pain keep you from your usual daily activities, or cause you to see a doctor?	$\square_0$ No or rarely $\square_1$ Yes	
31. Have you had your gallbladder removed?	$\square_0$ No → $\square_1$ Yes	Skip to question 33.
32. Did you have any severe or steady pain in the middle or right side of your abdomen since your gallbladder was removed?	$\square_0$ No or rarely $\square_1$ Yes	

* *Often* means that the symptoms were present during at least 3 weeks (at least one day in each week) in the last 3 months.

Question	Answer

Anorectal Symptoms

33. In the last year, when you had constipation or diarrhea, did you accidentally leak or pass stool for more than
one occasion in a month?

  ☐$_0$ No ⟶   Skip to
  ☐$_1$ Yes   question 35.

34. How much stool did you accidentally
lose? Would you say . . .

  ☐$_1$ A small amount (it
     stains underwear)
  ☐$_2$ A moderate or large
     amount (2 teaspoons
     or more)

35. In the last year, did you have more
than one episode of aching pain or
pressure in the anal canal or rectum?

  ☐$_0$ No ⟶   Skip to
  ☐$_1$ Yes   question 38.

36. Did this pain occur frequently or
continuously in the last 3 months?

  ☐$_0$ No
  ☐$_1$ Yes

37. Which of the following 2 statements
better describes the aching, pain, or
pressure that you had in the anal
canal or rectum?

  ☐$_1$ Lasts from seconds to
     minutes and disap-
     pears completely
  ☐$_2$ Lasts more than 20
     minutes and up to
     several days or longer

* *Often* means that the symptoms were present during at least 3 weeks (at least one day
in each week) in the last 3 months.

Question	Answer
38. In the last 3 months, when you were having bowel movements, did you. . . (*check all that apply*)	❏₁ Feel as if you had to strain to pass your stool on at least one quarter of the time ❏₂ Feel as if you were unable to empty the rectum at least one quarter of the time ❏₃ Have difficulty relaxing or letting go to allow the stool to come out at least one quarter of the time ❏₄ None of the above
End of Questionnaire	

Codes for Rome II Modular Questionnaire

Esophageal Disorders

Globus	Q1 = Yes	Q2 = No	Q8 = No
Rumination Syndrome	Q3 = Yes	Q4 = No	Q5 = Yes
Functional Chest Pain of Presumed Esophageal Origin	Q6 = Yes	Q7 = No	Q8 = No
Functional Heartburn*	Q8 = Yes	Q9 = No	
Functional Dysphagia[†]	Q9 = Yes	Q8 = No	

Gastroduodenal Disorders

Functional Dyspepsia[††]	Q10 = Yes Q14b = No	Q8 = No	Q13 = No	Q14a = No
Ulcer-like Dyspepsia	Functional dyspepsia *and* Q11 = pain			
Dysmotility Dyspepsia	Functional dyspepsia *and* Q11 = non-painful discomfort			
Aerophagia	Q15 = Yes	Q16 = Yes		
Functional Vomiting	Q17 = Yes	Q18 = No	Q19 = No	Q3 = No

Bowel Disorders

Irritable Bowel Syndrome (IBS)	Q20 = Yes, + 2 of (Q21 or Q22 or Q23) = Yes[†††]
Diarrhea Predom. IBS	IBS

+ 1 or more of
  [Q24(2) or Q24(4) or Q24(6)],
and none of
  [Q24(1) or Q24(3) or Q24(5)]

or + 2 or more of
  [Q24(2) or Q24(4) or Q24(6)]
and not more than 1 of
  [Q24(1) or Q24(5)]
and Q24(3) = No

---

*Gastroesophageal reflux must be excluded.

[†]Note, functional heartburn and functional dysphagia are mutually exclusive in the suggested algorithms. It is important to note that if both are present, neither will show up in the data.

[††]Some of the editors prefer that 2 or more of [Q13 = Yes; Q14a = Yes; Q14b = Yes] (i.e., full criteria for IBS) are needed to exclude these upper abdominal symptoms from the category of Functional Dyspepsia.

[†††]Respondents who do not fulfill these criteria but who endorse Q10 = Yes, + 2 of (Q13 or Q14a or Q14b) = Yes should also be considered to have IBS.

Constipation Predom. IBS	IBS
	+ 1 or more of
	  [Q24(1) or Q24(3) or Q24(5)]
	and none of
	  [Q24(2) or Q24(4) or Q24(6)]
	
	or + 2 or more of
	  [Q24(1) or Q24(3) or Q24(5)],
	and not more than 1 of
	  [Q24(2) or Q24(4) or Q24(6)]

Functional Abdominal Bloating	Q24(9), excluding IBS and Dyspepsia
Functional Constipation	Two or more of [Q24(1), Q24(3), Q24(5), Q24(7), Q24(10), Q24(11)] = Yes, and Q24(4) = No, excluding IBS
Functional Diarrhea	Q25 = Yes, Q10 = No, Q20 = No
Unspecified Functional Bowel Disorder	Bowel symptoms, but not sufficient to diagnose any other functional bowel disorder

Functional Abdominal Pain

Functional Abdominal Pain Syndrome	Q26 = Yes *and* Q27 = Yes, excluding IBS/dypsepsia
Unspecified Functional Abdominal Pain	Q26 = Yes *and* Q27 = No, excluding IBS/dyspepsia or fails to meet full criteria

Biliary Disorders

Gallbladder Dysfunction	Q28 = Yes *and* Q29 = Yes, Q30 = Yes *and* Q31 = No Q21 = No, Q22 = No, Q23 = No, [Q12 = 4 (only if Q10 = Yes and Q11 = Discomfort)]
Sphincter of Oddi Dysfunction	Q28 = Yes *and* Q29 = Yes *and* Q30 = Yes *and* Q31 = Yes *and* Q32 = Yes Q21 = No, Q22 = No, Q23 = No, [Q12 = 4 (only if Q10 = Yes and Q11 = Discomfort)]

687

Anorectal Disorders

Functional Incontinence	Q33 = Yes
Soiling	Q33 = Yes *and* Q34 = 1
Gross Incontinence	Q33 = Yes *and* Q34 = 2
Functional Anorectal pain	
Levator Ani Syndrome	Q35 = Yes Q36 = Yes Q37 = 2
Proctalgia Fugax	Q35 = Yes Q37 = 1
Pelvic Floor Dyssynergia	Functional Constipation + all of [Q38(1) + Q38(2) + Q38(3)]

Research Diagnostic Questions for Functional Gastrointestinal Disorders:

Rome II Integrative Questionnaire

Information for Investigator

This questionnaire has been developed primarily for epidemiological surveys, though it may also be used in clinical practice. It contains the Rome II criteria in addition to other symptom-related items that can be used in clinical research.

To make a diagnosis, the questionnaire criteria must be fulfilled as indicated in the coding form. The clinician or investigator must also determine that structural disease(s) that would explain these symptoms are excluded.

Note that the Rome II criteria require that symptoms must be present for at least 12 weeks (at least one day in that week) over the past year. However, the committee accepts that for survey purposes, symptoms might only be present in the previous three months. This questionnaire will allow for 1 year and in some cases 3 months for certain categories (functional gastroduodenal, functional bowel).

Information for Respondent

The purpose of this survey is to provide a better understanding of health problems specifically related to the gastrointestinal system. Your participation is entirely voluntary. This survey will take approximately 15 minutes to complete. You may find that some questions do not apply to you. Please follow the instructions that tell you which questions require your answer and which questions you can skip.

To answer each question, you need to mark the appropriate response box. For example:

Do you have stomach pain?

Yes . . . . ❑
No . . . . ❑

If you are not sure or can't remember the answer to a question, just choose your best guess. It is easy to miss questions, so please check that you haven't left any out as you go.

When we say belly or abdomen pain or discomfort, we mean any pain or discomfort in the areas labelled A, B, C or D as shown in Diagram 1 on page 692 (Please do not count cramps or pain with menstrual periods and do not count pain in your chest).

A1. In the *last year* have you had discomfort or
pain in your belly or abdomen?

Not at All or Rarely . . . . ❏
Occasionally . . . . ❏
Often . . . . ❏
Very Often . . . . ❏
Almost Always . . . . ❏

A2. In the *last three months* have you had discomfort or
pain in your belly or abdomen?

Not at All or Rarely . . . . ❏
Occasionally . . . . ❏
Often . . . . ❏
Very Often . . . . ❏
Almost Always . . . . ❏

If you answered *Not at All or Rarely* to Question A1 or A2 please go to
Question B1.

Occasionally: more than one tenth of the time   *Often:* more than one quarter of the time
Very Often: more than one half of the time

A3. How does the discomfort or pain you had in the *last three months* compare to what you had in the *last year?* Would you say it was ...

Better in the last three months . . . . ❑
Worse in the last three months . . . . ❑
About the same. . . . . ❑
Didn't have pain or discomfort in the last three months . . . . ❑

A4. In the last year when you had this discomfort or pain in your belly or abdomen was it continuous or nearly continuous (without breaks)?

Yes . . . . ❑
No . . . . ❑

A5. How old were you when this discomfort or pain first began (as close as you can recall)?

Age in years. . . . .

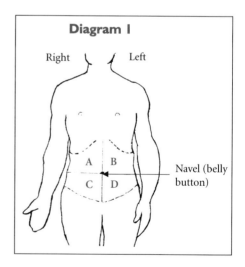

Diagram I

Right   Left

A   B
C   D

Navel (belly button)

Occasionally: more than one tenth of the time   *Often:* more than one quarter of the time
Very Often: more than one half of the time

A6. Where is your belly or abdomen pain located, according to the diagram on the previous page (areas A, B, C, or D)? You can mark more than one answer.

A. .... ❏
B. .... ❏
C. .... ❏
D. .... ❏

A7. If you have more than one pain, where was the location of your most troublesome pain. Choose only *one* area (A, B, C, or D) from Diagram 1.

A. .... ❏
B. .... ❏
C. .... ❏
D. .... ❏

A8. In the last year, were your daily activities affected by any discomfort or pain in your belly or abdomen?

Not at All or Rarely .... ❏
Occasionally .... ❏
Often .... ❏
Very Often .... ❏
Almost Always .... ❏

Occasionally: more than one tenth of the time   *Often:* more than one quarter of the time
Very Often: more than one half of the time

> The following questions refer to **any** belly or abdomen discomfort or pain (Areas A, B, C or D on Diagram 1) you may have had **in the last year.**

A9. In the last year, how bad was the discomfort or pain in your belly or abdomen?

Very Mild. . . . . ❏
Mild . . . . ❏
Moderate. . . . . ❏
Severe. . . . . ❏

A10. In the last year, did this discomfort or pain in your belly or abdomen get better or stop after having a bowel movement (passing stool)?

Not at All or Rarely . . . . ❏
Occasionally. . . . . ❏
Often. . . . . ❏
Very Often . . . . ❏
Almost Always . . . . ❏

A11. In the last year, did you have more bowel movements (stools) than usual when this discomfort or pain began?

Not at All or Rarely . . . . ❏
Occasionally. . . . . ❏
Often. . . . . ❏
Very Often . . . . ❏
Almost Always . . . . ❏

Occasionally: more than one tenth of the time   *Often:* more than one quarter of the time
Very Often: more than one half of the time

A12. In the last year, did you have fewer bowel movements (stools) than usual when this discomfort or pain began?

Not at All or Rarely . . . . ❏
Occasionally. . . . . ❏
Often. . . . . ❏
Very Often . . . . ❏
Almost Always . . . . ❏

A13. In the last year, did you have looser bowel movements (stools) than usual when this discomfort or pain began?

Not at All or Rarely . . . . ❏
Occasionally. . . . . ❏
Often. . . . . ❏
Very Often . . . . ❏
Almost Always . . . . ❏

A14. In the last year, did you have harder bowel movements (stools) than usual when this discomfort or pain began?

Not at All or Rarely . . . . ❏
Occasionally. . . . . ❏
Often. . . . . ❏
Very Often . . . . ❏
Almost Always . . . . ❏

A15. In the last year, was this discomfort or pain made better by belching?

Not at All or Rarely . . . . ❏
Occasionally. . . . . ❏
Often. . . . . ❏
Very Often . . . . ❏
Almost Always . . . . ❏

Occasionally: more than one tenth of the time   *Often:* more than one quarter of the time
Very Often: more than one half of the time

A16. In the last year, did this discomfort or pain occur after meals?

Not at All or Rarely .... ❏
Occasionally .... ❏
Often .... ❏
Very Often .... ❏
Almost Always .... ❏

A17. In the last year, did this discomfort or pain ever
wake you up from your sleep?

Not at All or Rarely .... ❏
Occasionally .... ❏
Often .... ❏
Very Often .... ❏
Almost Always .... ❏

A18. In the last year, did this discomfort or pain ever
spread to your back or shoulders?

Not at All or Rarely .... ❏
Occasionally .... ❏
Often .... ❏
Very Often .... ❏
Almost Always .... ❏

A19. In the last year, was this discomfort or pain
made better by bending forward?

Not at All or Rarely .... ❏
Occasionally .... ❏
Often .... ❏
Very Often .... ❏
Almost Always .... ❏

Occasionally: more than one tenth of the time   *Often:* more than one quarter of the time
Very Often: more than one half of the time

A20. In the last year, when you had this discomfort or pain,
did it last for more than 20 minutes?

Not at All or Rarely . . . . ❏
Occasionally . . . . ❏
Often . . . . ❏
Very Often . . . . ❏
Almost Always . . . . ❏

A21. If you have discomfort or pain in the *upper* belly or abdomen
(the areas marked A or B on Diagram 1) is it relieved
by having a bowel movement (passing stool)?

Yes . . . . ❏
Not at All or Rarely . . . . ❏
I do not have this pain . . . . ❏

A21.1. When you had this discomfort or pain in the *upper* belly
or abdomen did you have more bowel movements (stools)?

Yes . . . . ❏
Not at All or Rarely . . . . ❏

A21.2. When you had this discomfort or pain in the *upper* belly
or abdomen did you have fewer bowel movements (stools)?

Yes . . . . ❏
Not at All or Rarely . . . . ❏

A21.3. When you had this discomfort or pain in the *upper* belly
or abdomen did you have harder bowel movements (stools)?

Yes . . . . ❏
Not at All or Rarely . . . . ❏

Occasionally: more than one tenth of the time   *Often:* more than one quarter of the time
Very Often: more than one half of the time

A21.4. When you had this discomfort or pain in the *upper* belly or abdomen did you have looser bowel movements (stools)?

Yes . . . . ❑
Not at All or Rarely . . . . ❑

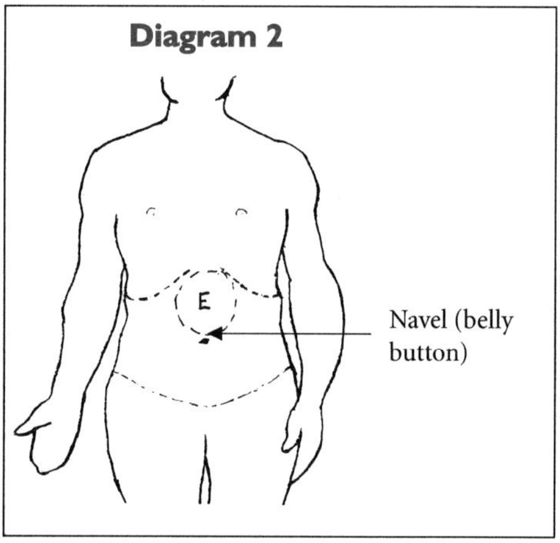

Diagram 2

E

Navel (belly button)

A22. In the last year, when you had discomfort or pain, was it usually in a single small area that you could point to with one or two fingers? (the area marked E on Diagram 2 above).

Yes . . . . ❑
No . . . . ❑

A23. In the last year, when you had this discomfort or pain was it steady and constant (it did not come and go in waves)?

Yes . . . . ❑
No . . . . ❑

Occasionally: more than one tenth of the time   *Often:* more than one quarter of the time
Very Often: more than one half of the time

A24. In the last year, have you been affected by episodes of steady severe pain (in the center of your upper belly or abdomen or in your right upper belly or abdomen) that lasted for 30 minutes or more?

Not at All. . . . . ❑
1 or 2 episodes of this pain. . . . . ❑
More than 2 episodes of this pain . . . . ❑

A25. Have you ever had an operation where your Gall Bladder was removed?

Yes . . . . ❑
No . . . . ❑

> **Please check that you have answered all of the appropriate Questions in Section A. Please begin Section B.**

Rome II Integrative Questionnaire

> ## Section B
> We would like to ask you some questions about other belly or abdomen problems you may have had **in the last year.**

B1. In the last year, did you feel uncomfortably full soon after starting to eat so that you could not finish your normal meal?

Not at All or Rarely .... ❏
Occasionally .... ❏
Often .... ❏
Very Often .... ❏
Almost Always .... ❏

B2. In the last year, after having normal meals, did you get an unpleasant feeling of food staying in your belly or abdomen?

Not at All or Rarely .... ❏
Occasionally .... ❏
Often .... ❏
Very Often .... ❏
Almost Always .... ❏

B3. In the last year, did you feel nauseated (wanting to vomit, but didn't)?

Not at All or Rarely .... ❏
Occasionally .... ❏
Often .... ❏
Very Often .... ❏
Almost Always .... ❏

Occasionally: more than one tenth of the time   *Often:* more than one quarter of the time
Very Often: more than one half of the time

Rome II Integrative Questionnaire

B4. In the last year, have you had vomiting that was not self-induced or caused by a drug or medication?

Not at All or Rarely . . . . ❏
Occasionally . . . . ❏
Often . . . . ❏
Very Often . . . . ❏
Almost Always . . . . ❏

B5. In the last year, did you vomit on at least three separate days in a week over a three month period?

Not at All or Rarely . . . . ❏
Occasionally . . . . ❏
Often . . . . ❏
Very Often . . . . ❏
Almost Always . . . . ❏

B6. In the last year, did you have retching (heaving as if to vomit, but not vomiting)?

Not at All or Rarely . . . . ❏
Occasionally . . . . ❏
Often . . . . ❏
Very Often . . . . ❏
Almost Always . . . . ❏

B7. In the last year, have you had the feeling of abdominal fullness or bloating or swelling?

Not at All or Rarely . . . . ❏
Occasionally . . . . ❏
Often . . . . ❏
Very Often . . . . ❏
Almost Always . . . . ❏

Occasionally: more than one tenth of the time   *Often:* more than one quarter of the time
Very Often: more than one half of the time

B8. In the last year, have you seen your belly or abdomen swell up?

Not at All or Rarely .... ❏
Occasionally .... ❏
Often .... ❏
Very Often .... ❏
Almost Always .... ❏

B9. In the last year, what has been your *most troublesome*
upper belly or abdomen symptom (areas marked A or B on
Diagram I on page 692). (Choose only one answer).

a. Belly or abdomen pain. .... ❏
b. Belly or abdomen burning .... ❏
c. Belly or abdomen discomfort (*not* pain) .... ❏
d. Bloating. .... ❏
e. Nausea. .... ❏
f. Food staying in belly or abdomen. .... ❏
g. Fullness .... ❏
h. Uncomfortably full soon after starting to eat .... ❏
i. I have no upper belly or abdomen symptoms .... ❏

Please check that you have answered all of the appropriate Questions in Section B. Please begin Section C.

Occasionally: more than one tenth of the time   *Often:* more than one quarter of the time
Very Often: more than one half of the time

Rome II Integrative Questionnaire

> **Section C**
> We would like to ask you some questions about some other health problems you may have had **in the last year.**

C1. In the last year, have you been troubled by repeated burping or belching?

Not at All or Rarely . . . . ❏
Occasionally . . . . ❏
Often . . . . ❏
Very Often . . . . ❏
Almost Always . . . . ❏

C2. In the last year, have you swallowed excess air?

Not at All or Rarely . . . . ❏
Occasionally . . . . ❏
Often . . . . ❏
Very Often . . . . ❏
Almost Always . . . . ❏

C3. In the last year, have you had the feeling of a lump in your throat when you were not swallowing?

Not at All or Rarely . . . . ❏
Occasionally . . . . ❏
Often . . . . ❏❏
Very Often . . . . ❏❏
Almost Always . . . . ❏❏

Occasionally: more than one tenth of the time   *Often:* more than one quarter of the time
Very Often: more than one half of the time

C4. In the last year, have you had difficulty swallowing solids
or liquids (food or drinks sticking or passing down abnormally)?

Not at All or Rarely . . . . ❑
Occasionally . . . . ❑
Often . . . . ❑
Very Often . . . . ❑
Almost Always . . . . ❑

C5. In the last year, have you had to bring up food, chew it again,
and either spit it out or swallow it again?

Not at All or Rarely . . . . ❑
Occasionally . . . . ❑
Often . . . . ❑
Very Often . . . . ❑
Almost Always . . . . ❑

> If you answered *Not at All or Rarely* to Question C5 please go on to
> Question C6.

C5.1. Did this happen at times when you felt nauseated
or had been vomiting?

Yes . . . . ❑
No . . . . ❑

C5.2. Did you stop this when the food you brought up tasted acidic or sour?

Yes . . . . ❑
No . . . . ❑

Occasionally: more than one tenth of the time   *Often:* more than one quarter of the time
Very Often: more than one half of the time

Rome II Integrative Questionnaire

C6. In the last year, have you had heartburn, by that we mean a
burning pain or discomfort behind the breastbone rising up towards the
throat? (Do not count if the pain was from angina or heart trouble)

Not at All or Rarely . . . . ❏
Occasionally . . . . ❏
Often . . . . ❏
Very Often . . . . ❏
Almost Always . . . . ❏

C7. In the last year, have you had pain or discomfort
in the center of your chest?

Not at All or Rarely . . . . ❏
Occasionally . . . . ❏
Often . . . . ❏
Very Often . . . . ❏
Almost Always . . . . ❏

**Please check that you have answered all of the appropriate Questions in
Section C. Please begin Section D.**

Occasionally: more than one tenth of the time   *Often:* more than one quarter of the time
Very Often: more than one half of the time

Rome II Integrative Questionnaire

Section D

We would like to ask you some questions about any bowel problems you may have had **in the last year.**

D1. In the last year have you been troubled by any bowel problems?

Not at All or Rarely . . . . ❏
Occasionally . . . . ❏
Often . . . . ❏
Very Often . . . . ❏
Almost Always . . . . ❏

D2. In the *last three months* have you been troubled by any bowel problems?

Not at All or Rarely . . . . ❏
Occasionally . . . . ❏
Often . . . . ❏
Very Often . . . . ❏
Almost Always . . . . ❏

D3. In the last year, have you had more than 3 bowel movements each day?

Not at All or Rarely . . . . ❏
Occasionally . . . . ❏
Often . . . . ❏
Very Often . . . . ❏
Almost Always . . . . ❏

Occasionally: more than one tenth of the time   *Often:* more than one quarter of the time
Very Often: more than one half of the time

D4. In the last year, have you had fewer than
3 bowel movements each week?

Not at All or Rarely .... ❏
Occasionally .... ❏
Often... ❏
Very Often .... ❏
Almost Always .... ❏

D5. In the last year, have you had lumpy or hard bowel movements (stools)?

Not at All or Rarely .... ❏
Occasionally .... ❏
Often... ❏
Very Often .... ❏
Almost Always .... ❏

D6. In the last year, have you had loose, mushy or
watery bowel movements (stools)?

Not at All or Rarely .... ❏
Occasionally .... ❏
Often... ❏
Very Often .... ❏
Almost Always .... ❏

D7. In the last year, have you found that after finishing a bowel movement
you felt that there was still stool which needed to be passed?

Not at All or Rarely .... ❏
Occasionally .... ❏
Often... ❏
Very Often .... ❏
Almost Always .... ❏

Occasionally: more than one tenth of the time   *Often:* more than one quarter of the time
Very Often: more than one half of the time

D8. In the last year, have you needed to strain
a lot to have a bowel movement?

Not at All or Rarely . . . . ❑
Occasionally . . . . ❑
Often . . . . ❑
Very Often . . . . ❑
Almost Always . . . . ❑

D9. In the last year, have you experienced an urgent need to have
a bowel movement that made you rush to a toilet?

Not at All or Rarely . . . . ❑
Occasionally . . . . ❑
Often . . . . ❑
Very Often . . . . ❑
Almost Always . . . . ❑

D10. In the last year, have you noticed mucus
(white slimy material) in your stools?

Not at All or Rarely . . . . ❑
Occasionally . . . . ❑
Often . . . . ❑
Very Often . . . . ❑
Almost Always . . . . ❑

D11. In the last year, have you had the sensation that your anus
(back passage) was blocked when having a bowel movement?

Not at All or Rarely . . . . ❑
Occasionally . . . . ❑
Often . . . . ❑
Very Often . . . . ❑
Almost Always . . . . ❑

Occasionally: more than one tenth of the time   *Often:* more than one quarter of the time
Very Often: more than one half of the time

D12. In the last year, have you needed to press your finger in or around the anus (back passage) or vagina (front passage) to help the bowel movement come out?

Not at All or Rarely . . . . ❑
Occasionally . . . . ❑
Often . . . . ❑
Very Often . . . . ❑
Almost Always . . . . ❑

D13. In the last year, have you had continual or recurring aching pain or pressure in the anus or rectal area?

Not at All or Rarely . . . . ❑
Occasionally . . . . ❑
Often . . . . ❑
Very Often . . . . ❑
Almost Always . . . . ❑

> If you answered *Not at All or Rarely* to Question D13 please go on to Question D16.

D14. When you had this continual or recurring aching pain or pressure in the anus or rectal area, did it usually: (Choose only one answer)

Last from seconds to minutes and disappear completely. . . . . ❑
Last for 20 minutes or longer . . . . ❑

D15. Were there periods of at least two weeks between episodes of pain or pressure in the anus or rectal area?

Yes . . . . ❑
No . . . . ❑

Occasionally: more than one tenth of the time   *Often:* more than one quarter of the time
Very Often: more than one half of the time

D16. In the last year, when you had constipation or diarrhea, have you leaked or passed bowel movements (stools) or soiled yourself when you did not want to?

Never. . . . . ❏
One occasion in any one month. . . . . ❏
Two occasions in any one month . . . . ❏
More than two occasions in any one month . . . . ❏

D17. Did this (passing bowel movements when you did not want to) happen mostly when you felt constipated?

Yes . . . . ❏
No . . . . ❏

D18. Did this (passing bowel movements when you did not want to) happen mostly when you had diarrhea?

Yes . . . . ❏
No . . . . ❏

Please check that you have answered all of the appropriate Questions in Section D.

THANK YOU.

Occasionally: more than one tenth of the time   *Often:* more than one quarter of the time
Very Often: more than one half of the time

Codes for Rome II
Integrative Questionnaire

The coding assumes organic disease has been excluded by appropriate testing.

A. Esophageal Disorders

A1. Globus QC3 = often or very often or almost always, QC4 = not at all, QC6 = no

A2. Rumination Syndrome QC5 = often or very often or almost always, QC5.1 = no, QC5.2= yes

A3. Functional Chest Pain of presumed esophageal origin QC7 = often or very often or almost always, QC6 = not at all, QC4 = not at all

A4. Functional Heartburn* QC6 = often or very often or almost always, QC4 = not at all

A5. Functional Dysphagia† QC4 = often or very often or almost always, QC6 = not at all

B. Gastroduodenal Disorders

B1. Functional Dyspepsia†† QA1 = often or very often or almost always + QA6 = A **and/or** B, QA21 = Not at all or rarely, I do not have this pain, QA21.1 = Not at all or rarely, QA21.2 = Not at all or rarely, QA21.3 = Not at all or rarely, or QA21.4 = Not at all or rarely

B1a. Ulcer-like dyspepsia Functional Dyspepsia + QB9a or QB9b = yes

B1b. Dysmotility-like dyspepsia Functional Dyspepsia + QB9c or QB9d or QB9e or QB9f or QB9g or QB9h = yes

*Gastroesophageal reflux must be excluded.

†Note, functional heartburn and functional dysphagia are mutually exclusive in the suggested algorithms. It is important to note that if both are present, neither will show up in the data.

††Some of the editors prefer that 2 or more of [QA21 = Yes], or [QA21.1 = Yes, QA21.2 = Yes], or [QA21.3 = Yes, or QA21.4 = Yes] are needed to exclude these upper abdominal symptoms from the category of Functional Dyspepsia.

B2. Aerophagia   QC1 = often or very often or almost always
and QC2 = often or very often or almost always

B3. Functional   QB4 = often or very often or almost always,
     Vomiting   QB5 = often or very often or almost always,
QC5 = not at all

C. Bowel Disorders

C1. Irritable Bowel   QA1 = often or very often or almost always + 2 or more of
Syndrome   • [QA10 = often or very often or almost always] and/or

     • [QA11 = often or very often or almost always;
     or QA12 = often or very often or almost always]

     • [QA13 = often or very often or almost always *or* QA14 =
often or very often or almost always].

Diarrhea   IBS + [one or more of
Predominant IBS   QD3 = often or very often or almost always,
     QD6 = often or very often or almost always,
     QD9 = often or very often or almost always
+ none of
     QD4 = often or very often or almost always,
     QD5 = often or very often or almost always,
     QD8 = often or very often or almost always]
or [two or more of
     QD3 = often or very often or almost always,
     QD6 = often or very often or almost always,
     QD9 = often or very often or almost always
+ one of
     QD4 = often or very often or almost always,
     QD8 = often or very often or almost always]
and QD5 = not at all

Constipation Predominant IBS

IBS + [one or more of
QD4 = often or very often or almost always,
QD5 = often or very often or almost always,
QD8 = often or very often or almost always
+ none of
QD3 = often or very often or almost always,
QD6 = often or very often or almost always,
QD9 = often or very often or almost always]
or [two or more of
QD4 = often or very often or almost always,
QD5 = often or very often or almost always,
QD8 = often or very often or almost always
+ not more than one of
QD3 = often or very often or almost always,
QD6 = often or very often or almost always,
QD9 = often or very often or almost always]

C2. Functional Abdominal Bloating

QB7 = often or very often or almost always,
excluding IBS and Functional Dyspepsia.

C3. Functional Constipation

Two or more of
QD4 = often or very often or almost always,
QD5 = often or very often or almost always,
QD7 = often or very often or almost always,
QD8 = often or very often or almost always,
QD11 = often or very often or almost always,
QD12 = often or very often or almost always,
+ QD6 = not at all, excluding IBS.

C4. Functional Diarrhea

QD6 = almost always + QA1 = not at all

C5. Unspecified Functional Bowel Disorder

Bowel symptoms, but not sufficient to diagnose any other functional bowel disorder.

D. Functional Abdominal Pain

D1. Functional Abdominal Pain Syndrome

QA1 = almost always + QA4 = yes
+ QA9 = moderate or severe,
excluding IBS and Functional Dyspepsia,
QA8 = often or very often or almost always

D2. Unspecified Functional Abdominal Pain

QA1 = almost always, and failure to meet any of the other criteria for Functional Abdominal Pain Syndrome

E. Biliary Pain

E1. Gallbladder Dysfunction

QA24 = [(1 or 2 episodes of pain) or (more than 2 episodes of pain)],
QA25 = no,
QA8 = often or very often or almost always,
QA21 = no, QA21.1 = no, QA21.2 = no,
QA21.3 = no, QA21.4 = no, QC6 = no,
QB9b = no, QB9c = no, QB9d = no,
QB9e = no, QB9f = no, QB9g = no,
QB9h = no.

E2. Sphincter of Oddi Dysfunction

QA24 = [(1 or 2 episodes of pain) or (more than 2 episodes of pain)],
QA25 = yes,
QA8 = often or very often or almost always,
QA21 = no, QA21.1 = no, QA21.2 = no,
QA21.3 = no, QA21.4 = no, QC6 = no,
QB9b = no, QB9c = no, QB9d = no,
QB9e = no, QB9f = no, QB9g = no,
QB9h = no.

F. Anorectal Disorders

F1. Functional Incontinence

QD16 = yes (1 or more occasion)
+ either QD17 or QD18 = yes

F2. Functional Anorectal Pain

F2a. Levator Ani Syndrome

QD13 = often or very often or almost always
+ QD14 = lasts for 20 minutes or longer

F2b. Proctalgia Fugax

QD13 = often or very often or almost always
+ QD14 = lasts from seconds to minutes
+ QD15 = yes

F3. Pelvic Floor Dyssynergia

Functional constipation
+ QD7 = often or very often or almost always
+ QD8 ≥ often
+ QD11 ≥ often

Appendix D

Clinical Diagnostic Questionnaire for Pediatric Functional Gastrointestinal Disorders

The purpose of the Pediatric Diagnostic Questionnaire[*] is to provide physicians with a clinical aid to diagnose pediatric functional gastrointestinal disorders during the patient interview. The diagnostic criteria are presented in the form of questions grouped by disorder. There is a check box for either yes or no before the diagnostic item. Items indicated in italics require additional clinical information (e.g., results of diagnostic procedures, response to treatment, etc.).

Scoring requires that each item be addressed and when indicated marked in the appropriate box. When all items within a diagnostic category are checked, the patient meets criteria for the functional GI disorder.

The following criteria apply only if (1) symptoms are chronic or recurrent for at least the amount of time indicated, and (2) based on adequate medical evaluation the symptoms are not attributable to other gastrointestinal disease.

* Developed by Lenore Schwantkovsky, Ph.D., and Paul E. Hyman, M.D.

G1. Vomiting

G1A. Infant Regurgitation

1. ❑ Yes   For at least 3 weeks, has your child regurgitated 2 or more times per day?

2. Has your child had any of the following symptoms:
   - ❑ No   Retching
   - ❑ No   Blood in the spit-up
   - ❑ No   Aspiration
   - ❑ No   Poor weight gain
   - ❑ No   Apnea

3. How old is your child?
   - ❑ Yes   1 to 12 months of age
   - ❑ Yes   Is your child otherwise healthy?
   - ❑ No   *Is there evidence of metabolic, gastrointestinal, or central nervous system disease to explain the symptom?*

G1B. Infant Rumination Syndrome

1. ❑ Yes   For at least 3 months, when not vomiting, did your child often bring up food, rechew it, and either spit it out or reswallow it?

2. ❑ Yes   Did this start when your child was between 3 and 8 months of age?

3. ❑ No   Does this occur during sleep?

4. ❑ No   Does this occur when the infant is interacting with family or friends?

5. ❑ No   Does your baby seem distressed by this?

6. ❑ No   *Has the baby responded to management for gastroesophageal reflux disease, anticholinergic drugs, hand restraints, formula changes, and gavage or gastrostomy feedings?*

G1C. Cyclic Vomiting Syndrome

1. ❏ Yes   Has your child had 3 or more periods of intense, acute nausea and vomiting lasting hours to days?

2. ❏ Yes   Between episodes, does your child have symptoms-free intervals lasting weeks to months?

3. ❏ No   *Is there metabolic, gastrointestinal or central nervous system structural or biochemical disease?*

2G. Abdominal Pain

G2A. Functional Dyspepsia

1. ❏ Yes   Is the child mature enough to give an accurate pain history?

2. ❏ Yes   For at least 12 weeks (*need not be consecutive*) in the past year, has your child had persistent or recurrent pain or discomfort centered in the upper abdomen (above the umbilicus)?

3. ❏ No   Is the pain or discomfort relieved by defecation?

4. ❏ No   Is the pain or discomfort associated with the onset of a change in stool frequency or stool form?

5. ❏ No   *Is there clinical, biochemical, endoscopic, or ultrasonographic evidence that organic disease is likely to explain the symptoms?*

To distinguish type of dyspepsia, examine the answers in the following three categories: ulcer-like dyspepsia, dysmotility-like dyspepsia, and unspecified (non-specific) dyspepsia.

G2A1. Ulcer-like Dyspepsia

1. ❏ Yes   Is the pain centered in the upper abdomen the predominant, most bothersome symptom?

G2A2. Dysmotility-like Dyspepsia

1. ❏ Yes   Is the unpleasant or troublesome non-painful sensation (discomfort) centered in the upper abdomen the prominent symptom?

718

2. Is this sensation characterized by (*any of the following*)?
   ❏ Yes Feeling full after eating very little
   ❏ Yes Upper abdominal fullness
   ❏ Yes Bloating
   ❏ Yes Nausea.

G2A3. Unspecified (nonspecific) Dyspepsia

1. ❏ No *Does the patient fulfill criteria for either ulcer-like or dysmotility-like dyspepsia?*

G2B. Irritable Bowel Syndrome

1. ❏ Yes Is the child old enough to provide an accurate pain history?

2. ❏ Yes For at least 12 weeks (need not be consecutive) in the past year, has your child complained of abdominal discomfort or pain?

3. Is this discomfort or pain (*two out of three*):
   ❏ Yes Relieved by a bowel movement
   ❏ Yes Associated with a change in frequency of bowel movements
   ❏ Yes Associated with a change in the form (appearance) of bowel movements

4. ❏ No *Are there structural or metabolic abnormalities to explain the symptoms?*

5. Is this discomfort or pain accompanied by: (*Symptoms that cumulatively support the diagnosis of IBS but are not necessary for diagnosis. Any of the following:*)
   ❏ Yes Abnormal stool frequency (greater than 3 BMs per day or fewer than 3 BMs per week)?
   ❏ Yes Abnormal stool form (lumpy/hard or loose/watery stool)?
   ❏ Yes Abnormal stool passage (straining, urgency, or feeling of incomplete evacuation)?
   ❏ Yes Passage of mucus?
   ❏ Yes Bloating or feeling of abdominal distension?

G2C. Functional Abdominal Pain Syndrome

1. ❏ Yes   For at least three months has your school-aged child or adolescent had continuous or nearly continuous abdominal pain?

2. ❏ No or only occasionally   Is the pain related to eating, menses, or defecation?

3. ❏ Yes   Has this pain interfered with your child's daily activities (ability to go to school or social activities)?

4. ❏ No   *Is the pain is feigned?*

5. ❏ No   *Does the child meet criteria for other functional gastrointestinal disorders that would explain the abdominal pain?*

G2D. Abdominal Migraine

1. ❏ Yes   For at least one year has your child complained of three or more episodes of intense, acute midline abdominal pain lasting from 2 hours to several days?

2. ❏ Yes   Does your child have symptom-free intervals lasting weeks to months?

3. Does your child complain of any of the following (*at least two*):
   a. ❏ Yes   Headache during episodes?
   b. ❏ Yes   Photophobia during episodes?
   c. ❏ Yes   Family history of migraine?
   d. ❏ Yes   Headache confined to one side only
   e. ❏ Yes   An aura or warning period consisting of either visual disturbances (e.g., blurred or restricted vision), sensory symptoms (numbness or tingling), or motor abnormalities (slurred speech, inability to speak, paralysis).
   f. ❏ No   *Is there evidence of metabolic, gastrointestinal, or central nervous system structural or biochemical diseases?*

G2E. Aerophagia

For 12 weeks (*need not be consecutive*) or more in the past year has your child (*two of the following*):

1. ❑ Yes   Swallowed air
2. ❑ Yes   Had a bloated stomach
3. ❑ Yes   Belched or passed gas repeatedly

G3. Functional Diarrhea (also called Toddler's Diarrhea, chronic non-specific diarrhea, irritable colon of childhood)

1. ❑ Yes   For at least 4 weeks, has your child had 3 or more large, painless, unformed bowel movements each day?

2. ❑ Yes   Did this symptom begin between 6 and 36 months of age?

3. ❑ Yes   Does your child have bowel movements only when awake?

4. ❑ Yes   Is your child growing and thriving?

G4. Disorders of Defecation

G4A. Infant Dyschezia

1. ❑ Yes   Does your baby strain and cry at least 10 minutes before having a bowel movement with soft stool?

2. ❑ Yes   *Is the infant less than 6 months of age?*

3. ❑ Yes   *Is the infant otherwise healthy?*

G4B. Functional Constipation (*Either 1 or 2 and 3*)

1. ❑ Yes   For at least 2 weeks has your child had pebble-like, hard stools most of the time? *or*
2. ❑ Yes   For at least 2 weeks has your child had firm stools two or fewer times per week?
3. ❑ No   *There is no evidence of structural, endocrine or metabolic disease.*

G4C. Functional Fecal Retention

1. ❏ Yes   For at least the past 3 months, has your child or adolescent passed large diameter stools less than 2 times per week?

2. ❏ Yes   Does your child try to avoid having a bowel movement by squeezing the legs or buttocks together?

3. *Accompanying symptoms may include the following and disappear immediately following passage of a large stool.*
   ❏ Yes   Fecal soiling
   ❏ Yes   Irritability
   ❏ Yes   Abdominal cramps
   ❏ Yes   Decreased appetite
   ❏ Yes   Early satiety

G4D. Functional Non-Retentive Fecal Soiling

1. ❏ Yes   For a week or more for the last 12 weeks, has your child had a bowel movement into places and at times inappropriate to the social situation?

2. ❏ Yes   *Is the child older than four years?*

3. ❏ No   *Is there evidence of structural or inflammatory disease?*

4. ❏ Yes   *Are signs of fecal retention absent?*

Photographs of the Rome II Working Team Participants

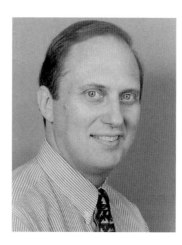

Douglas A. Drossman, M.D.
Chair, Coordinating Committee
  for FGID
Chair, Psychosocial Factors of
  the FGID
Member, Functional Bowel
  Disorders and Functional
  Abdominal Pain

Enrico Corazziari, M.D.
Member, Coordinating Com-
  mittee for FGID
Chair, Functional Biliary and
  Pancreatic Disorders

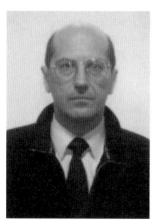

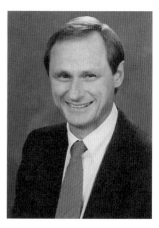

Nicholas J. Talley, M.D., Ph.D.
Member, Coordinating
  Committee for FGID
Chair, Functional
  Gastroduodenal Disorders
Co-Chair, Design of Treatment
  Trials for FGID

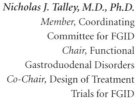

W. Grant Thompson, M.D.
Member, Coordinating
  Committee for FGID
Chair, Functional Bowel
  Disorders and Functional
  Abdominal Pain

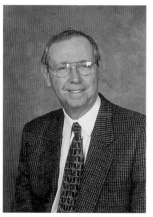

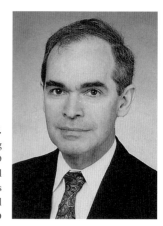

William E. Whitehead, Ph.D.
Member, Coordinating
  Committee for FGID
Chair, Functional
  Anorectal Disorders
Member, Psychosocial
  Factors of the FGID

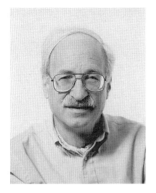

David H. Alpers, M.D.
Co-Chair, Basic Science:
 Brain-Gut

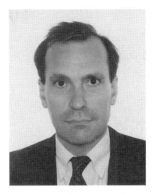

Fernando Azpiroz, M.D., Ph.D.
Member, Physiology:
 Motility/Sensation

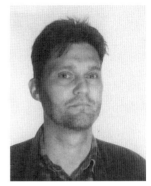

Peter Bytzer, M.D.
Member, Design of Treatment
 Trials for the FGID

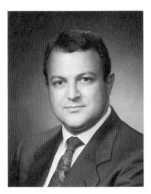

Michael Camilleri, M.D.
Member, Physiology:
 Motility/Sensation

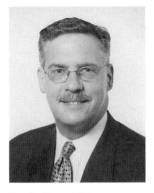

Ray E. Clouse, M.D.
Chair, Functional Esophageal
 Disorders

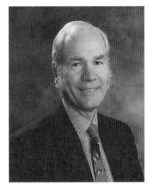

Francis H. Creed, M.D.
Co-Chair, Psychosocial Factors
 of the FGID

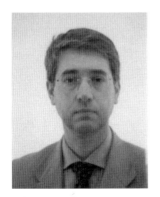

Salvatore Cucchiara, M.D.
Member, Childhood FGID

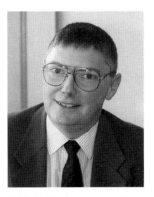

Michel M. Delvaux, M.D., Ph.D.
Co-Chair, Physiology:
 Motility/Sensation

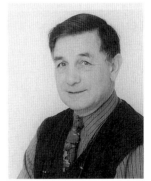

Nicholas E. Diamant, M.D.
Member, Functional Anorectal
 Disorders

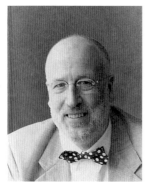

Paul Enck, Ph.D.
Member, Functional Anorectal
Disorders

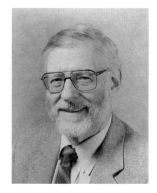

David R. Fleisher, M.D.
Member, Childhood FGID

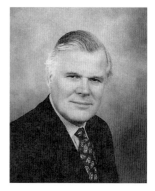

Robert C. Heading, M.D.
Member, Functional
Gastroduodenal Disorders

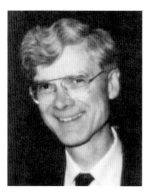

Kenneth W. Heaton, M.D.
Member, Functional Bowel Disorders and Functional Abdominal Pain

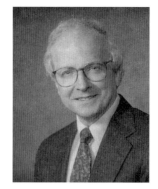

Walter J. Hogan, M.D.
Member, Functional Biliary and
Pancreatic Disorders

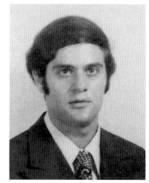

Jeffrey S. Hyams, M.D.
Member, Childhood FGID

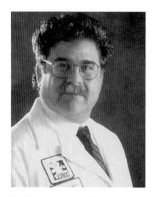

Paul E. Hyman, M.D.
Chair, Childhood FGID

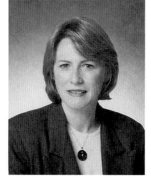

E. Jan Irvine, M.D.
Member, Functional Bowel Disorders
and Functional Abdominal Pain

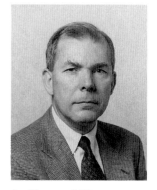

Jozef Janssens, M.D.
Member, Functional Esophageal
Disorders

726

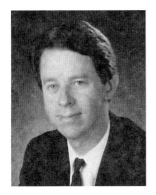

John E. Kellow, M.D.
Chair, Physiology:
  Motility/Sensation

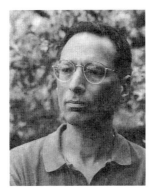

Kenneth B. Klein, M.D.
Member, Design of Treatment
  Trials for FGID

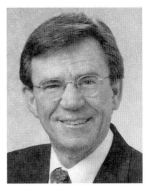

Kenneth L. Koch, M.D.
Member, Functional
  Gastroduodenal Disorders

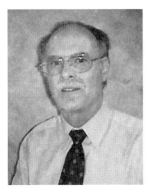

George F. Longstreth, M.D.
Co-Chair, Functional Bowel Disorders and Functional Abdominal Pain

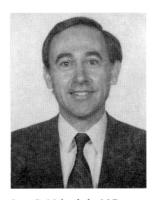

Juan-R. Malagelada, M.D.
Member, Functional
  Gastroduodenal Disorders

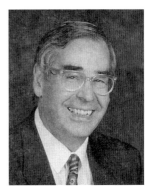

Peter J. Milla, M.D.
Member, Childhood FGID

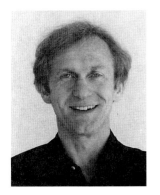

Stefan Muller-Lissner, M.D.
Member, Functional Bowel Disorders
  and Functional Abdominal Pain

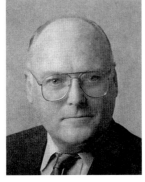

Kevin W. Olden, M.D.
Member, Psychosocial Factors
  of the FGID

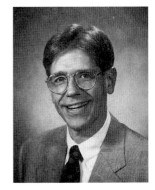

John H. Pemberton, M.D.
Member, Functional Anorectal
  Disorders

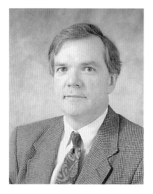

Eamonn M. M. Quigley, M.D.
Member, Physiology:
   Motility/Sensation

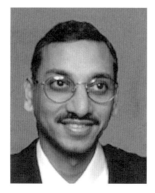

Satish S. C. Rao, M.D., Ph.D.
Member, Functional Anorectal
   Disorders

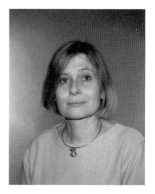

Andree Rasquin-Weber, M.D.
Co-Chair, Childhood FGID

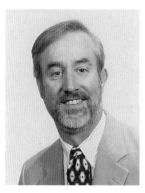

Joel E. Richter, M.D.
Co-Chair, Functional Esophageal
   Disorders

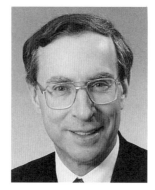

Eldon A. Shaffer, M.D.
Co-Chair, Functional Biliary and
   Pancreatic Disorders

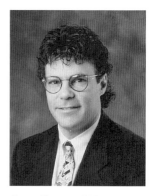

Stuart Sherman, M.D.
Member, Functional Biliary and
   Pancreatic Disorders

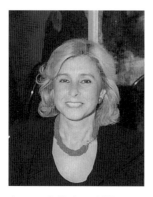

Annamaria Staiano, M.D.
Member, Childhood FGID

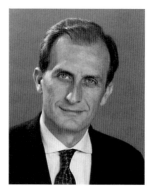

Vincenzo Stanghellini, M.D.
Co-Chair, Functional
   Gastroduodenal Disorders

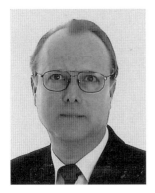
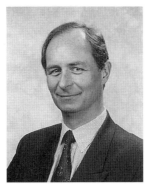
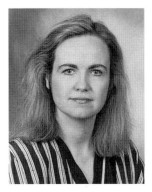

Jan Svedlund, M.D.
Member, Psychosocial Factors
of FGID

David G. Thompson, M.D.
Member, Physiology:
Motility/Sensation

Brenda B. Toner, Ph.D.
Member, Psychosocial Factors
of FGID

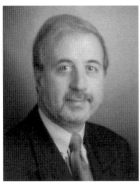
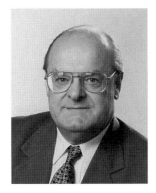
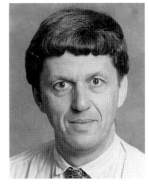

James Toouli, M.D.
Member, Functional Biliary and
Pancreatic Disorders

Guido N. J. Tytgat, M.D.
Member, Functional
Gastroduodenal Disorders

*Sander J. O. Veldhuyzen van
Zanten, M.D. Ph.D.*
Chair, Design of Treatment Trials
for FGID

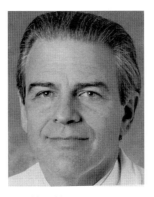
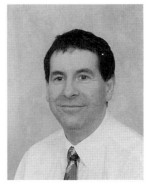

Arnold Wald, M.D.
Co-Chair, Functional Anorectal
Disorders

Peter J. Whorwell, M.D.
Member, Design of Treatment
Trials for FGID

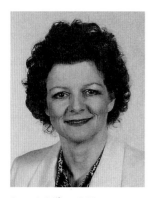

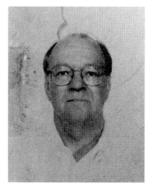

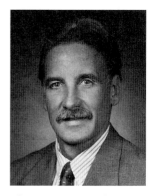

Janet A. Wilson, M.D.
Member, Functional Esophageal
  Disorders

Jackie D. Wood, M.D., Ph.D
Co-Chair, Basic Science:
  Brain-Gut

Alan R. Zinsmeister, Ph. D.
Member, Design of Treatment
  Trials for FGID

Not pictured:
Paul L. R. Andrews, Ph.D.
Member, Basic Science:
  Brain-Gut

Appendix F

Manuscript
Reviewers

We are grateful to the following consultants for their careful review of the Working Team Committee manuscripts.

Achem, Sami	Mayo Clinic, Jacksonville	Jacksonville, Florida, USA
Allescher, Hans Dieter	II Medizinische Klinik und Poliklinic Technischen Universitat München	München, Germany
Axon, Anthony	The General Infirmary at Leeds	Leeds, England, UK
Boyle, Tim	Rainbow Babies and Children's	Cleveland, Ohio, USA Hospital
Buddeberg, Claus	Universitätsspital Zürich	Zürich, Switzerland
Colletti, Richard	University of Vermont College of Medicine	Burlington, Vermont, USA
Corazziari, Enrico	Università "La Sapienza"	Roma, Italy
Crowell, Michael	Johns Hopkins Bayview Medical Center	Baltimore, Maryland, USA
Delvaux, Michel	CHU Rangueil	Toulouse, France
Diamant, Nicholas E.	Toronto Western Hospital	Toronto, Canada
Drossman, Douglas A.	The University of North Carolina	Chapel Hill, North Carolina, USA
Everhart, James	National Institutes of Health	Bethesda, Maryland, USA
Falk, Gary W.	The Cleveland Clinic Foundation	Cleveland, Ohio, USA
Fava, Giovanni A.	Università di Bologna	Bologna, Italy
Festi, David E.	Università di Chieti	Chieti, Italy
Fleshman, James W.	Washington University	St. Louis, Missouri, USA
Frieling, Thomas	Heinrich Heine Universität	Düsseldorf, Germany
Galmiche, J. P.	Centre Hospitalier, University de Nantes	Nantes, France
Grundy, David	University of Sheffield	Sheffield, England, UK
Holtmann, Gerald	University of Essen	Essen, Germany
Husebye, Einar	Ulleval University Hospital	Oslo, Norway

Johnston, Brian T.	Down Lisburn Trust	Lisburn, County Antrim, Northern Ireland
Jones, Roger	King's College	London, England, UK
Kahrilas, Peter J.	Northwestern Universtiy	Chicago, Illinois, USA
Katz, Philip O.	Graduate Hospital Department of Medicine	Philadelphia, Pennsylvania, USA
Kellow, John E.	Royal North Shore Hospital	Sydney, Australia
Kruis, Wolfgang	Evangel Krankenhaus Kalk	Köln, Germany
Kuijpers, Hans C.	Koloproktologische Klinik	Recklinghausen, The Netherlands
Lembo, Anthony	Harvard Medical School	Boston, Massachusetts, USA
Lennard-Jones, John E.	St. Mark's Hospital	Suffolk, England, UK
Levenstein, Susan	Studio Medico Internazionale	Rome, Italy
Levy, Rona L.	University of Washington	Seattle, Washington, USA
Li, B. Ulyssis K.	Ohio State University College of Medicine	Columbus, Ohio, USA
Loening-Baucke, Vera	University of Iowa	Iowa City, Iowa, USA
Mawe, Gary	University of Vermont College of Medicine	Burlington, Vermont, USA
Moser, Gabriele	University Klinik	Vienna, Austria
Paterson, William G.	Queens University	Kingston, Ontario, Canada
Patrick, Donald L.	University of Washington	Seattle, Washington, USA
Phillips, Sidney F.	Mayo Clinic	Rochester, Minnesota, USA
Portincasa, Piero	Policlinico di Bari Semeiotica Dipartimento Medicina Interna e del Lavoro (DIMIL)	Bari, Italy
Quigley, Eamonn M. M.	Cork University Hospital	Cork, Ireland
Sandler, Robert	The University of North Carolina	Chapel Hill, North Carolina, USA

Schuster, Marvin M.	Johns Hopkins Bayview Medical Center	Baltimore, Maryland, USA
Sharkey, Keith	University of Calgary	Calgary, Canada
Slivka, Adam	University of Pittsburg	Pittsburg, Pennsylvania, USA
Spiller, R.C.	University Hospital	Nottingham, England, UK
Summers, R.W.	University of Iowa	Iowa City, Iowa, USA
Svanvik, Joar	Sahlgrenska University Hospital	Goteborg, Sweden
Tack, Jan	University Hospital Leuven	Leuven, Belgium
Talley, Nicholas J.	University of Sydney	Penrith, NSW, Australia
Thompson, W. Grant	University of Ottawa	Ottawa, Ontario, Canada
Treem, William	Duke University Medical Center	Durham, North Carolina, USA
van Zanten, Sander J. O. Veldhuyzen	Victoria General Hosiptal	Halifax, Nova Scotia, Canada
Walker, Lynn	Vanderbilt University Medical Center	Nashville, Tennessee, USA
Wexner, Steven D.	Cleveland Clinic Florida	Fort Lauderdale, Florida, USA
Whitehead, William E.	University of North Carolina	Chapel Hill, North Carolina, USA
Whorwell, Peter J.	The University of South Manchester	Manchester, England, UK
Wienbeck, Martin	Krankenhauszweckverband	Augsburg, Germany
Wilcox, C. Mel	University of Alabama at Birmingham	Birmingham, Alabama, USA
Zeltzer, Lonnie	University of California at Los Angeles School of Medicine	Los Angeles, California, USA

Index